دكتور/مايكل إليوت
إستشارى أمراض العظام
Dr. Michael J. Elliott
Consultant Orthopaedic Physician

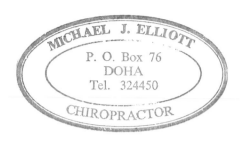

R. C. Schafer, DC, FICC
L. J. Faye, DC, FCCSS (c) Hon.

MOTION PALPATION
AND CHIROPRACTIC TECHNIC
—Principles of Dynamic Chiropractic

FIRST EDITION

MOTION PALPATION AND CHIROPRACTIC TECHNIC
—Principles of Dynamic Chiropractic

FIRST EDITION

R. C. Schafer, DC, FICC
WITH CONTRIBUTIONS AND CLINICAL COMMENTARIES BY
L. J. Faye, DC, FCCSS (c) Hon.

Developed by
ASSOCIATED CHIROPRACTIC ACADEMIC PRESS

Published by
THE MOTION PALPATION INSTITUTE
21541 Surveyor Circle • P.O. Box 6100 • Huntington Beach, CA 92615

Library of Congress Catalog Number: 88-93050

ISBN: 0924889-00-4

Copyright 1989
THE MOTION PALPATION INSTITUTE
21541 Surveyor Circle • P.O. Box 6100
Huntington Beach, California 92615

Printed in the United States of America.

Photography Credits: Photos of Dr. Faye's demonstrations by Michael J. Faye

Dedication

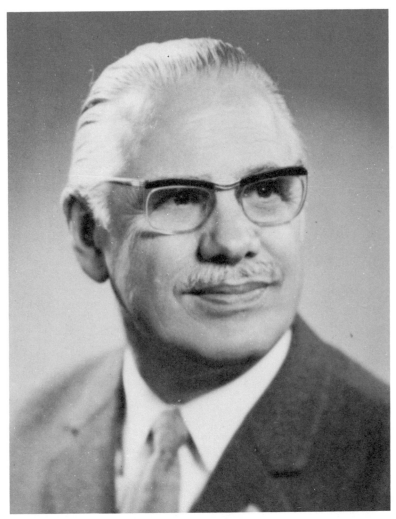

Henri J. Gillet, DC

This book is dedicated to Henri J. Gillet, DC—founder of the Belgian Chiropractic Research Association, the Belgian Chiropractic Association (1924), and the European Chiropractors Union (1935)—

and to M. Liekens, DC, and the other members of the Belgian Chiropractic Research Association whose many years of unselfish devotion to chiropractic science led to the development of the principles inherent within and associated with the study of the evaluation and correction of spinal and extraspinal articular mobility restriction (fixation).

Foreword

The shift from the dependency of static concepts to the dynamic functional model of chiropractic has created a demand for a new type of technic textbook. This book, *Motion Palpation and Chiropractic Technic*, is designed and written to fulfill this gap in the *paradigm shift*.

After being very disappointed in static x-ray listings as an indicator for a chiropractic adjustment, Dr. Henri Gillet developed methods of motion palpation that related to kinematics of the articulations of the spine and pelvis. During the early 1960s, I had the good fortune of hearing Gillet speak and was strongly motivated to pursue an in-depth study of his methods. My development of the skills of motion palpation led to great clinical success. The result was that the predictability of a patient's response had become a new-found joy in my practice. In addition, once the complexities of joint function were understood, the neuromusculoskeletal model depicted by Dr. A. E. Homewood took on a whole new meaning.

As I taught more classes and became more involved in the development of the Anglo-European Chiropractic College, the *chiropractic subluxation complex paradigm* was developed. So many previously dichotomous techniques, examination procedures, and theories gradually fit the complex. Others remained a mystery and were discarded for lack of confirmation. The volume of work and the effort needed to expand our understanding of the subluxation complex were more than enough to occupy my full attention. The task was complex. It became a matter of learning (1) biomechanical principles, (2) the neurobiologic mechanisms associated with manipulation, (3) the *functional* interpretation of orthopedic and neurologic tests, (4) the rational management of acute and chronic inflammation, and (5) how to enhance the skills necessary for motion palpation and the application of the chiropractic high-velocity low-amplitude adjustment, as well as various soft-tissue techniques.

The most pressing problem I had as a clinician and lecturer was in finding the time to develop the skills of a professional writer so that I could produce a textbook based on my lectures and demonstrations. Dr. Donald Petersen, the organizational man of the Motion Palpation Institute (MPI), recognized my dilemma and suggested the services of Dr. R. C. Schafer to develop a quality manuscript that would do justice to the importance of this work. Our collaboration has been a rewarding experience for me, and I have developed great respect for Dr. Schafer's ability to be so pragmatic. This book reflects the excellent teamwork that has been prevalent from ideation to creation.

This manual is dedicated to Dr. Henri Gillet, however, I also wish to express special thanks to my wife, Bernadette, who was even more committed than I at times to the paradigm shift with which we set out to challenge the chiropractic profession.

We hope this book, which is the product of many years of clinical testing, will help remove the necessity for chiropractic colleges to teach the obsolescent concept of static listings. The perpetuation of this myth is undoubtedly a response to Chiropractic Licensing Boards that insist on such listings in their technic examinations. Chiropractic adjustments restore joint function; they occasionally change initial listings. That is the bottom line. Healing is the result of the body's adaptation to renewed function.

— Leonard J. Faye, DC

Preface

It was a welcomed challenge when I was approached by Dr. Petersen, editor of *Dynamic Chiropractic*, to develop this text for I have long held a deep interest in motion palpation and its approach to adjustive therapy. The concepts uncovered and taught by the Motion Palpation Institute do not comprise an "empiric system" in the usual sense where much must be assumed on faith. Each precept is based on principles well established in clinical literature and can be proved by personal experience. Essentially, it is a complementary clinical approach to basic chiropractic applications that any doctor of chiropractic may apply regardless of his or her personal preferences in technique or philosophy.

This manual has been developed for the chiropractic physician and advanced student. Thus, it is assumed that the reader has a well-established knowledge of the basic sciences and the procedural standards of (1) physical and differential diagnosis; (2) orthopedic and neurologic workups; (3) supportive radiographic and clinical laboratory services; and (4) traditional chiropractic spinal and extraspinal adjustive methodology. To avoid duplication with texts that describe these procedures in detail, these standard routines are rarely described herein except for short mention when pertinent to a topic. Our major purpose here was to describe motion palpation, the adjustment of articular fixations, and the major ancillary procedures associated. Although chiropractic health care has proved itself time and again as more efficient in the treatment of many neuromusculoskeletal disorders than traditional allopathic care, the concepts described in this manual will offer an even broader viewpoint and deeper insight into the treatment of human dysfunction.

The general work of Henri Gillet and his associates within the Belgium Chiropractic Research Association are vaguely familiar to most chiropractic practitioners. Papers and reports authored by Gillet have appeared for 4 decades within *The Belgium Notes on Fixation* and in our national and numerous state periodicals. His research findings have been reported frequently within *The Digest of Chiropractic Economics, The Journal of Clinical Chiropractic, The Annals of the Swiss Chiropractors Association, The European Chiropractic Bulletin, The Brussels' Chiropractor*, and sundry chiropractic publications of Canada, Australia, New Zealand, and South Africa.

Because of the impact Gillet's findings and Faye's development of the subluxation complex concept have had and are having on the definition and scope of the term *subluxation complex* and its correction within the practice of chiropractic, my goal in developing this book was to bring the essence of Gillet's half-century study under one cover and to resolve the confusion sometimes associated with misinterpretations resulting from inappropriate translations, abstracted reports, and addresses reported from notes or recall. We have also included the marriage of joint-play palpation and extremity adjusting as developed by Faye in the mid-1960s.

The concepts of motion palpation and dynamic chiropractic are not based on on a proprietary system. As with all truly scientific principles, their use and development are open to all to apply and refine. The word *science* is defined in my *Webster's Dictionary* as (1) the study and theoretical explanation of natural phenomena; (2) a systematic activity requiring study and method; and (3) knowledge that has been acquired especially through experience. Herbert Spencer said "Science is organized knowledge," and Stanislaus is reported to have stated "Science when well-digested is nothing but good sense and reason." In all these viewpoints, the principles and methodology described herein meet all these definitions in being a significant contribution to chiropractic science. They should not be considered as an end in our quest to relieve human suffering; rather, a door through which we may find the answers to many problems.

The first two chapters of this book are general, nonregional in nature. Chapter 1, which lays the foundation for this study, introduces the dynamic chiropractic paradigm. It offers an overview of the clinical approach used and describes the normal movements of spinal articulations. Different types of fixation, significant physiologic and biomechanical mechanisms, and practical points in differentiating joint dysfunction from joint disease are described. Practice approaches, pertinent biomechanical terminology, and the fundamentals underlying chiropractic adjustive technics are also explained.

Chapter 2, establishes the basic principles delineated by Dr. Gillet and his associates within the Belgium Chiropractic Research Association. An overview of dynamic chiropractic clinical protocols and general considerations underlying palpation are portrayed. Some viewpoints regarding roentgenographic analyses, hygiene, and physical fitness are briefly represented in the context of this study.

The following four chapters are specific for each region of the spine, and they emphasize method. "Art and science have their meeting point in method," stated the great English author and diplomat Sir Henry Bulwer. Chapter 3, which concerns the cervical spine, depicts the relevant applied anatomy, biomechanical, diagnostic, and therapeutic considerations of this region of the spine. Chapter 4 does the same for the thoracic spine; Chapter 5, for the lumbar spine; and Chapter 6, for the pelvis. Chapter 7 briefly describes Gillet's experiences in delineating certain spinal fixation complexes, which are often the basis of problem situations in the clinical setting.

The remaining two chapters pertain to the extraspinal articulations. Chapter 8 embraces the subject of extraspinal axial and upper extremity joints, and Chapter 9 concerns the joints of the lower extremity. The text concludes with a comprehensive index that has been designed as a quick reference guide.

In closing, I wish to express my appreciation to Drs. L. John Faye and Donald M. Petersen for their cooperation, contributions, and encouragement during the development of this text. Without their recognition of the need for this book, its publication would not have been possible.

—RCS

Note: On the very day this manuscript was completed, word was received of the death of Dr. Petersen. It is our hope that this book will be received as one tribute to his many years of service to his beloved profession.

Table of Contents

Epilog

MISSION POLICY OF THE MOTION PALPATION INSTITUTE

Statement

The Motion Palpation Institute (MPI) is a nonprofit independent international organization with no political affiliations. It is dedicated to offering pertinent and diverse assistance to the profession of chiropractic as a whole. Along with its dedication to provide quality educational opportunities to the profession of chiropractic, MPI endeavors to earn recognition as a center for higher education in chiropractic science. The educational and research emphasis is on those neurobiomechanical mechanisms that influence the restoration and maintenance of health along with the psychomotor and clinical skills required to provide quality chiropractic care. Accordingly, MPI will initiate cooperation with colleges recognized by the Council on Chiropractic Education for the development of these skills. In addition, MPI will make information on chiropractic health care services available to the public so that informed and prudent judgments can be made.

Goals

To accomplish the Mission Statement described above, the MPI will seek to fulfill the following goals:
• To raise funds to advance scholarly pursuits and research in the biological sciences as they apply to the philosophy, science, and art of the profession of chiropractic as adopted by MPI.
• To provide continuing education programs to the profession of chiropractic to aid its members in maintaining competency and quality of practice.
• To seek recognition of MPI as an institute of higher education in chiropractic science.
• To provide opportunities for qualified doctors of chiropractic to pursue postgraduate education in chiropractic clinical science as offered by MPI.
• To maintain a tradition of cooperation with colleges recognized by the Council on Chiropractic Education in the pursuit of academic, clinical, and professional excellence.
• To provide a forum for doctors of chiropractic to deliberate and search for a consensus on matters of unity and progress.
• To encourage the availability of quality chiropractic care to all people by the dissemination of knowledge through creative teaching and professional activity by the profession of chiropractic.
• To clearly state and periodically review the mission goals and objectives of the MPI.

Basic Objectives

The mission objectives of the MPI are as follows:
1. To develop programs and facilities for the conduct of research into the science and practice of chiropractic.
2. To provide funds to qualified persons within the chiropractic profession and its educational institutions to research the vertebral subluxation and its neurobiomechanical complexities.

3. To prepare a thorough study of current MPI continuing education courses and develop or upgrade a complete syllabus for each.

4. To include within MPI continuing education courses lectures on rational office procedures and standards of practice (patient bill of rights) to encourage proficiency and professionalism in providing chiropractic health care.

5. To conduct an ongoing review all MPI continuing education course manuals for quality and accuracy of content and integration to course syllabuses.

6. To develop a competency-based evaluation system to measure motion palpation/adjustive skills and clinical proficiency outcomes as taught in all MPI courses.

7. To develop and implement an MPI faculty-evaluation system.

8. To determine what additional continuing education courses (along with syllabuses, manuals, and audiovisual aids) should be developed according to need.

9. To obtain higher education status for MPI in the State of California as either a freestanding institution or an affiliate of an accredited liberal arts/sciences college or university.

10. To develop an MPI postdoctoral program for selected chiropractors to pursue advanced studies in chiropractic clinical science with emphasis on neurobiomechanical mechanisms, including the need to conduct a supervised research project as a major component toward certification.

11. To begin the MPI postdoctoral fellowship program within 1 year after receiving higher education status.

12. To conduct a feasibility study on how MPI will cooperate with CCE-affiliated colleges.

13. To implement an MPI approved plan of cooperation with CCE-affiliated colleges within 1 year after completion of this study.

14. To develop a questionnaire for all chiropractors that when completed will result in a list of the major issues facing the profession.

15. To publish the questionnaire in *Dynamic Chiropractic* within 3 months of its preparation for distribution to all chiropractors for 3 consecutive months.

16. To analyze the information provided by the responses to the questionnaire with the goal of developing a list of concerns to be published within *Dynamic Chiropractic* within 3 months to stimulate intraprofessional communication.

17. To plan an international conference that will have as its theme: RESEARCHING A CONSENSUS FOR THE STATE-OF-THE-ART OF THE PROFESSION OF CHIROPRACTIC within 3 years after analysis of the analyzed information.

18. To develop patient education programs that will explain the importance of chiropractic care for the restoration and maintenance of health.

19. To promote to the profession of chiropractic the use of MPI patient education programs designed to distribute information on chiropractic health care in and through their practices.

20. To retain a public relations firm to develop a program that will explain to the general public the subluxation complex and chiropractic care for the restoration and maintenance of health.

21. To raise funds from the chiropractic profession to be used for presentation of the public information program on a national scale and in selected media.

22. To appraise the MPI Mission Policy each year for its accuracy and clarity.

MPI Definitions

Chiropractic Philosophy

The human body is endowed with certain inherent qualities that provide for the protection, maintenance, and restoration of health, of which the normal function of the nervous system is a major integrating force. It is reasoned that when normal transmission and expression of nerve energy is interfered with, particularly in the spine, pathophysiologic processes may develop.

Chiropractic Science

Chiropractic science is concerned with the relationship between structure, primarily the spine, and function, primarily the nervous system, of the body as that relationship may affect the restoration and preservation of health.

Chiropractic as a Health Discipline

Chiropractic is that discipline within the healing arts especially concerned with the etiology, pathogenesis, diagnostics, therapeutics, and prophylaxis of functional disturbances, pathomechanical states, pain syndromes, and other neurophysiologic effects related to the statics and dynamics of the neuromusculoskeletal system, particularly those related to the spine and pelvis.

Chiropractic Practice

Use of the phrase *the practice of chiropractic* by MPI refers to any professional service provided by a chiropractor, within the scope of his or her license to practice, whose aim is to restore and maintain health.

THE SUBLUXATION COMPLEX

MOTION PALPATION ⟶ PATHOPHYSIOLOGY ⟶ PATHOLOGY

AXIOM — Correction of a subluxation restores normal physiologic processes and the reversible pathology reverses.

SUBLUXATION — A complex clinical entity comprising one or more of the following:

1. NEUROPATHOPHYSIOLOGY

- Irritation ⟶ Facilitation
  - ⟶ Anterior Horn ⟶ Muscles Hypertonic
  - ⟶ Lateral Horn ⟶ Sympathetic Vasomotor
  - ⟶ Posterior Horn ⟶ Sensory
- Degeneration ⟶ Degeneration
  - ⟶ Atrophy
  - ⟶ Sympathetic Atonia
  - ⟶ Anesthesia
- Decreased Axoplasmic Flow

2. KINESIOPATHOLOGY

- Hypomobility   — Fixation Theory — H. Gillet
- Hypermobility   — Illi
- Loss of Joint Play   — J. Mennel

Compensation
- ⟶ Hypermobility + Hypomobility = Normal
- ⟶ Hypomobility and Hypermobility can be in the same motion unit

Change of axis of movement

3. MYOPATHOLOGY

- Spasm
  - ⟶ Compensation
  - ⟶ Facilitation ⟶ Visceromotor Reflex
  - ⟶ Hilton's Law
- Atonia

4. HISTOPATHOLOGY

- Cellular flow of inflammatory process
- Edema within intervertebral foramen, impeding flow of circulating fluids

5. BIOCHEMICAL CHANGES

- L.A.S. (Selye) from local tissue damage or further G.A.S.
- Histamines
- Prostoglandanines   Stress Syndrome
- Kinines   ∴ Proinflammatory

CHIROPRACTIC THERAPEUTIC APPROACH

Adjustive Procedures ⟶ Thrust, Recoil, Toggle, etc
Reflex Technics
Exercise
Diet, Supplementation   Produces a specific movement
Postural Advice   ↓
Modalities   ∴ Effects the movement component
Socio-occupational Advice   of a subluxation complex directly
Other   and others indirectly

RATIONALE FOR THE ADJUSTMENT

(A) Find the hypomobility; (B) use adjustive procedure to mobilize the fixation; (C) recheck to confirm that movement has improved. Therapeutic approach is then applied to other components of the subluxation complex and their causes; therefore, a holistic, multicausal interdisciplinary approach for each patient's health problems. The prognosis depends on the reversibility of the pathology, the restoration of normal function, and the ability to keep the joints free of subluxation-fixations and other causes of malfunction.

PREVENTION — Regular motion palpation examinations to discover early aberrant motion, especially fixations to prevent the subluxation complex from developing.

Chapter 1

Introduction to the Dynamic Chiropractic Paradigm

This chapter presents an overview of the background and basic concepts of *Dynamic Chiropractic*. The normal motions of spinal and related articulations, general considerations of spinal fixations, the different types of fixations, the significant physiologic mechanisms associated, a comparison of traditional and modern definitions of the vertebral subluxation complex, and other basic concepts are summarized.

OVERVIEW OF THE DYNAMIC CHIROPRACTIC APPROACH

In 1936, a small group of Belgium chiropractors began what was to be a long research project. Its aim was to study what chiropractors refer to as a *subluxation*, which is traditionally defined as an incomplete dislocation, a displacement in which the articular surfaces have not lost contact, or a partially reduced (spontaneously) dislocation.

Outstanding within the Belgium group were Drs. H. Gillet and M. Liekens. These investigators, who have been involved in this study for more than half a century, soon found that the clinical phenomenon of subluxation was a great deal more complicated than the effects of the oversimplified picture of "a bone out of place" that has been commonly proposed since the turn of the century. Their findings reported in the

Belgium Research Notes are a testimony to their skillful observations. Although the theory of "a displaced vertebra" contained enough truth within it to constitute a basic therapeutic approach that could be justified by large numbers of positive benefits witnessed empirically, it was not sufficient to serve as a scientific hypothesis.

This investigative group did not have the advantage of any but personal funding and their own office facilities, it was decided to concentrate their studies on the normal and abnormal mobility of articular segments, especially those of the vertebral column and pelvis. As the findings of their investigations were reported, some basic assumptions of the profession were confirmed and others had to be discarded in light of the new knowledge obtained. For example, it was found that two basic concepts withstood the assault of the knowledge obtained year after year. These concepts involved vertebral *position* and *motion:*

1. *Facts of Position.* It was determined that a subluxated vertebra has not "slipped out of place." It is not displaced from its physiologic boundary, nor has it exceeded its normal limits of motion. Thus, when a "subluxation" is adjusted, it is not really replaced, relocated, or reduced in the same context as would be a complete or partial dislocation for it is usually "freed" to function normally (made mobile).

2. *Facts of Movements.* Vertebral movements describe an arc around a center of

motion, from one extreme to the other. It was found that the basic movements of spinal segments are rotation about the longitudinal axis, lateral flexion (side bending, tipping) toward the right or left, posterior-anterior flexion, anterior-posterior extension, and long-axis distention. Factors may arise that can inhibit movement within any one or more of these directions, setting up a state of abnormal biomechanical translation and rotation leading to biomechanical and subsequent physiologic dysfunction.

Introduction to Fixation Terminology

The design of the spinal column's bony processes and its ligaments tend to stop the zygapophyses from exceeding their inherent range of motion. When this range is exceeded (eg, severe trauma, predisposing gross pathology), the articular surfaces lose contact and are in a state of dislocation.

Bones Do Not Subluxate

A single vertebra cannot become subluxated or fixated. Only an articulation can subluxate or become fixated. As fixation-subluxations occur between two normally articulating surfaces, we speak about adjusting or mobilizing vertebral motion units (two apposing vertebral segments), not a single vertebra. Thus, articulations subluxate, not bones.

The Perpetuation of a Misnomer

A state of "subluxation," in the surgical sense of the word, is difficult to achieve in gliding joints, and all zygapophyseal joints are gliding in nature. This is said to be one reason given why chiropractic theory has had such a difficult time being accepted by the general scientific community. It is thus paradoxical that the term *subluxation*, in the chiropractic sense, has forced its presence on all the health-care professions and is becoming widely used in circles beyond the chiropractic profession, while at the same time chiropractors have begun to understand that the term is a misnomer when all its pathophysiologic components are considered. For example, a vertebra may be in a hypomobile state of "fixation," unilaterally or bilaterally, that is well within its normal range of motion during the resting position yet be considered an articular aberration that can cause or contribute to many pathologic expressions.

Articular Fixation Defined

For an articulation to remain in an abnormal state of "subluxation," something must be holding it there to restrict its mobility—otherwise it would spontaneously reduce itself and produce little clinical concern. This "holding" or "mobility hindrance" mechanism is commonly called a "fixation." Thus, (1) if a subluxation (a malfunction less than that produced by a dislocation) exists, a fixation also exists, and (2) a fixation can exist even when the articular surfaces are in an ideal relationship during the static resting posture.

Although this holding mechanism is commonly called a *fixation*, this term too can be the cause of confusion if it infers a state of complete immobility. In this text, the term *fixation* is used in its traditional sense in motion palpation—referring to any physical, functional, or psychic mechanism that produces a loss of segmental mobility within its normal physiologic range of motion. Thus, *ankylosis* would be considered a fixation in its purest sense—a 100% fixation. However, most fixations found clinically will be far less (eg, in the 20%—80% range of normal mobility).

Dr. Henri Gillet's Fixation Theory

The ability of a doctor of chiropractic to detect restricted articular motion or hypermobility may mean the difference between success and failure with many patients. The study of motion palpation offers the examining physician far greater insight and confidence in why, where, when, how, and how often to administer appropriate therapy—especially a corrective adjustment.

In evaluating the state of the periarticular and intra-articular soft tissues (eg, muscles, ligaments, capsules, synovia, articular cartilages) involved in an articular fixation, it will generally be found that it is some abnormal state of these soft tissues that is preventing the articular surfaces from moving in a particular plane. Common examples are muscle spasm and fibrosis, ligament shortening, intra-articular adhesions, scar development, cartilage hardening and malformation, cartilaginous chips and fragmented loose bodies, and cartilage erosion that restrict motion. Subsequent bone erosion and exostoses may also be involved. Osteopaths established many years ago that the soft tissues involved in a "vertebral lesion" can vary from the simplest muscle contraction to degenerative fibrosis of the muscles or even further to complete ossification of the involved ligaments and bursae.

After years of study, Gillet and his associates concluded that abnormal spinal muscle tone and changes within periarticular ligaments and intra-articular soft tissues were the primary factors responsible for the subluxation complex. These elements were also found to be the ones most influenced by the "chiropractic adjustment." Gillet showed that the dynamic chiropractic adjustment does not replace a vertebra or realign a bone; rather, it tends to eliminate the reason for its so called "abnormal position." Once adjusted (mobilized), the vertebral motion unit readapts itself, rapidly or slowly depending on its state of adaptability, to its full range of motion—often without further necessity of the doctor's intervention.

Because bony segments have not actually slipped out of place, an explanation is offered on why postadjustment static x-ray films frequently fail to show anatomical changes after the patient becomes symptom free. A freely mobile joint will rest in its most ideal midrange of motion possible—a position of readiness. If structural changes have occurred that have altered the articular surfaces or otherwise impaired its dynamic motion and/or static position in anyway, the adaptive or compensating resting position may appear as a misalignment during roentgenographic analysis. This is the typical "malpositioned vertebra" so often described in chiropractic literature.

Gillet's studies of vertebral fixation do not amend basic chiropractic concepts regarding the potential effects of subluxation complex (eg, neurologic, myologic, circulatory, inflammatory, and/or cerebrospinal and axoplasmic fluid changes). They only place them in a more dynamic perspective. This will become clearer within the following sections of this chapter.

Spinal Dynamics

In general, it would seem that a spine will not remain normal if it is not kept in a good state of mobility. This supports the necessity for voluntary exercise of normal joints as a prophylaxis to disease.

During normal spinal motion, cineroentgenographic and surgical animal studies have shown that (1) the superior and inferior posterior articular facets constantly glide on one another, establishing a barrage of complex proprioceptive signals to higher central nervous system (CNS) centers; (2) the intervertebral foramina (IVFs) are constantly opening and closing, and thus compressing and stretching the contents of the IVFs (viz, the spinal nerves, recurrent meningeal nerves, arteries, and veins). This dynamic action is also thought to help "milk" cerebrospinal fluid both around the spinal cord and peripherally along the spinal nerves. Normally, these dynamic compressing and stretching actions only occur for a few seconds at each event of movement and only within physiologic limits. These momentary actions, which can be likened to mild massage, should not be confused with prolonged or severe compressing and stretching actions.

Acute vs Chronic Spinal Fixations

The physiologic stretching, compression, and stimulation of the contents of the IVFs is normal and quite necessary to maintain a healthy state of the structures involved. To not occur would produce in the spine or any extraspinal synovial joint effects similar to those seen following prolonged immobilization of a limb such as disuse atrophy, ligament shortening, circulatory stasis, neurotrophic changes, etc. It is well recognized that the atrophy of disuse is one of degeneration; it is a pathologic state that produces *minimal* nerve excitability (irritation). This is undoubtedly why we find that an acute subluxation-fixation produces far more clinical expressions than a chronic subluxation-fixation and its effects tend to reflect signs of hyperactivity (eg, spasm, warmth, hyperesthesia, visceral hyperfunction). On the other hand, a chronic subluxation-fixation tends to express signs of hypoactivity (eg, weakness, coolness, numbness, visceral hypofunction, musculoskeletal degeneration).

Some authorities relate these changes with either the effects of neural facilitatory or inhibitory effects within the anterior, lateral, and posterior columns of the spinal cord. For example, facilitation would respectively manifest as motor excitation (eg, hypertonicity, spasm), sympathetic vasomotor excitation (eg, warmth), and sensory excitation (eg, pain, hyperesthesia). In contrast, inhibition would exhibit as motor depression (eg, hypotonicity, weakness), sympathetic vasomotor depression (eg, coolness, trophic changes), and sensory depression (eg, anesthesia).

The Compensatory Factor

Whenever an articulation is deprived of carrying out its normal function (motion), at least one other articulation is forced to take upon itself the burden of compensatory excessive motion, which may include eccentric and/or out-of-plane movement. This additional role within the counterpart joint or an adjacent articulation in the kinematic chain leads to irritation to the degree of inflammation once its homeostatic reserves are surpassed. Therefore, it is often seen that a site of fixation is asymptomatic, while the compensating hypermobile joint is highly expressive. In such a situation, it would be contraindicated to adjust the already hypermobile segment even if it is the focal site of clinical symptoms and signs.

Because of this compensatory factor, vertebral position derangements are often only of the *dynamic* variety; ie, they only exist in compensation to motion stress applied to an adjacent articulation. If the

stress applied on the compensatory hypermobile segment is prolonged, the greater the degree of related neuromuscular stress. We often see this with the neuromuscular complaints of someone who has engaged in an unaccustomed activity such as shoveling, painting the ceiling, weekend gardening, or after exercise by an unconditioned person.

The question arises that if this is true, why have results appeared to have been achieved in adjusting the symptomatic joint when it was not the basic cause of the symptoms? One possible answer is because a specific contact is extremely difficult to obtain on a specific vertebra as three motion units have been shown to be affected by a specific thrust. If a broader contact is used, the force of the adjustment is undoubtedly distributed to a larger number of neighboring fixated segments. Another possible explanation is that a major function of all perispinal ligaments is to serve as straps to prevent excessive motion; thus, if a force is applied to one end of these straps, they tend to move the adjacent structures to which they are attached (eg, a fixated adjacent articulation). Other biomechanical and possibly somatosomatic reflex mechanisms may also be involved.

It is important to remember that a partial unilateral fixation (eg, muscular, early ligamentous) produces symptoms on the opposite side because of the induced compensatory hypermobility. Thus, contrary to previous thought, correction is made by applying the adjustment (mobilizing the fixation) on the contralateral side of symptom expression.

The Interrelationship of Fixations

Many speculations have been made in chiropractic of what has appeared to be certain vertebrae or areas in the spine having a dominating influence on the spine as a whole. Such topics as primary subluxations, secondary subluxations, "key" vertebrae, majors vs minors, etc have been discussed since the early years of chiropractic. Many DCs have been taught that because the sacrum is the base of the spine, it is almost solely responsible for the mechanical state of the whole spinal superstructure. Conversely, many others have been taught that because of its unique position near the brain stem, once the atlas is correctly adjusted the whole spine will automatically realign itself. Lieb, a dentist, shows pre- and post-therapy full-spine radiographs exhibiting that correction of a TMJ syndrome has resulted in the spontaneous correction of overt scoliosis, kyphosis, and lordosis. There is no doubt that there is both truth and some misinterpretations in these concepts. Nevertheless, they do, in part, help to explain many commonly witnessed clinical phenomena.

Gillet often observed that so-called lesser fixations frequently became spontaneously mobile after he adjusted what was felt to be the most fixated segment in the spine and/or extremities. It has also been the observation of Gillet and his associates that, as a general rule, any correction made in any part of the spine will help the whole spine to correct itself to a degree in relation to the importance of the local correction. A hypothesis for this phenomenon will be given later in this chapter.

Normal Intervertebral Relationships

Because of our training in postural analysis, many of us have developed the habit of mentally picturing a healthy spine as one in which each vertebra is stacked upon its neighbor, with the ends of the spinous processes representing a dotted vertical line when the patient is standing or sitting and facing forward. While this is generally true, this viewpoint of the spine in such static attitudes is far removed from its role in daily living in which the spinal segments (motion units) are constantly rotating, bending, flexing, and extending. Except for possibly a few seconds at a time, the spine and its associated tissues are never at rest.

In any given movement, a joint will assume the position demanded of it by its anatomical plane and the gravitational and muscular forces directed on it. This is obvious in a "short leg" syndrome when the spine is examined in the upright position, where the hip, sacroiliac, and lumbar articulations must attempt to accommodate themselves functionally to compensate for the unlevel base of support. This mechanism is evident during all normal body motions, for a movement of any body part requires a compensatory reciprocal action by other body parts to maintain equilibrium. The same biomechanical process is true in every case in which a vertebra is fixed at or near its extreme range of normal motion, causing other articulations to "displace" themselves in adaptation to the fixation during some or all motions, depending on the site and extent of the fixation. Thus, an "abnormal segmental position" by itself is not pathognomonic of subluxation. It is for this reason that the editor of the ACA's *Basic Chiropractic Procedural Manual* chose to take several pages to just summarize the criteria indicative of a subluxation.

Effects of Common Trauma

Ligaments are never tender unless they are in a pathologic state. Trauma far less than that causing fracture or dislocation produces an inflammatory reaction similar to that caused by a bacterial invasion. The reaction to bacterial invasion is designed to contain and wall off the bacteria to prevent further spreading of the infection. After trauma, localization serves to contain the products of the injured tissues. Unfortunately, the resolution of inflammation (scarring) can be especially harmful if the joint has not returned to normal mobility. This occurs because normal periarticular soft tissues are flexible, elastic, plastic, and generally richly vascular. Scar tissue, on the other hand, tends to be stiff, unyielding, and poorly vasculated. For this reason, reinjured joints that were not properly attended initially are extremely slow to heal. Every individual has sustained numerous bumps, strains, and sprains within his life.

Acute inflammation can develop into chronic inflammation that may continue for decades. Therefore, it is necessary to treat each trauma until all pain, tenderness, swelling, immobility, etc, are eliminated. Partial treatment is not adequate.

The diagnosis should be accurate and comprehensive. More than one tissue is usually affected by a single traumatic incident, and the treatment should be specific for each tissue affected. Determining the cause is not an easy task. For example, tender hypertonic perivertebral tissues found in the upper thoracic region of the spine may be from (1) overworked tissues (eg, unaccustomed activity of chopping wood or shoveling), (2) unusual sustained postures (eg, prolonged spinal extension as in painting a ceiling), (3) a viscerosomatic reflex (eg, heavy smoking, lung or heart disease), (4) excessive compensatory segmental hypermobility owing to one or more fixated lower cervical or midthoracic vertebral motion units, or (5) a combination of two or more of these factors.

The basic direction of case management can be considered as progressing through two phases. The first goal is to reduce the swelling and relieve the associated pain and soreness by R-I-C-E (rest, ice, compression, and elevation) and other physiotherapeutic measures when appropriate. The second objective is to promote healing and movement (eg, by manipulation, massage, stretching, passive and active exercise, and other standard regimens. It is also imperative to relieve any attending neurologic disorder in the spine, as this often cuts the reflex feedback cycle that facilitates prolonging the effect and also eliminates a possible source of a secondary or contributing subluxation complex.

Joint Play and Its Restrictions

In addition to the normal active and passive ranges of motion, there is a third type of motion called "joint play." This small but precise accessory movement within synovial joints cannot be influenced except passively. Although joint play is necessary for normal joint function, it is not influenced by a patient's volition. Thus, joint play can be defined as that degree of end movement or distention allowed passively that cannot be achieved through voluntary effort. In other words, total joint motion is the sum of the voluntary range of movement plus or minus any joint play exhibited.

Joint play occurs because normal joint surfaces do not appose tightly. Because joint surfaces are of varying radii, movement cannot occur about a rigid axis. The capsule must allow some extra play for full motion to occur. In addition to translatory and rotational joint play, a degree of distraction must exist. If any one of these involuntary movements is impaired for some reason, the articular surfaces become closely packed (compressed) and motion will be restricted. Added to this is the factor that there are small spaces created by articular incongruence necessary for hydrodynamic lubrication. Prolonged compression would lead to poor lubrication and possible ischemia, likely progressing to degenerative joint disease due to abrasion irritation.

Joint play cannot be produced by phasic muscle contraction. However, voluntary action is greatly influenced by normal joint play. The loss of joint play results in a painful joint that becomes involuntarily protected by secondary muscle spasm. Thus, motion palpation to detect restricted joint play is an important part of the biomechanical examination of any painful and spastic axial or appendicular joint. Pain and spasm result when a joint is moved (actively or passively) in the direction in which normal joint endplay is lacking. Once normal joint play is restored, the associated pain and spasm subside.

Joint play should exist in *all* ranges of motion that are normal for a particular joint. That is, if a joint functions in flexion, extension, abduction, and adduction, the integrity of joint play in all these directions plus distraction should be evaluated. It is not unusual for joint play to be restricted in some planes but not others.

A common cause of articular fixation and the resulting motion restriction is disuse. Many occupations require that certain joints move only in one or two planes but not all planes available. For example, a joint that is continually flexed but rarely extended will exhibit normal or abnormal joint play in flexion and frequently restricted joint play in extension. A similar situation occurs in a joint that is frequently abducted but rarely adducted or frequently rotated toward the left but rarely to the right.

The importance of freeing articular fixations (eg, by chiropractic adjustments, mobilization) is brought out by Mennell. Normal muscle function depends on normal joint function, and vice versa. If joint motion is not free, the involved muscles that move it cannot function and cannot be restored to normal. Thus, impaired muscle function leads to impaired joint function, and, conversely, impaired joint function leads to impaired muscle function. In this clinical cycle, muscle and joint function cannot be functionally separated from each other.

In summary, Faye emphasizes the following major points of joint play:

1. Total joint movement is the voluntary range of movement plus or minus the joint play present.

2. Voluntary action depends on normal joint play, but voluntary motion and exercise cannot produce or restore joint play. The presence or absence of joint play can only be demonstrated by an examiner; ie, passively.

3. Loss of joint play produces pain on testing; ie, whenever that direction of joint play is challenged. When restricted joint play is restored by manipulation, the related pain abates. A painful joint produces secondary muscular changes; ie, spasm, which is nature's way of preventing injurious joint movement. If painful joint movement occurs because of joint play restriction, the joint play must be restored to near normal to obtain a permanent reduction of the spasm. [See Clinical Comment 1.1]

4. Muscles that move a joint with joint dysfunction become hypertonic in response to the pain from irritation; therefore, the active range of motion is also restricted.

5. Joint play can only be restored by a mobilizing force (maneuver, thrust, impulse) delivered satisfactorily; ie, in line with the plane of articulation and against the motion resistance (fixation).

NORMAL MOVEMENTS OF SPINAL ARTICULATIONS

Although the gross movements of the spine and pelvis have been the subject of numerous studies, information about typical movements between individual segments was relatively obscure (except for the findings of Gillet) until Kapandji, White, and Punjabi reported their findings.

To fully appreciate the concepts of motion palpation, the mental picture of the spine being a straight, vertical, static structure (as viewed on a radiograph) must be discarded. The spine is a living, dynamic, segmented organ that is in constant motion during locomotion, work, and with every breath taken during rest. As most organs of the body, during day or night, work or rest, the spine never rests—it is in constant motion, constantly *dynamic*.

Because a force may act along a single line in a single plane or in any direction in space, this factor must be considered in any reference system. Such a reference system is necessary if we are to effectively communicate with each other about joint position and motion. Thus, this section will review pertinent terms and principles that will enhance our communication skills as well as deepen our understanding of *spinal dynamics*.

The Planes of the Body and Related Considerations

Many basic considerations in biomechanics involve time, mass, center of mass, movement, force, and gravity—which operate in accordance with the laws of physics. However, while numerous parameters of movement are interrelated, no one factor is capable of completely describing movement by itself.

DR. FAYE'S CLINICAL COMMENT #1.1

The pain experienced by the patient when joint play is restricted is sharp and only lasts as long as the doctor presses into the restriction during the examination. This must not be confused with the joint pain associated with an inflamed joint that produces a lingering type of pain when challenged.

The force of gravity is always directed toward the earth's center. Thus, the gravity line of action and direction are constants. In the upright "rigid" body posture, the gravitational force on the entire mass can be considered a single vector through the center of mass that represents the sum of many parallel positive and negative coordinates (Fig. 1.1).

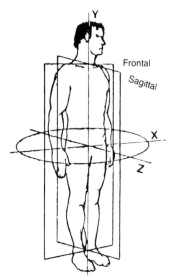

Figure 1.1. The planes of the body as they are related to the line of gravity. The X (frontal) axis passes from side to side (horizontally) and perpendicular to the sagittal plane. The Y (vertical) axis passes perpendicular to the transverse plane and the ground. The Z (sagittal) axis is perpendicular to the frontal plane, passing horizontally from front to back (Courtesy ACAP).

Describing Positions in Space

In a two-dimensional reference system, the plane is simply divided into four quadrants by a perpendicular vertical ordinate line (Y axis) and a horizontal abscissa line (X axis). A third axis (usually labeled Z) can be used to locate points in three dimensions. The Z axis crosses the origin and is perpendicular to planes X and Y.

There are several reference systems. This particular system is the *Cartesian coordinate system* in which: (1) flexion/extension

rotation is rotation about the X axis, (2) axial rotation is rotation about the Y axis, and (3) lateral flexion rotation is rotation about the Z axis.

All Z points in front of the X-Y plane are positive, while those behind are negative (Fig. 1.2). By using X, Y, and Z coordinates, any point in space can be located and depicted. However, a minimum of six coordinates is necessary to specify the position of a rigid body (eg, a vertebra).

In biomechanics, the body's reference origin is located at the body's center of mass. This is usually just anterior to the S2 segment. When this point is known, gross body space can be visualized as being in the sagittal (right-left) Y-Z plane, frontal or

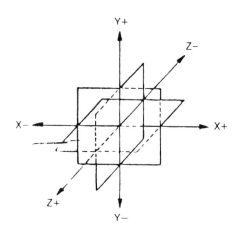

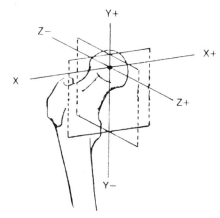

Figure 1.2. *Top,* positive and negative X, Y, and Z axes. *Bottom,* system of coordinates pertinent to the mechanical axis of the hip (Courtesy ACAP).

coronal (anterior-posterior) X-Y plane, or horizontal or transverse (superior-inferior) X-Z plane. With such a reference system, movement of any body segment in these planes can be described by placing a coordinate system at the axis of a joint and projecting the action lines of the muscles involved.

Axes

An axis is a straight line around which an object rotates, a line serving to orient a space or object (about which the object is symmetrical), or a reference line in a system of coordinates. Most body movements are rotations about joint axes and are rarely confined to a simple arc. Such motions vary to compensate for muscle-joint restrictions, bones twisting about their axes, and the transfer of power from one set of muscles to another within the range of movement. The joint surfaces of spinal joints are usually convexo-concave in design; ie, the convex surface is larger than the concave surface. This relationship is exaggerated in all extraspinal ball-and-socket joints.

If the anatomical position is used as a reference point, joint movements occur in a definite plane and around a definite axis. Flexion, extension, and hyperextension are movements in the sagittal plane about a frontal axis. Abduction and adduction are movements in the frontal plane about a sagittal axis. Rotation, pronation, and supination are movements in the transverse plane about a vertical axis. And circumduction is movement in both the sagittal and frontal planes. See Table 1.1.

Linear and Circular Motion

The two basic types of body movement are *linear movement* and *circular movement*. *Linear movement* is that in which the body as a whole or one of its parts can be moved as a whole from one place to another in a straight line. One example of linear (sliding, gliding, translation) movement without any circular motion is long axis distraction of a finger joint.

Circular movement (angular, rotational) is that in which the body or a part can be moved around the arc of a circle. An example of circular motion is seen between the long bones of the extremities and in the spinal column. Circular movements occur in definite planes and around a definite axis (center of rotation). They comprise an important diagnostic viewpoint in musculoskeletal disorders, and, as previously described, each of these three axes of rotation is perpendicular to the plane in which motion occurs.

Structural Motion

From a clinical viewpoint, structural motion can be defined as a body segment's relative change of place or position in space within a time frame and about some other object in space. Thus, motion may be determined and illustrated by knowing and showing its position before and after an interval of time. While linear motion is readily demonstrated in the body as a whole as it moves in a straight line, most joint motions are combinations of translation and

Table 1.1. Joint Movement Planes and Their Axes

Movement	Plane	Axis
Flexion	Sagittal	Frontal
Extension	Sagittal	Frontal
Abduction	Frontal	Sagittal
Adduction	Frontal	Sagittal
Rotation	Transverse	Vertical
Pronation	Transverse	Vertical
Supination	Transverse	Vertical

angular movements that are more often than not diagonal rather than parallel to the cardinal planes. For example, a vertebra cannot move in the A-P plane because its articulating facets are slanted obliquely. In addition to muscle force, joint motion is governed by factors of movement freedom, axes of movement, and range of motion.

Degrees of Joint Movement Freedom

The body is composed of numerous uniaxial, biaxial, and multiaxial joints. Joints with one axis have one degree of freedom to move in one plane such as pivot and hinge joints, joints with two axes have two degrees of freedom to move in two different planes, and joints with three axes have three degrees of freedom to move in all three planes (eg, ball-and-socket joints). Thus, that motion in which an object may translate to and fro along a straight course or rotate one way or another about a particular axis equals one degree of freedom.

To know the actual degrees of freedom (ranges of motions) available to a part of the body, one must sum the degrees available of adjacent joints to appreciate the amount of free motion of one part about another part. The degrees of freedom of a fingertip about the trunk, for example, are the sum of the degrees of freedom of all the joints from the distal phalanges to the shoulder girdle. While the distal phalanges have only one degree of freedom (flexion-extension), the entire upper extremity has 17 degrees in total. This summation process is an example of a living, *open kinematic chain.*

Combined Movements

Simple translatory motions of a body part invariably involve movements of more than one joint. This requires reciprocating actions of three or more segments at two or more joints if parallel lines are to be followed. For example, a fingertip cannot be made to follow the straight edge of a ruler placed in front when the wrist, elbow, and shoulder joints are locked. The fingertip must follow an arc and not a straight line. Thus, human

motion can be described as translation that gains major contributions from linear, angular, and curvilinear motions. The terms *general* or *three-dimensional body motion* infer that a body part may move in any direction by combining multidirectional translation and multiaxial rotation.

Plane Motion

Any motion in which all coordinates of a rigid body move parallel to a fixed point is referred to as *plane motion.* Such motion has three degrees of freedom (ranges of motions); viz, (1) moving toward the anterior or posterior, (2) laterally moving toward the right or left, and (3) spinning in one direction or the other. In other words, plane motion has two translatory degrees of motion along two mutually perpendicular axes and one rotational degree of motion around an axis perpendicular to the translatory axes. Thus, when an individual flexes his spine forward, the vertebrae flex and rotate in a single plane about an axis that is perpendicular to the sagittal plane. In such plane motion, various points on a particular vertebra will always move in parallel planes.

The Instantaneous Axis of Rotation

Plane motion is described by the position of its *instantaneous axis of rotation* and

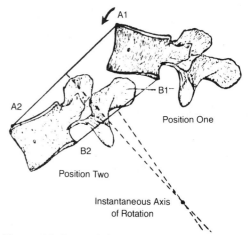

Figure 1.3. Determining the instantaneous axis of rotation of a vertebra from one position to another (Courtesy ACAP).

the motion's rotational magnitude about this axis. In the above example of spinal flexion, for instance, as a vertebra moves in a plane, there is a point at every instant of motion somewhere within or without the body that does not move. If a line is drawn from that point so it perpendicularly meets the line of motion, the point of intersection is called the instantaneous axis of rotation for that motion at that particular point in time (Fig. 1.3). Most joint movement is to a great extent rotational motion, but the axis of motion may change its location and/or its orientation during a complete range of motion.

Out-of-Plane Motion

As contrasted to plane motion, *out-of-plane motion* is a type of general body motion with three degrees of freedom: two rotations about mutually perpendicular axes and translation perpendicular to the plane formed by the axes. Thus, in out-of-plane motion, the body as a whole or a segment can move more than in a single plane. For example, if a person bends laterally, a mid-thoracic vertebral body translates from the sagittal plane towards the horizontal plane (Fig. 1.4). This is not plane motion because various points on the vertebra do not move in parallel planes.

Motion Barriers and Their Significance in Manipulation

All types of joint manipulation impose static and dynamic forces across joint surfaces. Within its anatomical range of motion, a normal joint exhibits in all planes of motion (1) a large voluntary active range, (2) an involuntary stress-less passive range, and (3) a slight paraphysiologic range that is determined by ligamentous plasticity, elasticity, and viscoelasticity (joint play). These ranges are used in voluntary exercise, mobilization, and adjustive techniques, respectively. To appreciate this more fully, an understanding of the barrier concept is necessary.

If a joint is tested passively to determine its range of motion, the examiner will note increasing end resistance to motion referred to as a "bind," the *physiologic motion bar-*

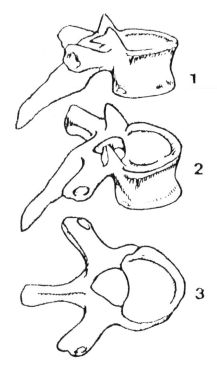

Figure 1.4. Schematic of vertebral out-of-plane motion (Courtesy ACAP).

rier, or the elastic barrier. If the joint is slowly carried past this point, the added motion becomes uncomfortable to the patient. If carried still further to a point just short of injury, this point is the *anatomical motion barrier*. That slight range of motion between the elastic barrier and the anatomical limit is the involuntary paraphysiologic space or range, the area of passive joint play. At the end of joint play, the anatomical barrier, the joint tissues are stretched to their structural limits.

The gross evaluation of passive joint movement is normally conducted to or within the elastic barrier (Fig. 1.5). Thus, joint motion evaluation is accomplished by passively carrying the joint through a range of motion until the physiologic motion barrier is firmly encountered, and then noting the degrees of movement achieved.

Active motion normally swings between the neutral position to the point of tissue resistance, while passive motion extends past this to within the elastic barrier. The usual objective of most *mobilization* tech-

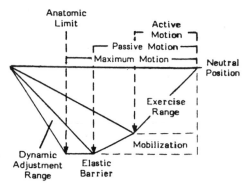

Figure 1.5. Comparative ranges of movement during exercise, mobilization, and dynamic adjustive techniques (Courtesy ACAP).

niques is to restore the normal range of passive joint motion from the neutral position to the normal elastic barrier. Thus, it is slightly longer in range than that of active motion and to the maximum point of slow passive motion. The objective of most *stretching* techniques is to restore motion from the neutral position to the elastic barrier. Many osteopathic "leverage" techniques are conducted within this range, as are many chiropractic extremity techniques. In contrast, specific dynamic chiropractic *adjustments* are usually carried a step further deep into the paraphysiologic range, often to the anatomical limit, but the duration of the application of maximum force is only a fraction of a second.

Wyke has shown that forced active motion on a joint whose mobility has been restricted will rapidly become painful and its periarticular muscles will be hypertonic or spastic. For example, loss of joint play in the sacroiliac joints can cause the gluteals and hamstrings to tighten. If a sudden strong contraction is required by the quadriceps, the unrelaxed antagonistic hamstrings are likely to tear if the primary motion is accomplished. Various degrees of this phenomenon are seen in sports and occupational injuries associated with fixations.

THE DIFFERENT TYPES OF FIXATIONS

A spinal fixation has been previously defined as some abnormal factor that blocks or inhibits passive motion. It has also been described that the term *fixation* is not synonymous with the term *subluxation;* fixation is only one, but highly necessary, characteristic of the subluxation complex.

There are four general types of fixations: (1) muscular, (2) ligamentous, (3) articular, and (4) bony. It is clinically important to attempt to judge the degree of fixation and the nature of the fixative element to evaluate the minimum amount of force necessary during an adjustive thrust to "break down" the fixation if it is logical to do so (breaking an ankylosis, for example, would usually be contraindicated). This is true whether the cause is a spasm, a shortened ligament, an interarticular adhesion, or some other ameliorable factor.

Muscular (Class I) Fixations

In relation to spinal fixations, the term muscular *spasm* is used by Gillet to describe the state of a muscle or muscles that fixate vertebrae and hinder their normal movement. Yet, he does this with misgivings because he states that such contractions are somewhat different from the spasms and cramps which occur in other muscles of the body. For example:

1. Spasms and cramps that occur in other parts of the body (eg, calf "Charley horse," intestinal colic, diaphragmatic spasm of "windedness") are acute contractions that are extremely painful. In contrast, the spasms associated with spinal fixations are usually only sensitive to deep pressure and otherwise go unnoticed by the patient.

2. Except for spastic paralysis (eg, poststroke), spasms in other parts of the body have a short duration. In contrast, the spasms associated with spinal fixations may endure for months or years without change. In spite of the chronicity, the muscles involved do not necessarily degenerate or become fibrotic as other muscles normally do under such conditions.

There is no doubt that these perivertebral spasms exist because they can be palpated. The most common ones found are of the rotatores, multifidi, interspinales, intertransversarii (cervical), obliquus capitis (atlas-axis), levatores costarum, spinalis groups, and different portions of the quadratus lumborum. While areas of spasm can sometimes be palpated in the large-long muscles of the back, they are rarely found to be responsible for individual fixations. Gillet's findings to date have tended to confirm Palmer's concept of a single segmental subluxation (the "major" concept) rather than Carver's hypothesis of abnormal curves of the spine (summation of the whole area) being the focus for pathologic expression. Regardless, further research is necessary for uncontested confirmation of either theory.

Muscle Tonicity vs Phasic Contractions

In all healthy skeletal muscles, there is a combination of two major neurologic factors at work: (1) The sustaining or resting tone (tension, firmness) of a muscle (an involuntary mechanism) is controlled by the sympathetic nervous system through low-frequency asynchronous impulses from the spinal cord. Its purpose is to keep the muscular system in a neurochemical and functional state of readiness to act and maintain static postural equilibrium (sustained by the stretch reflex). It is active during both rest and work, and is especially developed in the antigravity muscles. (2) The voluntary and involuntary gross contraction of a muscle, under the control of both the cerebrospinal motor system and cord reflexes, directs all postural, ballistic, and tension movements. It is electrically silent during rest and relatively silent during the relaxed upright position if the body is well balanced over weight-bearing joints. Voluntary muscle contraction is always superimposed on the involuntary intrinsic tone of the muscles involved in any musculoskeletal action.

Gillet postulates that the palpable spasm associated with a vertebral fixation could be an involuntary state of abnormal hypertonus rather than a cord reflex initiating a spasm via a phasic contraction as seen in typical spasms and protective "splinting." This theory could explain why the hypertonic muscles associated with fixations are tender to palpation but not otherwise painful.

Gillet's Theory of the Cause of Fixation-Related Hypertonicity

It is empirically evident that "subluxations" are often caused by trauma (direct or indirect) such as in blows, falls, and strains or indirect microtrauma such as from the various effects of biomechanical imbalance. The neuromuscular response to trauma is either contraction to a degree that varies with the severity of the trauma—either a strong rapid contraction or a slow contraction of long duration. In this context, paraphrasing Gillet, let us suppose that as soon as the contraction goes beyond a certain limit in force or duration the autonomic fibers controlling muscle tonicity become abnormally stimulated. As any neural stimulation of high intensity tends to "jump" impulses from sensory to motor tracts, via internuncial neurons in the spinal cord, instead of or before traveling up the cord, it is possible that such a mechanism could be established as a fixed pattern of behavior, a vicious self-perpetuating neuromuscular cycle.

If such a hypertonicity is sufficient enough and if it is unilateral, the motion unit involved will tend to be pulled into a sustained position of action. This appears likely as each vertebral segment is "balanced" at rest in a state of physiologic equilibrium between its extremes of motion. The spine is not a stiff column of segments. The structural properties of its discs, ligaments, and cartilages are relatively plastic, flexible, elastic, and viscoelastic. We can now add to this picture the neurologic mechanism of *reciprocal inhibition;* viz, phasic agonist contractions are accompanied by a reciprocal decrease in action in its antagonists. For example, when flexors act, extensors relax, and vice versa. Reciprocal inhibition is usually thought of as a temporary mechanism, but is this always true?

General Characteristics of Muscular Fixations

Muscular fixations are the most numerous type of fixation, and their potential number may appear great in any given patient. They are, however, usually minor or secondary. Although all possible muscular fixations will not necessarily exist in each patient, they are all possible and should be recorded with each patient. If no ligamentous or articular fixations are found, muscular fixations can be corrected. However, if a secondary muscular fixation is adjusted before mobilization of its primary focus, it will return quickly (in minutes) because it is an adaptation to the site of primary ligamentous or articular fixation.

The major characteristics of perivertebral muscular fixations are as follows:

• They are usually palpated as taut tender muscle fibers underneath hyperesthetic skin. If the overlying skin and subcutaneous tissues near the related spinous process are rolled between the skin and index finger, acute tenderness will be reported by the patient.

• They exhibit restricted mobility from the start when challenged, and the end feel exhibits a little "give" and a rubbery end block.

• They are completely released and almost immediately become nontender, relaxed, and the segment to which they are attached becomes mobile with the proper adjustment.

• They are usually secondary to another area of fixation or the result of a reflex (somatosomatic or viscerosomatic); thus, they will likely recur if the primary fixation or some other focus of irritation is not corrected.

Unilaterality and Acuteness Factors. Besides being the most numerous, muscular fixations are the most pathognomonic of overt symptoms yet the most open to change by either direct or indirect methods according to Gillet. They also are the type in which the "displacement" factor is the most visible because the spasm or hypertonicity involved is usually unilateral. This can often be seen with the axis, where unilateral hypertonicity of an obliquus capitis inferior muscle pulls the spinous of the axis laterally. This unilaterality is frequently a sign of its acute state. The more acute the condition, the less degeneration will be found in the muscle responsible and the greatest change can be observed after an adjustment—either locally or through the correction of more chronic major fixations.

Remote Effects. Muscular fixations are frequently secondary facilitated "reflex" responses to more chronic fixations elsewhere or an activated viscerosomatic reflex. If the result of a somatosomatic reflex, many of them disappear spontaneously after the correction of primary ligamentous and articular fixations. Furthermore, Gillet reports that there seems to be an important specificity between primary chronic fixations and acute muscular (reflex) fixations. This specificity is often surprising in its remote location, sometimes going from L5 to the lower cervicals without an apparent neurologic or biomechanical explanation. Another common example is an upper-cervical major fixation that produces low-back muscular fixations which, in turn, results in low-back pain and dysfunction.

Postural Changes Related to Muscular Fixations

These secondary reflex fixations just described appear to be primarily due to hypertonicity of the short spinal muscles, but certain long muscles are sometimes involved. When they are, they produce the characteristic postural distortions and antalgic positions that are so often seen in clinical practice and measured by grids, plumb line analyses, etc. Certain methods of spinal examination use these abnormal postures to deductively reason to the causative fixation, and some therapeutic techniques work on the long muscles in an attempt to bring the body back into normal balance. Such procedures may easily lead to erroneous conclusions and misinterpretations. [See Clinical Comment 1.2]

It is possible to change human posture by working on these long muscles because it is almost always possible to provide a centripetal effect on a primary condition by influencing the secondary half of the cycle. This can often be seen in the effects of medical treatment, and it is true with many chiropractic procedures. To perpetuate this effect, however, will require a greater repetition of the therapeutic agent. It can be stated as a general rule that each time a correction has to be repeated several times within a short period, this attempt at correction is being applied to an abnormality which is secondary to another located somewhere else, originating either within the body or its immediate external environment.

Another difficulty in using gross posture as a sign of fixation is that not all fixations produce a related hypertonus of long body muscles capable of altering gross posture. This effect is a characteristic of fixations that produce irritation of the cerebrospinal nerves and far less of those which can irritate the sympathetic nerves. Specific long muscles that are involved in postural changes and fixations will be described in subsequent chapters.

Etiologic Questions. The inquiry commonly arises: Which comes first, fixation or postural distortion? There are two general answers (possibilities) to this question:

1. Muscular contraction can pull a vertebra out of normal resting alignment.

2. Because the spine is forced to remain for long periods in a position of "unrest," the soft tissues of the spine will slowly adapt to the action demanded by the patient's daily activities and positions. The vertebrae involved can be considered to be "normally" misaligned as long as the reason for this malposition exists.

The first type (1 above) takes in all traumatic subluxations in which one or more muscles react to the trauma by a vigorous defensive contraction (nociceptive reflex). If this contraction exceeds an individual's limits, a noxious nerve-muscle cycle can be established that tends to remain until a counteracting force (eg, adjustment) interrupts the cycle. This type of fixation-malplacement syndrome would also include situations resulting from a feedback mechanism from a unilateral peripheral irritation (eg, a viscerospinal reflex), including those of the upper cervical area from excessive mental-emotional stimulation, visual fatigue, and other reflex fixations. As these fixations are of a muscular nature, they are usually unilateral, or predominantly so, and acute.

The second type of fixation-subluxation (2 above) is of the *spinal balance* class, including any vertebral articulation that would be forced to adapt itself to (1) a short leg, (2) malformed vertebrae, (3) the imbalancing effect of acute subluxations, (4) poor posture caused by unusual working conditions, and (5) unilateral imbalancing "specialized" movements in work. In all these conditions, we would have what could be called "microtraumatism," the most typical being the anatomical short-leg syndrome in which the associated lumbar scoliosis is a normal adaptation as long as the scoliosis is flexible to the degree that the spine will straighten in the sitting and recumbent positions. On this subject, Faye mentions that Lynton G. Giles has shown that a leg-length difference of approximately 15 mm is necessary before appreciable adaptation occurs.

Thus, we have two possible etiologies: (1) the fixation comes first, or (2) the "displacement" is the primary element. Both types may sometimes be found in the same area, in which case it is more often the acute type that adds itself to the chronic type. In the chronic type, states Faye, degenerative changes within the three-joint complex of the motion unit must be present for true displacement to exist.

Effects of Adjustive Therapy

If two spinal motion segments are in a state of "malposition" because of unilateral hypertonicity or spasm of one or more intervertebral muscles, the structures to which the involved muscles have their origin and insertion will be drawn towards one another during most types of adjustments. Thus, a dynamic thrust that has as its objective

---

DR. FAYE'S CLINICAL COMMENT #1.2

Most patients have more than one major ligamentous or articular fixation. We try to adjust the most fixated (least "springy") motion unit first. As the muscular fixations spontaneously normalize, a second or third motion unit is adjusted to influence other muscular fixations. As the biomechanics improve and there are less aberrant joint insults to the spine and locomotor system, the inflamed joints begin to heal.

"realignment" of the segments will obviously stretch the contracted muscles (increase the distance between muscle origin and insertion). It is probably for this that a chiropractic dynamic thrust, as contrasted to a simple slow pull or push, has proved to be more successful in practice.

While Gillet does not propose that this hypothesis offers a complete explanation, he does believe that it answers more questions than others projected in the past. In addition, this explanation is only rational for those muscular fixations that remain in a state of prolonged abnormal function and which are not associated with myodegeneration. He also adds that for some still unknown reason, other fixations (possibly those in which we have two or more hypertonic muscles between adjacent vertebrae) sometimes do undergo the usual degenerative process in a fixation-subluxation syndrome.

Ligamentous (Class II) Fixations

One early physiologic change seen with chronically fixated vertebral articulations is the shortening of ligaments. This is true because ligaments always tend to adapt themselves to the range of motion used. That is, they will shorten to the degree necessary to remove any slack. Thus, in complete or multimuscular fixations, the associated ligaments and related soft tissues will have distinctively shortened. The type of thrust used here must be one designed to lengthen ligamentous tissues (eg, repeated nontraumatic traction on the insertions of the involved ligaments). Total multimuscular and multiligamentous fixations are frequently found at the sacroiliac joints and the occipital-atlantal area and are associated with the thoracic spine.

The most pertinent characteristics of ligamentous fixations, which are often major fixations, are that they are usually:

• The reflection of a degenerating chronic muscular fixation or the effect of ligament trauma.

• Overlaid with atrophied subcutaneous tissues.

• Palpated as an abrupt, hard block within the normal range of motion that exhibits no end play.

• Bilateral (with one side tighter than the other) or else are in the median line.

• Improved only slightly immediately after each corrective treatment.

Shortening of Capsular Ligaments

Gillet and associates have found few spinal fixations that can be explained by shortening of the capsular ligaments, although practically all the other spinal ligaments seem to be involved in fixations.

When apophyseal capsular shortening occurs, one might think that it would result in an articular-like fixation. However, this has not been found to be true: there is still a certain amount of torsion possible. This is especially evident in the extraspinal joints; eg, when there are many fixations in the feet involving the calcaneus, tarsals, and metatarsals. Similar fixations can frequently be found in the proximal articulation of the fibula with the tibia, in sternoclavicular and acromioclavicular joints, and among the metacarpals. Such extraspinal fixations can have noxious effects either locally or in the spine (reflex fixation). These manifestations will be described in Chapters 8 and 9.

Musculotendinous Fixations Resembling Ligamentous Fixations

In certain purely muscular fixations, the spastic or hypertonic muscles involved tend to degenerate and become fibrotic. For all practical purposes, such fibrotic muscles resemble ligaments in function and structure. As most of the deep spinal muscles are underlaid and/or overlaid with ligaments, it is often difficult to determine which structure is responsible for the fixation. Fortunately, the type and direction of a corrective thrust is nearly the same, and even the amount of demonstrable change that can be expected from a fibrosed muscle or a shortened ligament is the same. Thus, from a clinical viewpoint, a fibrotic muscle fixation can be classed as a ligamentous fixation. Gillet believes that this type of fixation is the most common but not the most irritative.

Several authors have described the shortening or tension found in certain fascia and tendons as being responsible for the restriction of joint motion, either by themselves or by hindering the action of their associated muscles. One example of this is the fascia lata in fixations of the proximal femur. The Belgium researchers, however, have not been able to confirm this as yet.

Muscular vs Ligamentous Postadjustment Effects

While the adjustive technique need be modified only slightly with either muscular or ligamentous fixations, the postadjustive reaction is quite different. In muscular fixations, an immediate near-normal range of motion should be expected. In ligamentous fixations, however, the immediate gain in mobility is only slight with each treatment. This does not mean, however, that the increased movements during everyday activities between office visits are not another important factor in restoring mobility. [See Clinical Comment 1.3]

The Intervertebral Discs

Gillet gives no more importance to the intervertebral disc (IVD) in the production of spinal fixations than any other ligamentous structure. He believes the integrity of the IVD is generally more of a passive factor than an active factor. A few exceptions to this general rule will be described in subsequent chapters, but motion palpation studies have not confirmed that true IVD lesions are as common as generally accepted in the medical community and to a great extent within our own profession. Faye states that disc degeneration, with its internal disruption and posterior joint gapping, causes more hypermobility and instability.

Articular (Class III) Fixations

True articular or total fixations are common manifestations in the human spine, and they have been the subject of several studies that arrive at conflicting conclusions. Regardless of cause, they appear to be the result of intra-articular joint "gluing" similar to that seen in adhesive capsulitis and multiple ligamentous shortenings. Overt pathology does not appear to be related as the fixation is eventually made mobile by repeated chiropractic adjustments.

In any total articular fixation, one lateral pair of articulations (inferior and superior facets) of the bilateral posterior articulations may be the seat of fixation and the other not. The contralateral pair may be normal initially, but as the inferior and superior zygapophyses become more immobilized because of the fixation of their contralateral counterparts, they also become functionally incapable of motion. In time, the pathologic effects of disuse can be expected in the initially normal pair of articulations.

In total fixations in which the fixative element is the product of degeneration of the interarticular and periarticular soft tissues, with the probable development of "adhesions," the major corrective effect of the chiropractic adjustment is produced by the forced opening of the apposed facets.

Gillet points out that this type of unilateral *total* fixation can be demonstrated when reflex-fixations are searched for and found. This procedure will be described in a following chapter. It should be mentioned, however, that total unilateral fixations in the spine function differently than total unilateral fixations in the sacroiliac joints. In total unilateral fixation of a sacroiliac joint, the contralateral articulation is not restricted in movement and typically adapts by becoming *hypermobile* and acutely overstressed in a prolonged attempt to serve the role of both joints.

DR. FAYE'S CLINICAL COMMENT #1.3

During this phase of treatment, stretching exercises at home should be recommended to the patient. A 30-second stretch into the fixation, just short of inducing pain, is my suggestion. This stretching should be repeated two or three times a day. The last few seconds of the stretch is done while exhaling.

This reciprocity of immobility and hyper-mobility is found in all types of fixations. In total fixations found between vertebrae, Illi states that the adaptive hyperkinesis takes place in the articulation above and below, or in the opposite articulations exceptionally. In partial fixations, it takes place on the still mobile side of segments unilaterally fixated (Figs. 1.6 and 1.7).

In summary, the major characteristics of articular (total) fixations are that they:

• Are motion palpated as being complete-ly immobile in all directions and asympto-matic.

• Are painful when challenged by the palpator.

• Progress to ankylosis; thus, irreversible in the terminal stage.

Articular fixations, which are always considered major faults, should usually be corrected first, and ligamentous fixations should be given priority consideration over muscular fixations because the latter are often secondary (compensatory, reflexively produced). [See Clinical Comment 1.4]

Bony Restrictions

Bony outgrowths may be obvious, but if they are near the periphery of a joint, they may be recognized only by the sudden arrest of an otherwise free motion. In true anky-losis, there is no mobility whatever and adja-cent joints are often hypermobile in compen-sation. Roentgenography is usually neces-sary for diagnosis.

During physical examination, bony out-growths within a joint are sometimes recog-nized by the sudden arrest of an otherwise free joint motion at a certain point. That is, an abrupt hard halt in motion usually signi-fies bone-to-bone contact, signifying that fur-ther movement should not be conducted. Such an approximation will be felt before the end of normal motion occurs when hypertro-phic bone growth (eg, an osteophyte, a mal-united fracture, or myositis ossificans) has developed. If force that is continued beyond the point of a bony block is painless, neuro-pathic arthropathy is likely.

True bony ankylosis is one type of total fixation. It has been Gillet's experience that

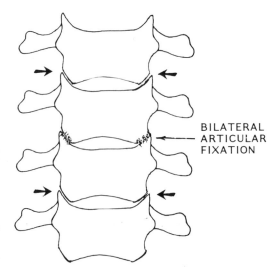

BILATERAL ARTICULAR FIXATION

Figure 1.6. Typical reciprocal actions in total articular fixation in the midcervical spine. Bold arrows show hypermobile articulations (Courtesy ACAP).

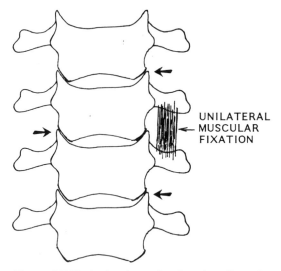

UNILATERAL MUSCULAR FIXATION

Figure 1.7. Typical reciprocal actions in unilateral muscular fixation in the midcervical spine. Bold arrows show hypermobile articulations (Courtesy ACAP).

ankylosis is invariably the result of a local bone disease process or severe trauma and practically never correctable by adjustive therapy. On the other hand, he feels that a fibrous type of *pseudoankylosis* is far more frequent, especially in the midthoracic area during middle age or in the elderly. This is likely the result of a general degeneration of the perivertebral muscles and ligaments. Although this fibrous condition can be manipulated, it takes months or years to produce a pale picture of normal motion. Gillet also states, "Unfortunately, as long as it exists, the rest of the spine will never remain free from recurrent fixations." [See Clinical Comment 1.5]

Muscle spasm is distinguished from bony outgrowth as a cause of limited joint motion by several features. Bony outgrowths allow perfectly free motion up to a certain point, after which motion is arrested suddenly, completely, and without great pain. Muscular spasm, on the contrary, checks motion slightly from the onset. Resistance and pain gradually increase until the examiner's efforts are arrested at some point.

Adaptive Therapy

We have described that there are four different types of fixations: muscular, ligamentous, articular, and bony. Granted, these are crude classifications and closer evaluations made in subsequent chapters will show that these phenomena are much more complicated than they appear on the surface. Each region of the spine, nearly each motion unit, has its peculiar characteristics in a fixation-subluxation complex. Certain muscles and ligaments have a greater tendency to become hypertonic or shortened than others, while certain articular soft tissues also have a greater probability of becoming atrophied or eroded by articular pressure. Furthermore, some of these fixations show a greater

predisposition toward degeneration than others.

It should also be evident to the reader that chiropractic adjustive technics should be adapted to the type(s) of fixation present if a maximum corrective effect in quality and duration is to be achieved. An understanding of the various types of fixation possible will also help to explain why certain other physical or medical forms of treatment may have a direct or indirect influence on the spine. In this context, we are in a better position to appreciate the effects that rest, warmth, counterirritation, acupuncture, mental relaxation, biofeedback training, or even psychotherapy may have on enhancing muscle relaxation (hypotonus) and indirectly encouraging the spontaneous correction of muscular fixations, which, according to Gillet, are the more irritative ones.

SIGNIFICANT PHYSIOLOGIC AND BIOMECHANICAL MECHANISMS

The Mechanisms of Equilibrium

Most practitioners will agree that many patients will present with one lower limb anatomically shorter than the other limb. Although the term *short leg* is used to describe this phenomenon, the length of all structures contributing to the structural distance between the head of the femur and the floor is being considered. Thus, more structures can contribute to this "shortness"

DR. FAYE'S CLINICAL COMMENT #1.4

I have found it a clinical advantage to adjust one major at one office visit. However, I attempt multiple adjustments in different ranges of motion in the motion unit selected. Some will produce audible releases, others will effect only a mobilization.

DR. FAYE'S CLINICAL COMMENT #1.5

It has been my clinical experience that if chronic changes are present the gross ranges of motion can be restored to the spine with repeated mild adjustments directed to the least fixated areas. Gradually, over a long period of time (often 12—16 months), the doctor can adjust the most fixated areas. The change of flexibility is greatly appreciated by the older patient. I see these patients twice a week for 1—2 years and have recorded many remarkable improvements in range of motion.

than just the weight-bearing tibia of the leg; viz, the pelvis, femur, ankle, and foot.

When a short leg exists, the crests of the pelvis will not be level and the superimposed spine will try to adapt through various curvatures in an attempt to keep the eyes level and at the same time keep various body parts balanced relative to the body's line of gravity. This usually occurs in the same manner as the biomechanical adaptation of a person walking on the side of a hill.

All people do not adapt to walking on a horizontally slanted surface in the same manner, nor do all people adapt to a short leg in the same manner. Some spines will regain an equilibrium imbalance due to a short leg within a few lumbar segments (eg, L3), while others will not achieve this until the upper cervical area is reached. The reasons for this variance may be structural, functional, or just habitual.

Cabot, the famous diagnostician, constantly admonished his students that "to recognize the abnormal, one must be completely familiar with the normal and its many variations." Several mechanisms will be described in this section that are normal responses to the commonly seen anatomical short leg.

The "Flatfoot" Factor

Some authorities consider a unilateral flattened longitudinal arch in the foot to be one factor that will cause a measurable lowering of one femur. Gillet feels that this is true in a way, but not in the oversimplified manner that is often given in explanation. When the Belgium researchers measured the influence of the height of the arch on the total length of a lower extremity, they found it to be not more than 1 mm. As anatomical short legs usually have a discrepancy of at least 5 mm, it is obvious that other causes must be found.

It has been the experience of Gillet that a fallen arch frequently appears on the side of the *long leg*. After adding a heel lift on the short side, the fallen arch may spontaneously correct itself within a few days to become near normal. He offers the following possible explanations for this phenomenon.

Flatfoot. The flattening of the arch (pes planus or valgus) on the long extremity could be a natural adaptation process to diminish the leg of the relatively long leg. If we examine pelvic equilibrium, it will be found that the long extremity has rotated externally because of movement of the related ilium, when the weight of the body during gait falls abnormally at an angle over the arch of the foot (forcing it downward). When such a mechanism occurs, it would appear to be contraindicated to attempt to raise the compensatory fallen arch with an arch support.

Foot Eversion. Another mechanism, which in a way is part of the one described above, is foot eversion. This usually occurs simultaneously on the side of the fallen arch and also tends to bring the head of the femur (and the structures supported) a little closer to the ground. Gillet contends that the wearing of a wedge-shaped heel in such a case could aggravate the situation because it would hinder intrinsic adaptation mechanisms from shortening the long extremity, thus forcing the pelvis and superimposed spine to distort further. Such foot eversion (toe-out, ankle pronation) is also part of other adaptive mechanisms.

Other Efforts to Achieve Equilibrium with an Anatomical Short Leg

The Trochanter Phenomenon. The trochanter phenomenon, a term coined by Illi, refers to the lateral sway of the whole pelvis towards the side of the short leg. Gillet explains that this mechanism would not be able to influence pelvic level if the lower extremities were simply straight vertical structures and if the feet were placed exactly beneath the heads of the femurs because this would constitute a parallelogram in which the upper horizontal arm would always be parallel to the floor. The influence of lateral sway is achieved because the femoral head projects at an angle from the surgical neck and, as the femur is usually slanted exteriorly, each femur slants to a different degree during lateral sway. This makes one femur shift slightly superior on the long side and the other slightly inferior on the short side.

Compensatory Sacroiliac Rotational Misalignment. The next articulations that try to align themselves in an abnormal fashion to achieve equilibrium in a short-leg syndrome are the sacroiliac joints. Even with the compensatory trochanter phenomenon, the whole pelvis will still be tilted downwards on the side of the short leg so the ilia attempt to rotate anteriorly and superiorly on the low side to lift its articulation with the sacrum and rotate posteriorly and inferiorly on the high side to lower its articulation (Fig. 1.8). This is possible because the sacroiliac joints lie somewhat posteriorly in relation to the head of the femur. This motion permits another gain of 1—2 mm, but unfortunately, it is achieved at the expense of other joints.

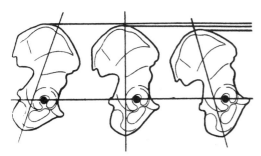

Figure 1.8. Changes of apparent iliac crest vertical height produced by normal rotation. *Left,* anterior iliac rotation; *center,* neutral position; *right,* posterior iliac rotation. The pivot point around the femoral head is represented by the black dot. These normal motions during gait also occur at rest in compensation to a short leg (Courtesy ACAP).

Compensatory Sacral Tilt. Intrinsic adaptive mechanisms also attempt to tip the sacrum itself into a position normally seen during lateral bending; ie, upward on the short-leg side and downward on the long-leg side in order to provide a more stable base for the spinal column.

Compensatory Inferior-Superior Sacroiliac. At times, in addition to the iliac rotation and sacral tilting described, inferior translation of the sacrum on the ilium on the long side and superior translation of the ilium on the side of the short leg may be found as an aid to sacral leveling.

Compensatory Lumbar Rotation. The area where postural deformation and compensation is greatest is within the lower lumbar region. The vertebral bodies and IVDs of the lumbar vertebrae are thicker anteriorly than they are posteriorly, exhibiting the shape of a wedge. During adaptation to a short leg, the lower lumbars rotate posteriorly on the shortened side in an attempt to compensate for the slanted sacral base. Unfortunately, this rotation produces a prolonged deformation of the lower lumbar IVFs that tends to encroach on the nerve roots on the side of posteriority and add tension on the nerve roots on the contralateral side. Although the sacrum also tries to rotate to adapt to the position of the rotated L5, the attempt is in vain because the sacrum is held in a vise-like grip by the ilia assisted by the strong sacroiliac ligaments and superimposed body weight. The lumbar vertebrae above L5 also rotate and laterally bend in accordance to their respective base of support. In a typical spine, it is rare to find levelness achieved below the interface of the disc of L2 and the superior surface of L3.

Compensatory Thoracic Rotation. The mechanisms of pelvic sway and lumbar rotation described above attempt to swing L3 sideward for 1—3 cm, but this cannot be tolerated because it places greater weight on that side. The long muscles of the legs and lower back are forced to remain tensed to restrain this sway from increasing. So it is at this point that equilibratory forces begin to return the spine toward the median line, which it usually reaches in the region of the lower thoracic spine, to distribute body weight more equal bilaterally. While the perimeters of the lumbar vertebrae may appear to have rotated considerably, it should be noted that the vertebral canal has only distorted slightly because each vertebra has rotated only slightly in relationship to its adjacent vertebrae: the spine is not only designed for segmental motion, it is also designed for protection of the contents of the vertebral canal. Furthermore, if the lumbar spine is normally flexible, the lower thoracic vertebrae are progressively less so because of their attachment to the thoracic cage. The necessary counterrotation of the thoracic vertebrae, in compensation to the contralateral lower lumbar rotation, is usually complete by the level of T8, at which point the vertebrae thereafter rest on a relatively level plane. Another curve is then produced to return the spine to the midline near the level of C7 or C6.

Although the compensatory shifting mechanisms described above are slight, each in its own way attempts to contribute a benefit to the overall adaptation to an anatomical short leg (Fig. 1.9). It should also be noted that the mechanisms described and their effects are the ideal and the result of an extremity deficit likely acquired at birth or during childhood when the spine was supple enough to regain balance easily and completely. Such ideal adaptation could also be achieved during puberty or early adulthood if the spine is supple enough.

Maladaptation Attempts. During the aging process, connective tissues tend to lose their youthful degree of flexibility, elasticity, viscoelasticity, and plasticity. The rib cage especially tends to become tough and tight, and the spine is forced to use whatever compensatory mechanisms are available. When the forces of adaptability are meager, we may see the unfortunate picture of a cervical spine that has had to distort itself to a great degree to "catch up" the lost balance which stopped at the lower thoracic spine. Fortunately, like the lumbar vertebrae and discs, the cervical segments are also wedge shaped and this helps considerably. There is also the biologic necessity to maintain, if possible, level eyes. This sometimes forces a high degree of lateral flexion at the occipitoatlantal articulations—with all the danger of nerve compression and/or irritation that we know is possible in this highly vulnerable area of the spine.

The spine is always subject to the trauma of daily living (stumbles, jars, falls, blows, strains, chronic biomechanical microtrauma, psychic tension, etc), and it is disturbing to see the spine of a patient in which the mechanisms of adaptation are continually being overtaxed and overthrown by fixation-subluxations. These deficiencies add to the noxious process and introduce new causes of imbalance that force adaptive reserves to start new efforts at several stages. It is this poorly adaptable spine that we see so frequently within our respective practices.

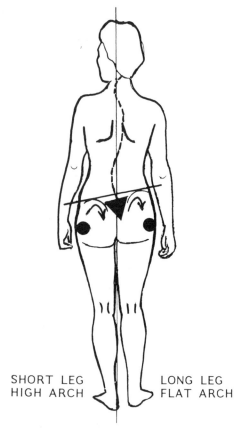

SHORT LEG
HIGH ARCH

LONG LEG
FLAT ARCH

Figure 1.9. Typical adaptive mechanisms to an anatomical short left leg (Courtesy ACAP).

But let us not forget that even a perfectly rebalanced spine can and will, sooner or later, become functionally inadequate as mechanisms of rebalancing lose their ideal properties.

Adding the Factor of Fixation. We should not insist that all the compensations described are seen only in the standing position and disappear in positions that eliminate the basic factor of imbalance such as the influence of an anatomical short leg. Ideally, they should not exist in the sitting and recumbent postures. However, such adaptive forces necessary in the erect position will, little by little, tend to become *fixed* and remain in the state of compensation regardless of the position assumed, whether it serves a beneficial purpose or not.

In the situation of adaptation to a short leg, such fixation is especially true in an individual whose occupation requires prolonged hours of standing, for it is in the standing position that the involved muscles, ligaments, and cartilages have been forced to change their architecture. The ligaments especially on the concave side of a spinal curve tend to shorten and those on the convex side of the curve stretch to conform to the demands upon them. Then, and only then, will the lumbar curve, the sacral adaptation, the iliac rotation, the thoracic counterrotation, the trochanter phenomenon, and the flattened longitudinal arch become static, *fixated*. As such, they must not be "replaced" but *mobilized*. Thereafter, the role of the doctor of chiropractic changes from therapeutic to preventive. And unless the reason for the focal imbalance is found and corrected (eg, a short leg), all the fixations associated will recur.

Testing a Patient's Spinopelvic Adaptability. The following test will demonstrate to the student of *dynamic chiropractic* a patient's ability to adjust to imbalancing factors: First, position the patient in front of a plumb line and dot the back with a skin pencil where the vertical line falls. Second, place a piece of wood or a book about 2-cm thick under a patient's foot. Observe the changes of the plumb line relative to the patient's spine and pelvis, and mark with a different color the points at which the line crosses the patient's cervicals, thoracics, lumbars, and sacrum or buttocks. Then place the block or book under the other foot of the patient and mark the patient again with a different color. If this test is first conducted with many supple spines, the examiner is likely to be astonished to see how much imbalancing a normal spine can withstand. Sometimes, it does not appear to react with any difficulty to even a 3 cm foot raise. Then compare this to the reactions viewed with typical adult patients. Some spines will not be able to adapt to even 1 cm of change, and some changes witnessed will be abnormal. Although this test will not be of benefit in localizing the specific sites of fixations, it will show the diverse changes that can take place within an individual's spine that are due to imbalancing influences.

The Mechanisms of Irritation

Gillet's studies continually verified several major characteristics of fixations, one being that the *pathogenicity of a fixation varies inversely to the degree of fixation existing*. In a unilateral nontotal fixation, for example, signs of irritation will be found on the movable (contralateral) side of the vertebra and not on the side of fixation. In a partial bilateral fixation in which some movement occurs on the A-P plane, the signs of irritation will be bilateral and often of the same degree on both sides. In a total fixation, there are rarely any signs of irritation at the level of the involved segments—with one notable exception: the occipitoatlantal articulation.

Another finding of Gillet was that if the area of the spine in fixation was actively or passively flexed or rotated several times, skin temperature readings tend to immediately increase and then decrease upon rest. This supports the hypothesis that the site of fixation, especially if degeneration has occurred, will exhibit signs and symptoms of *hypofunction* (eg, anesthesia, paresthesia, vasodilation, stasis). This would explain why a total fixation (eg, an ankylosed articulation) is not painful but important clinically because of the extraordinary motion it forces on adjacent mobile articulations in the kinematic chain and by the secondary fixations it produces.

When a unilateral fixation exists that allows some contralateral movement, that motion will occur around an abnormal axis which, if forced, causes a distinct pivoting-type of aberrant joint separation rather than the normal translatory gliding or sliding of the articulating surfaces. Oblique x-ray films of the spine, for example, will reveal reduced facet mobility on the side of fixation and separation of the facets contralaterally—which will widen further when the patient's spine is forced into flexion or rotation.

Although there is a tendency of many within chiropractic to narrow their practices to the treatment of musculoskeletal disorders, Gillet strongly believes that a subluxation complex is involved in many functional disorders of the viscera. He also proposes that many of these disorders are due more to faults in autonomic innervation than to irritation or compression of the cerebrospinal nerves. The question then arises why a subluxation should affect the smaller sympathetic and parasympathetic nerves without seemingly producing greater harm to the extremely larger motor and sensory nerves. He answers this by calling attention to the *position* of the vertebra in fixation, whose motion may be blocked either *within* or *beyond* the normal range of motion. The latter occurs when an articulation is forced into a compensatory movement that it would not normally take.

This type of subluxation was frequently described in pioneer chiropractic literature. In has been absent in more recent years because it has not conformed to the data about *normal* vertebral motion. Gillet contends, however, that when such abnormal motion is forced to occur, the facets *are* displaced, the intervertebral foramen *is* abnormally closed, the IVF contents *are* impinged, and processes leading to neurologic, circulatory, and osseous degeneration in this area *are* formed that involve the most vulnerable tissues first. If occurring in the thoracic spine, for example, we could have visceral symptoms but no intercostal neuralgia associated. This could be called a *pathologic subluxation* in contrast to the *physiologic subluxation* in which motion is restricted within the normal range of motion. In the latter, we would expect to find minimal compression on or stretching of the involved IVF contents. Fixations producing sympathetic abnormalities appear to produce far less secondary contractions in the long spinal muscles and, therefore, far less postural distortion.

Potential Effects of the Summation of Irritation

It has been perplexing to many chiropractors of a narrow school of thought why doctors of chiropractic using widely divergent techniques, medical doctors, doctors of osteopathy, physiotherapists, Christian Science practitioners, etc, frequently obtain comparable results on seemingly the same types of cases. Typical rationalizations either deny the allegations of others or attribute the benefits achieved to suggestion or a placebo effect. Our competitors have done the same when the benefits to our form of chiropractic are described. Obviously, there are several factors at work during a healing process that can be activated either directly or indirectly through a wide variety of approaches.

Individual Responses to Adverse Conditions

Every practitioner who has been in practice for several years has seen patients with frightful compensations that exhibit little handicap and few symptoms. There are also those patients in whom only minor, recently acquired fixation-subluxations produce grotesque manifestations. In each situation, the fixation-subluxations found may be either a cause or an effect of some other disturbing focus.

We have previously described how an articular correction made in any part of the spine (or anywhere in the skeletal system) has an influence on the neuromusculoskeletal system as a whole. This is especially true with partial muscular-type fixations. Thus, the correction of an atlas fixation will have an affect on the sacrum and possibly as distal as the feet, and the correction of a metatarsal or sacral fixation will have an affect on the atlas. This fact does not mean that one fixation is necessarily the *cause* of the remote effect; it just means that it can be *one* factor within the causal picture.

There is, however, far more to consider in the analysis of the cause of disease than articular fixations and their correction. The effects of pathogenic microbes, parasites, toxins, poisons, excessive heat or cold, malnutrition, poor habits, physical and psychologic stress, etc, should not be overlooked. Any one of these factors can produce illness in itself, but more frequently each plays a variable contributing share or predisposing role in the health status of the patient at hand. See Table 1.2.

Gillet believes that the pathogenicity of any agent or act that is detrimental to health

Table 1.2. Assaults of Daily Living

Type of Stress	Examples	
Mental	Anger	Divorce
	Anxiety	Emotional overexertion
	Changes in lifestyle	Frustration
	Changes in sex life	Loss of a job
	Constant tension	Loss of social status
	Death of a loved one	Mental exhaustion
	Depression	Phobias
Physical	Biomechanical microtrauma	Insufficient rest or sleep
	Changes in environment	Obesity
	Dislocation	Overexertion, prolonged
	Fixation-subluxations	Postural imbalance
	Fracture	Sprain
	Homeostatic malfunction	Strain
	Inadequate exercise	Structural distortion
	Inherited impairments	Surgery
Thermal	Abrupt temperature changes	Frostbite
	Burns	Heatstroke
	Dehydration	Temperature extremes
Chemical	Caustic chemical contact	Food additives
	Chemical depressants	Herbicides
	Chemical stimulants	Malnutrition
	Denourished foods	Pesticides
	Drugs	Poisoning
	Endotoxins	Pollution
	Environmental anoxia	Radiation
	Exhaust fumes	Toxicosis

is summed with others present until they accumulate to the point where the reserve forces and defenses (eg, neurologic, hormonal, immunologic) of the body become overpowered. He proposes that each individual has a certain hereditary or acquired *health-index* (ie, a threshold of dysfunction).

Neural Stimulation vs Irritation

The physiologists of Europe make a subtle differentiation between biologic *stimulation* and *irritation*. They consider stimulation to be any circumstance that sets up a normal action or response in a tissue or function. Thus, the sight and smell of tempting food to a hungry person does not irritate the optic and olfactory nerves, higher CNS centers, or the salivary glands; rather, the visual image and odor just *stimulate* certain tissues to act in a normal manner that is beneficial to an individual's health and well being. It is usually a subtle yet precise reaction, adapted to the needs of the moment. In contrast, any situation that is dangerous to the life or integrity of a body is considered to be *irritative* to the tissues responding. It is usually a more violent reaction such as when drawing the hand away from a hot or otherwise dangerous object, but it may be subtle such as during the development of antibodies to fight an invasion. Unfortunately, this differentiation between stimulation and irritation is not made in North America: here biologic stimulation and irritation are considered to be synonymous.

The Physiologic Stress Factor in Illness

We are indebted to Hans Selye for his descriptions of the nonspecific mechanisms that the body initiates to defend itself against danger and stress (Fig. 1.10). Unfortunately, he did not differentiate between normal and abnormal defensive reactions in time or degree. We can, however, divide diseases into two categories for study in which: (1) the symptoms are overanxious reactions of the body to rid itself of a new or chronic irritation; and (2) the manifestations reflect degeneration of diseased tissues. According to

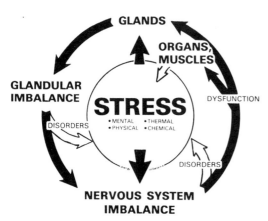

Figure 1.10. Stress in any form can disrupt the proper function of the body's intricately balanced homeostasis. The forms of stress are interrelated and cumulative. Stress frequency, intensity, and duration are important factors in determining the degree of systemic functional overload, leading to impairment and the resulting loss of resistance that may predispose, contribute to, or cause overt pathology. Thus, the effects of stress can play an important role in most any disease process. Any disorder is a stress in itself; hence, a vicious cycle has been established (adapted from a chart developed by Steven P.L. Young, DC).

this classification, a majority of symptoms belong to the first category. Normal defensive reactions (eg, fever, tachycardia, hypertension) may become so poorly integrated or out of control that the overreaction progresses to an action that kills the individual.

In this context, we can consider a subluxation complex as being one possible effect of an excessive normal defensive mechanism. Gillet hypothesizes that the deep short muscles of the spine were the slowest to adapt to the upright biped posture, therefore in a constant state of alert readiness or preparedness for danger. In this functional state, he believes that an overreaction to a threat of danger is likely and that, once the danger has passed, a noxious self-perpetuating nerve-muscle cycle manifesting as contraction can be established.

From another viewpoint, Gillet believes that subclinical subluxations may so pre-irritate spinal nerves and lower their firing threshold that a minor peripheral irritation will produce reactions far out of proportion to the extent or severity of the lesion. In such a case, either peripheral or spinal therapy would likely be beneficial—at least temporarily until the *summation factor* of circumstances detrimental to neurologic, musculoskeletal, circulatory, glandular, or psychic health arise again.

Let us suppose that an individual has a health index that is capable of withstanding a moderate degree of debilitating factors before dysfunction appears in the most vulnerable tissues. If smoking, drinking too much, infrequently exercising, chronic worry, having poor nutritional habits, and the irritation from subclinical subluxations deplete his or her reserves to just below the threshold of dysfunction, it would not require much additional stress (in whatever manner) to so overtax his systems reserves that one or more vital organs fail. A chill, unaccustomed exertion, a fright, loss of a job, or a mild infection may be all that is necessary for functional collapse to occur. Conversely, correcting existing subluxations and offering logical counsel regarding rest, diet, and exercise, even if wise counsel is followed only partially, may be all that is necessary to have the patient become symptom free and feeling well.

The same principles can be applied strictly from a spinal-health viewpoint. If a patient's health index is being depleted from cervical, pelvic, and some extraspinal fixation-subluxations and manifesting as neuromusculoskeletal complaints in tissues with a low threshold to stress, correction of any one or more of these factors may be enough to make the patient symptom free and feeling well.

In discussing this concept with students, Gillet admonishes that "truth is always complex; all generalizations are false, including this one."

The Hereditary Factor

Patients who are born into families whose members have lived long lives for generations often appear to come into this world with an intrinsic genetic makeup for longevity in spite of some adversities that would lead to the early death of another. Many extremely heavy drinkers and smokers who overeat and avoid exercise long outlive their doctors who neither drink or smoke, are careful in their diet, and exercise frequently. Population statistics are useless in predicting the actions and reactions of an individual. We must learn to deal with the patient and circumstances at hand—not on our subjective expectations, regardless of how valid they might be when related to humanity as a whole.

The Psychic Factor

When a patient enters a doctor's office, he or she does so for two reasons: the disorder existing and the disorder feared. Both must be treated and treated with skill, compassion, thoroughness, and confidence. Also, it should not be forgotten that (1) the patient's faith in the doctor's ability/honesty and (2) psychotherapeutic *suggestion* designed to enhance the patient's hope in achieving rational goals are two therapeutic components in every act of healing, whether it be chiropractic, medical, or whatever.

Although women appear to have a higher threshold for pain than men, Gillet points out that nature appears to also have provided them with a compensatory lower threshold for worry. It is likely for this that females seem to suffer with cancer phobia more than males.

DIFFERENTIATING JOINT DYSFUNCTION FROM JOINT DISEASE

Joint dysfunction implies the loss of one or more movements within the normal range of motion and associated pain, but it is only one possible problem that must be differentiated from other causes of joint pain. There may be many clues within a history of joint pain that point to the diagnosis of joint disease and many may strongly suggest joint dysfunction. This may represent separate overlapping problems or one complex problem. For example, joint pain may be the chief complaint in such systemic diseases as polyarteritis nodosa, systemic lupus erythematosus, dermatomyositis, erythema nodosum, and scleroderma. It is also sometimes associated with kidney or pulmonary diseases, ulcerative colitis, acromegaly, and hemorrhagic dyscrasias. It should be remembered that gout may occur in any limb joint and is occasionally found in the spine. It is not always associated with tophi or limited to the feet and hands.

Primary joint dysfunction is usually the product of intrinsic joint stress that occurs at an unguarded moment when the joint is active within its normal range of motion. Another cause is that of extrinsic joint stress following a definite but minor trauma and often classified as sprain and/or strain.

Secondary joint dysfunction is often overlooked in traditional medicine. Yet joint dysfunction is, according to Mennell, "the most common cause of residual symptoms after severe bone and joint injury and after almost every joint disease when the primary pathological condition has been eradicated, has healed, or is quiescent." Immobilization after surgery, immobilization from a fracture cast even if the fracture is far from a joint, and immobilization from a taped sprain all cause residual symptoms of joint dysfunction. Such symptoms also follow joint inflammation or resolution of systemic joint disease with or without internal adhesions. When joint dysfunction causes residual symptoms after so-called joint disease recovery, the symptoms change from those of joint disease to those of joint dysfunction; ie, during the active process, rest increases joint pain and stiffness. During the residual dysfunction, rest relieves and action aggravates the pain. These points should be brought out during the case history.

Specific features elicited in the history can point directly to certain diseases. For instance, migrating joint pain following systemic illness suggests rheumatic fever. A tubercular joint is often a single joint offering mild complaints yet associated with marked muscle atrophy. An acute gonococcal joint presents a single acutely painful joint that is protected by the patient as if it were a boil. Hemarthrosis has a history of trauma and is characterized by slight but rapid swelling from the blood pool; the joint is hot and acutely painful. Synovitis may also have a history of trauma, but the swelling due to excess synovial fluid may not occur for many hours. The joint may feel warm rather than hot, aching rather than acutely painful.

In the hand(s), the location of joint involvement offers a general rule that aids the diagnostic process: (1) gout affects the metacarpophalangeal joints, (2) rheumatoid arthritis involves the proximal interphalangeal joints, and (3) osteoarthritis affects the distal interphalangeal joints. Mennell feels that osteoarthritis by itself does *not* cause joint pain; rather, he projects that the pain is from the associated joint dysfunction rather than the disease process itself.

The key history points of primary joint dysfunction are: (1) the pain has a sudden onset and is sharp, (2) it usually follows stress at some unguarded joint motion, (3) the pain is limited to one or adjacent joints, (4) the pain is aggravated by movement and usually is at some particular area of motion, (5) rest relieves the pain and doesn't produce stiffness, and (6) marked swelling or warmth is not associated.

Keep in mind that while the major problem may be of joint dysfunction, persistent pain following normally adequate treatment may show the presence of a secondary low-grade asymptomatic infection or irritation in spite of blood reports to the contrary. In such cases, suspicion should be directed toward a distant focus of infection such as the gastrointestinal or genitourinary tracts, the teeth, sinuses, or tonsils. In food preparation, adequate cooking heat will kill pathogenic bacteria, but it has little affect on toxins and spores.

In summary, (1) joint dysfunction pain does not occur at night and is relieved by rest, (2) usually one joint is involved in the major complaint, (3) joint swelling is not associated, (4) the onset is sudden, (5) the pain occurs when doing the same action the same way, and (6) the pain is not relieved by aspirin.

PRACTICING THE MODERN SUBLUXATION COMPLEX PARADIGM

The word *paradigm* means a pattern, model, or viewpoint. In pioneer chiropractic, this viewpoint was usually restricted to considering a subluxation complex as being the result of a static articular displacement; viz, a bone out of place. This concept has led to frequent puzzlement when a patient became symptom free and yet posttherapy static radiographs of the spine showed little change in the original static malpositioning of certain segments. It also failed to explain why patients with well aligned segments in a static radiograph were expressing obvious signs and symptoms of a subluxation complex. In modern chiropractic, the emphasis is on some factor that is interfering with normal articular mobility; thus, a dynamic impairment of mobility rather than a static positional impairment.

In the modern context, there are two categories of significance in the rationale of joint manipulation: (1) the hypermobile state, which obviously needs no further mobilization, adjustment, or manipulation; (2) the hypomobile (restricted, fixated) state, which requires mobilization to return the joint to normal function.

The objective of studying motion palpation and the related concepts of *dynamic chiro-*

practic is to know with confidence (1) where to adjust, (2) when to adjust, (3) why adjust, (4) how to adjust, and (5) how often to adjust. Thus, one major reason for mastering the art of motion palpation is to determine the quality of existing fixations. After such areas have been found and classified as muscular, ligamentous, articular, or bony fixations, a rational approach to adjustive therapy can be outlined. During this process, in which the doctor should be constantly attempting to verify whether a fixation is primary or secondary, the following general rules should be kept in mind:

• Only primary and possibly minor nonsecondary fixations require adjustment, and they should be mobilized in all directions of restricted mobility.

• Primary fixations feel the most blocked, and restricted mobility is demonstrable in more than one direction. Primary fixations are not particularly tender in contrast to secondary fixations except when they are stressed by an examiner into the direction of restriction.

• The adjustment of a secondary fixation will exhibit short-lived benefits or possibly an adverse reaction unless the primary fixation is corrected first.

• The adjustment of a primary fixation will produce changes both locally and elsewhere in the spine (eg, normalization of signs and symptoms expressed at the site of a secondary fixation).

If the primary fixation(s) have been correctly determined and adjusted, the treated articulation(s) should exhibit increased mobility on the next office visit, and fixations judged as secondary should have spontaneously improved or disappeared. There should be general improvement in general spinal mobility, equilibrium, and related symptomatology. However, if the site of a primary subluxation was misdiagnosed, the patient will likely report no improvement or an increase in symptoms on the next visit, and the fixations previously adjusted will be found to be in the same state as they were during examination on the previous visit. When this latter situation occurs, a determination must be made whether the previous diagnosis was correct or not.

If a fixation palpates as being completely cleared on one visit and is found to recur on the subsequent visit, it should not be readjusted. Rather, its cause (a primary fixation elsewhere) should be sought. If, however, the fixation does not clear completely during the office visit, it should be adjusted on the next and subsequent visits until full mobility is achieved. [See Clinical Comment 1.6]

PERTINENT BIOMECHANICAL TERMINOLOGY

Movement Terms

Motion. A continuous change (displacement) of position.

Degrees of Freedom. Vertebrae have six degrees of freedom (ranges of motions); ie, translation along and rotation about each of three orthogonal axes. Any motion in which an object may translate to and fro along a straight course or rotate one way or another about a particular axis equals one degree of freedom. For example, joints with one axis have one degree of freedom to move in one plane (eg, pivot and hinge joints). Joints with two axes have two degrees of freedom to move in different planes, and joints with three axes have three degrees of freedom to move in all planes (eg, ball-and-socket joints).

Range of Motion (ROM). ROM refers to the difference between two points of physiologic extremes of motion. Rotation is measured in degrees. A vertebra has six

---

DR. FAYE'S CLINICAL COMMENT #1.6

It has been a common experience for me to treat a chronically fixated spine in patients over the age of 35 on a twice-a-week schedule over a period of 6—18 months. The constantly imposed demand of spinal manipulation being applied to the most fixated motion units eventually is met by a specific adaptation of joint motion and elastic connective tissue.

degrees of freedom as it moves in three-dimensional space; eg, translations along and rotations about each of the three cardinal axes (x, y, and z). If passive distraction is considered a motion, seven degrees of freedom exist.

Translation. Linear motion that occurs when all parts of an object at a given time have the same direction of motion about a fixed point is called *translation*. This commonly occurs in a train moving along a track, the body moving as a whole during gait, or a facet that glides or slips across a relatively fixed surface. Translation is measured in millimeters.

Coupling. Coupling is a motion of translation or rotation occurring along or about an axis as an object (eg, a vertebra) moves about another axis.

Instantaneous Axis of Rotation (IAR). The IAR is that fixed point which does not move but about which rotation occurs. It can exist inside or outside the object moving and is subject to change at any given instant.

Kinetics. Kinetics is the study of the rate of change of a specific factor in the body that disregards the cause of the motion; ie, the study of the relationship between a force acting on a body or body segment and the changes produced in body motion. Kinetic actions are expressed in amounts per units of time.

Kinematics. Kinematics is the complex study of motions of body parts and forces causing motion (with emphasis on displacement, acceleration, and velocity) that is mainly the result of muscle activity.

Closed Kinematic System. This phrase refers to a series of body links or a chain of joints in which segments are interdependent on each other for certain movements in order that each joint can function properly in a coordinated movement; eg, the movement of the first costotransverse joint necessary for the cervical spine to extend and laterally flex.

Orthogonal Coordinates. These coordinates are points of position described around three axes (x, y, and z). Typical vertebral motions and their coordinates are shown in Table 1.3.

Flexion and Extension. Generally, when the joint angle becomes smaller than when in the anatomical position, it is in *flexion*. For example, when the elbow is bent, it is flexed. The opposite of flexion is *extension*. Thus, when the elbow is straight, it is extended. Most joints are able to flex and extend. When motion exceeds the normal range, it is called hyperflexion or hyperextension; eg, as in instability of the elbow or knee.

Abduction and Adduction. When a part is farther away from the midline than it is in the anatomical (zero) position, it is in *abduction*. The opposite of abduction is *adduction*. Abduction and adduction occur at the shoulder, metacarpophalangeal, hip, and metatarsophalangeal joints.

Elevation and Depression. Raising a part from its normal (zero) position is called *elevation*. *Depression* means to lower a part from its normal position. Good examples of both can be seen in the shoulder.

Circumduction. Movement of a bone circumscribing a cone such as at the shoulder or hip is called *circumduction*. Such motions usually comprise at least flexion, extension, abduction, and adduction.

Rotation. If a bone of a joint is capable of

Table 1.3. Vertebral Movements and Their Coordinates

Motion	Coordinate
Flexion	+X
Extension	- X
Right rotation	- Y
Left rotation	+Y
Right lateral flexion	+Z
Left lateral flexion	- Z

angular motion or turning on its longitudinal axis (spinning), the motion is called *rotation*. The motion of turning an anterior surface of a part toward the midline of the body is called inward or *internal rotation*. The motion of turning out is called outward or *external rotation*. The axis may be located outside or inside the rotating body. The classic example of internal-external rotation is at the shoulder.

Pronation. The word *pronation* refers to the act of assuming the prone position or the state or condition of being prone. When applied to the hand, it refers to the act of turning the hand backward, posteriorly, or downward by medial rotation of the forearm. When applied to the ankle or foot, it refers to a combination of eversion and abduction movements taking place in the tarsal and metatarsal joints that result in lowering the medial margin of the foot and thus the longitudinal arch.

Supination. *Supination* is the opposite of pronation. It is the act of turning the palm forward or upward or of raising the medial margin or longitudinal arch of the foot. Pronation and supination movements are seen at the forearm (rotation of forearm between the wrist and elbow, palm turning up or down, respectively) and in the foot. However, inversion and eversion are better terms to use for actions of the foot than pronation and supination.

Dorsiflexion and Plantar Flexion. Backward flexion or bending such as of the hand or foot is called *dorsiflexion;* movement toward the dorsal surface. *Plantar flexion* or *palmar flexion* is the opposite of dorsiflexion: movement toward the plantar surface or palm. In the hand or foot, the midline is an arbitrary line drawn through the middle finger or toe. Dorsiflexion movements are seen at the ankle and wrist, toes and fingers.

Inversion and Eversion. A turning inward, inside out, or other reversal of the normal relation of a part is called *inversion*. Inversion is a type of adduction of the foot where the plantar surface is turned inward relative to the leg. *Eversion* is the opposite of inversion, referring to a turning outward of a part. Eversion of the foot means to turn the plantar surface outward in relation to the leg.

Arthrokinematic Terms

Angular Motion. This term is used to indicate an increase or decrease in the angle formed between two bones; eg, flexion-extension at the elbow or knee.

Roll. The term *roll* refers to movement in which points at intervals on a moving joint surface contact points at the same intervals on an apposing surface.

Slide. When one bone slides over another with little rotation or angular movement, the action is referred to as a *sliding motion;* eg, carpal motion. It is motion in which a single contact point on a moving articular surface contacts various points on the apposing surface.

Spin. Any rotational, sliding movement in which a bone moves but its mechanical axis remains stationary is called a *spin*. In the shoulder, for example, spin is accomplished by flexion combined with some abduction because the glenoid cavity faces slightly forward. With spin, one half of the articular surface slides in one direction, while the other half slides in the opposite direction; ie, the moving joint surface rotates about some point on the apposing articular surface.

Impure Swing. This is a type of motion in which the mechanical axis follows the path of an arc about an appositioned ovoid surface of a joint.

Pure (Chordate) Swing. The term *pure swing* refers to movement of a bone in which an end of the mechanical axis traces the path of a chord about the ovoid formed by an appositioned joint surface.

Conjunct Rotation. This motion refers to the element of spin that accompanies impure swing or the rotation that may occur with a succession of swings.

Compression. The approximation of joint surfaces is called *compression;* eg, motion occurring when joint surfaces are moving toward a packed or jammed position.

Distraction. This term refers to separation of joint surfaces, usually by traction.

Accessory Movements. These are secondary movements that are necessary for a primary motion to occur. They occur with most all joint movements. Secondary movements may include such actions as rolls, slides, spins, distractions, and/or compressions. They usually occur to prevent undue articular cartilage jamming or capsule stress. Lateral rotation of the tibia during extension of the knee is a typical example.

Notation Symbols Used in Motion Palpation

See Figure 1.11.

FUNDAMENTALS OF CHIROPRACTIC ADJUSTMENT TECHNICS

It may come as a surprise to some that there is no standardization of chiropractic technic. Many of us have assumed that the chiropractic adjustive procedures we were taught in chiropractic college were similar to those taught in other chiropractic colleges.

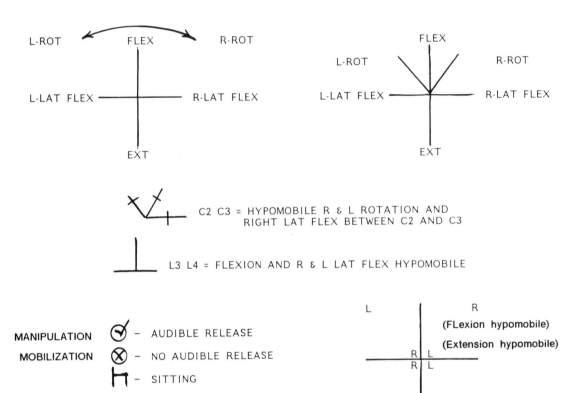

Figure 1.11. Notation symbols used in motion palpation. Any two vertebrae involved in a fixation are listed and recorded in the direction that is hypomobile. This is done with a star or modified star diagram, as illustrated in the uppermost diagrams. The listing(s) found during motion palpation are recorded in symbolic form and show the directions of movement that require manipulation to increase the range of motion.

In the sacroiliac four-quadrant diagram above (lower right), the letters represent the side of the leg raised during the motion palpation test and the side of the flexed hip during side posture adjusting. The outer letters are contacts on the posterior-superior iliac spines. The centralized letters near the crossed lines indicate sacral hypomobility between the innominates, and the sacrum is contacted on the down side, which is on the opposite side of the flexed hip.

This assumption is false. There is a wide variance in instruction among chiropractic colleges, and this instruction varies when one instructor is replaced by another at the same college. This is not unusual in teaching a manual art. Chiropractic technic, like a surgical skill, is an art and not a science. Regardless of the variance in methodology, each method taught is valuable; and the more variances we know, the more we can refine, expand, and diversify our personal applications. Perfection of an art is a constantly expanding process. The quest of perfection in our profession is the basis of the diligent *practice* of chiropractic.

This section will attempt to briefly define certain general principles that underlie most all chiropractic adjustive technics, yet few apply in all instances. These principles must be amended to the situation at hand and the individual making the application. For example, technics must be adapted to the size, strength, and skill of the doctor; the age, sex, health status, and pain tolerance of the patient; and the type of adjusting table used. Obviously, a doctor of relatively short height treating a senior citizen on a high table may find difficulty in applying the same contact or technic that might be applied by a tall doctor treating a lean young adult on a low table. The variables that can arise are too numerous to list, and each must be adapted to when encountered as conditions and personal skill permit.

A technic is only a method, *one method of many*, that must be adapted to the situation at hand, clinical judgment, and personal preference. This is true for those technics described in this text or within any other book or seminar.

Background

The goal of any therapy must be based upon a rational hypothesis. According to its founder, the primary objective of chiropractic therapy is to restore normal "tone" to the nervous system. This goal has not varied over the years, but the primary and secondary methods (technics and techniques) used to achieve this goal have undergone and will continue to undergo constant refinement.

This is true for the therapeutic procedures used within all health-care professions. Although some practitioners achieve this by "nonthrust" means (eg, the application of somatosomatic reflexes), objectives are *generally* achieved by dynamic manual articular mobilization unless such a technic is contraindicated in a specific situation.

Terminology

The terms *technique* and *technic* are generally considered to be synonymous outside the profession of chiropractic. In chiropractic, however, the term *technic* has been historically restricted to the application of a manually applied adjustive force, while the term *technique* is used in reference to the application of any other procedure (therapeutic or diagnostic).

Chiropractic *treatment* or *therapy* should be differentiated from chiropractic *technic*, which is one form of treatment. Case management includes the application of a primary method plus all ancillary procedures incorporated to achieve the clinical objective. These ancillary procedures often include such procedures as physiotherapeutic modalities, heat, cold, nutritional supplementation, diet control, therapeutic exercise, meridian therapy, biofeedback, psychotherapy or other counseling, or other forms of justifiable therapy in the most efficient manner.

Bergmann has stated that the most specialized and significant therapy employed by the chiropractor involves the adjustment of the articulations of the human body, especially of the spinal column, manually or mechanically, actively or passively, for the purpose of restoring normal articular relationship and function, restoring neurologic integrity, and influencing physiologic processes.

Although the "adjustment" has always been the foundation of chiropractic therapeutics, few have tried to define it and most who have were met with severe criticism.

Sandoz states that an "adjustment" is a passive manual maneuver during which the three-joint complex (IVD and apophyseal joints) is suddenly carried beyond the normal physiologic range of movement without exceeding the boundaries of anatomical integrity. Swezey, an allopath, refers to a dynamic chiropractic adjustment as the high-velocity short-arc-inducing passive movement of one articulating surface over another. Few would strongly object to either of these attempts to define the purely structural effect induced; ie, if the objective is solely to mobilize a fixation or realign a subluxation. Unfortunately, such purely mechanical concepts are limited; eg, they fail to consider the induced neurologic stimulation upon the cord, root, axoplasmic flow, and mechanoreceptors of the area and the local and remote "spillover" effects of such stimuli.

A recent trend by some authors and editors is to lump what a chiropractor does during an "adjustment" under the general category of *spinal manipulative therapy* (SMT). This appears to be a term originated by the allied health professions for it was rarely seen in chiropractic literature before the late 1970s. Schafer is uncomfortable with such a generalization because he believes that what a chiropractor attempts to do is far removed from the general "mobilization" and gross "manipulation" procedures commonly conducted by physiotherapists and many osteopaths, which typically are passive attempts to increase a restricted gross range of movement of a joint by stretching contractures. While the term SMT may be appropriate for a large variety of low-velocity extraspinal adjustive techniques or the application of a stretching maneuver to improve a joint's gross range of motion, it can be argued that its use is a clear misnomer in most instances when applied to the application of scientific chiropractic during spinal therapy.

The function of a robot can be explained in electrical and mechanical terms. This is not true for the human organism. Purely biomechanical explanations will not suffice for every situation. More than 20 years ago, Levine had the foresight to warn those who defined the chiropractic adjustment *solely in structural terms* without considering the *neurologic overtones* involved:

"In discussing chiropractic techniques, it is only proper to note that chiropractic holds no monopoly on manipulation. Manipulation for the purpose of setting and replacing displaced bones and joints, including spinal articulations, is one of the oldest therapeutic methods known. It has been and still is an integral part of the armamentarium of healers of all times and cultures.

"What differentiates chiropractic adjusting from orthopedic manipulations, osteopathic maneuvers, massage, zone therapy, etc? In one sentence, it is the dynamic thrust! The use of the dynamic thrust is singularly chiropractic. And it is the identifying feature of chiropractic techniques.

"However, chiropractic's rationale is hardly based on the fact that its adjustive techniques are applied with a sudden impulse of force. It is the reasons why these techniques are applied, and why they are applied in a certain manner, that distinguish chiropractic from other healing disciplines, manipulative or not. In fact, some chiropractic techniques of recent vintage are *not* characterized by sudden application. We are thinking of those techniques which have been named 'non-force,' though strictly speaking, the term is a misnomer. What makes them also part of chiropractic is that they are designed to serve the same purpose as the dynamic thrust, though whether they are equally efficient is a moot question."

The Articular Snap

Skilled spinal adjustments often involve the breaking of the synovial seal of the apophyseal joints, which results in an audible "snap." While some feel this is of little significance, most authorities feel that breaking the joint seal permits an increase in mobility (particularly that not under voluntary control) from 15—20 minutes—allowing the segment to normalize its position and functional relationships. Unsuccessful manipulations that result in increased pain rarely produce an audible joint release, while successful adjustments usually produce an immediate sense of relief (even though some pain and spasm remain), a reduction in palpable hypertonicity, and an improvement in joint motion, and are typically followed by a gradual reduction in symptoms.

The General Oval Posture

The original adjusting table was primarily designed to position the patient's spine in an "oval posture" (mild flexion). In general terms, it can be said that without an abdominal support that can be arched, it is difficult to open the thoracolumbar foramina and facets. It also avoids postural compression of the discs, permits free movement at the posterior articular processes, reduces muscular tension, and enhances the corrective forces of a properly applied adjustment. Without an abdominal support that can be lowered and released of tension, it would be contraindicated to adjust a pregnant woman in the prone position. Today, this primary objective of achieving an "oval posture" has been sustained and a large number of other optional mechanical adjustments and automatic mobilization devices can be incorporated that enhance the application of chiropractic technics. The two most important instruments for a chiropractic adjuster are his or her hands and adjusting table.

Contact Points and Their Options

Each chiropractor has a number of contact points he or she uses, but usually one or two are used whenever possible because of personal preference. The most commonly applied contact points are shown in Figure 1.12.

All contact points are optional at some time. For example, if the site of contact is to be upon a thoracic transverse process, the use of a pisiform, thenar, palm heel, or thumb contact could all meet the same objective, essentially depending on doctor-patient positions and the segmental position of fixation.

Stance and Spinal Zones

The principles of stance and spinal zones were originally developed in pioneer chiro-

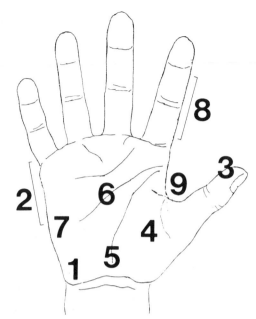

Figure 1.12. Contact points: 1, pisiform; 2, medial knife-edge (or edge); 3, thumb-pad; 4, thenar; 5, palm heel; 6, palm; 7, hypothenar; 8, lateral knife-edge (or interphalangeal); 9, web.

practic when a recoil thrust was almost the sole type of adjustive thrust used in chiropractic. At that time, stance and its relationship to the spinal zones were religiously adhered to. This is no longer true in modern chiropractic, but the principles of proper stance still are applicable in the delivery of recoil and other types of adjustive thrusts. Proper stance allows the line of drive to be delivered in the most efficient direction.

The term *spinal zones* refers to four zones of the spine: Zone One, T2—L3; Zone Two, C6—T1 and L4—L5; Zone Three, C2—C5; and Zone Four, the atlas. Some classic stances for Zone One are shown in Figure 1.13.

Table Height

It has often been stated that the ideal adjusting table height is 18 inches for an adjuster of average stature. Of course, other variables would be the thickness of the patient and the type of adjustment to be given. If the table is too high, a mechanical disad-

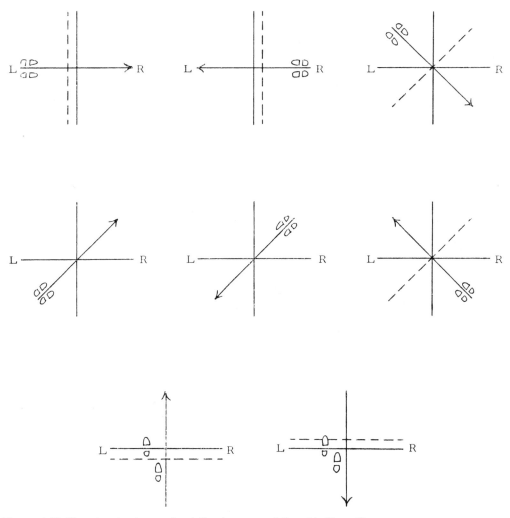

Figure 1.13. The classic stances for delivering a recoil thrust in Zone One.

vantage occurs. If too low, overstress on the adjuster's spine results when several patients must be treated.

Securing the Contact (Active, Nail) Hand

Precautions should always be taken when applying an adjustment to avoid *slipping* and *pounding*, as both can bruise the patient, induce unnecessary pain, and result in an inefficient correction attempt. Slipping results from not having the contact point properly anchored. Pounding is generally produced by administering an adjustment when the contact is lifted from the patient's skin just prior to applying the adjustive force or delivering a recoil adjustment when the elbows are not completely relaxed.

As an example of proper contact, the following describes anchoring the pisiform to deliver a recoil thrust: Once the vertebra to be adjusted has been located, the index finger of the palpating (nonactive) hand comes to rest on the exact point where the contact will be taken. The patient's skin is then drawn taut in the direction of drive. Next, all fingers except the palpating finger are withdrawn and the wrist of the palpating hand is dropped or lowered. In applying contact with the active hand, the wrist of the nail hand is extended and the fingers are flexed to form an arch. The fingers of the nail hand should contact the patient's skin first, drawing the skin further taut to insure a secure (anchored) contact. The pisiform contact (nail point) is then slid into the exact position previously occupied by the palpating (pointing) finger, while simultaneously withdrawing the palpating finger. The higher the arch of the active hand, the smaller the contact point at which the force of the adjustment will be concentrated. This may or may not be an advantage.

The palpating hand is then used to reinforce and further stabilize the active hand. This supporting *hammer hand* is placed over the contact hand (nail hand) during recoil thrusts. The fingers of the hammer hand grasp the wrist and lower forearm of the contact hand so that the pisiform of the hammer hand is directly over the pisiform of the nail hand.

Direction of Drive

The direction of drive should be against (through) the fixation, in the direction of blocked mobility, and in line with the articular plane. As in any generality, there are a few exceptions to this rule that will be described in subsequent chapters.

Movement of the segment being adjusted is determined by the direction of drive and the plane of articulation. To understand this, let us take as an example a midthoracic vertebra whose apophyseal joints have a plane of articulation almost at a 45° angle. A P-A force directed against both transverse processes will move the segment anteriorly and superiorly. A P-A force directed against the right transverse process will rotate the vertebra in a counterclockwise direction (anterosuperiorly on the right, posteroinferiorly on the left) while a P-A force applied against the left transverse process will rotate the segment in a clockwise direction (anterosuperiorly on the left, posteroinferiorly on the right).

If the contact is taken on the left side of the spinous process and a force is delivered toward 2 o'clock, the vertebra will rotate in a counterclockwise direction, and vice versa if the contact is applied against the contralateral side of the spinous process.

A spinous process contact taken in the midline or a double transverse contact will flex the vertebra if a P-A force is delivered and the subjacent segment is stabilized. However, if the superior segment is stabilized and the inferior segment is forced to extend, the same intersegmental motion is achieved. Once the mechanical principles behind this concept are grasped, there need be little argument in the effectiveness of one technic over another. Likewise, a P-A thrust against a right transverse process or a thrust against the left side of the spinous process will both rotate the vertebra in a counterclockwise direction. The choice of contact is solely a matter of clinical judgment and personal preference. The direction of drive, however, is not optional if the best mechanical advantage is to be assured. The direction of drive is determined by the site of fixation.

Different Types of Adjustive Technics

Thrust technics applied to an articulation can be divided into two categories: low-velocity technics (LVTs) and high-velocity technics (HVTs), and each has various subdivisions depending upon the joint being treated, its structural-functional state, and the primary and secondary objectives to be obtained. The term *adjustment velocity* refers to the speed at which the adjustive force is delivered.

In either low-velocity or high-velocity technics:

• The force applied may be low, medium, or high.

• The duration of the force may be brisk or sustained.

• The amplitude (distance of articular motion) may be short, medium, or long.

• The direction of the force may be straight or curving and/or perpendicular, parallel, or oblique to the articular plane.

• Overlying soft-tissue tension may be mild, medium, or strong.

• Primary or secondary leverage may be

applied early, synchronized, or late.
• Contralateral stabilization may or may not be necessary.
• Thrust onset may be slow, medium, or abrupt.

Fixations may be produced by perivertebral fascial adhesions, ligamentous contractures, IVD dehydration, fibrosed muscle tissue, spondylosis, or meningeal sclerosis and adhesions. An excessively forceful dynamic thrust to these conditions may result in increased mobility by stretching shortened tissues and breaking adhesions, but there is always some danger of osseous avulsion or tearing of meninges as scar tissue has a much higher tensile strength than osseous or nerve tissue. Because of this, professional training is mandatory.

Low-Velocity Technics (LVTs)

In the category of low-velocity adjustments fall the many applications that apply slow stretching, pulling, compression, or pushing forces. Sustained or rhythmic manual traction or compression and procedures to obtain proprioceptive neuromuscular facilitation (PNF) are typical examples. Many of the leverage techniques advocated by Spears, Cox, Markey-Steffensmeier, and others to reduce IVD protrusions and functional spondylolisthesis can be placed in this category.

High-Velocity Technics (HVTs)

Within the category of high-velocity adjustments fall the many applications of classic *dynamic-thrust* (direct, rotary, or leverage) chiropractic adjustment technics that are applied to a vertebra's transverse or spinous process or a lamina, with various degrees of counterleverage and/or contralateral stabilization. Contact pressure is usually firm, if the underlying tissues are not acutely painful, when the contact is to be maintained at a specific point and the thrust delivered in a precise direction.

The objective of almost all HVTs is to release the fixated articulation (increase joint mobility). *How* this is achieved has not been specifically determined because more is involved than the application of a mechanical force against a resistance. The most common theories are briefly described below:
• *The mobilization of fixated articular surfaces.* The apophyseal joints can become fixated because of the effects of joint locking (eg, traumatic), muscle spasm, degeneration, an entrapped meniscoid or other loose body, capsular fibrosis, intra-articular "gluing" or adhesions (eg, postsynovitis, chronic rheumatoid conditions), bony ankylosis, facet tropism, etc.
• *The relaxation of the perivertebral musculature.* While a high-velocity force that suddenly stretches muscles spindles in primary muscle spasm *increases* the spasm, the same force applied to a segment where the related muscles are in secondary or protective spasm tends to produce relaxation if the thrust succeeds in removing the focal stimulus for the reflex.
• *The shock-like effect on the CNS.* Shock-like forces (1) are known to frequently have a normalizing effect on self-sustaining CNS reflexes; (2) are stimulative to the neurons involved, resulting in increased short-term neural and related endocrine activity; and (3) set up postural and muscle-tone-normalizing cerebellar influences via the long ascending and descending tracts.

Indirect (Functional) Approaches

Manual mobilization and thrust techniques are direct approaches to relieving articular fixations. Indirect functional approaches are often used when the cause for fixation has been determined to be essentially muscular in origin or when any form of manipulation would be contraindicated. Within this category fall many manual light-touch cutaneous reflex techniques, trigger-point therapy, electrotherapy, transverse massage, traction, therapeutic vibration, isometric and isotonic contraction, etc. It is theorized that these procedures produce much of their effects because of their influence on the gamma-loop system and/or by the superiority of mechanoreceptor input upon nociceptive input.

Different Types of Adjustive Thrusts

Impulse Thrusts

Faye describes an impulse thrust as coming from the diaphragm, like coughing or spitting. The hands adopt a preset tension in the direction of the impulse, and the impulse is characterized by a high-velocity low-depth thrust.

Recoil Thrusts

A thoracolumbar recoil adjustment delivered to a patient in the prone position should not be applied on a firm table. Injury to the patient's chest or abdomen may result because of the velocity and force associated with this type of thrust. The table should have a spring support in which the tension is released, yet there must be resistance under the thighs and upper thorax of the patient.

The classic recoil thrust, stated Firth, is applied against a spinous process in Zone One. After the contact has been accurately taken and secured, the correct stance must be assured and the elbows must be completely relaxed. At the instant of maximum patient exhalation, the adjuster's extensor muscles of the arms and pectorals are suddenly and simultaneously contracted. As the elbows are in line with each other and in the same plane, this spasmodic-like contraction will adduct the elbows and produce the thrust. So that the force of the adjustment will not go in the opposite direction (ie, toward the ceiling), the adjuster must contract the abdominal, thoracic, and neck muscles at the same time the adjustment is delivered. This will maintain a rigid trunk and the adjuster's body weight will concentrate the force upon the spinous process being adjusted.

The force of the adjustment should be applied equally with both arms at the same instant after the adjuster positions the trunk so that the force of the adjustment will be applied in a straight line from the episternal notch to the point of contact. The proper position, therefore, is to have the episternal notch directly over the point of contact. Another factor of importance is for the adjuster to position the elbows at right angles to the line of drive and bent only to the extent that allows the entire force of the adjustment to be delivered in a short, swift manner. Immediately after the adjustment is delivered, the adjuster's hands should "recoil" away from the patient's spine.

Body Drop Thrusts

A body drop thrust is usually associated with Carver's technic, as described by Beatty. It consists of centering the adjuster's trunk weight over the contact hand(s) and raising the body between the shoulders using straight arms. The adjuster's trunk is then dropped with a short sharp impulse, and the force is delivered through straight arms. This method is not to be confused with that of dropping the body by bending the knees as is occasionally used in lumbar side-posture adjusting.

The Carver body drop has to be used cautiously with children, the elderly, osteoporotics, etc.

Leverage Moves

The term *leverage move* refers to the use of counterpressure or contralateral stabilization. It is applied to prevent the loss of applied force, secure the most work with the least amount of energy expenditure, and concentrate the movement or force at the directed point of contact. Only enough counterpressure is used to balance the force of the adjustive thrust.

Multiple Thrusts

The objective of multiple thrusts is to permit a gradual increase in force, prolong the relief on compressed discs and articular cartilage, allow time to compensate for the applied force, and permit the application of a force that can be equal to or greater than that used in a single thrust, thus reducing patient discomfort.

A specific example of a multiple-thrust

technic would be the application of Spears' double-transverse contact, which is applied to the spine with thenar contacts in a deep, low-velocity, alternating, rhythmic fashion to obtain patient relaxation and to stretch perispinal and intersegmental adhesions and other tightened tissues prior to more specific spinal therapy. It has been described as a "down light, down heavy, and down deeper" multiple thrust in which each nonjerky thrust (without retraction) applies progressive pressure after tissue adaptation.

Extension Thrusts

The term *extension thrust* should not be confused with that for an extension fixation. An extension (distraction) or separation of joint surfaces and elongation of shortened soft tissues, states Beatty, should be a component of every thrust so that articular pressure is reduced to a minimum at the moment of joint movement. In this manner, articular friction with its accompanying trauma and pain will be reduced and taut tissues contributing to the fixation will be stretched. Instruction in adding intersegmental traction to all adjustive procedures was a fundamental principle in pioneer chiropractic.

Rotatory Trusts and Rotatory Breaks

A *rotatory thrust*, with accompanying joint distraction, is administered for the purpose of correcting either local or area rotatory fixations. A *rotatory break*, commonly applied in the cervical area, is the addition of a lateral force on the contralateral side of an accompanying lateral flexion fixation (eg, as in unilateral disc wedging along the concavity of a scoliosis).

Test Thrusts

Test thrusts are mild preliminary thrusts applied before the actual corrective thrust is delivered. They have a twofold purpose: first, to acquaint the adjuster with the structural resistance present and patient response to the pressure applied; second, to acquaint the patient with what to expect.

Different Approaches to Adjusting

Most all chiropractic adjustive technics have the common objectives of freeing restricted mobility and releasing impinged or stretched nerves. Added factors are the expansion or compression of abnormal IVFs and IVDs, the elongation of shortened tendons and ligaments, and the release of adhesions.

General Adjusting

General adjusting means nonspecific adjustments applied in different general areas of the spine. Such general adjustment are usually applied in postural distortions (eg, scoliosis, lordosis, kyphosis) to affect groups of vertebrae, muscles, and ligaments rather than specific segments. Many practitioners apply a general adjustment to relax the patient before adminstering specific adjustments.

Specific Adjusting

Specific adjusting means to deliver an adjustment to a specific vertebrae to alter specific symptomatology.

The biomechanical objective in specific chiropractic adjustments is to restore motion throughout the active, passive, and paraphysiologic range of motion (refer to Fig. 1.5). Because of the dynamic forces involved, such techniques must carefully consider the exact geometric plane of articulation (normal or abnormal), asymmetry, the force magnitude to be applied, the direction of force, torque, coupling mechanisms, the state of the holding elements (eg, spastic muscles, articular fixations, stiffness and damping factors), the integrity of the check ligaments (eg, stretched, shortened), and any underlying pathologic processes (eg, infectious, neoplastic, sclerotic, arthrotic, osteoporotic) of the structures directly or indirectly involved. As local tissue temperature, trabeculae arrangement, density, elasticity, flexibility, plasticity, nutrition, etc, are variables that affect the material properties of tissues, these factors must also be considered. The application of any clinical procedure without consideration of the cause-and-effect forces anticipated is not within the confines of scientific chiropractic.

It can generally be stated that joints and nerves become painful only when nociceptors are stretched, compressed, or chemically irritated. In adjusting acute lesions, proper analysis consists of the localization of fixations as well as the determination of which of these conditions exist to produce the nociceptive input experienced by the patient in pain.

Major Adjusting

Major adjusting refers to the correction of a priority motion unit to relieve a presenting complaint. Once this major (primary) consideration has been corrected, the next motion unit in importance to the patient's condition becomes the major.

Bibliography

Balduc HA: Overview of contemporary chiropractic science for the Chiropractic Association of Oklahoma. Northwestern College of Chiropractic, Convention notes, April 24, 1983.

Baltzell LG, Mackey RH (eds): *Firth's Technic Notes.* Publishing data not shown, 1967, pp 7-11, 34-40. Distributed by National College of Chiropractic.

Beatty HG: *Anatomical Adjustive Technic*, ed 2. Denver, published by author, 1939, pp 25-39, 133-186.

Bergmann T: Integrated chiropractic methods. Compilation of notes presented to the convention of the Oklahoma Chiropractic Association; April 23, 1983; in cooperation with Northwestern College of Chiropractic.

Burns L, Chandler LC, Rice RW: *Pathogenesis of Visceral Disease Following Vertebral Lesions.* Chicago, American Osteopathic Association, 1948, pp 11-27.

Cassidy JD, Kirkaldy-Willis WH, McGregor M: Spinal manipulation for the treatment of chronic low back and leg pain: an observational study. In Buerger AA, Greenman PE (eds): *Empirical Approaches to the Validation of Spinal Manipulation.* Springfield, MO, Charles C. Thomas, 1985.

Chicoine EP: The place of chiropractic in sports. *MPI's Dynamic Chiropractic*, 6(10):14-16, May 15, 1988.

Cox JM: *Low Back Pain: Mechanism, Diagnosis and Treatment.* Baltimore, Williams and Wilkins, 1985.

Dishmann R: Review of the literature supporting a scientific basis for the subluxation complex. *Journal of Manipulative and Physiological Therapeutics*, 8(3):163-172, September 1985.

Elftman H: Biomechanics of muscle. *Journal of Bone and Joint Surgery*, 48A:363-377, 1966.

Elftman H: The action of muscles in the body. *Biological Symposium*, 3:191-209, 1941.

Faye LJ: Before the Consultation (Patient Education Film) [Videotape]. Dynaspine, Inc, 10780 Santa Monica Blvd, Suite 400, Los Angeles, CA 90025.

Faye LJ: Before the Report of Findings (Patient Education Film) [Videotape]. Dynaspine, Inc, 10780 Santa Monica Blvd, Suite 400, Los Angeles, CA 90025.

Faye LJ: Chiropractic Subluxation Complex [Cassette tapes]. Huntington Beach CA, Motion Palpation Institute, 1986, tapes 1 and 2.

Faye LJ, et al: *Spine II: Motion Palpation and Clinical Considerations of the Cervical and Thoracic Spine.* Huntington Beach, CA, Motion Palpation Institute, 1986, p 3.

Faye LJ: Introduction, Rationale, Review of Clinical Examination; Causes, Treatment, and Management of Joint Dysfunction [Videotape]. Dynaspine, Inc, 10780 Santa Monica Blvd, Suite 400, Los Angeles, CA 90025.

Faye LJ: *Motion Palpation and Clinical Considerations of the Lower Extremities.* Huntington Beach, CA, Motion Palpation Institute, 1986, p 2.

Faye LJ: Patient Education [Cassette tape]. Huntington Beach, CA, Motion Palpation Institute, date not shown.

Faye LJ: *Spine I: Motion Palpation and Clinical Considerations of the Lumbar Spine and Pelvis.* Huntington Beach, CA, Motion Palpation Institute, 1987, pp 2-4.

Faye LJ, Weary B, Hooper P: *Motion Palpation and Clinical Considerations of the Upper Extremities.* Huntington Beach, CA, Motion Palpation Institute, 1986, p 2.

Giles LG: Leg length inequalities associated with low back pain. *Journal of the Canadian Chiropractic Association*, 20(1):25-32, 1976.

Giles LG: Lumbosacral facetal joint angles associated with leg length inequality. *Rheumatology and Rehabilitation*, 20:233-238, 1981.

Giles LG, Taylor JR: Lumbar spine structural changes associated with leg length inequality. *Spine*, 7(2):159-162, 1982.

Giles LG, Taylor JR: Low back pain associated with leg length inequality. *Spine*, 6(5):510-21, 1981.

Gillet H: A definition of the subluxation. *The Texas Chiropractor*, February 1974.

Gillet H: Gillet of Belgium: a definition of the subluxation. *Digest of Chiropractic Economics*, 15(6):14-17, 1973.

Gillet H: The history of motion palpation. *European Journal of Chiropractic*, 31(4):196-201, 1983.

Gillet H, Liekens M: *Belgian Chiropractic Research Notes.* Huntington Beach, CA, Motion Palpation Institute, 1984, pp ii-iv, 1-4, 11-35, 65-70, 78-81, 123-125; 165.

Gillet H, Liekens M: A further study of spinal fixations. *Annals of the Swiss Chiropractors Association*, 4:41-46, 1969.

Gillet H: Spinal and related fixations. *Digest of Chiropractic Economics*, 14(3):22-24, 1971.

Glasgow EF, Twomey LT, Scull ER, Kleynhans AM, Idczak RM: *Aspects of Manipulative Therapy*, ed 2. New York, Churchill Livingstone, 1985, pp 109-115.

Goodman CE: Pathophysiology of pain. *Archives of Internal Medicine*, 143:527, 1983.

Gowitzke BA, Gowitzke MM: *Understanding the Scientific Bases of Human Movement*, ed 2. Baltimore, Williams & Wilkins, 1980, pp 3-10.

Grecco MA: *Chiropractic Technic Illustrated*. Jarl, New York, 1953, pp 9-24, 51.

Grice AS: A biomechanical approach to cervical and dorsal adjusting. In Haldeman S (ed): *Modern Developments in the Principles and Practice of Chiropractic*. New York, Appleton-Century-Crofts, 1980, pp 338-339.

Homewood AE: *The Neurodynamics of the Vertebral Subluxation*, ed 3. Place of publication not shown, published by author, 1981, pp 51, 71.

Illi FW: *The Vertebral Column: Life-Line of the Body*. Chicago, National College of Chiropractic, 1951, pp 19-21, 25-40.

Janse J: History of the development of chiropractic concepts: Chiropractic Terminology. In Goldstein M (ed): *The Research Status of Spinal Manipulative Therapy*; NINCDS Monograph No. 15, US Dept of HEW. Washington, DC, U.S. Printing Office, 1975, pp 25-32.

Kellgren JH, Samuel EP: The sensitivity and innervation of the articular capsule. *Journal of Bone & Joint Surgery*, 32(B):84-92, 1950.

Kendall HO, Kendall FP, Wadsworth GE: *Muscles Testing and Function*, ed 2. Baltimore, Williams & Wilkins, 1971, pp 18-22, 28.

Kern DP: Preface. In Gillet H, Liekens M: *Belgian Chiropractic Research Notes*. Huntington Beach, CA, Motion Palpation Institute, 1984, p iv.

Kessler RM, Hertling D (eds): *Management of Common Musculoskeletal Disorders*. Philadelphia, Harper & Row, 1983, pp 18-19, 75-104, 107-109, 178-181.

Kirkaldy-Willis WH: Manipulation. In Kirkaldy-Willis WH (ed): *Managing Low Back Pain*. New York, Churchill Livingstone, 1983, pp 175-177.

Korr IM (ed): *The Neurobiologic Mechanisms in Manipulative Therapy*. New York, Plenum Press, 1978, pp 5-6, 44-45.

Levine M: *The Structural Approach to Chiropractic*. New York, Comet Press, 1964, p 85.

Lieb MM: Oral orthopedics. In Gelb H (ed): *Clinical Management of Head, Neck, and TMJ Pain and Dysfunction*. Philadelphia, W.B. Saunders, 1977, pp 32-71.

McCole GM: *An Analysis of the Osteopathic Lesion*. Great Falls, MT, published by author, 1935, pp 10-11, 23-30.

Mennell JMcM: *Joint Pain*. Boston, Little, Brown, 1964, pp 1-10, 12-31, 134-136, 156-157, 167.

Palmer DD: *Textbook of the Science, Art and Philosophy of Chiropractic*. Portland, OR, Portland Printing House, 1910, pp 69, 77.

Rosse C, Simkin PA: Joints. In Rosse C, Clawson DK: *The Musculoskeletal Sycstem in Health & Disease*. Hagerstown, PA, Harper & Row, 1980, pp 77-80.

Salter RB: *Textbook of Disorders and Injuries of the Musculoskeletal System*. Baltimore, Williams & Wilkins, 1970, pp 22-26.

Sandoz R: Some physical mechanisms and effects of spinal adjustments. *Annals of the Swiss Chiropractors' Association*, 6:91, 1976.

Schafer RC: *Chiropractic Health Care*, ed 3. Des Moines, IA, The Foundation for Chiropractic Education and Research, 1979, pp 35, 41-44.

Schafer RC: *Clinical Biomechanics: Musculoskeletal Actions and Reactions*. Baltimore, Williams & Wilkins, 1983, pp 44-46, 57-59, 74-81, 136-137, 246-247, 468.

Schafer RC (ed): *Basic Chiropractic Procedural Manual*, ed 4. Arlington, VA, American Chiropractic Association, 1984, pp 5-8.

Schafer RC (ed): *Chiropractic State of the Art*. Des Moines, IA, American Chiropractic Association, June 1979, pp 9-13.

States AZ: *Spinal and Pelvic Technics*, rev ed 2. Lombard, IL, National College of Chiropractic, 1968, pp foreword, 1-7.

Stephenson RW: *Chiropractic Textbook*. Davenport, IA, published by author, 1927, pp 308, 322-325.

Swezey RL: The modern thrust of manipulation and traction therapy. *Seminars in Arthritis and Rheumatism*, 12(3):326, 1983.

Tehan PJ: Functional technique: A different perspective in manipulative therapy. In Glasgow EF, Twomey LT, Scull ER, Kleynhans AM, Idczak RM: *Aspects of Manipulative Therapy*, ed 2. New York, Churchill Livingstone, 1985, pp 94-96.

Travell JG, Simons DG: *Myofascial Pain and Dysfunction: The Trigger Point Manual*. Baltimore, Williams & Wilkins, 1983, pp 18-19, 21-24.

Vladef T, Hardy M: The theory of fixation points, *National Chiropractic Journal*, June 1945.

Watkins RJ: Subluxation terminology since 1964. *ACA Journal of Chiropractic*, 2(9):S65-70, 1968.

White AA, Hirsch C: The significance of the vertebral posterior elements in the mechanics of the thoracic spine. *Clinical Orthopaedics*, 81:2-41, 1971.

Will TE: The biochemical basis of manipulative therapeutics: hypothetical considerations. *Journal of Manipulative and Physiological Therapeutics*, 1(3):153-156, September 1978.

Wyke BD: Articular neurology and manipulative therapy. In *Aspects of Manipulative Therapy*. Proceedings of Multidisciplinary International Conference on Manipulative Therapy. Melbourne, Lincoln Institute of Health Sciences, Carlton, Victoria, Australia, August 1979, pp 67-72.

Chapter 2

The Basic Clinical Approach in Dynamic Chiropractic

This chapter offers an overview of dynamic chiropractic protocols and describes the general concepts underlying the application of motion palpation and related procedures.

AN OVERVIEW OF DYNAMIC CLINICAL PROTOCOLS

The Interview

It is recommended that the interview be conducted as quickly and efficiently as possible, while assuring that all the details of a standard case history and systems review are covered.

Data gathering concerning the nature of the patient's problems may begin as early as when the patient calls for an appointment and attempts to describe the problem and onset to the receptionist. As the patient with low-back pain, for example, enters and navigates around the office, observe his ease of movement and posture. Is he bent laterally to one side or forward? Does he limp or shuffle when he walks? Does his facial expression reflect pain? Does he have difficulty straightening when rising from the chair? Can he sit down? Can he cross his knees? The answer to these and similar questions will help direct the consultation and examination to follow.

The History of Joint Pain

Investigating the history of joint pain such as its onset, character, and duration can offer significant clues (Table 2.1).

Features of a neuromusculoskeletal nature that cannot be linked to trauma are suspect of a chronic degenerative or organic process. Unfortunately, a history of stress or strain may not be remembered. Even severe trauma is easily put out of the mind during sports or other activities when emotions are high or forgotten once the pain and swelling have left. Whether pain is present or not, the history must be thoroughly investigated to help determine the cause of the dysfunction (eg, bone, periarticular soft tissues of the joint, or the motor apparatus involved in the joint motion).

Typical Signs and Symptoms in Musculoskeletal Disorders

Abnormalities that are commonly discovered in disorders of the neuromusculoskeletal system include: (1) pain on motion, (2) tenderness on palpation, (3) limitation of motion, (4) joint instability, (5) color changes such as ecchymosis and redness, (6) local heat, (7) soft-tissue swelling from synovial thickening, periarticular swelling, or nodules,

Table 2.1. Typical Questions Asked During the Investigation of Joint Pain

What seems to be the matter?
What do you think caused it?
Where exactly does it hurt?
Does it always hurt there?
Does the pain feel sharp, dull, burning, tingling, boring, or what?
Does it feel deep inside or near the surface?
Does its quality or intensity ever change?
Is it constant or does it come and go?
Does the pain seem to start at one place and spread to another?
Do you notice other things at the time the pain is severe?
When did the pain first arise?
Did it first occur gradually or rapidly?
Was an injury or some unusual activity involved?
At what time of day is the pain worse?
At what time of day is the pain better?
How long have you suffered with this condition?
Have you ever had this condition before and it appeared to go away?
If so, what did you do for it?
Does anything seem to precipitate an attack?
What aggravates the pain?
What relieves the pain?
What home remedies have you tried and what were their effects?
How has this problem affected your work, activities, or sleep?
How is your health otherwise?
Are you presently being treated for any other condition?
Are you taking any drugs or medications?
What illnesses have you had in the past?
What injuries have you had in the past?
Has anybody else in your family had a condition similar to this?
Do you have any opinion on what might have caused this problem?
Is there anything else you would like to add?

Note: Many of these questions would be pertinent to a complaint other than pain.

(8) swelling from bony enlargement, (9) bone deformity or subluxation, (10) wasting from atrophy or dystrophy, and (11) carriage and gait abnormalities.

A gradually arising pain is often associated with chronic nonspecific arthritis. A rapid onset is seen in acute sprain/strain, rheumatic conditions such as rheumatic fever, septic arthritis, and gout. A history of a recent injection of antitoxin or the administration of a new drug may suggest joint symptoms having an allergic basis. Severe throbbing pain is characteristic of gout and septic arthritis. A dull ache during rest that is aggravated by motion suggests inflammatory arthritis. Chronic meniscal derangement is always suspect when the patient's history indicates sudden joint locking during motion (eg, knee, jaw).

The pain from degenerative arthritis and muscular disorders is an aching type that is relieved by rest, aggravated by certain motions, and often accompanied by muscle splinting and paresthesias. A sharp severe pain (associated with muscle changes and sensory disturbances) radiating along the distribution of a nerve is characteristic of acute nerve compression. Fracture pain is severe, throbbing, and acutely aggravated by movement of the part. Bone pain resulting from tumor or aneurysm is usually deep, constant, boring, more intense at night, and rarely relieved by rest or a change in position. Referred pain is often associated with musculoskeletal disorders, as are many noxious somatosomatic, somatovisceral, viscerosomatic, somatopsychic, and psychosomatic reflexes. Clues in differentiating acute from chronic disorders are shown in Table 2.2.

Interpreting the History of Low-Back Pain

The three most common origins of low-back pain are (1) the lumbar facet syndrome, (2) the sacroiliac syndrome, and (3) the lumbar radicular syndrome, which may be either discogenic or biomechanical in origin (Fig. 2.1). These syndromes will be described in Chapters 5 and 6, but it is worthy to mention here that each of these syndromes can be acute or chronic, arise from trauma or spontaneously, and have varying degrees of concomitant pathomechanics involved. It should also be pointed

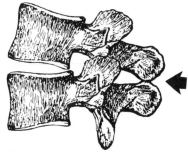

Figure 2.1. Schematic presentation of "kissing spines." Posterior apposition of spinous processes such as this are traditionally attributed to an unstable IVD. However, note that the same picture may result if the superior segment is locked in extension (Courtesy ACAP).

out that these syndromes are named according to the level of inflammation (eg, the pain-producing structures involved) and more than likely *not* the area in need of correction. Their common causes include sprain/strain from overuse, poor posture, disuse, a development abnormality, joint dysfunction (fixation, hypermobility, aberrant motion), or degenerative changes.

Table 2.2. Differentiation of Acute and Chronic Disorders

Clinical Finding	Acute Inflammation	Chronic Inflammation
Pain	Relatively constant; likely to be referred over a diffuse segmental area. In intrinsic disorders, pain is increased on movement in any direction; in periarticular disorders, pain is increased on movement only in certain planes. Pressure produces a lingering-type pain; ie, "springing test."	Increased by specific movements, relieved by rest; likely to be relatively localized near, but not necessarily over, the site of the lesion. Heavy pressure produces a lingering-type pain.
Passive motion	Muscle spasm or empty end-feel at the end of motion.	No muscle spasm or empty end-feel at the end of motion, possible blocking.
Tenderness	Severe.	From slight to moderate.
Skin temperature	Measurable increase.	No measurable increase.
Sleeping pattern	Difficulty in falling asleep, staying asleep, or both.	No sleeping difficulty unless a hip or shoulder is involved.

Clinical Rationale and Therapeutic Goal

When a disorder is determined to be of an articular disorder of the vertebral column, the basic rationale for a chiropractic adjustment is that a fixation-subluxation can lead to a pathophysiologic (altered function) state than can readily progress to a pathologic (altered structure) state. Correction of the fixation-subluxation encourages the restoration of normal function and tissue if it is reversible. A rational therapeutic approach should take a holistic multicausal approach to each patient's particular health problems (refer to Figure 1.10).

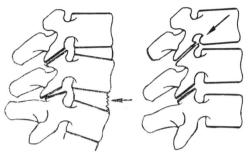

Figure 2.2. *Left,* extension subluxation encouraging impingement of the IVF as the result of a segment being fixed in extension or lax anterior fibers of the anulus. *Right,* osteophytic encroachment of the IVF in the superior segment, compared to a normal foramen in the inferior segment (Courtesy ACAP).

Review of the Clinical Fixation-Subluxation Complex

The clinical fixation-subluxation complex has been developed by Faye of MPI and consists of five major potential components:

1. A *neuropathophysiologic component.* This may express in one or two forms or both; eg: (a) irritation producing CNS facilitation in the anterior horn manifesting as hypertonicity or spasm, in the lateral horn manifesting as vasomotor changes (hypersympathicotonic vasoconstriction and pallor), and in the posterior horn manifesting as sensory changes; (b) pressure (compression) producing CNS degeneration manifesting as muscular atrophy, sympathetic atonia (hyposympathicotonic vasodilation and stasis), and anesthesia. See Figure 2.2.

At this point, it is well to remember *the Wallerian law:* After section of a posterior nerve root of a spinal nerve between the root ganglion and the spinal cord, the central portion degenerates. After division of the anterior root, the peripheral portion degenerates. Thus, *the trophic center of the posterior root is in the ganglion,* and the trophic center of the anterior root is in the *spinal cord.*

2. A *kinesiopathologic component;* eg, hypomobility, diminished or absent joint play, and compensatory segmental kinematic hypermobility (as described by Gillet, Mennel, and Illi, respectively).

3. A *myopathic component;* eg, hypertonicity or spasm (as the result of compensation, facilitation, and/or Hilton's law) or atonia and weakness. *Hilton's law* states: the trunk of a nerve sends branches to (a) a particular muscle, (b) the joint moved by that muscle, and (c) the skin overlying the insertion of that muscle.

4. A *histopathologic component;* eg, inflammation (pain, heat, swelling) as the result of hypermobile irritation or degeneration (numbness, coolness, circulatory stasis, atrophy) as the result of hypomobility (physiologic nonstimulation). We can, in time, also expect certain osseous changes according to two clinical principles:

• *Wolff's law:* Every change in the form and functions of a bone, or in its function alone, is followed by certain definite changes in its internal architecture and secondary alterations in its external conformation.

• *Weigert's law (overproduction theory).* The loss or destruction of a part or element in the organic world is likely to result in compensatory replacement and overproduction of tissue during the process of regeneration or repair (or both). Typical examples are seen in the formation of callus when a fractured bone heals or marginal exostoses and other excrescences as the result of chronic inflammation and degenerative processes.

5. A noxious *biochemical component;* eg, hormonal and chemical imbalance owing to

the proinflammatory stress syndrome, histamine production, prostaglandin production, and bradykinin production—as described by Selye.

With these possible components in mind, the therapeutic approach may incorporate:

• Dynamic adjustive procedures designed to release sites of fixations directly or indirectly (reflexively).

• Other procedures designed to enhance the healing process such as reflex technics, exercise, physiologic therapeutics (modalities), nutritional supplementation, biofeedback, and counsel about exercise, posture, diet, relaxation, stress reduction, etc.

The prognosis will be determined by the potential reversibility of the pathologic process at hand depending on the restoration of normal physiologic processes, the ability to keep the spine free of subluxations and the body from other factors that tend to deplete systemic physiologic reserves, and the significance of *Spallanzani's law:* The younger the body the greater is the regenerative power of its cells. Besides the standard routines of physical diagnosis, optimal preventive and maintenance care should incorporate regular motion palpation examinations to discover early sites of fixation and aberrant motion.

General Examination Procedures

The principles of dynamic chiropractic are not built on guesswork or mechanical formulas. If an articular disorder of the spine has been determined to exist that can account for the patient's symptoms and signs, patient improvement will coincide with increased segmental spinal mobility, and, conversely, conditions not responding to therapy will usually coincide with a failure to achieve increased segmental spinal mobility.

In developing the skill of motion palpation, the physician will acquire the knowledge to know where, why, when, and how a correction to a site of hypomobility should be made. Skill develops from practice: palpating, adjusting, and verifying the results. Once this skill becomes developed to a high level, your self-confidence and the patient's confidence in you are greatly enhanced.

Dynamic chiropractic uses the standard procedures of physical, laboratory, roentgenographic, neurologic, and orthopedic diagnosis as taught in accredited chiropractic colleges. As these procedures are professional standards, reference to them will only be brief in this manual.

The Main Steps of the Examination Process. It is rarely good policy to project a diagnosis on the basis of one finding. All pertinent symptoms and signs should confirm and validate each other.

1. *Inspection.* Note any signs of abnormal skin discoloration, pigmentation, texture, erythema, moisture or dryness, nodules, masses, scars, hair patches, skin lesions, swelling, etc. Seek signs of regional biomechanical distortion (eg, ear level and rotation, shoulder level and rotation, hip level and rotation, knee and ankle posture).

2. *Static palpation.* Seek signs of abnormal heat or coolness, edema, mass, muscle spasm or hypertonicity, atrophy, and tissue texture (eg, sinewy, boggy). Keep in mind that bent spinous processes and asymmetrical bony structures are common in both healthy and unhealthy spines. Extra vertebra, absent vertebra, hemivertebra, and spina bifida occulta are not infrequently found, and these may contribute contradictory data.

3. *Motion palpation.* Note motion restriction and type of end block in every plane of normal motion for each segment by carrying the segment through its normal ROM. Your palpating fingers should be on the active and at least one adjacent segment. Never force motion beyond patient tolerance, and always maintain open communications with the patient during the examination process.

Plumb Line and Grid Analyses. Although plumb line and similar postural analytical devices will not determine the site of spinal fixations, they sometimes do offer a gross indication for pre- and post-adjustive mensuration once the sites of fixation have been found. One obvious fault in such analyses is that they will fail to suggest any change in a site of fixation that has formed in the "at rest" or "neutral" position. In most chronic cases, however, even these may be reflected in some type of compensatory effort that, in time, has become fixed.

Specific examples will be given in later chapters of this phenomenon.

Painful Joints

During the examination of any synovial joint (Fig. 2.3), the following tissues should be visualized as they are often the site of injury and/or pathology:

• Articular cartilage or intra-articular fibrocartilage (if normally present)
• Blood vessels
• Capsule
• Lymphatics
• Nerves
• Periarticular ligaments
• Periarticular muscles
• Periosteum
• Synovium
• Tendon sheaths (if normally present)
• Tendons

Pain may arise from any joint tissue containing nociceptors such as ligaments, tendon insertions, periosteum, fibrocartilages (slightly), capsules, and vascular walls. Authorities differ in whether the synovium contains nociceptors; most believe that it does not. Some basic clues in differentiating synovial from mechanical causes of joint pain are shown in Table 2.3.

Muscle Pain. Muscle pain has its peculiar characteristics. The pain that arises from myositis or an injury to muscle tissue may be elicited by making the muscle contract against resistance without allowing it to shorten; ie, preventing movement of adjacent joints. This test, although it may be of help in differentiating myalgia from the pain of other etiologies, is not absolute because it is not always possible, even with great care, to avoid some indirect pressure on or movement of adjacent structures. An additional feature is that sometimes the pain which arises from a chronic contraction of the involved muscle is not increased by contracting the muscle further.

Tendon Pain. The pain of true tendinitis is often superficial, resulting from a tenosynovitis. It is evoked by passively moving the tendon to and fro within its sheath. Pain from injured tendons usually arises when the attached muscle is contracted. The torn tendon fibers will usually not cause pain when the muscle is relaxed; but, with the least muscle shortening, pain arises.

Ligamentous Pain. Ligament pain especially develops when a joint is under extremely prolonged tension, and a restricted joint should be the first suspicion in such cases. Inflamed ligaments become painful by stretching and deep pressure. When accessible to palpation, an irritated ligament will be tender; and if it can be squeezed, pain will be evoked. Chronic pain arising from ligaments usually comes on slowly after assuming some posture in which the involved joint(s) are held at a limit of motion. The ache arises from the stimulation of intraligamentous and periosteal receptors near the insertion. Ligaments are normally painless upon moderate pressure.

Bone Pain. Compact bone is, for the most part, insensitive to painful stimuli. Most of the pain sensitive fibers within the medullary portion of bone are those few located within vascular walls. The periosteum, how-

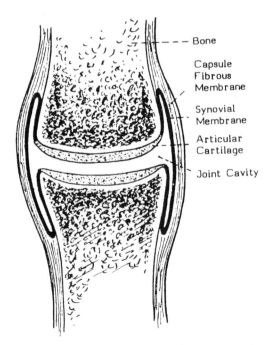

Figure 2.3. Schematic of the major components of a typical synovial joint that has been cut across the longitudinal midline. The synovial cavity has been exaggerated laterally to depict the potential space (Courtesy ACAP).

Table 2.3. Synovial vs Mechanical Causes of Joint Pain

Feature	Synovitic Lesions	Mechanical Lesions
Onset	Symptoms fairly consistent, during use and at rest.	Symptoms arise chiefly during use.
Location	Any joint may be involved.	Primarily involves weight-bearing joints.
Course	Usually fluctuates. Episodic flares are common.	Persistently worsening progression. No acute exacerbations. May produce acute episodes elsewhere.
Stiffness	Prolonged in the morning.	Little morning stiffness.
Anti-inflammatory effect	Aided by cold and other anti-inflammatory therapies; eg, 80—120 Hz interferential current.	Responds to 1—20 Hz interferential current, according to Faye.
Major pathologic features	Negative radiographic signs or diffuse cartilage loss, marginal bony erosions, but no osteophytes.	Radiographic signs of cartilage loss and osteophyte development.

ever, is richly supplied with nociceptors. Bone pain is often perceived as a "sick pain;" the patient will feel ill.

Painful Adhesions. Adhesions do not contain nociceptors. During movement, however, pain may arise when they stretch or occlude adhering, connecting, or congruent pain-sensitive tissues (eg, periosteum, vascular walls, joint or visceral capsules). The cause of pain from joint adhesions may be from direct compression or tensile forces or be the product of ensuing stasis, ischemia, or distention. The pain is immediate in onset. Another diagnostic clue is that there is pronounced hypomobility when adhesions are present. A common condition encountered is the painful adhesions that develop after surgery or major trauma. However, adhesions may develop naturally as the result of adhesive capsulitis, rheumatoid arthritis, and septic arthritis. The pain originating in capsules tightened by adhesions occurs immediately when the capsule is stretched. If the adhesions are stretched further, a sharp pain ensues, leaving the surrounding muscles flaccid. The intensity of such a pain varies with the site and size of the adhesions. For the most part, pain arising from adhesions is only momentary because motion is quickly halted as soon as the sharp pain is felt.

Cartilaginous Pain. As with adhesions, pain arises from most cartilaginous tissues only when they are displaced or swollen and stretch or pressure is applied on adjacent pain-sensitive receptors. The periphery of most fibrocartilages (eg, IVDs, menisci of the knee and jaw) contain some nociceptors, but the degree that they are involved in a patient's report of pain is difficult to determine. A cartilaginous loose body will certainly produce pain if it is caught between two apposing pain-sensitive articular surfaces. Cartilaginous thickening and even chondrophytes at articular sites have been shown to be impregnated with sensory fibers; thus, pain can arise when they are compressed. If adjacent tissues are inflamed, then both compression and tensile forces will produce pain.

Painful Nerves. Pain arising from nerve lesions manifests within the involved nerve's distribution, on the surface or deep, and it usually radiates. Pain of intrinsic neurologic origin is generally accompanied by paresthesias and root signs. There is an excessive response to stimulation. It is difficult for the patient to describe its character as it is unlike any other type of pain and usually is a combination of painful sensations. It is provoked by any peripheral stimulation in the involved zone, and stimulated trigger points cause spontaneous paroxysms. The patient vigilantly guards the involved part and shows great apprehension. Pain that is accentuated by heat points to neuritis or congestion. In contrast, pain that is relieved by heat suggests something producing abnormal myotonia.

Hyperalgesia. The term *hyperalgesia* means an excessive sensitivity to pain. A painful tenderness produced by external pressure frequently results from trigger points, traumatic lesions of sensitive subdermal tissue, the development of a toxic accumulation, or a deep-seated inflammatory irritation. Hyperalgesia of soft tissues is not rare in the areas that have been the seat of reflex sensory pain. For example, subcutaneous soreness within the shoulder and upper arm muscles is often associated with inflammatory diseases of the lungs. Overlying cutaneous hyperalgesia is also a common finding in many other visceral diseases. Zones of hyperalgesia (often associated with precapillary vasoconstriction and hypermyotonia) are more commonly associated with acute and subacute visceral disease than with chronic disorders. The level of facilitation in the subluxation complex is often determined by the patient's response to a sharp pin prick applied to the skin or during a skin rolling test.

Joint Clicks

The importance of atmospheric pressure and surface tension of synovial fluid in joint stability is readily demonstrated during the action of knuckle cracking or the audible click accompanying a chiropractic adjustment. A relaxed loosely packed joint may be moved several degrees to prove that its collateral ligaments are relaxed. When the joint is distracted to the degree that a sound is heard, it is at this point that the articular surfaces suddenly separate and a bubble of carbon dioxide forms within the joint cavity that can often be shown in roentgenographs.

A distraction force applied to a synovial joint is resisted by both surface tension and atmospheric pressure. The adhesiveness of synovial fluid attempts to maintain articular juxtaposition; but, once it is overcome, the intra-articular pressure is suddenly reduced to a level below atmospheric pressure so that gas is audibly released from the fluid. The larger the joint, the greater the force necessary for distraction. This is not only because of the proportionately greater contributions of surface tension and atmospheric pressure but also because of the stronger stabilizing muscles and ligaments.

The sound produced can reflect some important clinical data. When tension is applied to a joint so that motion is just beyond the elastic barrier of resistance, a sudden yielding is perceived, a cracking sound is heard, and the range of motion is increased into the paraphysiologic space. The joint click so often heard during an adjustment is thus an indication that the elastic barrier has been exceeded and motion within the area of joint play has been achieved. When the tension is relaxed following the "click," the joint surfaces will be further separated at rest than before the tension was initially applied.

Such normal "clicks" will be absent, however, if the muscles are so splinted around the joint that adequate distraction is prevented, if the intra-articular space is swollen, or if the bubble of gas does not form during the distraction for whatever reason. Thus, while a "click" demonstrates wide intra-articular separation, its absence does not prove a lack of separation.

Sandoz has demonstrated that a *manipulation* produces a "click" or "crack" and maximum separation. A *mobilization* stretches the elastic barrier but produces much less separation and fails to influence the interarticular joint space during rest.

Surface Signs of Peripheral Nerve Dysfunction

As previously described, *Hilton's law* states that an overstressed nerve trunk (irritated, stretched, compressed) will manifest signs of abnormal innervation in particular muscles, the joints moved by those muscles, and the skin overlying the insertion of those muscles. Thus, as the posterior ramus of a spinal nerve supplies both the perispinal musculature and the overlying dermatome, it can be expected that changes in these overlying tissues may reflect an IVF lesion. Granted, changes in these tissues may be the result of other lesions, but volumes of empiric reports appear to link many of these changes with an IVF lesion.

Tenderness. The term *tenderness* refers to pain on pressure. Certain fixations are invariably accompanied by either spontaneous pain or that brought out by palpation or some other type of pressure. As a general rule, partial spinal fixations are associated with perivertebral tenderness because muscle tissue becomes tender when in a state of prolonged contraction. Whether this state of hypersensitiveness is the result of vascular engorgement, the accumulation of lactic acid or other metabolic by-products, potassium leakage, or some other factor is controversial. Regardless, in the context of perispinal tenderness, we should keep in mind two clinical principles that will aid the final diagnosis:

1. *van der Kolk's law:* In any mixed nerve (eg, posterior rami of a spinal nerve), the sensory fibers are distributed to parts moved by the muscles controlled by the motor nerves.

2. *Sherrington's law:* Every posterior spinal nerve root supplies a special territory of the skin (dermatome), which is, however, invaded above and below by fibers from adjacent spinal segments. Thus, tenderness does not point assuredly to one specific nerve root.

If degenerative processes have not progressed to a state of anesthesia, Gillet describes two types of shortened ligaments that are almost always tender to pressure or stretching: (1) the interspinous ligaments in segmental lordosis and (2) the anterior longitudinal ligaments in segmental kyphosis. Tender interspinous and intertransverse ligaments and muscles can best be palpated when the spine is flexed forward. Positive findings, however, do not amend the precept that acute minor fixations are the result of chronic major fixations that are characteristically accompanied by diminished sensation.

Reflexogenicity. It has been Gillet's experience that hypertonic muscles throughout the back will react with a short rapid contraction when tapped with a reflex hammer. This reaction, however, is difficult to elicit in obese patients.

Vasomotor Changes. For about the last 60 years, chiropractic investigators have strived to link various vasomotor changes occurring in the skin overlying the spine with the possibility of an underlying subluxation complex. Typical examples of such changes are heat abnormalities measured by bipolar and unipolar skin temperature recording devices and thermographic procedures, circulatory abnormalities measured by infrared photography, and electrical resistance abnormalities measured by various types of ohm meters.

Thermographic Changes. Gillet has used a heat measuring device in which one detector is held in an unsymptomatic palm of the patient to serve as a constant or norm while another detector is placed on the skin of the back to obtain a comparative value. His findings have been that many abnormal readings are bilateral, especially in the upper cervical area. Some spinal readings were areas of coolness (relative hypothermia) and some of abnormal warmth (relative hyperthermia) in contrast to the skin temperature of surrounding areas. However, no firm diagnostic criteria on the significance of these changes could be established.

Electrical Resistance Changes. The Belgium researchers also developed an instrument that was designed to detect the sites of variant electrical resistance and measure their degree of abnormality. Readings were taken before and after adjustments were administered. The general conclusion was that abnormal local readings reduced as did readings throughout the spine. Again, no firm conclusions or relationships could be established.

Many claims have been made for the efficacy of skin-property-measuring procedures, but few, if any, have been objectively collaborated by controlled studies. Although the subject is highly controversial, there is no doubt that such data are helpful if placed in proper perspective and collaborated by several other signs and symptoms. It is hoped that future research will be able to arrive at some significant correlation between vertebral lesions and various dermatographic temperature, electrical, exocrine, and vasomotor changes. We can add to this the significance of local hyperesthesia, hypoesthesia, capillary filling rate after stripping, nerve tracing, skin texture changes, thermesthetic alterations, scratch tests, local areas of diminished subcutaneous fat, trophic blotches and blemishes, and on and on.

The Gillet Routine in Chronic Cases

In the method used by Gillet, an attempt to make a *complete* examination of spinal mobility on the first visit is not attempted (especially not at the beginning of therapy). The first few visits are given to searching for total and possibly important partial fixations. One reason for this is that the passive movements necessary to determine a site of fixation are in themselves irritating to the patient who is likely already in pain. Once the major fixations are corrected, many minor fixations will spontaneously disappear. Palpation on subsequent visits will reveal major fixations still present requiring correction.

The type of adjustive technic used is not important as long as it is a standard taught in an accredited chiropractic college. Any type of adjustment that will mobilize the fixed articulation (ie, directed against the motion restriction) will be effective. The least painful to the patient will be an adjustment delivered that is parallel to the plane of articulation. The objective is to free the restricting soft-tissue factors and allow normal function of the involved perispinal muscles and ligaments, bursae, and articular cartilage to "realign" the segments according to the degree of reversibility present. [See Clinical Comment 2.1]

Gillet describes the management of a typical case exhibiting several sites of chronic fixation as follows:

First visit. Seek and correct any total occipitoatlantal fixation found. Nothing more is done this visit because at least a few hours or days are necessary to permit the changes that will take place in the remainder of the spine. It is sometimes possible to achieve a complete correction of a total occipitoatlantal fixation (immobility in all planes) with one adjustment, but usually the first correction is only partial.

Second Visit. The atlas is re-examined. If the atlas is still partially fixed, leave it alone. This partial fixation is ignored until the effect of other corrections on the upper cervical spine can be determined. Examine the caudad aspect of the spinal chain; ie, seek and correct total sacroiliac fixation if found. Occipitoatlantal and sacroiliac fixations are usually coexisting. Unlike heavily fibrotic chronic upper-thoracic fixations, a total sacroiliac fixation can frequently be corrected with one treatment that successfully manipulates or adjusts each ROM fixated.

Third Visit. If the atlas and sacroiliac adjustments have restored mobility, seek the most fixed motion unit remaining in the spine such as an upper dorsal major (eg, T1 anterior-body fixation) and adjust. It will commonly be found that multiple motion units (eg, involving 3—5 vertebra) in the area will be affected rather than just a single motion unit. Once such an area is felt, it is easy to repalpate to localize the specific site(s) of fixation.

Fourth Visit. If the previously adjusted motion unit has remained mobile, seek other sites of fixation such as a lower lumbar interspinous fixation (eg, L4—L5) and correct if found.

Fifth Visit. If the previously adjusted motion unit has remained mobile, seek other possible sites of total fixation such as a vertebrocostal fixation (eg, T3). If the pre-

---

DR. FAYE'S CLINICAL COMMENT #2.1

The second and most important objective is to create an imposed demand for motion in the motion unit. Any biologic system given a regular demand will adapt specifically to the demand. Salter proved in his studies joint hyaline cartilage would even regenerate given an environment of motion instead of the immobilization of casts. Thus chiropractic adjustments often need to be repeated long after the pain subsides to act as an imposed demand. Exercise is ineffective until the intersegmental motion is normal.

viously adjusted fixation is only partially eliminated, it is best to temporarily move on to the next major total fixation.

Sixth Visit. If the previously adjusted fixation is now mobile, seek and correct any other site of fixation found such as an intercostal fixation (eg, 7th ribs).

Seventh Visit. Re-examine all sites of previous fixation. If all are mobile, seek sites of extraspinal fixation such as in the feet and correct if found.

The above examples are only generalizations. Each patient will require an individualized approach depending on the situation at hand.

If several sites of fixation are found, it is usually preferable to correct the most inferior one first and only one motion unit per office visit to allow for natural compensating mechanisms to adapt. The correction of more than one area of major fixation at a time has not appeared to offer any beneficial effects (but possibly add some detrimental effects) to either the patient's spinal mechanics or symptoms. Each time a fixation is released, the entire spine must readapt to a new state of equilibrium. This requires a multitude of changes in scores of ligaments, muscles, and cartilages that may not have been so positioned or worked for many years. If structural pathologic changes have occurred in the spine, it may take many months for the diseased tissues to regenerate or remold even moderately. However, it is often surprising how symptom free a patient can become while static roentgenographic evidence of change is lacking. Kinematic radiographic studies, however, will show increased mobility.

It will generally be found that each subsequent fixation localized during motion palpation can be released with greater ease. Conversely, if a fixation is resistant to correction, some point in this routine has likely been missed. If this occurs, complete re-examination and re-evaluation of the case are necessary.

Gillet believes that there is a tendency by many chiropractors to overtreat. "Once a fixation has been released, even partially, leave it alone." No further therapy of any type is necessary on that visit. If overtreatment occurs, he recommends that the atlas (which he calls the therapeutic "barometer") be re-examined at the end of therapy: overtreatment (even prophylatic exercise) can be reflected by increased fixation at the atlas level. If the patient leaves the office with an iatrogenic-created atlas fixation, he or she will undoubtedly return with a report of new or increased symptoms.

It is recommended that accurate progress records be kept of every preadjustive motion palpation, correction, and postadjustive motion palpation made on the first and subsequent visits. A complete examination of segmental dynamics need only be conducted on the last visit before anticipated dismissal.

Posttraumatic Treatment

Because of the vascularity in well-conditioned muscles, which is enhanced during exercise, interstitial hemorrhage following severe strains tend to be quite profuse. While rest, ice, compression, and elevation are standards in the treatment of acute injury of any individual, the factor of increased vascularity in a physically active individual underscores the need for the immediate application of R-I-C-E. During this initial healing period, manipulation is contraindicated. Various forms of nontraumatizing electrotherapy, however, may be applied to speed the healing process. At this stage, the goal is to remove inflammatory exudates, remove any stasis present, tone the vasculature, enhance venous and lymph drainage, and control the pain with any one of the many modalities available for this purpose.

After the acute stage of an injury has passed, attention should be given to more microscopic considerations. Invariably, the greater the bleeding, the more acute and diffuse the inflammatory stage, and the greater induration and fibrous thickening can be anticipated if the condition is not well managed. [See Clinical Comment 2.2]

After the stage of likely recurrent bleeding has passed and the injured tissues begin to toughen, manipulation can be conducted, if indicated by signs of hypobility, and a gradual rehabilitation program can be initiated to encourage the remaining inflammatory reaction of resolution to pass quickly—thus reducing the buildup of subsequent fibrous thickening. This program may be accelerated once the initial stage of fibrous thickening exhibits—as noted through inspection and palpation and a reported lessening of pain.

The Stages of Healing

Nothing should be done during the complicated healing stage that might disrupt the natural process or restimulate bleeding. [See Clinical Comment 2.3] The injury itself is all the local stimulation necessary for maximum response. Direct massage, forms of heat, whirlpool baths, ultrasonics, enzymes, and hormones, etc are usually contraindicated as they only add additional stimulation to an already maximally stimulated part.

The optimal procedure is to expect each step in the healing process and provide the opportunity for natural processes to express themselves—offering aid only when necessary. This is not to say that if a variation in the process is seen at a normal stage of healing that treatment should not be enhanced or directed accordingly. For example, increased local swelling and tenderness during a late stage strongly suggest an infectious process.

After bleeding stops, resolution of the injured tissues begins by organizing minute thrombi to form the richly vasculated granulation tissue that allows:

1. The *inflammatory stage*, where the white blood cells dissolve extravasated blood elements and tissue debris, characterized by swelling and local tenderness.

2. The *reparative stage*, where the network of fibrin and the fibroblasts begin the reparative process, characterized by local heat, redness, and diffuse tenderness.

3. The *toughening stage* of fibrous deposition and chronic inflammatory reaction, characterized by palpable thickening and induration in the area of reaction, with tenderness progressively diminishing.

Professional care during healing requires repeated inspection and external support: (1) Periodic and regular appraisal can usually be made simply through inspection, palpation, function studies, and patient reports. When dealing with many traumatic injuries, one becomes astute in seeing and feeling the various stages of healing. (2) Continuous support during the resolution stage should be provided by external measures without impairing the natural healing process. The common means are through tapes, bandages, splints, foam-type braces, etc.

Since the effects of injury and the body's efforts to defeat them are constantly changing, the doctor cannot rely on one observation or one outstanding symptom in evaluating the condition of the patient, especially one seriously injured. Repeated observations must be made and indications of the patient's circulatory condition, neural expression, temperature, blood pressure, pulse, respiration, color, strength, vitality, and emotional status must all be considered to obtain as clear a picture as possible of the patient's holistic condition and what treatment may be required at the moment the particular observation is made.

DR. FAYE'S CLINICAL COMMENT #2.2

I find that interferential therapy is best because I can create a therapeutic field in the center of the four electrodes. It is not a polarized current and if used at the higher Hz setting and a low Ma intensity it has very positive anti-inflammatory and anti-edematous effects.

DR. FAYE'S CLINICAL COMMENT #2.3

The injury itself is enough local stimulation for a natural response. Direct massage, forms of heat, whirlpool baths, ultrasonics, and hormones are usually contraindicated as they risk overstimulating an already maximally stimulated part. However, clinicians have found full field interferential and ordinary interferential therapy properly applied can greatly speed up the recovery from a trauma. Soccer teams in Europe have known this for many years with respect to sprained ankles. Patients low in vitamin C also respond less quickly and supplementation should always be considered if signs of C deficiency are present.

Two important clinical paradoxes deserving mention here are those of posttherapy immobilization following trauma and heat versus cold. Following an acute joint injury, short-term immobilization tends to offer the affected tissues a period of rest to promote healing and prevent further inflammation from activity. Applications of cold will usually be necessary within the first 72 hours to reduce pain and swelling. On the other hand, extended immobilization tends to weaken periarticular muscles (disuse atrophy), encourage circulatory stasis and the accumulation of metabolic debris, and promote shortened ligaments and stiff capsules, which would encourage the formation of soft-tissue fixation. At this stage, heat and exercise will usually be necessary to soften taut tissues and enhance circulation.

Considerable atrophy, muscle weakness, and fibrous induration can be eliminated by applying progressive rehabilitative mobilization as soon as possible. Naturally, timing must be coordinated with the type of injury; ie, bone injuries often require longer support and rehabilitation procedures than do less severe soft-tissue injuries. However, once bone heals, it is usually stronger; once soft-tissue heals, it is usually less pliable thus prone to reinjury.

No injury is static: it continues to produce harmful effects on the injured person until either the injury or the person is defeated. As these effects are both systemic and local, the response to injury is also both systemic and local. Thus, injuries and their effects must be evaluated from the standpoint that the whole person is injured and not from the view that an otherwise well-off person is afflicted with a local disability or that only a part of the total system is affected.

Faye believes that "It is best to treat soft-tissue injuries excessively. 'That's good enough' will not suffice, and minor pains and dysfunction will persist."

Early Mobilization: The Key to Optimal Soft-Tissue Healing

While prolonged immobilization of an injured limb may assure a less painful recovery in most instances, it always carries with it a promise of related fibrosis and atrophy. On the other hand, quickly but logically initiated and gradual applied rehabilitation speeds the reduction of swelling and tenderness, and minimizes fibrosis and atrophy. [See Clinical Comment 2.4]

Prolonged inactivity following major surgery has been shown to leave an indurated scar of thick fibrous tissue that remains tight and uncomfortable for a long time after surgery. Likewise, major joint and skeletal injury inevitably results in overabundant scar tissue from necessary immobilization. Even minor disorders treated with long-term immobilization develop large scar masses that can permanently restrict function. On the other hand, uncomplicated surgery, wounds, and sprains followed by ambulation in a few days result in a cicatrix that is not tight, but soft and pliable.

The standard allopathic treatment for a sprained ankle several years ago was 3 days in a plaster boot, followed by 3—4 days of radiant heat and whirlpool baths, and then crutches for another week, all totaling about 2 weeks of therapy. The result was an individual exhibiting a distinct limp for 2—4 weeks and an indurated leather-like ankle where motion was restricted in all normal arcs. It was common to take several months before the ankle was considered functionally normal. Today the procedure and results are much different. For instance, the Athletic Department of Yale University found that the same type of injury put on a regimen of straps and cold packs for 1 or 2 days, supported walking the 2nd day, and jogging to tolerance the 4th day will exhibit a normal-

---

DR. FAYE'S CLINICAL COMMENT #2.4

When I am present as a team physician or presiding at a track meet and someone sprains their ankle; as soon as my diagnosis is established I exert mild but steady long axis distraction. This gentle mobilization relieves the sense of compression and often one or more audible releases occur spontaneously. No thrust is applied. After this maneuver R.I.C.E. is the routine unless interferential therapy is handy.

looking ankle on the 5th or 6th day with subsiding tenderness (localized only) and no evidence of edema. With external support, the athlete is able to return to competition. It would appear to be a worthy objective within and without athletics, if not mandatory, to carefully control rehabilitation towards full return of function with minimal scar tissue and thus minimal motion restriction.

Adjustive Therapy

One major MPI objective is to teach doctors of chiropractic how to locate specific fixations and develop the necessary skills to restore mobility to every fixated joint in the body; ie, (1) find the fixation, (2) adjust (mobilize) the fixated site, and (3) recheck mobility to confirm that a correction has been made. It does not matter what particular technique you wish to use in your practice; that is a matter of personal preference and clinical judgment (Fig. 2.4). But whatever technique is used, remember *Hooke's law:* The stress applied to stretch or compress a tissue is proportional to the strain, or change in length thus produced, so long as the limit of elasticity of the tissue is not exceeded.

The Correction of Fixations

To produce a therapeutic adjustment, it is first necessary to evaluate the degree of joint motions and end plays present. Once motion restrictions have been found, the joint should be adjusted with the force directed *into* the restriction. In any joint exhibiting a fixation, it is often necessary to adjust in more than one direction if more than one plane of motion is restricted or blocked.

A dynamic thrust at the point of resistance is an effective method of imposing the force necessary to produce adequate mobility to initiate the recovery process. Especially when leverage is applied before the application of a corrective impulse, considerable skill and caution are necessary to avoid iatrogenic trauma. The same is true if motion beyond the physiologic limit (eg, overextension, overflexion) is applied.

Note: It was once taught by Gillet that a

slow stretch will induce contraction via the stretch reflex, while a quick stretch (eg, a recoil thrust) would not. This assumption is not correct. It is true that the stretch reflex is usually associated with slow stretches such as in postural changes, but his reference was probably to a slow stretch inducing a *nociceptive protective reflex contraction* rather than a *stretch reflex.* A dynamic thrust *will* start a momentary myotactic stretch reflex even faster than a slow stretch, via the low-threshold stretch circuit, but, if delivered properly, a dynamic thrust will also excite the higher threshold Golgi tendon apparatus that will initiate the *inverse myotatic reflex* to cause the contracted muscle to suddenly give way (clasp-knife reflex). If you were to hold a finger near a colleague's contact hand while a dynamic adjustment is given to a patient, you will be able to feel the quick contraction followed by relaxation of the underlying musculature. This phenomenon is called *autogenic inhibition,* and has many applications in *dynamic* and *traditional chiropractic* in correcting muscular fixations and relaxing splinted muscles.

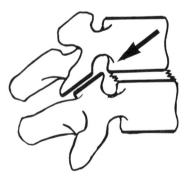

Figure 2.4. Anterosuperior subluxation of a superior process into the IVF. This may be the result of a superior segment being locked in extension, an inferior segment being fixed in flexion, a weakened anterior longitudinal ligament, degenerative disc disease, or stretched anular fibers, or a combination of all these factors. Such a fixed malposition may be influenced by a force directed anteriorly on (a) the spinous process above or (b) bilaterally upon the transverse processes. An instability will exist to allow this pathologic subluxation (Courtesy ACAP).

The application of dynamic chiropractic has empirically proved that to manipulate further after a fixation has been released often produces a new defensive contraction and therefore predisposes to the development of a new fixation. Thus, the pioneer chiropractic axiom of "find it, fix it, and leave it alone" is still often pertinent. Nerves and other tissues that have suffered stress and irritation need time to heal. To manipulate further, without good cause, is only a hindrance to natural healing processes. In addition, Schafer believes that to manipulate a segment that is pain-free and not in a state of fixation is not clinically justified, it only adds iatrogenic irritation (induced trauma) to a functional joint. [See Clinical Comment 2.5]

Overt signs of restored segmental function in chronic cases takes time. It may take months or even years for the ligamentous straps and IVDs to adapt to the remobilized state of the segment and for the vertebra(e) to appear "realigned" on an x-ray film, even though the patient becomes symptom free within a short duration. When rapid restoration of function occurs, it is most likely that a muscular fixation has been corrected. It should also be remembered that fixations do not occur only between apophyseal articular surfaces. They can occur between vertebrae and ribs, between vertebrae and the longitudinal ligaments, and between vertebrae and the perispinal ligaments and muscles.

Articular, ligamentous, and muscular fixations found in specific regions of the body will be described in subsequent chapters. However, a few general points will be made in the following few pages.

Articular or Total Fixations

Aside from those of the occipitoatlantal and sacroiliac joints, total fixations are rare.

Gillet states that they are very rare in the lumbar spine, slightly less rare in the mid and lower cervical spine, and slightly more frequent in the thoracic spine.

In total fixations, attention need not be given to relaxing specific muscles. The primary concern here is the degenerative shortening and toughening of perivertebral ligaments and the joint capsules, and possibly the development of intra-articular adhesions.

Technic Suggestions. As with muscular fixations, the least irritation-producing type of thrust is a short, rapid, dynamic maneuver directed against the restricted plane of motion so that the "frozen" facets are forced open. Regardless of the technic used and the articulation on which it is applied, *never use more force than is necessary to produce mobility.* Any force applied past the point of achieving mobility constitutes induced trauma to some degree. The ideal amount of force used is that amount which is just enough to produce mobility and no more. Usually, a mild thrust followed by a moderate thrust is sufficient. An audible "click" is not necessary to achieve; ie, mobilization, determined by postadjustment motion palpation, can be achieved with or without an audible release. Faye points out that, "As the joint responds, an audible release will assure that a manipulation has occurred and a greater ROM will be induced."

Managing Degenerative Disorders. Many advanced states of degeneration cannot be repaired to a completely normal state, but they can, with proper treatment, be halted in their progress and considerable function can be restored. The more chronic a ligamentous-related condition, the longer adjustive therapy will be necessary. Once the asymptomatic stage occurs, maintenance care every 3—6 weeks or more is usually necessary to keep the involved joint(s) optimally mobile. In time, joints that are chron-

---

DR. FAYE'S CLINICAL COMMENT #2.5

I have however confirmed the procedure of Dr. Ray Sandoz of utilizing passive motion in order to stimulate the mechanoreceptors and proprioceptors in the manipulated joints. I find the continuous passive y-axis distraction of the motorized Leander Table causes a reduction of pain and muscle spasm and is not contraindicated in any area of the spine. It is common for my patients to receive 10 minutes of y-axis distraction after a manipulation of a motion unit.

ically swollen, painful, crepitant, and immobile often return to normal or near-normal function with appropriate extended management—yet radiographs may show no or little change in joint space narrowing or hypertrophic alterations. This adds credence to the hypothesis that most joint complaints are the result of joint dysfunction rather than pathologic processes.

Ligamentous Fixations

Ligamentous fixations (including those caused by muscular atrophy) are numerous and can be located most anywhere in the spine. They are second in importance to, yet far more prevalent than, total fixations. In many spines, ligamentous fixations are the only chronic fixations that will be found.

Technic Suggestions. The recommended adjustive thrust used for ligamentous fixations is similar to that used for muscular and total fixations with essentially two differences: (1) the slack taken in the overlying tissues is less than with total fixations and even more so than with muscular fixations; (2) the thrust is much shorter than that used for muscular fixations because the tissues acted on are not as elastic. Nevertheless, the amount of postadjustment change can be surprising yet less than that following a correction of a muscular fixation. This initially slight postadjustment improvement is optimally followed by continual slight improvement visit after visit, resulting in a slow carefully monitored progress. In such situations, slow, carefully specified, stretching exercises are beneficial to case management. Faye recommends a 30-second stretch and hold (with the last 5 seconds during exhalation) as being the best procedure.

Muscular Fixations

Muscular fixations are extremely labile, variable, and dependent on the individual's general state of "nervous tension." It is for this reason, most likely, that muscular fixations often disappear after a remote total fixation in the spine has been corrected. Thus, any therapy (eg, dynamic thrust, reflex, medicinal, exercise, counseling, biofeed-

back, cold, heat, electrostimulation, detoxification, etc) that will ease a state of excessive tension in the body, appears to have a beneficial effect on muscular fixations—at least for a short time. This also appears to be true when the fixation is the result of a peripheral irritation (eg, a viscerosomatic reflex). Unfortunately, such acute subluxations tend to continually recur until the predisposing condition or chronic fixations are corrected.

At times, it may appear that just examining a muscular fixation by putting the involved segments through their ROMs is enough to correct the condition: as substantiated by a report from the patient that the area feels much better after the examination. The opposite of this can also occur; ie, too vigorous an examination or too much probing in the involved area may enhance the irritation already present—thus aggravating the patient's discomfort.

Etiology. Gillet believes that just about anything that has a beneficial or noxious effect on the body (whether it be mechanical, thermal, chemical, or emotional overstress) will have a similar effect on the spine to some degree. This appears to be especially true with the development of muscular fixations.

Stubborn Muscular Fixations. Once all total and ligamentous fixations have been corrected, there are times when a few true muscular fixations have not spontaneously disappeared. Some typical examples are listed below:

1. *The coccygeus muscle.* Prolonged unilateral coccygeus contraction tends to pull the sacral apex laterally. Extensive bilateral coccygeus contraction tends to pull the ischia together. Gillet reports that if all other local fixations have been corrected, especially those of the inferior sacroiliac ligaments, restriction found during passive lateral bending of the trunk can be attributed to the coccygeus contracture.

2. *The lumbar spine.* The intertransversarii, quadratus lumborum, rotatores, or psoas group may still be hypertonic after all lumbar and pelvic articular and ligamentous fixations have been released. Unilateral contraction of the intertransversarii and/or quadratus lumborum tends to laterally flex the lumbars. Bilateral contraction tends to

alter the normal lumbar lordosis. Prolonged contraction of the rotatores, usually unilateral, tends to extend and rotate the segments to which they are attached to the opposite side. Bilaterally shortened psoas muscles tend to increase the normal lumbar lordosis, with a compensating thoracic hyperkyphosis; unilateral contraction produces a lumbar scoliosis toward the side of contraction, with a compensating thoracic scoliosis to the other side.

3. *Lower thoracic spine.* The intertransversarii and serratus (posterior and inferior) muscles may be stubbornly contracted in the lower thoracic spine. Shortening of these serratus muscles, which is usually bilateral, tends to pull the lower ribs inferior and posterior.

4. *Midthoracic spine.* Although serratus posterior shortening is often found in the midthoracic area, levator costorum hypertonicity is far more common. Shortening of the rib elevators tends to pull the ribs out and up; ie, the patient's thoracic spine will resemble the normal state of deep inspiration when in the resting position. The serratus superior muscles may also be involved. Midthoracic interspinous fixations (muscles or ligaments) tend to flatten the normal thoracic kyphosis (eg, ram-rod spine), while shortening of the anterior longitudinal ligaments tend to increase the thoracic kyphosis.

5. *Upper thoracic spine.* The upper thoracic spine is a favorite site of rotatores shortening. The effect is the same as that seen in the lumbar spine: segmental extension and rotation to the opposite side.

Technic Suggestions. With all the examples given above, a thrust directed perpendicular to the belly of the hypertonic muscle will correct the fixation or a contact can be taken on the involved segment and a thrust made that will stretch the shortened muscle. A short dynamic thrust appears to be the most efficient approach in correcting muscular fixations. Technic will have to be adapted somewhat if the muscles involved have degenerated to a state resembling ligamentous fixations.

Acute vs Chronic Spasticity. When muscles become acutely spastic or indurated, normal movement is impaired and the foci for referred pain and noxious somatosomatic reflexes are established. Even with proper conditioning and warmup procedures, myalgic syndromes are commonly seen when treating athletes or stoic individuals because they habitually ignore the warning signals of pain. The degree of impairment is essentially determined by the severity of spasm, the amount of induration, and the extent of functional disability. Both spastic and indurated muscles are characterized by circulatory stasis, which is essentially the effect of compressed vessels. This leads to tissue nutrition impairment and the accumulation of metabolic debris. During the early stages of degeneration, palpation will often reveal tender areas that feel taut, gristly, ropy, or nodular.

Majors vs Minors

In motion palpation terminology, a *major* is the most fixed motion unit. A minor is a secondary (usually muscular) fixation. During motion palpation, always attempt to discern which fixations are primary and which are secondary. Primary fixations will feel the most blocked, usually in more than one direction. Secondary fixations will exhibit the greatest tenderness. Following are some general guidelines that can be applied whenever planning a therapeutic approach towards mobilizing articular fixations:

1. Adjusting a primary fixation will cause palpable changes elsewhere in the spine, and offer symptom relief at the site of a related secondary fixation even though the secondary fixation is not adjusted. When a primary fixation is adjusted, it tends to show some immediate improvement and progressive improvement with time.

2. Adjusting a secondary fixation before its primary fixation is corrected offers only momentary improvement, quickly returning to its preadjustment state and often with an adverse reaction reported by the patient.

The Biomechanical Approach to Manipulation

The key biomechanical principles described by Faye in MPI's Spine 1 Course are

Table 2.4. Phases of Vertebral Unit Degeneration

Features	Dysfunction ——>	Instability ——>	Stabilization
History	Strain/sprain	Strain/sprain with likely history of previous injury	Chronic episodes of pain
Features	Perivertebral muscle splinting, pain (usually local, unilateral) that is aggravated by certain movements (eg, "catches"), tenderness of hypertonic erectors, lateral flexion unilaterally restricted, painful extension from flexion, antalgic scoliosis with muscle contraction on concave side of lateral bending.	Similar to those of dysfunction, except feelings of weakness and periodic tendency toward collapse are usually reported; a segmental shift may be seen during extension from flexion. Faye includes here "catches" and "locks"; patient unable to change posture.	Radicular pain, area stiffness, incapacitating attacks after minor trauma, muscle weakness.
Biomechanics	Rotation or compressive overstress leading to subluxation complex.	Hypermobile joint motion with frequent subluxation, facets likely open and malpositioned.	Hypomobile joint motion.
Pathology	Small anular disc tears, possible disc bulging or herniation, possible nuclear displacement, synovitis leading to facet fixation due to intraarticular adhesion and/or articular cartilage degeneration, probable facet displacement (subluxation).	Lax anulus and posterior joint capsules, coalesced disc tears, degenerated nucleus with probable displacement, circumference bulging of disc at periphery, probable abrupt change in pedicle height, possible A-P shift of unit during flexion and extension, possible tilt of unit on rotation, possible nipping of a synovial fold.	Fibrosis, loss of nuclear substance, severe disc-space thinning, apophyseal osteophytes, centrum osteophytes, possible ankylosis, probable root entrapment, resorption.

worthy of mention here. They are:

1. Each vertebra moves in six voluntary planes, which often is accompanied by coupled reactions (eg, lateral flexion is accompanied by rotation, and vice versa). From L5 to T8, the spinous processes rotate to the concavity during lateral flexion; from T8 to C1, the spinous processes rotate to the convexity.

2. The hips joints must allow lateral sway, flexion, extension, and rotation.

3. The sacroiliac joints allow the sacrum to move independently of the illia and/or allow the illia to flex and extend independently—obviously, also moving at the symphysis pubis.

4. During gait, the lumbars remain fairly immobile unless pelvic biomechanics are disturbed (eg, fixation exists).

5. Hypomobility (fixation) of an articulation causes a shift of the normal axis of rotation, producing an adaptive compensatory motion that may be aberrant in character. If aberrant, it often becomes a focus for pathologic changes (eg, arthritis, facet syndrome, IVF-content alterations, spondylosis).

The phases of vertebral degeneration are shown in Table 2.4. These points have been adapted from the writings of several authorities but especially those of Kirkaldy-Willis.

Physical Therapy

If physical therapy is to be employed, whatever modality selected should be chosen for specific indications. Some examples are shown in Table 2.5.

General Considerations

Adjunctive therapy is often helpful to normalize continuous motor nerve firing, dislodge the collections of metabolic debris, and improve circulation and drainage. Regardless of the modality or manual procedure used, its intensity should be maintained below the threshold of pain to prevent a protective reflex contraction of the involved musculature. Stretching, heat (superficial or deep), cryotherapy, sine-wave muscle stimulation, galvanism, high-volt therapy, interfer-

ential current, pulsating vibration, and massage have all proved themselves effective under certain conditions.

Contrary to popular belief, the effects of cold are not exactly opposite to those of heat. Several responses are similar. A comparison of the effects of heat and cold in the treatment of various complaints and conditions is shown in Table 2.6.

When deep mechanical vibration is used, several reports state that pressure across muscle fibers tends to release accumulated metabolic byproducts, while pressure parallel to muscles fibers (directed to the heart) enhances drainage. When spastic areas of partial fixations do not release adequately or conventional methods only offer temporary relief, a nutritional evaluation should be made. A calcium, vitamin B, vitamin D, and/or magnesium deficiency may be a contributing cause.

Cryotherapy

Cold is an important aspect in the therapeutic acronym RICE (rest, ice, compression, and elevation). It is the standard for treating almost any acute trauma and its associated pain and splinting or the acute phases of inflammatory conditions. Obviously, the initial primary physical characteristic of cold is that it cools body tissues: hypothermia. Tissue cooling decreases local tissue metabolism, arterioles begin to constrict (minimizing bleeding), the excitability of free nerve endings is reduced, nerve conduction velocity in both motor and sensory fibers is slowed, the response of muscle afferents are reduced, the perception of pain is reduced, the release of histamine responsible for vasodilation and exudate formation is reduced, and the body then acts reflexively by sending blood to the skin and musculature, which produce a secondary hyperemia.

Functional Changes. The general physiologic effects of cold include increased heart rate, respiratory rate, leukocytosis, and decreased fatigue. As most circulatory activities are reduced during cooling, there is a decrease in the delivery to and utilization of nutrients in the involved tissues, a decrease in phagocytic activity, and a decrease in the production of lymph. Skin color, occurring first as blanched skin, changes to red or blue-red in prolonged cold and is the result of a histamine release associated paradoxically with an increase in utilization of oxygen by local tissue. When cold is removed, the demand for tissue oxygen is increased and the vessels dilate in compensation to produce hyperemia.

Types of Application. Several different forms of cryotherapy can be applied. Common techniques include icebags, gel packs, cold packs, ice massage, cold immersion, vapocoolant sprays, cryokinetics, Priessnitz compresses, humid-cold boric alcohol or aluminum acetate compresses, and cold-clay packs. All these modalities can be considered to be *heat absorbent,* thus cooling agents.

Penetration. In comparing the effects of cold and heat, exposure of the skin to cold will penetrate deeper than exposure of the skin to the modalities of heat. The effect may even result in core temperatures lowering below normal. Studies in ice massage show that tissue temperature drops 18°F at a depth of 1 cm with effects lasting up to 3

Table 2.5. Brief Resume of Common Physical Agents and Their Effects

Physical Agent	Primary Effect	Secondary Effects
Hot water, hot air, radiant heaters, incandescent lamps, diathermy, microwaves	Thermal	Hyperemia, sedation of sensory or motor irritation, attenuation of microorganisms
Cryotherapy (vapocoolants, ice)	Hypothermal	Sedation, decongestion, ischemia
Ultraviolet (sun, heated metals, carbon arc, mercury vapor arc)	Photochemical	Erythemia, pigmentation, activation of ergosterol
Ultrasound	Mechanical, thermal, chemical	Cellular massage, heat, sedation
Low-volt galvanic currents	Electrochemical	Polar, vasomotor
Low-frequency, interrupted current, sinusoidal current, other alternating currents	Electrokinetic	Muscle stimulation, increase of venous and lymph flow, reflex stimulation
Medium frequency interferential currents, full field or frequency difference (Faye)	Electrochemical	Profound analgesia by depolarization of C fibers, nerve blocks, Wedensky inhibition, muscle stimulation, edema reduction, neural stimulation, enhances sodium-potassium pump and healing, serotonin response from CNS, local endorphin response.
Vibration, massage, traction (intermittent), therapeutic exercise	Kinetic	Muscle stimulation, increase of venous and lymph flow, tissue stretch, reflex stimulation

hours. Ice massage can reduce surface skin temperature to 60°—58°F, and no ill effects to normal skin is seen until skin temperature is reduced below 50°F. However, it takes considerable time for some applications of cold to penetrate. For example, when icebags whose water temperature is 32°F are continually placed on an extremity, the outside of the towel covering the bag will be about 40°F. It takes about 15 minutes for the skin temperature to drop from 84°F to 43°F, about an hour for subcutaneous tissue to drop from 94°F to 70°F, and about 2 hours for intramuscular temperature to drop from 98°F to 79°F.

The Hunting Reaction. When cooling is extreme (eg, immersion into ice water, ice massage), the body responds with regular "bursts" of vasodilation. These periodic reactions have come to be called the *hunting reaction* and are thought to occur in the area of arteriovenous anastomosis. This phenomenon is one of alternating vasoconstriction and vasodilatation in irregular repeated sequences in an apparent physiologic "hunt" for skin temperature equilibrium. This is a normal response, and failure of body tissues to react by vasodilation via an autonomic reflex may lead to injury of the local tissues from cryotherapy. Thus, cold must be used prudently to avoid secondary cold-induced swelling (a natural survival response) or prolonged cold-induced ischemia that can lead to necrosis.

The general indications for and contraindications to cryotherapy are shown in Table 2.7.

Table 2.6. Comparative Effects of Heat and Cold

Symptom/Sign	Heat	Cold
Cellular metabolism		
Enzyme activity	Increases	Decreases
Membrane diffusion	Increases	Decreases
Oxygen consumption	Increases	Decreases
Inflammatory reaction	Increases	Decreases
Joint response		
Connective tissue distensibility	Increases	Decreases
Contractures/adhesions	Softening	Less pain on stretching
Range of joint motion	Increases	Decreases
Synovial fluid viscosity	Decreases	Increases
Muscle spasm		
Spindle activity	Increases	Decreases
Fiber contractility	Increases	Decreases
Involuntary (reflex) contractions	Decreases	Decreases
Afferent activity		Decreases
Efferent activity		Decreases
Pain		
Nerve conduction velocity	Increases	Decreases
Enkephalins	Produced	Produced
Placebo effect	Positive	Highly variable
Psychic effect	Relaxation	May irritate
Skin tissue	Local vasodilation	Local vasoconstriction
Vascular response		
Consensual	Vasodilation	Vasoconstriction
Local	Vasodilation	Vasoconstriction
Capillary permeability	Increases edema	Decreases edema
Vascular wall tone	Decreases	Increases

Table 2.7. General Indications and Contraindications to Cryotherapy in Treating Musculoskeletal Disorders

INDICATIONS

Decrease blood flow to areas of acute inflammation	Reduce swelling
Inhibit bleeding after acute trauma	Relieve pain and reduce the accompanying reflex muscle spasm
Pressure sores (closed)	Sprains and strains
Spasms and spasticity	Varicose ulcers

CONTRAINDICATIONS

Chilblain (pernio)	Paroxysmal cold hemoglobinuria
Coma	Raynaud's phenomenon/disease
Cryesthesia	Rheumatoid or gouty arthritis

Note: This table is only a guide. Extreme caution must be used when any inflammatory condition is being treated. Each patient must be treated as an individual and in accord with high standards of professional judgment as directed by the diagnosis.

Muscle Re-education

According to *Starling's law*, a normal long muscle is a strong muscle; a normal short muscle, is a comparatively weak muscle. Thus, any type of therapy that tends to elongate an abnormally shortened muscle will be clinically indicated in most cases. How this is accomplished is not as important than that it is accomplished. Such procedures as proprioceptive neuromuscular facilitation and the postisometric relaxation technique are especially effective.

Integrated Treatment Approach

Once a logical tentative diagnosis can be arrived at with the information gathered so far, it is well to consider it as a *working diagnosis*. A working diagnosis is usually confirmed or replaced in a few weeks if all the necessary data can be gathered during that period.

The first therapeutic concern is often the control of pain and inflammation. The most effective methods of reducing inflammation also reduce pain. For example, cryotherapy and electrotherapy are usually effective dur-

ing the early stages of case management. Restoring joint mobility also has a great pain-relieving effect.

In acute cases, the cause of the trauma must be differentiated: traumatic vs nontraumatic and if traumatic (Fig. 2.5), invasive (eg, physical assault, bacterial, neoplastic) or biomechanical. While manipulation is usually contraindicated in situations of invasive trauma, it is usually appropriate in cases of trauma produced by biomechanical insult. In biomechanical situations, the primary area requiring manipulation is often not at the level of apparent dysfunction (eg, site of inflammation).

PALPATION: GENERAL CONSIDERATIONS

Static Bony Palpation

The major purpose of static bony palpation is to assess bony relationships to determine if structural malalignment is present and/or to note hypertrophic changes. The palpation should be conducted in the various planes of reference of one bony structure to another and compared bilaterally. When structural abnormalities are suspected (eg, dislocation, fracture, osteophytes), they should be confirmed by roentgenography.

An involved joint should be palpated for masses and points of tenderness that may suggest osteoarthritis, synovitis, or a torn ligament or meniscus. Palpation should be conducted for tenderness, masses, muscle tone, fasciculations, and spasm. A suggestion of bone inflammation or fracture is enhanced when the bone is percussed at a site distant from the point of tenderness and pain is felt at the site of tenderness rather than at the site of percussion.

The Art of Motion Palpation: General Considerations

Healthy articulations can be moved through their planes of normal motion actively and passively without causing pain; ie, until they reach their anatomical limit. A general rule of thumb holds that pain emanating from compressed tissues will be relieved by traction and aggravated by compression. Conversely, pain arising from tensile lesions will be relieved by compression and aggravated by traction.

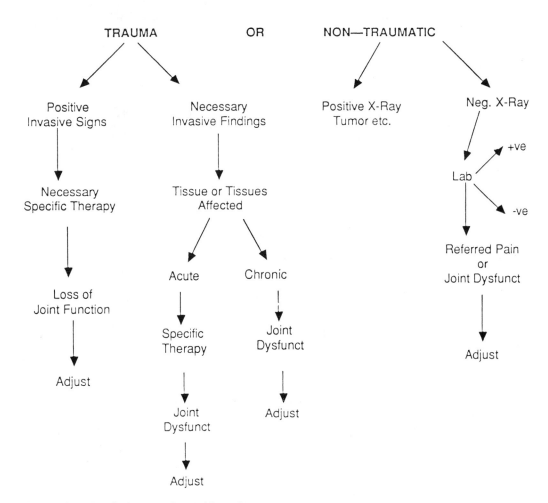

Figure 2.5. Faye's therapeutic goal flow chart.

Biomechanical Adaptation

During our studies of neurology, we have been taught *Meltzer's law of contrary innervation:* All living functions are continually controlled by two opposite forces: augmentation or action on the one hand, and inhibition on the other. There is a similar maxim used in dynamic chiropractic concerning biomechanical adaptation in articular lesions: if there is local segmental hypermobility without a history of overt trauma (eg, severe sprain resulting in instability), there is also the causative site of primary fixation; in joint disorders, there is almost always hypomobility in one area and compensatory hypermobility in another.

The General Spinal Survey (Scan)

Specific motion palpation of the various regions of the spine will be explained in following chapters. Our purpose here will be to describe some basic underlying principles in how a basic motion palpation examination is conducted. Once the basic principles, positions, and contacts are understood, a general scanning examination can be conducted with confidence in less than a minute. The purpose of a general scan is to isolate general areas that will require more specific motion palpation later. This saves conducting a specific ROM test of each spinal segment in all three planes of freedom.

General Survey Position. With both the patient and the examiner in the sitting position, the examiner sits behind, slightly diagonally, and stabilizes the patient with the nonexamining hand. If you are right handed, it is usually done by placing your left elbow on the patient's left shoulder and extending your forearm horizontally behind the patient's neck so that the patient's right shoulder can be firmly grasped with your left hand (Fig. 2.6). This allows the patient to be held firmly with your stabilizing hand while your examining hand conducts the general survey. In examining children and small adults, you may find it more convenient to have the patient cross their arms in front and then you can reach around anteriorly so your left hand can grasp the patient's right shoulder

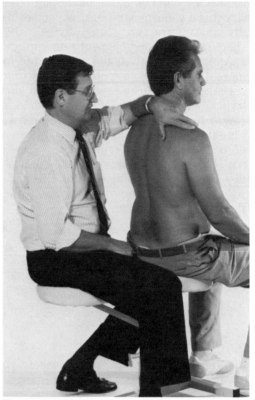

Figure 2.6. Position for general survey.

from the front. The best procedure is the most efficient procedure. There are few hard rules in health care.

General Survey Procedure. With the patient sitting, thus stabilizing the pelvis, and your left arm and hand stabilizing the patient's shoulder girdle, the patient's spinal segments will be functionally "floating" between these two points. The actual scan begins by placing the back of your right (palpating) hand (fingers pointing downward) on the patient's sacrum and pushing your hand inward, translating the sacrum forward (Fig. 2.7). Quickly relax the pressure, and the patient's spine will automatically return (extend) to the neutral position. Do this two or three times in succession at a moderate speed. This will allow you to sense the freedom of the sacrum during flexion and extension. This push—relax maneuver is similar to a "pumping" motion. Next, close your palpating hand into a fist (fingers

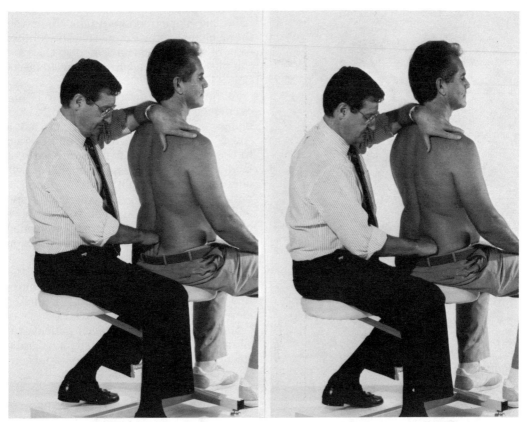

Figure 2.7. Positions for pelvic scan.

open), and with the back of your fingers check the freedom of the patient's superior and inferior sacroiliac joints bilaterally with the same type of push—relax maneuver.

Next, turn your hand horizontally so that the back of your fingers are across the patient's lumbosacral area (eg, fingers of the right hand pointing to the left, parallel to the floor). Instruct the patient not to attempt to help with assisted motions while you are conducting this test. Maintain stabilization of the patient's shoulder girdle and, with your examining hand, push forward smoothly (1—1½ inches) and relax your pressure (Fig. 2.8). Do this two or three times to sense the induced spinal extension and automatic flexion motion to the neutral occurring in this area. This same procedure is continued up to the upper thoracic spine as you slide your examining hand cephalad two or three segments and repeat the process (Figs. 2.9 and 2.10). At each position, you will be able to

sense how the motion units under the back of your examining fingers are responding to this induced extension and the resulting relaxation-flexion to neutral as the "push" pressure is released. These motions are rhythmically executed and flow up the levels of the spine.

Once the upper thoracic region is reached, some examiners have the patient interlock the hands behind the neck, elbows pointing medially. Raise and lower the patient's elbows a few times while your palpating hand feels the motion of the upper thoracic segments.

To scan the patient's cervical spine, place your stabilizing hand on the patient's forehead, holding the neck in the neutral position (Fig. 2.11). Starting at C7, place the thumb and middle finger of your examining hand on the lamina of each segment, push forward smoothly and relax your pressure, slide upward a segment or two and repeat,

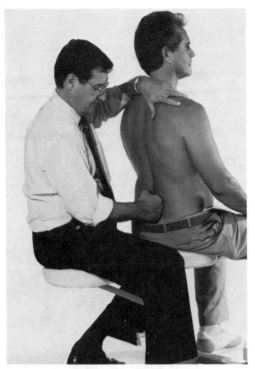

Figure 2.8. Position for lumbar scan.

continuing up to the occiput. This is essentially the same motion produced in the thoracolumbar scan except that the contact is more specific. Remain seated so that you can push upwards against the angled facets (Fig. 2.12).

At no time during the "scan" will your examining hand leave the patient's skin; doing so results in a "punch" rather than a "push" that offers no significant information to the receptors of your palpating hand. A medium examining pressure should be used; not too hard, not to light. If it is too hard, the patient will respond by contracting the spinal muscles. If it is too light, you will have difficulty in eliciting the information needed to appraise segmental extension-flexion movement.

"In the neutral posture," states Faye, "the discs have a zero coefficient of resistance. Any resistance perceived will be at one or more of the sites of possible fixation."

Maintain firm but not rough patient stabilization so that the patient's shoulder girdle is centered over the pelvis and hold your con-

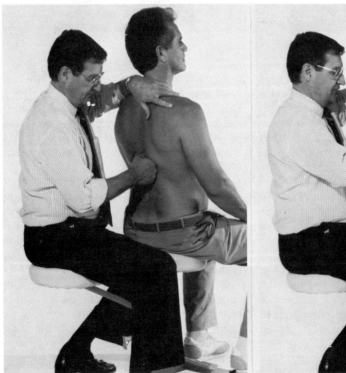
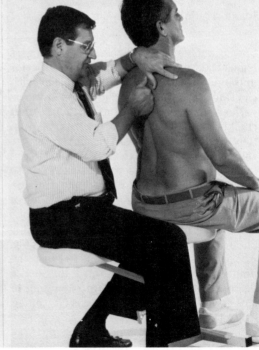

Figure 2.9. Scanning the lowerand mid-thoracic spine.

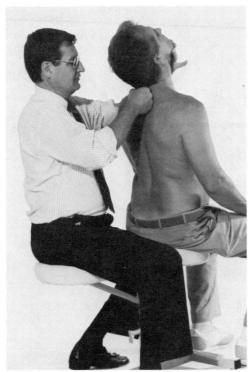

Figure 2.10. Position for upper thoracic scan.

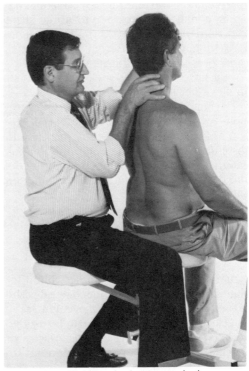

Figure 2.11. Position for lower cervical scan.

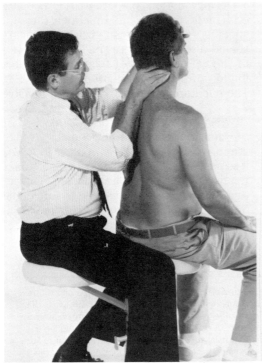

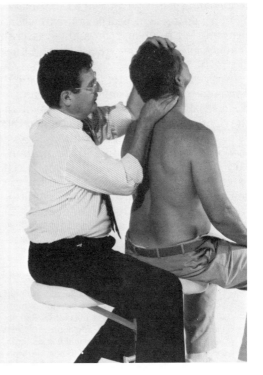

Figure 2.12 Positions for upper cervical scan.

centration by visualizing what you are sensing (viz, know the anatomy). With some patients, it may be necessary to apply slight backward pressure on the patient's shoulders to maintain centering the patient's trunk over the pelvis during your push (extension) pressure. Avoid rocking the patient on his or her buttocks.

The Spinal Research Corporation has promoted a custom two-seated palpation station to facilitate this procedure. It is not an absolute in conducting a proper motion palpation of the spine, but it is extremely helpful and decreases doctor fatigue during motion palpation of the spine.

Visualization During Scanning and Specific Motion Palpation

As each vertebra moves in six voluntary planes, a notation system has been devised to symbolically record these movements. The diagram shown in Figure 2.13 can be used to denote fixations during a general scan or specific motion palpation examination. In subsequent chapters, it will be described how, in basically the same position just described for a general scan, you will be able to motion palpate segmental flexion, extension, right and left rotation, right and left lateral bending, and rib motion. [See Clinical Comment 2.6]

In review: The first step in motion palpation is to realize that each vertebra has six basic ROMs: flexion, extension, rotation to the right and left, and lateral bending to the right and left. These are voluntary, active motions. To these, we can add the involuntary motions of passive distraction (axial extension) and passive joint play at the extreme ROM. Daily activity normally utilizes these motions, which are often coupled, to various degrees—but all too often far less

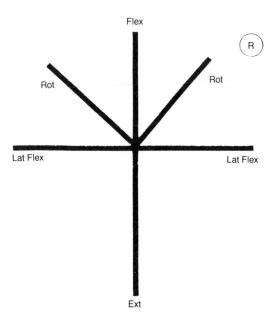

Figure 2.13 Star diagram, adapted from Maigne's star diagram.

than the extreme degrees of ROM with the possible exception of flexion.

During motion palpation, we visualize each motion as being unidirectional during a specific test. This visualization process should also incorporate the characteristics of the various types of fixation commonly found: muscular, ligamentous, or articular. These features are briefly reviewed in Table 2.8.

Whenever we feel a motion is blocked or see that it appears "misaligned" in a radiograph, we should always ask ourselves *why* is it so positioned? Is it a primary or secondary fixation? What type is it: articular, ligamentous, or muscular? Is it caused by functional or pathologic mechanisms? Acute or chronic? Reversible? To what extent? In what time?

DR. FAYE'S CLINICAL COMMENT #2.6

This past two years I have added the motion palpation procedure of y-axis translation. This procedure is conducted with the patient prone on a motorized mechanical flexion distraction table with the abdomen dropped to allow a normal lumbar lordosis to be present. This prevents the interspinous ligament from stretching taut, and confusing the procedure. As the pelvis and legs descend in flexion the interspinous space widens if normal flexion and y-axis translation occur. Spinous processes that fail to separate constitute a fixation. (Ref: Leander notes and video tape recording of a motion x-ray series.)

Table 2.8. Qualitative Degrees of Fixation

Type of Fixation	Major Characteristics
Muscular	Palpates as taut, tender fibers. Skin hyperesthetic over affected muscle. Motion exhibits rubbery end feel. Changes after adjustment are complete (eg, motion is normal, muscles no longer tender or taut), but improvement soon disappears if secondary to a primary fixation.
Ligamentous	Subcutaneous atrophy over involved ligaments. Abrupt hard end feel during motion palpation. Correction of fixation after adjustment is slight but steadily improves with time and further therapy.
Articular (Total)	Complete motion block; no motion in any plane. Pseudoankylosis or ankylosis; thus not always reversible, especially in late stage.

What are the other components of the subluxation complex (eg, involved nerves, muscles, inflammation, etc)?

Adapting Movement Palpation to Each Practice

Rational principles adapt themselves readily to all types of chiropractic practice whether it be that of a practitioner who specializes in uppercervical specific, meric—general—full spine adjustments, spinal-pelvic balance, and all the various combinations possible. Regardless of approach, the primary goal is to isolate fixations and mobilize them whenever possible.

One will often hear that a practitioner's personal preference in adjusting technique need not be altered by the application of *dynamic chiropractic* into his or her practice. The reason for this is found in the study of vertebral anatomy and biomechanics.

Each vertebra is a structural unit, two adjacent vertebrae comprise a vertebral motion unit (Fig. 2.14), and each motion unit has three articulations: the two posterior apophyseal joints and the "joint" formed at the interface of the two vertebral bodies (ie, the IVD). Just as hyaline cartilage serves as the articular surface between the facets, the fibrocartilaginous intervertebral disc serves (for one purpose) as the articular surface between the vertebral bodies. Although

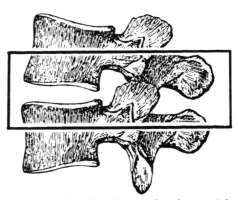

Figure 2.14 Functional area of an intervertebral motion unit (Courtesy ACAP).

healthy bone has considerable elasticity, it is not elastic enough to allow appreciable motion of one articulation of a vertebra without all three articulations moving reciprocally. Thus, from a mechanical viewpoint, which articulation is fixed, the point of contact, and the direction of drive need not be that specific to release a fixation within a specific vertebral segment. If segmental motion is induced, all articulations must move.

Thus, one's preference in technic is optional from a purely mechanical viewpoint. In health care, however, we are not dealing with purely mechanical principles. We are dealing with patients, sensitive human beings, who are often already in pain and we do not wish to induce any more discomfort during a correction than in necessary to achieve release of a fixation. To achieve this, the following principles should be kept in mind, especially when treating total fixations:

1. *Type of contact.* The type of contact used is optional in most situations. The broadest contact that is efficient should be used, because the force will be directed through a larger surface area. A force applied by an open palm against the skin is perceived by the patient far differently than a force applied by a pointed finger against the skin. Thus, a palm heel, thenar, or knife-edge (medial edge of the hand) contact produces less patient discomfort than a pisiform or thumb contact. There are times, however, when a pisiform or thumb contact is necessary to get the job done quickly and efficiency.

2. *Point of contact.* The point of contact is optional in most situations. For example, the choice of selecting a transverse process, a spinous process, or a lamina contact is optional. A mobilizing force directed against any of these structures will induce articular separation, tissue stretching, and the effected segmental motion, although one contact may be more efficient and less painful to the patient than another, depending on the situation at hand.

3. *Angle of drive.* The angle of drive is optional in many situations. If a motion unit is totally fixated, induced motion in almost any direction will separate the facets and release the fixation. That is the reason, states Gillet, "why the first adjustment given to a new patient is nearly always the most effective." This, however, is not to say that a force directed in line with the plane of articulation and perpendicular to the motion resistance is not usually the most efficient and less painful to the patient.

4. *Leverage through patient position.* If it is found that segmental lateral bending to the left is blocked, for example, it takes far less effort to achieve a correction if the patient can be placed in a position of lateral bending to the left before applying the corrective thrust. The same is true for flexion, extension, and rotational fixations. This is usually achieved by (a) table positioning (eg, raising or lowering the abdominal piece, (b) increasing or releasing the spring tension),

(c) patient position (prone, supine, lateral-recumbent), (d) positioning the patient with your stabilizing hand, or (e) using wedged-shaped pillows in various positions under a patient's shoulder, hip, or both. Some modern adjusting tables even provide for horizontal shifting positions. In such a manner, proper positioning can conduct a large portion of the correction because it encourages motion (through both extrinsic and intrinsic mechanisms) toward the direction desired. Proper preadjustment positioning that induces motion up to the point of "block," can therefore add leverage and the benefits of soft-tissue tensile forces. For this reason, a "rotary" type of technic delivered at the end of passive rotation is less traumatizing to the patient than a "recoil" type of adjustment with the patient in the neutral position.

ROENTGENOGRAPHIC ANALYSIS

The detailed study of roentgenographic analysis in chiropractic is beyond the scope of this book. To do so would require a book in itself, but some basic considerations will be described that will underscore some concepts described earlier.

Static Films

Joint abnormalities exhibit significant alterations in structure, symmetry, continuity, positional relations, length and breadth, cartilaginous joint space, and density. Radiographic findings can be used to confirm or dispose of suspicions arising during the history and physical examination, and not to be the sole basis of the diagnosis. Once relevant features have been found to classify an abnormality, a search should then be made for those details that enable it to be distinguished from others in the same class. This takes careful evaluation of frequently subtle soft-tissue changes that confirm osseous alterations. The examiner must be well acquainted with the nature of all substances visible on a film. In addition to roentgenography of distressed joint(s), spinal and chest films are almost always included if the possibility of referred pain or systemic symptoms are involved.

There is no doubt that static films have proved themselves to be of value in the study of advanced osseous pathology, several types of soft-tissue lesions, fractures, and dislocations. Used along with contrast media, they are often beneficial toward the diagnosis of alimentary tract and CNS lesions. In this context, films taken in the neutral A-P, lateral, and sometimes oblique positions are usually adequate.

Stress Films

Static films taken in the neutral resting positions, however, have little value in studying dynamic lesions unless comparative *stress films* (also called kinematic radiographic studies) are taken at the extreme ranges of motion (eg, full flexion and extension, full lateral bending to the right and left). Sites of fixation are often disclosed by such films in which it can be seen that certain areas are moving as a whole rather than as separate segments, with no significant intersegmental motion measurable. Aberrant motion, in which one or more segments are not moving in a smooth synchronized manner with an adjacent segment, can also be exhibited on such films. Keep in mind that in a total fixation of a single posterior vertebral joint, neither joint will show motion; but in a partial fixation of a single joint, the contralateral joint will be movable. When studying the sacroiliac joint, comparative A-P analyses can be conducted of films made with the patient in the sitting and standing position.

Joint-Space Alterations

The area between adjacent articular cartilages (spinal or extraspinal) in either static or stress films may be wide, thin, or unbalanced. The same is true of the space occupied by IVDs and other fibrocartilages (Fig. 2.15). Function has a considerable effect on joint cartilage thickness. The frequent movements and increased motions of athletes and vigorous physical laborers tend to thicken cartilage, while a lack of motion tends to decrease thickness by atrophy or underdevel-

opment. Joint imbalance in the extremities is commonly seen in the knee, for example, suggesting a derangement of the meniscus on the thin side, especially if there is no other feature except effusion. The medial side may appear thin, while the lateral side will be abnormally wide—or vice versa. Joint space may be reduced by compression (jamming), atrophy, cartilage underdevelopment, excessive conversion of cartilage to bone, fibrous degeneration, or destructive disease processes.

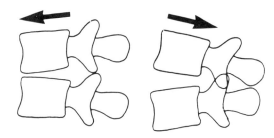

Figure 2.15. *Left,* flexion malposition, in which the superior segment of the motion unit is fixed in the normal state of flexion. *Right,* extension fixation malposition (Courtesy ACAP).

HYGIENE AND PHYSICAL FITNESS

Each health-care profession, including chiropractic, tends to judge itself with a magnified view—forgetting that there were and are other therapeutic sciences previously that did have and still have merit and there are likely others forthcoming. One of the most basic and beneficial of these is the practice of *hygiene* (the science of health and its preservation). It was not until late into the middle ages that hygiene and sanitary practices began to be slowly incorporated into the practice of medicine and public health.

Traditional medicine has always been slow in changing its preoccupation with cases and specific organs rather than with causes. When a gallbladder becomes diseased, for example, it is treated with various medications or surgically removed—with no concern for why it became diseased in the first place. When vertebral joints become fixated, they are adjusted by a chiropractor—often with no concern for why they became fixated in the first place. All health-care professions give lip service to "find the cause and fix it," but little more than lip service. Traditional approaches in allopathy, chiropractic, and osteopathy tend to treat effects with little concern for their cause. With the exception of immunology, it has only been within the last score of years that any licensed health-care profession as a whole has given much more than a token consideration to preventive health care.

We are now coming to realize that doctors must be more than healers, they must become teachers of four hygienic practices: (1) *personal hygiene* (cleanliness, good nutrition and elimination); (2) *environmental hygiene* (waste disposal, water purification, pollution control, etc); (3) *structural hygiene* (development of a fixation-free balanced musculoskeletal system); and (4) *mental hygiene* (development of healthy mental and emotional reactions and habits). The practice of these hygienes to perfection will not guarantee a disease-free world, but it will certainly help.

General Physical Fitness

Fitness is an attribute of the human organism at its best. The development of optimal physical fitness produces changes that increase physical capacity and produce changes in altered metabolism at the cellular level. A reduced level of fitness predisposes to injury, its extent, and modifies its healing at both its macroscopic and microscopic aspects.

The common human performance parameters are those of strength, flexibility, endurance, power, speed, coordination, balance, and agility. The quality of these factors is determined by neuromuscular and articular functions. Individual body type, intelligence, creativity, and motivation are also parameters that vary in importance to the individual and conditions at hand.

Patient Prescriptions

Comprehensive therapy cannot be restricted to the health-care office environment. Nutritional counsel and prescribed home exercises, for example, have been shown to be of extreme benefit in many musculoskeletal, neurologic, circulatory, hormonal, and visceral disorders.

The degree of vascularity of the capillary network between skeletal muscle fibers and in associated tissues depends greatly on the type of exercise to which a specific individual is exposed. The quantity of interstitial fat, most marked in atrophied muscle, is also determined by the degree of exercise.

Obviously, to be effective in enhancing a patient's rehabilitation, exercise must be conducted with sufficient warmup, frequency, duration, and intensity, and these factors must be based upon the individual patient's current functional and biomechanical status and need. Thus, explicit motivational instruction and patient compliance are often basic factors in arriving at a long-range successful outcome. [See Clinical Comment 2.7]

Miscellaneous Supportive and Rehabilitative Procedures

It has been Schafer's observation that many chronic musculoskeletal disorders seen in a chiropractic office present with two underlying periarticular muscle-ligament conditions: one or more muscle groups that

DR. FAYE'S CLINICAL COMMENT #2.7

I find if I use a 2500 Hz current at an intensity that causes a strong contraction for a period of ten seconds with a fifty second rest period producing ten contractions, the muscles in chronic areas respond to exercise at home better. This Russian Stimulation method should be applied in the office every other day for 6 or 8 visits once the pain has disappeared. The extension exercises especially can be executed during the electrostimulation treatment.

are in a weakened state and a shortened and spastic condition of their antagonists, or vice versa. It is presumed that this functional imbalance, which leads to both physiologic and biomechanical overstress, is one frequent cause of many articular disorders. Thus, adjunctive therapy in articular disorders directed to the involved joint(s) is often helpful in correcting this imbalance by strengthening certain muscles and ligaments, and stretching others. If not, the effects of primary therapy are likely to be effective only during the short term and recurrence of some problem (either locally or somewhere else in the kinematic chain) can usually be expected.

Reciprocal Soft-Tissue Compensation

If this hypothesis is often true, then the clinician can expect to find in joint disorders weak extensors associated with shortened and tight flexors, or vice versa, and weak abductors often associated with short tight adductors, and vice versa. These syndromes are common in many low-back pain cases where we find weakened abdominals associated with short spastic *deep* lumbosacral extensors. While light palpation may indicate normal tone of the superficial erectors, deep palpation will invariably reveal hard-inflexible tissues. Gross observation from the side will show in many cases a pot-bellied individual, an extremely sharp lumbosacral angle (due to an anteriorly rotated pelvis) and a flattened lumbar and thoracic spine above. This picture does not fit the overconcern in most textbooks with classic lumbar hyperlordosis and thoracic hyperkyphosis. Unfortunately, such an imbalance syndrome in the extremities such as in the shoulder, elbow, wrist, knee, and ankle is much more subtle. Yet, careful examination will show its presence. For example, it is rare to find a meniscus disorder of the knee not associated with a weak quadriceps (especially a vastus medialis) and tight hamstrings. Likewise, it is rare to find a case of shin splints not associated with weak anterior leg muscles and tight calf muscles.

Articular Degenerative Causes and Effects

Osteoarthritis is the most prevalent disorder within the animal kingdom. Even mature fish and foul are not excluded from widespread signs of this degenerative process. It was once thought this common disorder was the result of joint trauma and overwork, but evidence collected during recent years shows that degenerative bone disease is just as common in the sedentary individual as it is in the manual laborer or professional athlete. Thus, the explanation of prolonged overstress can no longer be held valid as a general assumption.

While the cause of osteoarthritis is still unknown, it is possible that it will be found within investigations of the nutrition of articular cartilage. We do know that fibrocartilage and hyaline cartilage are nourished by a pump-like action in which nutrients are pulled or sucked inward and metabolic products are exuded or expelled outward during reciprocatively opposite joint motions. If an articular fixation exists, this pump-like mechanism cannot be effective. If any tissue is not properly nourished, its power and reserves to withstand normal stress are diminished and lead to inflammation initially and degeneration when prolonged and tissue defenses are depleted. When degeneration is advanced, the structural design of the segment will additionally not allow normal function and normal proprioceptive input to the CNS is severely altered. Faye points out another factor involving joints required to move in abnormal ranges of motion; ie, long-term hypermobile or eccentric motions predispose the development of degenerative bone disease.

Bibliography

ACA Council on Physiological Therapeutics: Physiotherapy guidelines for the chiropractic profession, *ACA Journal of Chiropractic*, p S-68, June 1975.

Andrews FW: Discussion of ice therapy. *ACA Journal of Chiropractic*, April 1968.

Basmajian JV (ed): *Manipulation, Traction, and Massage*, ed 3. Baltimore, Williams & Wilkins, 1985, pp 157-163.

Bierman W, Friedlander M: The penetrative effect of cold. *Archives of Physical Medicine and Rehabilitation*, 21:585-592, 1940.

Brown A: Physical medicine in rehabilitation. *Maryland State Medical Journal*, 19:61, 1970.

Dishmann R: Review of the literature supporting a scientific basis for the subluxation complex. *Journal of Manipulative and Physiological Therapeutics*, 8(3):163-172, September 1985.

Eldred E, et al: The effect of cooling on mammalian muscle spindle. *Experimental Neurology*, 2:144-157, 1960.

Elftman H: The action of muscles in the body. *Biological Symposium*, 3:191-209, 1941.

Elftman H: Biomechanics of muscle. *Journal of Bone and Joint Surgery*, 48A:363-377, 1966.

Faye LJ: *Motion Palpation and Clinical Considerations of the Lower Extremities.* Huntington Beach, CA, Motion Palpation Institute, 1986, pp 3-7, 19.

Faye LJ: Motion Palpation of the Spine [Cassette tape program]. Huntington Beach, CA, Motion Palpation Institute, 1981, 6 tapes.

Faye LJ: Rationale for Motion Palpation and the Subluxation Complex [Videotape]. Dynaspine, Inc, 10780 Santa Monica Blvd, Suite 400, Los Angeles, CA 90025.

Faye LJ: The Rationale for the Chiropractic Adjustment [Cassette tape]. Huntington Beach, CA, Motion Palpation Institute, date not shown.

Faye LJ: *Spine I: Motion Palpation and Clinical Considerations of the Lumbar Spine and Pelvis.* Huntington Beach, CA, Motion Palpation Institute, 1987, pp 6-9, 21, 28-32.

Faye LJ, Weary B, Hooper P: *Motion Palpation and Clinical Considerations of the Upper Extremities.* Huntington Beach, CA, Motion Palpation Institute, 1986, pp 3-12.

Fox RH: Local cooling in man. *British Medical Bulletin*, 17:14-18, 1961.

Gillet H: A cineradiographic study of the kinetic relationship between the cervical vertebrae. *Bulletin of the European Chiropractic Union*, 28(3):44-46, 1980.

Gillet H, Liekens M: *Belgian Chiropractic Research Notes.* Huntington Beach, CA, Motion Palpation Institute, 1984, pp 35-40, 61-78, 92-101, 108-111, 115-116, 118-122, 126-127, 130-132, 144-146, 148-150, 166.

Gillet H, Liekens M: Fixation analysis—movement palpation. In Kfoury PW (ed): *Catalog of Chiropractic Techniques.* Chesterfield, MO, Logan College of Chiropractic, 1977, pp 101-102.

Gillet H: Movement palpation—measurements. *Bulletin of the European Chiropractors Union*, 23(2), 1974.

Goodman CE: Pathophysiology of pain. *Archives of Internal Medicine*, 143:527, 1983.

Hayden CA: Cryokinetics in an early treatment program. *Journal of the American Physical Therapy Association*, 44:990-993, 1964.

Hocutt JE Jr: Cryotherapy. *American Family Physician*, 23(3):141-144, March 1981.

Jaskoviak PA, Schafer RC: *Applied Physiotherapy: Practical Applications Within Clinical Chiropractic.* Arlington, VA, American Chiropractic Association, 1986, pp 217-219, 235, 278-279, 350, 361-364.

Kellgren JH: On the distribution of pain arising from deep somatic structures with charts of segmental pain areas. *Clinical Science*, 4:35-46, 1939.

Kirkaldy-Willis WH: *Managing Low Back Pain.* New York, Churchill Livingstone, 1983, pp 24-25, 73-91.

Lee JM, et al: Effects of ice on nerve conduction velocity. *Physiotherapy*, 64:2-6, 1978.

Liekens M: The Liekens method. In Gillet H: *Belgium Chiropractic Research Notes.* Huntington, CA, Motion Palpation Institute, 1973, pp 58-61.

Lowther DA: The effect of compression and tension on the behavior of connective tissue. In Glasgow EF, Twomey LT, Scull ER, Kleynhans AM, Idczak RM: *Aspects of Manipulative Therapy*, ed 2. New York, Churchill Livingstone, 1985, pp 16-21.

Maitland GD: The importance of adding compression when examining and treating synovial joints. In Glasgow EF, Twomey LT, Scull ER, Kleynhans AM, Idczak RM: *Aspects of Manipulative Therapy*, ed 2. New York, Churchill Livingstone, 1985, pp 109-114.

McMaster WC, et al: Laboratory evaluation of various cold therapy modalities. *American Journal of Sports Medicine*, 6:291-294, 1978.

Mennell JMcM: *Joint Pain.* Boston, Little, Brown, 1964, pp 1-10, 12-27, 134-136.

Miglietta O: Action of cold on spasticity. *American Journal of Physical Medicine*, 52:198-205, 1973.

Ng SY: Skeletal muscle spasm: Various methods to relieve it. *ACA Journal of Chiropractic*, 14:23, February 1980.

Nielsen AJ: Spray and stretch for myofascial pain. *Physical Therapy*, 58(5):567-569, May 1978.

Olson JE, Stravino VD: A Review of cryotherapy. *Physical Therapy*, 52:840-843, 1972.

Reddy MP: Peripheral nerve entrapment syndromes. *American Family Physician*, 28:5, November 1983, pp 133-143.

Rogoff JB (ed): *Manipulation, Traction, and Massage*, ed 2. Baltimore, Williams & Wilkins, 1980, pp 170-178.

Rollis C: Motion palpation procedure manual. In Gillet H, Liekens M: *Belgian Chiropractic Research Notes.* Huntington Beach, CA, Motion Palpation Institute, 1984, Appendix.

Rosse C, Simkin PA: Joints. In Rosse C, Clawson DK: *The Musculoskeletal System in Health & Disease.* Hagerstown, PA, Harper & Row, 1980, pp 77-80.

Sandoz R: Some physical mechanisms and effects of spinal adjustments. *Annals of the Swiss Chiropractors' Association*, 6:91, 1976.

Schafer RC: *Chiropractic Management of Extraspinal Articular Disorders.* Arlington, VA, American Chiropractic Association. In preparation.

Schafer RC: *Chiropractic Management of Sports and Recreational Injuries.* Baltimore, Williams & Wilkins, 1982, pp 166-167, 197-198, 230, 252-255.

Schafer RC: *Clinical Biomechanics: Musculoskeletal Actions and Reactions.* Baltimore, Williams & Wilkins, 1983, pp 155, 208-214, 263.

Schafer RC: *Physical Diagnosis: Procedures and Methodology in Chiropractic Practice.* Arlington, VA, American Chiropractic Association. In preparation; scheduled for release in 1988.

Schafer RC: *Symptomatology and Differential Diagnosis.* Arlington, VA, American Chiropractic Association, 1986, pp 327, 833-834.

Smythe H: "Fibrositis" and soft-tissue pain syndromes: The clinical significance of tender points. In Leek JC, Gershwin ME, Fowler WM Jr: *Principles of Physical Medicine and Rehabilitation in the Musculoskeletal Diseases.* Orlando, FL, Grune & Stratton, 1986, pp 515-527.

Soderberg GL: *Kinesiology: Application to Pathological Motion.* Baltimore, Williams & Wilkins, 1986, p 58.

Sola AE: Myofascial trigger point therapy. *Medical Times,* pp 70-77, January 1982.

Travell J: Ethyl chloride spray for painful muscle spasm. *Archives of Physical Medicine and Rehabilitation,* 33:291-298, 1952.

Travell J: Myofascial trigger points: clinical view. In Bonica JJ, AlbeFessard, D: *Advances in Pain Research and Therapy.* New York, Raven Press, vol 1, 1976.

Voss DE, et al: Traction and approximation. *Proprioceptive Neuromuscular Facilitation: Patterns and Techniques,* ed 3. Philadelphia, Harper & Row, 1985, p 294.

Chapter 3

The Cervical Spine

This chapter describes the basic biomechanical, diagnostic, and therapeutic considerations related to motion palpation and the cervical spine. Emphasis will be on relating the general concepts previously explained about the chiropractic fixation-subluxation complex to specific entities that can be revealed by motion palpation and frequently corrected by *dynamic chiropractic.* Some aids to differential diagnosis are also included.

APPLIED ANATOMY CONSIDERATIONS

There are seven sites of possible "articular" fixation in the cervical spine. They are at the bilateral apophyseal joints, the bilateral covertebral joints, the superior and inferior intervertebral disc (IVD) interfaces, and the odontal-atlantal articulation (Table 3.1).

The Apophyseal Joints of the Spine

Throughout the spine, paired diarthrodial articular processes (zygapophyses) project from the vertebral arches. The superior processes (prezygapophyses) of the inferior vertebra contain articulating facets that face somewhat posteriorly. They mate with the inferior processes (postzygapophyses) of the vertebra above that face somewhat anteriorly. Each articular facet is covered by a layer of hyaline cartilage that faces the synovial joint. The angulation of vertebral facets normally varies with the level of the spine and can be altered by wear and pathology.

In visualizing the motion of any joint, it is helpful to keep in mind that the hyaline-coated articulating surface is not the shape of the often flat bony surface exhibited on an x-ray film. Most apophyseal joints of the spine have a convex-concave shape.

Fisk states that the posterior joints of the spine are more prone to osteoarthritic changes than any other joint in the body: "Evidence of disc degeneration precedes this arthritis in the lumbar spine, but there is no such relationship in the cervical spine." However, most authorities agree with Grieve that the presence of arthrotic changes in the facet planes does not, of itself, necessarily have any effect on ranges of movement, neither does the presence of osteophytosis.

Regional Structural Characteristics

Nature has made many structural adaptations in the cervical region because of the relatively small weight-bearing structures, the required range of motion, and the enlarged spinal cord in this region as compared to other spinal regions. The laminae are slender and overlap, and this shingling design increases with age. The osseous elevations on the posterolateral aspect of most cervical vertebrae (that form the uncovertebral pseudojoints) tend to protect the spinal canal from lateral IVD herniation, but hypertrophy of these joints added to IVD degeneration can readily lead to intervertebral foramen (IVF) encroachment.

The IVDs are broader anteriorly than posteriorly to accommodate the cervical lordosis. It is helpful to know the location of the nucleus pulposus of a region because it indi-

Table 3.1. The 27 Sites of Possible Spinopelvic Articular Fixation

In the cervical spine (7 possible sites of fixation)

Bilateral apophyseal joints	2
Bilateral covertebral joints	2
Superior and inferior IVD interfaces	2
Odontal-atlantal articulation	1

In the thoracic spine (8 possible sites of fixation)

Bilateral apophyseal joints	2
Superior and inferior IVD interfaces	2
Bilateral costovertebral joints	2
Bilateral costotransverse joints	2

In the lumbar spine (4 possible sites of fixation)

Bilateral apophyseal joints	2
Superior and inferior IVD interfaces	2

In the pelvis (8 possible sites of fixation)

Bilateral superior sacroiliac joints	2
Bilateral inferior sacroiliac joints	2
Sacrococcygeal joint	1
Pubic joint	1
Bilateral acetabulofemoral joints	2
	27

cates the normal site of maximum load, but authorities differ on the normal location of the nucleus in the cervical region. Kapandji locates it centrally. Cailliet places it slightly posterior (further anterior than a lumbar nucleus), and Jeffreys says it is distinctly posterior from the midline. Thus, such conflicting reports are no better than no data at all. Because the atypical atlas has no centrum, there is no IVD between the occiput and atlas or the atlas and axis.

The Cervical Apophyseal Joints

The articular processes of the mid and lower cervical spine incline medially in the coronal plane and obliquely in the sagittal plane so that they are approximately at a 45° angle to the vertical. This is an important fact to remember when adjusting this region. The bilateral articular surface area of the segments, which shares a good part of head weight with the vertebral body, is about 67% of that of the vertebral body.

The short, thick, dense *capsular ligaments* bind the articulating processes together (Fig. 3.1), enclosing the articular cartilage and synovium. Their fibers are firmly bound to the periosteum of the superior and inferior processes and arranged at a 90° angle to the plane of the facet. This allows maximum laxity when the facets are in a position of rest. They normally allow no more than a few millimeters of movement from the neutral position per segment, and possibly provide more cervical stability than any other ligament complex of this region.

Capsulitis from overstretch in acute trau-

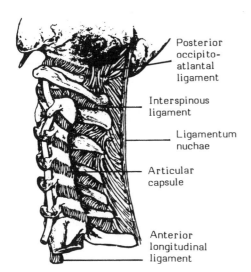

Figure 3.1. Posterolateral schematic of the ligaments of the cervical region (Courtesy ACAP).

matic subluxation complex or excessive compensatory hypermobility is common. Within the capsule, small tongues of meniscus-like tissue flaps project from the articular surfaces into the synovial space. They are infrequently nipped in severe jarring at an unguarded moment during the end of extension, rotation, or lateral bending, establishing a site of apophyseal bursitis.

The posterior joint capsules and the perivertebral supporting ligaments enjoy an abundance of nociceptors and mechanoreceptors, far more than any other area of the spine. The IVDs are almost void of such receptors.

The Cervical Intervertebral Foramina

The foramina in the cervical region are shaped more like rounded gutters than orifices, averaging 1 cm in length. There is no true IVF between the atlas and the occiput or between the atlas and the axis. The C1 nerve exits over the superior aspect of the posterior arch of the atlas in the vertebral artery sulcus (Fig. 3.2). The C2 nerve exits between the inferior aspect of the posterior arch of the atlas and the superior aspect of the pedicle of the axis. It then, in a vulnerable

position, transverses the lateral atlantoaxial joint, anterior to the ligamentum flava for a short while, then exits (Fig. 3.3). The C3—C8 nerves exit through short oval canals that increase in size as they progress caudally.

In contrast with the dorsal and lumbar regions, the boundaries of the cervical IVFs are designed more for motion than they are for stability. The greatest degree of functional IVF-diameter narrowing occurs ipsilaterally in lateral bending with simultaneous exten-

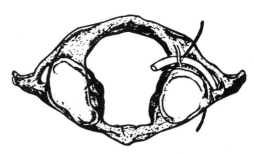

Figure 3.2. The C1 nerves leave the spinal cord behind the superior articular processes. The C1 nerve, shown only on the right, follows a groove on the upper surface of the posterior arch of the atlas, posteroinferiorly to the occipitoatlantal capsule and beneath the vertebral artery as it crosses the atlas (Courtesy ACAP).

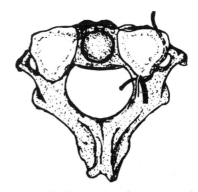

Figure 3.3. Similar to the C1 nerves, the C2 nerves leave the spinal cord behind the superior articular processes. The C2 nerves transverse the arch of the axis behind the articular process and in contact with the joint capsule. They exit the vertebral canal via a small opening in the ligamentum flavum, thus are especially vulnerable to ligamentous degenerative processes. Only the right nerve is shown in the diagram (Courtesy ACAP).

sion. Thus, this position should be avoided whenever possible during cervical adjustments and manipulation.

The Contents of the Intervertebral Foramina

Cervical nerves, especially, fill the transverse diameter of the their IVFs. Thus, any disorder that reduces this dimension structurally or functionally (eg, subluxation, osteophytes, disc herniation, edema, vascular engorgement) will undoubtedly compromise the integrity of the IVF contents (Fig. 3.4).

Each IVF of the cervical, thoracic, and lumbar spine is dynamic; widening and expanding with spinal motion, serving as a channel for nerve and vascular flow egress and ingress, and allowing for massage-like compression and expansion of the conduits and lipoareolar bed. From one-third to one-half of the foraminal opening is occupied by the spinal nerve root and its sheath, with the remaining portion filled essentially by fat, connective tissue, and various vessels. The following structures are found in the IVF:

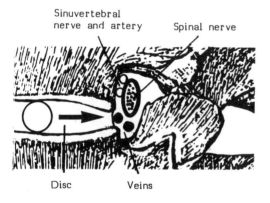

Sinuvertebral nerve and artery
Spinal nerve
Disc
Veins

Figure 3.4. Diagram showing the major contents of an IVF. An extension fixation of the superior segment of a motion unit, a flexion fixation of the inferior segment of a motion unit, a posterior IVD herniation, or exostoses near the IVF can readily encroach on the nerve root, the sinuvertebral nerve and artery passing anterosuperior to the nerve root, and the two veins passing below the nerve root (Courtesy ACAP).

- Anterior nerve root
- Posterior nerve root
- Part of the dorsal nerve root ganglion
- A bilaminar sleeve of dura and arachnoid membrane to the ganglion
- A short continuation of the subarachnoid space with cerebrospinal fluid that ends just after the ganglion
- Recurrent meningeal nerve
- Spinal ramus artery
- Intervertebral vein
- Lymphatic vessels
- Fat, fascia, and areolar tissue

The Cervical Nerves

The cervical nerves coalesce into the cervical plexus (C1—C4) and brachial plexus (C5—T1). See Table 3.2. The cervical nerves are named after the vertebra below; the IVDs, the vertebra above.

Dynamics of the Cervical Cord

During forward flexion of the neck, the cervical spinal canal is lengthened so that the posterior wall of the spinal canal lengthens relative to the anterior wall. The opposite occurs during backward extension. During flexion and extension, the cord itself does not appreciably ascend or descend, but the accordion-like folds within its dural sheath deepen during extension and almost disappear during forced flexion owing to the tension developed by the tensile force.

Dynamics of the Cervical Roots

It is highly controversial whether the nerve root sleeves normally adhere to the IVFs (ie, if they ingress or egress within the IVFs during spinal movements). See Figure 3.5. Most authorities, however, agree that the roots are normally held high within their respective IVFs in the neutral position and especially so during flexion. During extension, the dura mater and arachnoid around the spinal cord relax and the roots descend to a more mid-IVF position. It is well to keep this in mind when one or more segments are found to be severely locked in flexion or extension.

Table 3.2. Segmental Function of the Cervical Nerves

Segment	Function
	CERVICAL PLEXUS (C1—C4)
C1	Motor to head and neck extensors, infrahyoid, rectus capitis anterior and lateral, and longus capitis.
C2	Sensory to lateral occiput and submandibular area; motor, same as C1 plus longus colli.
C3	Sensory to lateral occiput and lateral neck, overlapping C2 area; motor to head and neck extensors, infrahyoid, longus capitis, longus colli, levator scapulae, scaleni, and trapezius.
C4	Sensory to lower lateral neck and medial shoulder area; motor to head and neck extensors, longus colli, levator scapulae, scaleni, trapezius, and diaphragm.
	BRACHIAL PLEXUS (C5—T1)
C5	Sensory to clavicle level and lateral arm (axillary nerve); motor to deltoid, biceps; biceps tendon reflex. Primary root in shoulder abduction, exits under the C4 vertebra.
C6	Sensory to lateral forearm, thumb, index and half of 2nd finger (sensory branches of musculocutaneous nerve); motor to biceps, wrist extensors; brachioradialis tendon reflex. Primary root in wrist extension, exits under the C5 vertebra.
C7	Sensory to second finger; motor to wrist flexors, finger extensors, triceps; triceps tendon reflex. Primary root in finger extension, exits under the C6 vertebra.
C8	Sensory to medial forearm (medial antebrachial nerve), ring and little fingers (ulnar nerve); motor to finger flexors, interossei; no reflex applicable. Primary root in finger flexion, exits under the C7 vertebra.
T1	Sensory to medial arm (medial brachial cutaneous nerve); motor to interossei; no reflex applicable. Primary root in finger abduction, exits under the T1 vertebra.

The nerve roots themselves occupy about a quarter of the contents of the IVF, the remaining area is occupied by the tissues previously listed. The motor root runs close to the clefts (the covertebral joints of Luschka) and the sensory root lies close to the articular processes. Soon after the nerves exit the IVF, their epineural sheaths become attached to the transverse processes, posterior longitudinal ligament, and scalenii fascia. Thus, the roots are not as free as some have reported. [See Clinical Comment 3.1]

Cutaneous Branches of the Cervical Plexus

Extensions of the cervical plexus divide into deep muscular (primarily motor) and superficial (primarily sensory) branches. These latter branches are frequently involved (tender) in subluxation syndromes of C1—C4, especially when the disorder is complicated by advanced spondylosis. The four common resulting neuralgias are:

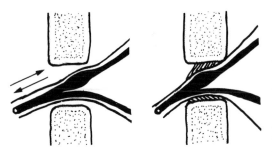

Figure 3.5. *Left,* ingress and egress of a nerve root during spinal motion if it is not attached to the borders of the IVF. *Right,* normal attachments or adhesions will place considerable traction on the root complex during normal movements, resulting in stretching the dural sheath and possibly its contents (Courtesy ACAP).

1. *Lesser occipital neuralgia,* which usually manifests in the occipitalis muscle, tissues around the mastoid process, and upper posterior aspect of the pinna.

2. *Greater auricular neuralgia,* which expresses over the front and back of the pinna, the skin over the parotid gland, and otherwise parallels the distribution of the auriculotemporal branch of the trigeminus and is thus often mistaken for trifacial neuralgia.

3. *Cervical cutaneous neuralgia,* which primarily involves the zone of the middle third of the platysma. It may spread to involve an area extending from the chin to the sternum.

4. *Supraclavicular neuralgia.* The anterior, middle, and posterior rami of the lower cervical plexus (C3—C4) have the following cutaneous distribution, respectively: (a) skin over the upper portion of the sternum, (b) skin over the pectoralis major, and (c) skin over the deltoid. Thus, C4 and/or C5 vertebral lesions may produce neuralgia in and refer hyperesthesia to these areas.

The Greater Occipital Nerve

The posterior primary divisions of C2 are by far the largest of all spinal nerve posterior rami. They divide into several terminal branches that ramify in the superficial fascia of the occiput and supply the skin of the scalp above the superior nuchal line as far as the vertex. Kinetic disturbances of the upper cervical segments are notorious in their contribution to mechanical etiologic patterns of cervical neuralgia (migraine), which is typically unilateral and referred along the distribution of the greater occipital nerve. This common disorder will be described later in this chapter.

The Brachial Plexus

The brachial plexus is formed by the anterior primary divisions of C1—T1. Chronic mid- and lower-cervical subluxation complexes and/or traumatic tensile or compression injuries may produce a wide variety of upper-extremity motor and sensory signs and symptoms that often lead to peripheral degenerative changes (eg, frozen shoulder, tendinitis, bursitis, cubital and carpal tunnel syndromes).

The Sympathetic Nerves

Two major components of the sympathetic nervous system are located in the neck: the bilateral sympathetic chains and the vertebral nerves. The vertebral nerves course along the vertebral arteries as they pass through the foramina of the cervical transverse processes—thus easily subjected to

---

DR. FAYE'S CLINICAL COMMENT #3.1

It is clinically very important to palpate over the roots and the scalenii fascia. If an anterior doorbell sign is present, it almost always is accompanied by an anterior-to-posterior rotation fixation and a flexion fixation of the same side; ie, A-P rotation and forward flexion will be hypomobile. This sign and these fixations are almost always present on the same side as tennis elbow, carpal tunnel syndrome, Adson's sign, scalenius anticus syndrome, migraine (hemicrania) and many other sympathetic symptoms of the cervical syndrome. This is my personal observation.

torsion and shear stresses. Although it is not fully understood how these sympathetic system components cause certain symptoms, the symptoms attributed to them are generally accepted.

The cervical cord contains neither lateral horn cells or preganglionic fibers. Preganglionic fibers of the neck arise from the upper thoracic spine and ascend to the cervical ganglia. Postganglionic fibers from the cervical ganglia course in three directions: (1) branches accompanying the distribution of the anterior roots; (2) branches that synapse into postganglionic fibers that travel with the cranial nerves and arteries of the neck and head and to the cardiac plexus; and (3) branches that re-enter the IVFs with the recurrent meningeal nerve to supply the dura and internal longitudinal ligaments. [See Clinical Comment 3.2]

The *superior cervical ganglion* is the largest of the cervical sympathetic chain and lies just below the base of the skull: in front of the axis and C3, between the internal jugular vein and the internal carotid artery. Thus, upper-cervical kinetic disturbances of any of the upper cervical vertebral joints may cause irritation of this important ganglion—leading to symptoms of hypersympathicotonia or to compression leading to Horner's syndrome.

The Vagus

In its bilateral descent through the neck, the vagus passes laterally to the superior cervical ganglion, lying in almost immediate contact with the transverse process of the atlas. Thus, upper-cervical kinetic disturbances (eg, atlanto-occipital and/or atlanto-axial fixations) may cause irritation leading to signs and symptoms of hypervagotonia or pressure leading to hypovagotonia.

Pertinent Neurovascular Considerations

The Recurrent Meningeal Nerve (Nervus Sinu Vertebralis)

The thread-like recurrent meningeal nerve is composed of unmyelinated sensory and sympathetic fibers. It is given off from each spinal nerve at a point just beyond the ganglion and returns through the IVF to supply the dural sheath of the nerve root, the vessels passing through the IVF, and the anterior surface of the dura mater of the spinal cord. Some authorities also state that it sends sensory fibers into the posterior aspect of the anulus of the IVD.

The Vascular Bed

The Vertebral Arteries. The vertebral arteries arise bilaterally from the subclavian arteries, pass through the foramina of the cervical transverse processes, and then ascend into the cranium. Each artery is surrounded by a plexus of sympathetic postganglionic neurons (the vertebral plexus) and a venous plexus formed by the vertebral vein. Any external factor that can obstruct a vertebral artery is thus likely to interfere with the drainage of the vertebral vein and the function of the sympathetic vertebral plexus. Typical examples are bony encroachments narrowing the transverse foramina; vertebral artery deflection, torsion, or tension as the result of severe degenerative changes and misalignment of the motion unit (especially the occipito-atlantal unit); severe upper-cervical muscle spasm; or an expanding space-occupying perivertebral mass. The most common cause of *intraluminal* ob-

---

DR. FAYE'S CLINICAL COMMENT #3.2

The (1) group are also palpated as per the doorbell sign as noted in the previous comment. Increased sympathetic activity according to Korr will inhibit healing and perpetuate or accentuate the inflammatory process of the tissues its facilitated fibers supply. Once again I wish to stress the importance of adjusting the cervicals from anterior to posterior and into forward flexion on the side of signs and symptoms.

struction is artherosclerosis. The resulting syndromes, which may forewarn an impending stroke, will be described later in this chapter.

The Vertebral Veins. The vertebral veins begin in the posterior vertebral venous plexus in the suboccipital triangle, from which it communicates with the internal vertebral venous plexuses.

The Deep Cervical Veins. These veins, larger than the vertebral veins, course down the neck behind the transverse processes of the cervical vertebrae. They begin in the posterior vertebral venous plexus, receive tributaries from the deep muscles of the neck, and communicate with the occipital veins by a branch that perforates the upper trapezius muscles. For this latter reason, prolonged spasm of the deep suboccipital muscles may produce a congestive stasis leading to a throbbing discomfort and suboccipital pain. Such symptoms, which may be unilateral or bilateral, are often associated with tender nodules within the suboccipital musculature.

Cerebrospinal Fluid Circulation: Pertinent Considerations

The intracranial pressure of the cerebrospinal fluid (CSF) system must be sustained within fine limits. An increase in pressure as in hydrocephalus leads to papilledema, cerebral pressure ischemia—necrosis, and cerebellar symptoms. A decrease in pressure such as follows a spinal tap of 5 cc or more may lead to intractable headache with possible convulsions and coma.

The posterior medullary velum, which forms the posteroinferior wall of the 4th ventricle and which is perforated by the foramina of Luschka and Magendie, extends well into the foramen magnum. It is separated from the posterior ramus of the foramen magnum by the subarachnoid space and the contained dura mater. It is at this point that one of two possible structural impediments to CSF circulation may occur because of fixed occipitoatlantal shifting, tilting, or rotation:

1. The cerebral subarachnoid space may become constricted, inhibiting the amount of cerebrospinal fluid flow into the spinal canal and ultimately to the spinal roots and cauda equina. This would result in increased intracranial pressure and possibly decreased intraspinal pressure.

2. An occipitoatlantal disrelationship may be sufficient enough to press the dura mater constituting the floor of the cisterna cerebellaris (subarachnoid space of the cerebellum) against the posterior medullary velum and partially occlude the exit of the foramina of Luschka and Magendie, thus interfering with CSF egress from the 4th ventricle and increasing intracranial pressure. Early symptoms may include intractable pressure headache, frequent and otherwise unexplainable feelings of nausea with tendencies toward projectile vomiting (especially on exertion), unpredictable protopathic ataxias, and/or bizarre visual disturbances.

BIOMECHANICAL CONSIDERATIONS

The head mechanically teeters on the occipitoatlantal joints, which are shaped like cupped palms tipped slightly medially. Because the line of gravity falls anterior to these articulations, an automatic force must be constantly provided in the upright posture by the posterior neck muscles to hold the head erect. Added to this gravitational stress is the action of the anterior muscles of the neck (essentially the masticatory, suprahyoid, and infrahyoid groups), which serve as a muscle chain to join the anterior cranium to the shoulder girdle.

The biomechanical efficiency of any one of the 26 vertebral motion units from occiput to sacrum can be described as that condition (individually and collectively) in which each gravitationally dependent segment above is (1) free to seek its normal resting position in relation to its supporting structure below, (2) free to move efficiently through its normal ranges of motion, and (3) free to return to its normal resting position after movement.

Flexion, extension, rotation, lateral flexion, and circumduction are the basic movements of the cervical region. Movements of the head on the neck are generally confined to the occiput-atlas-axis complex and can be described separately from movements of the neck on the trunk.

Action and Brake Mechanisms in the Spine as a Whole

Flexion

During flexion, the IVDs tend to compress at their anterior aspect, the inferior set of articular facets glide anterosuperiorly on the mating set of superior facets of the vertebra below, and the normal range of motion is checked by the posterior anulus of the disc, posterior longitudinal ligament, intertransverse ligaments, supraspinous ligament, nuchal ligament, and extensor muscle tendons. See Figure 3.6. Slight z-axis translation occurs anteriorly.

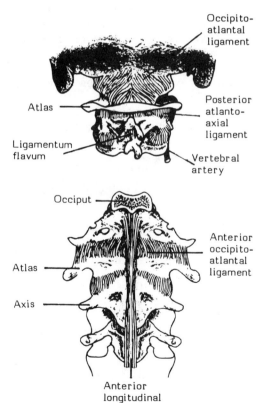

Figure 3.6. *Top,* the major postvertebral ligaments of the upper cervical area; *bottom,* the major prevertebral ligaments (Courtesy ACAP).

Extension

Extension has a much lower magnitude than flexion throughout the spine. The IVDs tend to compress and bulge at their posterior aspect, and the inferior set of articular facets glide posteroinferiorly on the mating superior facets below. The motion is checked by the anterior anulus of the disc, the anterior longitudinal ligament, all the anterior and lateral tendons that contribute in flexion, the anterior fascia and visceral attachments, and probably spinous process and/or laminae jamming at maximum extension. Slight z-axis translation occurs posteriorly.

Rotation

Spinal rotation is limited by the planes of the articular facets, the thickness of the associated IVDs, and the resistance offered by the fibers of the disc's anulus and the vertebral ligaments under torsion.

Lateral Bending

Sideward abduction involves a degree of tilting of vertebral bodies on their discs. The anterior aspect of the vertebral bodies in the upper spine also rotate toward the side of convexity, the posterior aspect swings in the opposite direction, and the facets tend to slide open on the convex side and override on the concave side. The motion is checked by the intertransverse ligaments and intercostal tissues on the convex side, behind the fulcrum, and the apposition of ribs on the concave side in the thoracic region.

Coupling and Related Effects

Some motions restrict other motions and enhance still others. For example, flexion and extension restrict rotation and lateral bending ranges. Rotation decreases A-P and P-A glide and is accompanied by a degree of lateral flexion. Lateral flexion inhibits A-P and P-A glide and enhances cervical rotation toward the concave side and lumbar rotation toward the convex side.

The Upper Cervical Region

All movements in the cervical spine are relatively free because of the saddle-like joints. The cervical spine is most flexible in flexion and rotation. The latter occurs most freely in the upper cervical area and is progressively restricted downward.

An understanding of the basic kinematics of the cervical spine is important to accurate clinical diagnosis and therapeutic applications. Our major concern in this section will be the motion between the occiput and the atlas and the atlas upon the axis. Normal ranges of motion are shown in Table 3.3. It should be noted that the specific ranges of cervical motion differ widely among so many authorities that any range described here should be considered hypothetical depending on individual planes of articulation, other variances in structural design (eg, congenital, aging degeneration, posttraumatic), and soft-tissue integrity. This wide variance in opinion is also true for the centers of motion described. Such guidelines should not prejudice your clinical findings.

The oblique cup-and-saucer occipitoatlantal joints are designed for a limited range of flexion-extension nodding movement (Fig. 3.7). Translatory movements are slight; most action is a rolling movement. The long axes of the joints are obliquely set, but a slight curve in the coronal plane allows some end play for lateral tilt.

The frontal plane angle of the joint axes for the occipital condyles can be determined on a radiograph by drawing lines that are parallel to the articulating surfaces of the condyles. Normally, this angle is 124° in males and 127° in females. However, anomalies (congenital or pathogenic) such as basilar impression or condylar hypoplasia will increase this angle. Faye points out that this angle does not really exist as the joint's hyaline cartilage (invisible on film) has a different contour than that of the bone shadows.

Occipitoatlantal Flexion

Much cervical motion is concentrated in specific spinal areas. For example, about half of flexion and extension occurs at the occipitoatlantal joints (Fig. 3.8), with the other half distributed among the remaining cervical joints. As the nucleus of the disc is nearer the anterior of a *complete* cervical vertebra, flexion-extension is more discernible at the spinous process than at the anterior aspect of the vertebral body.

Without any participation of the neck below the atlas, the head can be moved about 10° in flexion between the occiput and atlas. During strict upper neck flexion, the condyles roll backward and slide slightly posterior on the atlas while the atlas rolls anteriorly and somewhat superiorly on the occiput, with the atlas taking the odontoid of

Table 3.3. Normal Ranges of Upper Cervical Motion

Motion Unit	Movement	Degrees*
Occipitoatlantal	Flexion	10
	Extension	15
	Lateral bending	7
	Rotation	3
Atlantoaxial	Flexion	11
	Extension	1
	Lateral flexion	2
	Rotation	45

*These ranges are approximate. Authorities differ in several degrees in their reported findings. The above is a composite of findings.

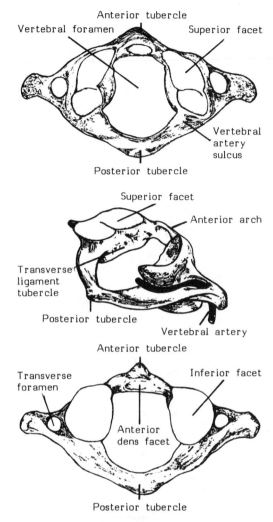

Figure 3.7. *Top,* the atlas, viewed from above; *middle,* viewed from the superolateral; *bottom,* viewed from below (Courtesy ACAP).

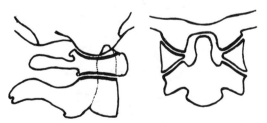

Figure 3.8. The occipitoatlantal joints, lateral view shown on the left and A-P view on the right. As the plane of articulation is less in the sagittal plane than in the frontal plane, traumatic A-P occipital subluxation or dislocation is more likely than lateral displacement (Courtesy ACAP).

the axis with it so that the dens slightly approaches the clivus of the basiocciput. As the atlas slides anteriorly from the condyles, the occiput and posterior arch of the atlas separate just slightly, but this is exaggerated if movement is virtually isolated at the occipitoatlantal joint (eg, in ankylosing spondylitis).

The prime mover of occipitoatlantal flexion is the rectus capitis anterior, aided by the longus capitis. The range is limited primarily by the elasticity of the posterior ligaments and by the tip of the dens meeting the bursa below the anterior rim of the foramen magnum. See Figure 3.9.

Occipitoatlantal Extension

Upper cervical flexion-extension usually occurs before any lower cervical motion; thus initial visual examination can often help to discern dysfunction of the upper cervical spine solely by observation of active motion. The skull can be extended on the atlas for about 15° without participation by any other cervical vertebra (Fig. 3.10). During normal extension of the neck, the condyles slide anteriorly on the atlas and the atlas rolls upward so that its posterior arch approximates the occiput. Slight opening of the inferior aspect of the atlanto-odontoid space occurs, but it is limited by the tectorial membrane.

Upper cervical extension is powered by the rectus capitis posterior group. Extension and lateral tilt of the upper cervical region is restricted by tension of the tectorial membrane and the posterior arch of the atlas becoming trapped between the occiput and the axis. During clinical observation, the chin should move before the neck moves in active cervical flexion and extension.

Occipitoatlantal Lateral Bending

Cervical lateral flexion is performed by the unilateral contraction of the neck flexors and extensors with motion occurring in the coronal plane. Such flexion is accompanied by rotational torsion below C2, distributed fairly equally in the normal cervical joints.

That is, when the cervical spine as a whole bends laterally, it also tends to rotate anteriorly on the side of the concavity so that the vertebral bodies arc further laterally than the spinous processes.

Normally, about a 45° tilt can be observed between the skull and the shoulder. About 7° of this occurs at the occipitoatlantal joint, following the arc of the condyles on the superior facets of the atlas (Fig. 3.11). As the occiput and atlas shift laterally as one unit towards the concavity during lateral bending, the space between the dens and lateral mass of the atlas widens on the concave side. At the same time, the occipital condyles translate slightly laterally on the superior facets of the atlas toward the convexity and the atlas slips slightly toward the side of concavity. These movements are slight unless there is a degree of instability involved. If the occipito-atlantal capsular ligaments are weakened, the condyle on the side of lateral

bending may strike the tip of the odontoid. The body of the axis tends to rotate towards the concavity while its spinous process shifts toward the convexity owing to the coupling mechanism.

Occipitoatlantal lateral bending is produced by the rectus capitis lateralis, which is helped by the semispinalis, splenius capitis, sternomastoideus, and trapezius. The range

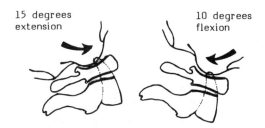

Figure 3.10. Occipitoatlantal flexion and extension (Courtesy ACAP).

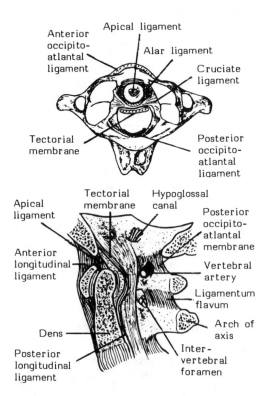

Figure 3.9. *Top,* upper cervical ligaments as viewed from above; *bottom,* sagittal section (Courtesy ACAP).

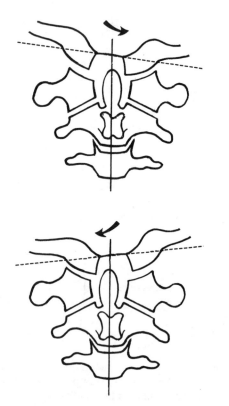

Figure 3.11. *Top,* occipital condyles fixed in lateral flexion to the right; *bottom,* condyles fixed in lateral flexion to the left (Courtesy ACAP).

is limited primarily by the alar ligaments. In mild coronal lateral flexion and transverse rotation of the head and neck, the occiput and atlas move as a unit because of the planes of the articular facets. Close observation will show that the occiput specifically abducts on the atlas without rotation about a vertical axis. Thus, the atlas is caught between trying to follow the motion of the occiput or the axis. See Fig. 3.12). This stress, according to Gillet, forces a slight amount of rotational end play of the occiput on the atlas even though the design of the condyles is not conducive to rotation.

Occipitoatlantal Rotation

During rotation, the occipital condyles and the atlas initially move as one unit on the axis. Approaching the end of the range of motion, the condyles can rotate a few de-

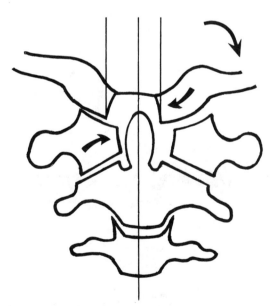

Figure 3.12. Occipitoatlantal and atlantoaxial lateral flexion. During lateral bending of the upper cervical spine, only slight movement is exhibited at the occipitoatlantal and atlantoaxial articulations. The occiput slips towards the convexity and the atlas slips toward the concavity. This creates shear forces at the superior articulations of the atlas and distortion of the odontoid space (Courtesy ACAP).

grees on the atlas in the direction of movement. Some authorities contest this fact, thus the range is often listed as 0°.

Atlantoaxial Flexion

In addition to the side-rolling motion of the atlas on the occiput, the atlas is capable of some tilting where the anterior ring of the atlas moves upward on the odontoid and the posterior arch rides downward, or vice versa. During severe flexion, there could be considerable separation of the anterior arch of the atlas from the odontoid, but it is checked by the weak transverse arms of the cruciate and by tension of the stronger tectorial membrane.

During cervical flexion, the inferior lateral masses of the atlas roll upward posteriorly and slide backward on the superior facets of the axis. Opening of the superior aspect of the atlanto-odontoid space is not appreciably restricted by the delicate transverse cruciate ligament (Fig. 3.13). Movement is restricted mainly by the apophyseal capsules, the ligamentum flavum, the interspinous ligament, the posterior nuchal muscles, and apposition of the chin against the sternum.

Atlantoaxial Extension

Similar to the motion described between the occiput and atlas during cervical ex-

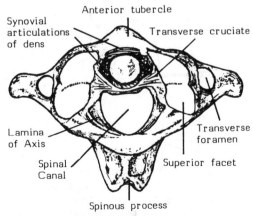

Figure 3.13. View of the atlanto-odontoid articulation, as seen from above (Courtesy ACAP).

tension, the posterior arches of the atlas and axis also approximate. The range of pure extension of C1 on C2 is minimal. The reason for this is that all other segments of the spine tip *and* translate posteriorly during extension from the neutral. The atlas cannot do this because of the odontoid process of the axis (Fig. 3.14). All that it can do during extension of the neck is tip downward at its posterior aspect and tip upward at its anterior aspect, a rotatory motion. During forced extension, the posterior arch of the atlas is caught as in a vise between the occiput and axis. Extension is even more resisted when the anterior arch meets the odontoid and the interarticular tissues compress. These facts are important to remember when someone speaks of extension of the atlas on the axis.

Atlantoaxial Lateral Bending

Some authors report that no motion occurs between C1 and C2 during lateral bending; however, motion palpation typically reveals slight motion (joint play) that follows the arc of the inferior facets of the atlas on the superior facets of the axis. Thus, if a major fixation is found at this point, it should be released because it is an extremely symptom-producing fixation.

When lateral flexion is restricted to the upper cervical area, the articulating facet

spaces open on the side of convexity and compress on the side of concavity. However, when lateral flexion is generalized throughout the cervical region, the lateral masses of the atlas sideslip towards the side of concavity so that the space between the lateral mass and the odontoid increases on the side of the concavity. Obviously, this is limited by the size of the bony crescent about the dens unless the cruciate is torn.

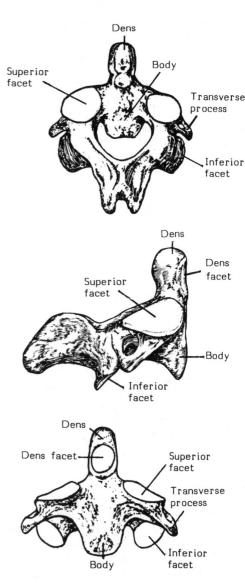

Figure 3.15. *Top,* the axis, viewed from the superoposterior; *middle,* viewed laterally; bottom, viewed from the anterior (Courtesy ACAP).

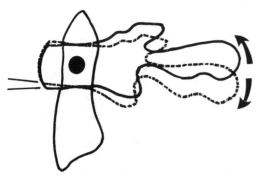

Figure 3.14. During atlantoaxial flexion and extension, the atlas slides up and down on the odontoid in relation to the instantaneous axis of rotation (black dot). The longer lever arm posteriorly produces far more motion posteriorly than anteriorly (Courtesy ACAP).

Atlantoaxial Rotation

During normal movement, the occiput and atlas move as one about the odontoid process of the axis (Fig. 3.15). [See Clinical Comment 3.3] Keep in mind that the odontoid of the axis is usually firmly attached to the occiput via the ligament complex. These ligaments (especially the alar ligaments, transverse cruciate, and the apophyseal capsules of the axis) tend to restrict C2 rotation on C3 as compared to the wide range allowed by the atlas. Although the inferior facets of the atlas and the superior facets of the axis may both be concave (as viewed on film), their articular cartilages are biconvex.

The inferior facets of the atlas are the flattest of any in the spine, and the superior facets of the axis are convex and slope slightly downward laterally. This pivotal design offers a gap anteriorly and posteriorly between the facets as much as 2—5 mm. In addition, the extremely loose and wide articular capsules of the C1—C2 joint, which enter the articular space on each side to form a meniscus-like fold of synovium, probably allow the greatest degree of inherent instability present in the cervical spine. It is for these reasons that misdiagnosis of axial instability is a common orthopedic error. During cineroentgenographic studies, the atlas appears to almost fall off the superior facets of the axis during maximum rotation.

About half of active cervical rotation takes place at the atlantoaxial joints about the odontoid process, with the remaining half distributed fairly evenly among the other cervical joints. During rotation, the odontoid represents a peg encased within an enclosed ring or a stake surrounded by a horseshoe. C1 rotation normally occurs about the dens of C2, which serves as a pivot.

As mentioned, 50% of total neck rotation occurs between C1 and C2 before any rotation is noted from C2 to C7 or at the occipitoatlantal joint. After about 30° of atlas rotation on the dens, the body of the axis begins to rotate (Fig. 3.16), followed by progressively diminishing rotation in the remaining cervical segments. Because the occipitoatlantal and atlantoaxial apophyseal articulations are not horizontal, rotation must be accompanied by a degree of coupled tilting.

Atlantoaxial rotation is powered by the obliquus capitis and rectus capitis posterior major, with help offered by the ipsilateral splenius capitis (Fig. 3.17) and the contralateral sternocleidomastoideus. During maximum atlantoaxial rotation in a supple spine, there is considerable kinking or stretching of the contralateral vertebral artery. Remembering this may save you from a malpractice suit.

If a complete fixation occurs between C1 and C2, the remaining cervical segments tend to become hypermobile in compensation. Thus, gross inspection of neck rotation (or other motions) should never be used to

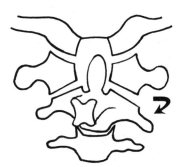

Figure 3.16. Rotatory fixation of the axis; right transverse rotated posterior on the right. The axis slips posteroinferiorly on the right and anterosuperiorly on the left, in accord with the planes of articulation (Courtesy ACAP).

DR. FAYE'S CLINICAL COMMENT #3.3

During normal movement Punjabi and White state the occiput and atlas move as one about the odontoid process of the axis (Fig. 3.15). However Kapandji states there is up to 11 degrees of rotation of the occiput on the atlas. With Gillet's method of palpation, we state that the occiput and atlas moving together is a fixation. As the occiput rotates around the y-axis, the tip of the atlas transverse should disappear from the palpator's finger. If Panjabi and White sources are correct we need a more accurate description of our atlas-occiput palpation methods.

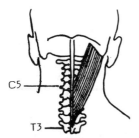

Figure 3.17. The splenius capitis (Courtesy ACAP).

evaluate the function of individual segments. Specific segmental motion palpation is always required. [See Clinical Comment 3.4]

The Lower Cervical Region

The IVDs of the lower cervical region normally contain an exceptional amount of elastin, which allows them to conform to the many possible planes of movement. Excessive flexion is limited by the ligamentous and muscular restraints on the separating posterior arches, and overextension is limited by bony apposition. Other factors include the resistance of the anular fibers to translation, the stiffness property of the anulus relative to its vertical height, and the physical barrier produced by the uncinate processes that are fully developed in late adolescence.

The Cervical Planes of Articulation

In the cervical region, the plane of articulation is almost perpendicular to the sagittal plane and inclined about 45° to the vertical plane. The lateral cervical gravity line extends from the apex of the odontoid process through the anterior portion of T2. The stable base between T1—T2 progressively changes upward so that the planes of articulation tend to be forced inferior, posterior, but not medially as in the thoracic and lumbar regions of the spine.

A horizontal locking-type base of support at the atlantoaxial articulation is similar to that found at the lumbosacral area. The inferior articular surfaces of the atlas offer a bilateral, medial, and inferior slant that forces the atlas to move inward toward the odontoid to allow rotary movements of the head. Excessive A-P and P-A movement is stabilized by the anterior and posterior rings and check ligaments. The posteromedially slanted cup-like superior articular surfaces of the atlas help stabilize the occipital articulating surfaces. These concave facets allow free rocking for flexion-extension nodding of the head.

From C3 to C7, the almost flat and thus freely mobile articular processes are found at the junction of the pedicles and laminae. The inferior facets face downward and forward, and glide on the superior facets of the vertebra below which face upward and backward. Maximum cervical A-P and P-A motions usually take place between C4 and C5. It should also be noted that it is almost impossible to actively flex the normal neck without causing some flexion in the upper thoracic region.

Facet Action

In the mid- and lower-cervical areas, A-P and P-A motion is a distinctly gliding translation because of the 45° facet planes and the biconcave vertebral bodies (Fig. 3.18). During flexion and extension, the superior vertebra's inferior facets slide anterosuperiorly during flexion and posteroinferiorly during extension on the inferior vertebra's superior facets. During full flexion, the facets may be almost if not completely separated. Thus, an adjustment force is usually contraindicated in the fully flexed position. The center of motion is often described as being within the superior aspect of the body of the subjacent vertebra.

DR. FAYE'S CLINICAL COMMENT #3.4

It is my hypothesis that many of the upper-cervical technique systems are more correctly explained from the biomechanical aspect than from the neurological interference theory. The mid- and lower-cervical hypermobilities cause a large percentage of cervical brachial syndromes. These hypermobilities are compensations to upper-cervical fixations in many cases.

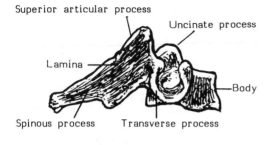

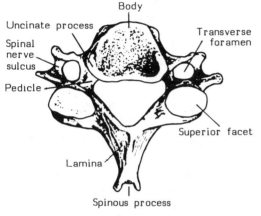

Figure 3.18. *Top,* side view of C4, showing major structural features; *bottom,* view of C4 from above (Courtesy ACAP).

Some pivotal tilting of the superior facets, backward in extension and forward in flexion, is also normal near the end of the range of motion. The facets also tend to separate (open) on the contralateral side of rotation and lateral bending. They appose (compress) during extension and on the ipsilateral side of rotation and lateral bending. Likewise, the foramina normally open on flexion, narrow on extension, close on the concave side of lateral bending, and open on the convex side of lateral bending. Because of the anterosuperior slant of the lower cervical facets, an inferior facet that moves downward must also slide posteriorly, and vice versa.

Any corrective adjustment must take into consideration the general extent of cervical lordosis, the *existing planes of articulation*, the *facet tilt present*, and the *amount of interfacet opening*, as well as any underlying pathologic process(es) involved, and applying just enough force during correction

to overcome the resistance of the fixation into the direction of the resistance.

Coupling Patterns

In the cervical spine, rotation about the Z axis is coupled to rotation about the Y axis, and vice versa; ie, during cervical lateral bending the cervical centra tend to rotate toward the concavity while the spinous processes swing in a larger arc towards the convexity. Note that this is exactly *opposite to the coupling action that occurs in the lumbar spine.* During cervical bending to the right, for example, the right facet of the superior vertebra slides down the facet plane and toward the posterior and the left facet slides up the facet incline and toward the anterior. This coupling phenomenon is exaggerated in circumstances in which an unusual ratio of axial rotation and lateral bending produces a subluxation or unilateral facet dislocation.

The amount of cervical rotation that is coupled with lateral flexion varies with the segmental level. At C2, for example, there is 1° of rotation with every 1.5° of lateral flexion. This 2:3 ratio changes caudally so that the degree of coupled rotation decreases. At C7, there is 1° of rotation for every 7.5° of lateral flexion, a 2:15 ratio.

Ranges of Motions

All cervical vertebrae from C2 to C7 partake in flexion, extension, rotation, and lateral bending, but some segments are more active in certain movements than others. In the C3—C7 area, flexion and extension occur as mild gliding translation of the upper on the lower facets, accompanied by appropriate disc distortion. The site of greatest movement in flexion is at the C4—C5 interface (Table 3.4), while extension movement is fairly well diffused. This fact probably accounts for the high incidence of arthritis at the midcervical area. Rotation below the axis is greatest near the C5—C6 level, slightly less above and considerably less below. Lateral bending in greatest at the C2—C5 levels and diminishes caudally. The arc of lateral

Table 3.4. Normal Ranges of Lower Cervical Motion

Motion Unit	Movement	Degrees	Motion Unit	Movement	Degrees
C2—C3	Flexion/extension	8	C5—C6	Flexion/extension	17
	Lateral bending	10		Lateral bending	8
	Rotation	9		Rotation	14
C3—C4	Flexion/extension	13	C6—C7	Flexion/extension	16
	Lateral bending	10		Lateral bending	7
	Rotation	12		Rotation	10
C4—C5	Flexion/extension	19	C7—T1	Flexion/extension	9
	Lateral bending	10		Lateral bending	4
	Rotation	12		Rotation	8

*These ranges are approximate. Authorities differ in several degrees in their reported findings. The above is a composite of findings.

motion is determined by the planes of the covertebral joints (if they are present). Faye points out that, for cervical lateral flexion, the first rib costotransverse joint must be mobile because it is an important component of the kinematic chain.

Lower Cervical Instability

Instability in the lower cervical region is rarely obvious in the ambulatory patient. The most important stabilizing agents in the mid- and lower-cervical spine are the anulus fibrosis, the anterior and posterior ligaments, and the muscles, especially, which serve as important contributing stabilizers. During dynamic palpation, states Faye, any segmental joint play found to be more than a "sponginess" should arouse suspicions of lack of ligament restraint. This is often accompanied by an audible click (similar to that heard during knuckle cracking).

Motion of the Transitional Cervicothoracic Area

In the cervicothoracic area, normal movement is somewhat similar to that in the lumbosacral area insofar as the type of stress (but not magnitude of load) to which both areas are subjected is similar. L5 has poor mobility on the sacrum and C7 has poor mobility on T1, with the major amount of movement in the cervicothoracic junction being at the C6—C7 interface and primarily that of rotation. Faye mentions that diminished cervicothoracic joint play is clinically significant in many chronic, stubborn cases.

Reversal of the Normal Cervical Curve

As opposed to the primary thoracic kyphosis which is a structural curve, the cervical and lumbar lordoses are functional arcs produced by their wedge-shaped IVDs (developed in the upright position). The cervical and lumbar curves normally flatten in the non-weight-bearing supine position. Likewise, they adapt comparatively fast to changes involving the direction of force. Adaptation in the thoracic spine takes much longer.

The force of gravity on the cervical lordosis normally falls just anterior to the support of the posterior cervical musculature. When the cervical curve flattens, a larger workload is placed on the musculature of the neck to maintain biomechanical integrity. A pathologic straightening of the normal anterior curve of the cervical spine, as viewed in a lateral weight-bearing x-ray film, results in mechanical alteration of normal physiologic and structural integrity. The normal vertical line of gravity, as viewed laterally, falls near or through the odontoid and touches the anterior border of T2. As the cervical spine tends to flatten in the erect position, the gravity line passes closer to the center of the cervical discs.

While the cervical curve is the first secondary curve to develop in the infant, its maintenance in the erect posture is primarily determined by the integrity of the lumbar curve when the spine is supple. Faye considers the angle of the thorax an equally important factor; ie, the sternum should face slightly upward. A flattened cervical spine that is not compensatory to a flattened lumbar spine is usually the result of a local disorder such as a subluxation syndrome caused by facets fixed in flexion, posterior shifting of one or more disc nuclei, hypertonicity of the anterior musculature, or anterior ligamentous shortening as the result of local overstress, inflammation, occupational posture, or congenital anomaly.

A flattened cervical spine in the erect posture resembles a normal spine during flexion. To appreciate the mechanisms involved, it is well to review the biomechanics involved: The nucleus of the disc serves as a fulcrum during flexion and return extension. When the spine is subjected to bending loads during flexion, half of the disc on the convex side suffers tension, widens, and contracts, while the other half of the disc on the concave side suffers compression, thins, and bulges. Concurrently, the nucleus bulges on the side of tension and contracts on the side of compression, which increases tension on the adjacent anulus. This creates a self-stabilizing counteracting flexion force to the motion unit that aids a return to the resting position.

In a reduced curve (cervical hypolordosis), Bergmann reminds us that more weight has to be born on the vertebral bodies and discs; while in an increased curve (hyperlordosis), more weight must be borne by the facets. The shape of the vertebra and angles of the facet and disc determine the degree of lordosis. If through degenerative changes and/or stress responses these are altered, the "normal" arc of the curve will be changed.

Numerous studies relating ideas of what the normal curve should be have been conducted, and most seem to be in agreement that the cervical lordosis extends down to T2, with C5 being the midpoint or "stress" vertebra (Fig. 3.19). Flattening of the cervical curve is often the result of perispinal spasm secondary to an underlying injury, irritation, or inflammatory process. The latter may be the result of a lower primary fixation.

Symptomatology. The acute clinical picture can be torticollis. Other manifestations may include headaches (occipital, occipitofrontal, or supraorbital), vertigo, tenderness elicited on lateral C4—C6 nerve roots, neuritis involving branches of the brachial plexus owing to nerve root irritation, hyperesthesia of one or more fingers, and loss or lessening of the biceps reflex on the same or contralateral side. In less frequent situations, the triceps reflex may be involved. One or more symptoms are frequently aggravated by an abnormal position of the head such as during reading in bed, an awkward sleeping position, prolonged typing, or long-distance driving.

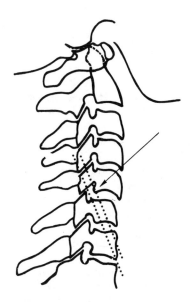

Figure 3.19. Film tracing of a flattened cervical curve. Enlargement of an IVF (with consequential stretching of attached dural sleeve) as the result of a flexion fixation of C5 on C4 (Courtesy ACAP).

Effect of Atlas Position. It has been postulated by several authorities that the cervical curvature directs the position of the atlas; ie, a hyperlordotic cervical spine is compensated by the atlas moving superiorly and that a flattened curve is compensated for by the atlas moving inferiorly. After studying the lateral cervical films of 109 patients, however, Ng has shown statistically that malposition of the atlas in the A-P plane does not necessarily accompany an alteration of the cervical curve. No significant correlation could be found between the atlantopalatal angle and the degree of cervical curvature, thus indicating that an anterosuperior atlas does not necessarily accompany cervical hyperlordosis or vice versa.

DIAGNOSTIC CONSIDERATIONS

Dynamic Palpation of the Cervical Region

The objectives of dynamic palpation are to note (1) normal and abnormal segmental motion and (2) motion restrictions, "jumps," erratic gliding, and motion smoothness. Bilateral motion quantity and quality are primary concerns because of their influence of the health of the individual, biomechanically and neurologically.

During motion palpation, *each* cervical motion unit is palpated during flexion, extension, rotation, and lateral flexion to assess segmental mobility and end play. The amount of motion in any particular joint primarily depends on (1) the shape of the joint surface, (2) the laxity or tautness of supporting ligaments, and (3) the tone of the related musculature. See Figure 3.20. The extent of movement below the axis is primarily dependent upon ligamentous and muscular laxity and the distortion and compressibility of the IVDs. On this point, Faye includes the joints of Lushka.

The "joints" of Lushka (or uncovertebral joints) are not found in a large percentage of the population. Jeffrey's points out that an academic controversy has existed for many years of whether these clefts on the cervical segments are true synovial joints. The current orthodox teaching is that they begin as stress fissues of the annular fibers, which appear in the second decade of life, and are later converted into cartilage-lined joint surfaces.

Cervical Muscle Considerations

Gillet's investigations have shown that several deep short muscles are found in the cervical region that have a tendency toward hypertonicity and therefore fixation. It must be emphasized, however, that most of them are reflexively influenced by lower primary fixations and, thus, not necessarily in need of manipulation. They often require trigger-point therapy and/or massage for the fibrotic changes, states Faye who adds that this is a difficult area for electrotherapy.

The Intertransversarii. The cervical muscles most involved in a muscular fixation, according to Gillet, are the anterior and posterior intertransversaii that assist lateral bending, usually working reciprocally. When hypertonic, however, they often act separately. Acting together unilaterally, they pull the top vertebra of a motion unit into lateral flexion with a certain amount of rotation because of the plane of articulation of the cervical segments. When acting bilaterally, they assist forward flexion. When fixed in flexion, they tend to produce a segmental or area hypolordosis or, at times, kyphosis.

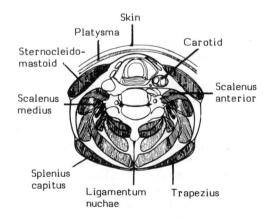

Figure 3.20. Diagram of a transverse section at the midcervical area showing the relative arrangement of the cervical musculature (Courtesy ACAP).

Chronic hypertonicity of the anterior intertransversaii forces flexion even when the spine is in the neutral resting position. The involved segments will be hypolordotic, hypermobility will be found at the extreme posterior elements of the vertebrae, and segmental extension will be restricted. The same state can occur in reverse when the posterior transversarii become fixed in extension; ie, flexion will be restricted. At times, intertransversaii fixation will be found both anteriorly and posteriorly. Both of these pairs of muscles can limit motion (lateral bending especially, and rotation partially), although they do so to a lesser degree than the rotatores and multifidi.

Because these muscles are so small, deep, and so close to each other, it is often difficult to determine which are responsible for any given restriction or dysfunction. Fortunately, hypertonic muscles can often be palpated as abnormal bulges, and this is especially true when they are put under tension. In many cases, they are secondary and recur if primary fixations in the subluxation complex are not adjusted.

The Multifidi and Rotatores. In the mid and lower cervical region, it seems that the multifidi muscles are more apt to be abnormal. Around the axis and C3, however, Gillet has found that the rotatores are often found to be responsible. Each type of fixation has, fortunately, its type of motion in which it is felt more easily during motion palpation. The multifidi arise from the transverse processes of the cervical vertebrae and insert on the spinous process of the segment above, assisting in extension and rotation. The rotatores are a series of small muscles that span deep in a groove between the spinous and transverse processes of each vertebrae, assisting in extension and rotation toward the opposite side.

The Interspinales. The interspinal muscles are short bands of well-developed muscle fibers that extend bilaterally between the spinous processes of contiguous vertebrae, assisting in extension. Hypertonicity contributes to hyperlordosis. This exaggerated lordosis may be short, and the hypertonic muscles involved are usually easily discernible. It becomes especially visible when the patient's neck is passively moved into maximum forward flexion. Although this type of fixation is common, Gillet believes it is rarely pathogenic.

The Oblique Muscles of the Head. The obliquus capitis superior arises from the transverse processes of the atlas and insert broadly on the occiput, helping to extend

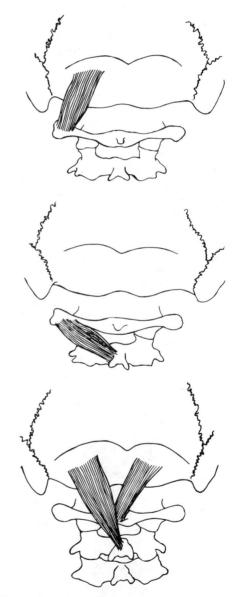

Figure 3.21. *Top,* left obliquus capitis superior muscle; *middle,* left obliquus capitis inferior; *bottom,* left rectus capitis posterior major and right rectus capitis posterior minor (Courtesy ACAP).

and move the head laterally. The obliquus capitis inferior arises from the spinous process of the axis and inserts on the transverse processes of the atlas, assisting in rotating the atlas and head. When these muscles are hypertonic on one side, the axis can be pulled laterally. See Figure 3.21.

The Rectus Capitis Group. The rectus capitis posterior major arises from the spinous process of the axis and inserts broadly on the occiput, assisting in extension of the head (Fig. 3.22). When hypertonic, the occiput is rotated backward upon the spinous process of the axis, obliterating the space over the posterior tubercle of the atlas and thus producing atlantal hyperlordosis. It is usually caused by a primary fixation found much lower in the spine, according to Gillet (eg, anterior thoracic body fixation). The rectus capitis posterior minor arises from the posterior tubercle of the atlas and broadly inserts on the occiput, assisting in extension of the head. The rectus capitis lateralis originates on the transverse process of the atlas and inserts on the jugular process of the occiput (Fig. 3.23), assisting in flexion and stabilization of the occiput on the atlas. The rectus capitis anterior arises from the lateral masses of the atlas and broadly insert on the basilar part of the occiput, also assisting in flexion and stability of the cranium.

The Longus Colli. The superior oblique portions of the long muscles of the neck arise from the C3—C5 transverse processes and insert on the anterior tubercle of the atlas, assisting in cervical flexion and stabilization. Spasm or chronic contraction of the cervical longus colli produces a clinical picture that is opposite to that of rectus capitis major fixations. The head is pulled down and forward, opening the space between the occiput and the axis, thus producing atlantal kyphosis.

The Longus Capitis. The long muscles of the head arise from the C3—C6 transverse processes and insert at the occiput, assisting in flexion of the head. Hypertonicity contributes to flattening of the cervical curve.

The Occipito-Atlanto-Axial Complex

The occipital condyles, atlas, and axis function as a unit with unique characteristics. The normally ball-and-socket-type artic-

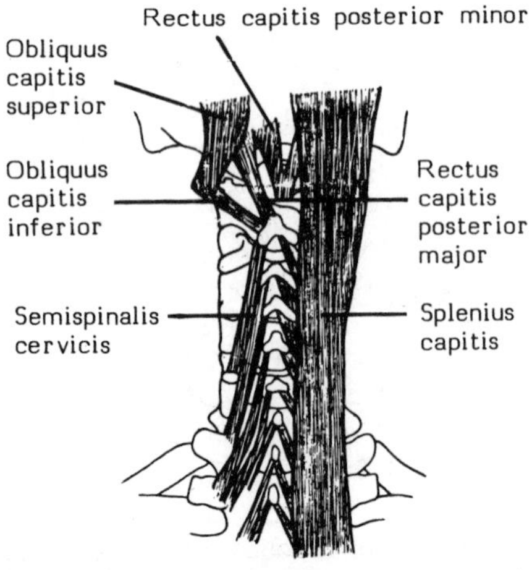

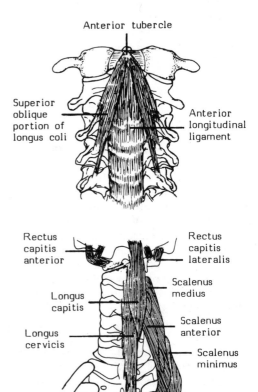

Figure 3.22. Some major posterior cervical muscles (Courtesy ACAP).

Figure 7.23. *Top,* the major prevertebral ligaments; *bottom,* the major prevertebral muscles (Courtesy ACAP).

ulations at the occipitoatlantal joint allow flexion, extension, slight lateral flexion, and rotation end play. The facets of the atlas and axis are both convex. This allows considerable rotation and minimal lateral flexion, and their loose capsules and ligamentous straps allow significant flexion and extension. The axis, however, has more ligamentous attachments with the skull than does the atlas. Dove describes how many of these attachments bypass the atlas as does the spinal dura. The muscles that attach to the axis extend widely to the skull and atlas above, and to all the lower cervicals, upper five thoracics, first rib, and scapulae.

Craton reports that differences in area size of the two condyle-glenoid groove surfaces results in different articular mobility. The least mobile articulation exhibits the least erosion of the cartilage plates, and he suggests that a condyle sideslip with a counterclockwise rotation is the cause of the variable erosion and size.

Occipital-Atlantal Palpation

The occipitoatlantal junctions are typically described as ball-and-socket-type joints, where the condyle "ball" is elipsoid and its axis is transverse. This, states Dove, permits flexion-extension and a slight amount of rotation and lateral flexion. However, Rude, a German investigator, has shown that the occipital condyles vary greatly in shape, and the specific design of the facets determines their movement. While typically convex, many condyles have been found to be square, rhomboidal, rectangular, flat, prismatic, concave (rare), and some have split forms. Flattened and angular condyle facets allow great slipping and tipping during motion. A convex condyle facet allows only rotary slippage if the corresponding atlantoid facet has a similar radius. These facts should be kept in mind during occipitoatlantal motion palpation.

Note: All motion-palpation procedures described in this chapter are conducted with the patient in the standard sitting posture and the doctor sitting directly behind the patient. As previously mentioned, a motion palpation station is used to allow the doctor to swing sideways for greater leverage and ease.

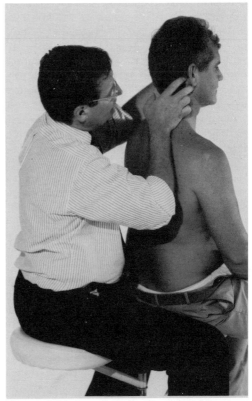

Figure 3.24. Locating the tip of the right transverse process of the atlas at the start of atlantal motion palpation.

Rotation of the Occiput on the Atlas. Place the pad of your palpating finger on the tip of a transverse process of the patient's atlas (Fig. 3.24). With your stabilizing hand on the patient's skull, rotate the patient's head slowly to one side, then to the other side (Fig. 3.25). Avoid any flexion, extension, or lateral bending of the patient's neck. This is enhanced by using your palpating finger as a fulcrum. Repeat with your palpating finger on the patient's contralateral transverse process. You will be able to feel the transverse process glide behind the mandible when the patient's head is fully rotated to the side of palpation. If the joint is fixed, this motion will be absent. Occipital rotational end play is sometimes a difficult motion to palpate because of the bulging of the sternocleidomastoideus tendon. Obviously, Gillet and Faye support those authors who report occipital rotation on the atlas because it is palpable.

Flexion-Extension of the Occiput on the Atlas. This is a remarkable two-phase process. During the first phase, the occiput anteflexes on the atlas. During the second phase of flexion, however, Snijders/Timmerman state that the occiput retroflexes relative to the atlas and axis during flexion-extension of the neck.

With your stabilizing hand supporting the patient's vertex, place your palpating finger into the small space between the lateral tip of a transverse process of the atlas and the ramus of the patient's jaw (Fig. 3.26). Push the patient's head with your stabilizing hand so that the patient's chin moves directly forward, parallel to the floor. Have patience in your practice of this palpation, as the skill can be difficult to master. If there is no unilateral fixation, you should feel the space between the transverse process and the jaw open wider. (The pushing hand on the crown of the patient's head should feel for the springy end feel, states Faye.) Then bring the

patient's occiput backward, tucking the patient's chin inward against the throat (Fig. 3.27). If there is no unilateral fixation in flexion, the space being palpated will narrow and sometimes become lost to the touch. Repeat this procedure on the contralateral side.

During this evaluation, the ramus of the jaw may be felt to flip distinctly superior rather than rolling anterior. Gillet believes that this hinge-type motion (rather than a rolling motion) is the result of hypertonicity of the rectus posterior minor muscle, either unilateral or bilateral, that produces restricted motion of the posterior atlas but free motion of the anterior atlas. If this is the case, forced motion will produce a shear force. On the other hand, if the anterior muscles are hypertonic, the anterior aspect of the condyle will be compressed against the anterior lateral mass of the atlas, while the posterior aspect opens. This can be palpated on forced motion by placing the palpating

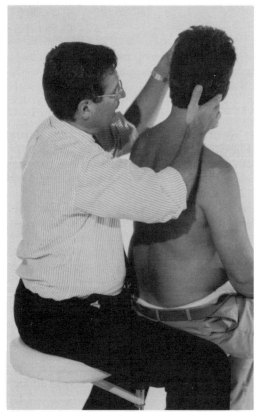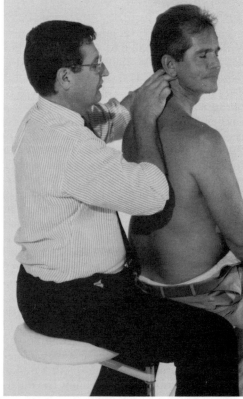

Figure 3.25. *Left,* checking right-to-left rotation of the occiput on the atlas; *right,* left-to-right rotation.

finger in the posterior aspect of the transverse mastoid space while the patient's head is moved into maximum extension and flexion.

Lateral Bending of the Occiput on the Atlas. Place your palpating finger over the tip of a transverse process of the patient's atlas. Place your stabilizing hand on the patient's vertex and flex the crown laterally (Fig. 3.28), first toward one side and then toward the other, taking care to localize motion at the occipitoatlantal level. Avoid midcervical motion by using your palpating finger as a fulcrum. If fixation is absent, you will be able to feel the space above the transverse process open and close as you laterally flex the patient's head away and toward your palpating finger. Again, states Faye, the hand stabilizing the patient's crown feels for joint end play.

Differentiating Occipitoatlantal Mus-

cular and Articular Fixations. The tip of the palpating finger is placed under the posterior occiput, midway between the occipital notch and the mastoid process (Fig. 3.29). Some examiners prefer to cup the atlas in the web of the palpating hand so that the thumb palpates one side while the middle finger palpates the other side. The supporting hand rocks the patient's head into flexion and extension. If a stubborn articular fixation exists, the fibrous tissues will feel like a hard mass that does not change texture during motion. This feeling is characteristic and different from the softness of the tissues surrounding a freely or partially movable atlas. You also have an opportunity here of changing hands and palpating the same spot on the other side. Keep in mind that if a *total* fixation is evident unilaterally, the atlas will not be able to move on the contralateral side even if all tissues there feel normal.

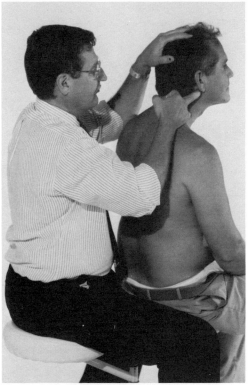

Figure 3.26. Palpating the depression anterior to the right transverse process of the atlas during evaluation of flexion-extension of the occiput on the atlas.

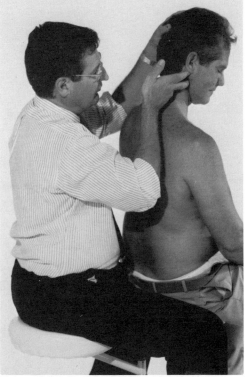

Figure 3.27. Position for checking A-P motion of the occiput on the atlas.

An important exception to the rule that the amount of irritation decreases with the degree of fixation is found with total fixation of the occipitoatlantal joints. Here, for some unknown reason, there is almost never degeneration in the soft tissues and the fixation remains in an acute stage, according to Gillet. Thus, in this disorder, the amount of signs of irritation increases with the degree of fixation.

Atlantal-Axial Palpation

Rotation of the Atlas on the Axis. The pads of the first three fingers are placed horizontally in the suboccipital space so that the first finger firmly presses against the occipital notch, the second finger rests in the space over the posterior tubercle of the atlas, and the third finger rests lightly on the tip of the C2 spinous process. The free hand is used to rotate the head. During passive rotation, sev-

eral degrees of atlas rotation should take place before the axis begins to move. Normally, the third finger will slip on the spinous process of the axis as the head is rotated because the head moves 1 cm or more prior to axial motion. Bilateral atlantoaxial fixation is indicated if the axis immediately follows the movement of the head (primarily the atlas), noted by the third finger not gliding over the process of the axis. If unilateral (pivotal) fixation is present, this situation will occur during rotation to one side but not to the other, and the center of movement will be at the point of fixation rather than at the odontoid. If the axis is fixed unilaterally, rotary movement will also be felt on the free side during A-P motion.

Faye also checks the mobility of atlas-axis rotation by placing the pads of the palpating fingers against the pillars of the upper cervical vertebra. He pronates his wrist and palm and holds his elbow horizontal during this palpation (Fig. 3.30). At the extreme of pas-

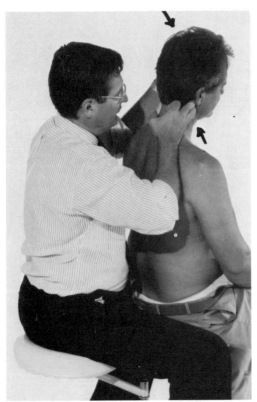

Figure 3.28. Position for checking lateral bending to the right of the occiput on the atlas.

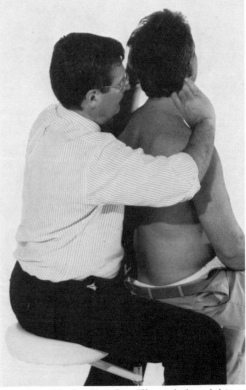

Figure 3.29. Position for differentiating right occipitoatlantal muscular and articular disorders.

sive rotation, he uses an end push to judge the integrity of end play. During atlantal-axial A-P rotation, facet translation is judged with the fingertips placed on the anterolateral aspect of the transverse process of the atlas (Fig. 3.31). These P-A and A-P motions, as all motions, must be checked bilaterally.

Lateral Bending of the Atlas on the Axis. Active lateral bending of the atlas on the axis is questioned by some authorities, but an important and distinct end play can be palpated in healthy spines. It has been Gillet's experience that abnormal lateral flexion of the atlas on the axis is affected most by hypertonicity of the intertransversarii and/or the upper part of the longus colli. Motion restriction can be determined by placing the tip of the palpating finger in the posterolateral space between the transverse processes of the atlas and axis and making contact on the atlas close to the rim of the occiput posterolaterally (Fig. 3.32). It

is often necessary to slip off the occiput to contact the atlas. The fulcrum for lateral bending is at the palpating finger, and a springy end feel is tested before any lower cervicals begin movement. Remember, in this type of motion palpation, we are palpating for fixation at the end of the passive range of motion. We are not palpating the gross motion available. Our palpation is a *joint challenge*, and we try to determine if the resistance is (1) more than normal but a springy muscular fixation exists, (2) more than normal with an abrupt end feel, or (3) abrupt with an end feel in all directions.

While intertransversarii hypertonicity restricts lateral bending, a small degree of lateral gliding of the atlas on the axis is usually allowed. This does not appear to be true when hypertonicity of the longus colli exists or if articular fixation is present.

Flexion-Extension of the Atlas on the Axis. Palpate between the transverse proc-

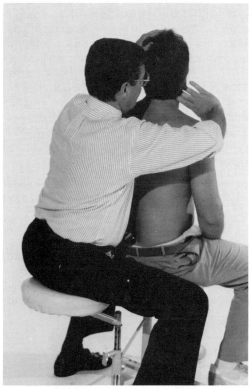

Figure 3.30. Position for checking atlas-axis motion during cervical rotation to the left.

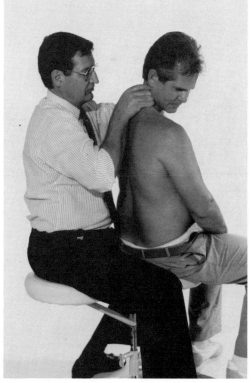

Figure 3.31. Position for checking facet translation during A-P atlantal-axial rotation to the posterior on the right.

esses of the atlas and axis during passive flexion-extension of the patient's head. During normal motion, you should feel the transverse process of the atlas glide forward (anteriorly) during flexion and return (posteriorly) to neutral during extension (Fig. 3.33). [See Clinical Comment 3.5] Keep in mind that there cannot be true posterior extension translation of the atlas on the axis from the neutral position because of the odontoid process. Only tipping can occur.

Another method is to place the palpating finger in the space between the posterior tubercle of the atlas and the spinous of the axis. This space should open on flexion and close on extension of the neck, and the posterior tubercle should become more apparent on flexion and be lost to touch on extension of the neck.

Occipital and Lower Cervical Relationships

The occiput and axis are not structurally adjacent, thus cannot articulate, but, as previously described, they are combined into a function unit by ligaments, fascia, and several deep cervical muscles, which, when shortened, pull the occiput and lower cervicals into hyperlordosis. This type of fixation is sensed by putting the pads of the palpating fingers into the interspinous spaces, placing your stabilizing hand on the patient's vertex, and then conducting the patient's head into full upper-cervical flexion and extension.

For example, hypertonicity of the rectus capitis posterior major and minor produces extension of the occiput toward the spinous process of the axis in the neutral resting position. The upper- and mid-cervical interspinous spaces will feel closed even during passive flexion of the neck. Hypertonicity of the superior oblique portion of the longus colli and/or rectus capitis anterior and lateralis pull the cervical spine into flexion. The interspinous spaces will feel open even on forced passive extension of the neck. [See Clinical Comment 3.6]

Lower Cervical Palpation

All cervical vertebrae from C2 to C7 partake in flexion, extension, rotation, and lateral flexion, but some segments (eg, C5) are more active than others. Refer to Table 3.4.

Lateral Flexion of C2—C7. The mid and lower cervicals are palpated in lateral bend-

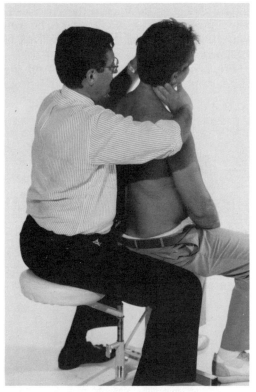

Figure 3.32. Position for evaluating lateral bending to the right of the atlas on the axis.

DR. FAYE'S CLINICAL COMMENT #3.5

I palpate the posterolateral portion of the posterior arch of atlas with my wrist pronated and push into extension when the head is extended. For flexion I palpate the anterior of the tip of the atlas transverse. To achieve this the wrist is supinated and the middle finger comes in from the ramus of the jaw to make very gentle contact on the atlas transverse tip. As the head is nodded gentle pressure posterior with the palpating finger determines if joint play is present. The loss of joint play here is very painful, and a cough reflex is elicited if too much pressure is exerted.

ing as moving away from the side of flexion. To evaluate lateral gliding, place your thumb or the pad of your pronated middle finger firmly against the posterolateral aspect of the spinous processes or on the articular pillars of the segments being evaluated, while your supporting hand moves the patient's head in wide lateral flexion (refer to Fig. 3.32). Laterally flex the patient's head over your palpating finger, which will serve as a fulcrum, and check for additional joint play at the end of passive motion.

The importance of palpable asymmetry in response to passive cervical sidebending has been clearly brought out by Johnston and associates who concluded that it appears to be an early indicator of a measurable impairment of cervical function, even in the absence of pain or other complaints. Thus, the role of segmental motion palpation in preventive health-care is underscored.

Segmental motion studies should not be confused with gross motion studies. When a motion-unit becomes dysfunctional, it exhibits asymmetric behavior that is palpable. In addition, secondary (compensatory) effects spread to adjacent units, usually within three segments, which does not necessarily

---

DR. FAYE'S CLINICAL COMMENT #3.6

The greatest relationship to upper-cervical fixation is a mid- or lower-cervical hypermobility. The neutral lateral radiograph will miss this finding; however, the lateral views of flexion and extension will elicit the hypermobility. More than 3 or 4 mm of stair-stepping is an instability and a sign of ligament pathology. This sign often occurs 6 months after a "whiplash" injury especially if pain occurred within 24 hours of the accident and even if the patient became pain free in less than 6 months. It is worth noting post-traumatic fixations of the upper thoracics; the upper costotransverse joints and the sternoclavicular joints can all contribute to the need for hypermobility of the middle and lower cervicals.

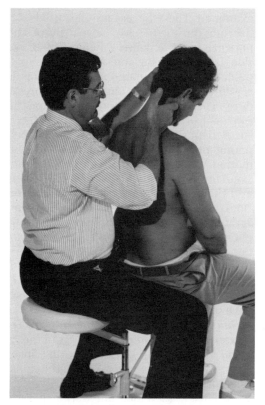 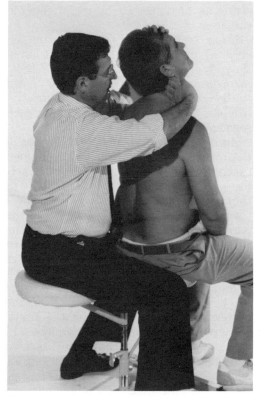

Figure 3.33. Palpating the transverse processes of C1 and C2 during flexion of the atlas on the axis: from the anterior during flexion *(left),* from the posterior during extension *(right).*

limit regional function. Only in advanced stages where multiple units are involved will overt regional motion be affected.

Flexion-Extension of C2—C7. To check P-A motion and joint play of any mid- or lower-cervical vertebra, place the pad of your pronated middle finger on the articular pillars of the motion unit being examined (refer to Fig. 3.33). With your other hand (the stabilizer), cup the patient's forehead in your palm. Place the patient's neck in full passive extension, using the palpating finger as a fulcrum at each level, and check for additional joint play at the end of each motion by applying a digital push with your contact finger. Also note the separation and closure of the spinous process on P-A and A-P motion. A-P motion is checked in a similar manner as P-A motion except that the pad of the palpating finger is placed against the anterolateral surface of the transverse processes and the patient's neck is flexed. You will have to pull the sternocleidomastoideus slightly back and lateral to make contact. Be gentle, as the tissues are normally tender in this area.

In the cervical spine, flexion and extension occur around a horizontal axis that lies in the body of the vertebra below. For C2, Bergmann locates it in the posteroinferior area of the body of C3 and states that it progressively moves anteriorly and superiorly for each segment caudally.

Anterior Rotation of C2—C7. Areas of P-A rotatory fixation are easily determined except in the individual with extremely heavy neck muscles. In evaluating rotation to the anterior, the palpating finger is slid down the posterolateral aspect of the neck as the patient's neck is passively rotated with the stabilizing hand. The palpation is made with the pad of the pronated middle finger after pushing the sternocleidomastoideus anterior and the upper trapezius backward (refer to Fig. 3.30). The palpation is against the posterolateral tissues between the transverse processes or along the apophyses. In checking motion, rotate the patient's head to one side and then to the other, checking for additional joint play at the end of full passive rotation. A firm "bulge" will be evident over the restricted transverse, and this is usually attributed to a hypertonic multifidus or in-

tertransversarii muscle. Palpation in the middle and lower cervical region can be difficult because the palpating finger can be against tender nerves. Because of this, some examiners prefer lamina palpation.

Posterior Rotation of C2—C7. In evaluating rotation to the posterior, the pad of the palpating finger is moved down the anterolateral side of the cervical transverse processes while the neck is rotated posteriorly on the same side by the stabilizing hand on the patient's crown (refer to Fig. 3.31). During this palpation, the palpating finger tugs slightly upward and backward to pull the sternocleidomastoideus muscle out of the way. Such palpation must be extremely gentle as the underlying tissues are normally highly sensitive. Avoid contact with the carotid artery.

Simultaneous Extension, Lateral Bending, and Posterior-to-Anterior Rotation of C2—C7. A posterior contact is taken with the pad of the middle or index finger against the articular processes being examined. These fingers are also used as a fulcrum during passive movement of the patient's head to control the level of extension, lateral bending, and rotation. The palpating hand is pronated, and the elbow is raised to the horizontal during this procedure. The stabilizing hand, placed on the forehead or vertex of the patient, extends the patient's neck backward while your palpating finger checks segmental extension motion. With the patient's head still in extension, the neck is rotated first toward one side and then toward the other to check posterior-to-anterior rotation. The patient's head is then returned to the neutral position, the palpating fingers are slid to an adjacent motion unit, and the procedure is repeated. This polymotion procedure should only be used after all standard cervical orthopedic, vertebral artery patency, and thoracic outlet tests have proved negative.

Simultaneous Flexion and Anterior-to-Posterior Rotation of C2—C7. Contact is taken with the pad of the palpating finger against the anterolateral aspect of the transverse processes being examined. This finger is also used as a fulcrum during passive movement of the patient's head to control the level of flexion-rotation. The stabilizing hand, placed on the forehead or vertex of the patient, rolls the patient's head down and forward, tucking in the patient's chin, to check segmental forward flexion. With the patient's head still in forward flexion, the patient's neck is turned toward the side of palpation to check A-P rotation. During this maneuver, the palpating finger must be controlled by bringing it backward and upward, tugging against the sternocleidomastoideus muscle so that it will not hinder the palpation. After a motion unit has been checked, the patient's head is returned to the neutral position, the palpating fingers are slid to an adjacent motion unit, and the procedure is repeated.

Long-Axis Tension (Elongation). To evaluate the degree of distraction available between the facets of the segments of the cervical spine and the adaptability of the IVDs to tensile forces, place the patient in the supine position. Stand or sit facing the head of the table. Take a bilateral index or middle finger contact on the lamina of each segment, one at a time, and apply moderate traction, keeping the patient's neck in the neutral position by avoiding flexion or extension. The patient's skull should be supported by your palms. You should be able to feel a slight separation at each level.

Common Types of Mid- and Lower-Cervical Fixations. The two most common types of fixation in this area, states Faye, are those involving (1) simultaneous extension, lateral bending, and P-A rotation, and (2) simultaneous flexion and A-P rotation. [See Clinical Comment 3.7]

Interspinous fixation. Hypertonicity of one or more extensors tends to bind spinous processes together so that a segmental lordosis is formed. This condition, often found at the C3—C4 level, is palpable when the spinous processes refuse to open during passive flexion. It is also often evident on lateral stress films during forward flexion where two or more vertebrae do not follow the curve of the neck as a whole.

Covertebral articular fixation. Fixation is common at the lips of the joints of Luschka by longus colli hypertonicity, ligamentous shortening, and exostosis. See Figure 3.34. If it is found during passive motions that the patient's neck stops sharply at a point far short of normal motion, Gillet refers to this "brick wall" sign of strong restriction as an indication of cervical osteophytes. This is a classic sign of chronic degeneration found in the cervical joints of the elderly exhibiting a "dry" cervical spine. These fixations often produce chronic brachialgia.

The joints (or fissures) of Luschka (the uncovertebral joints of the cervical spine)

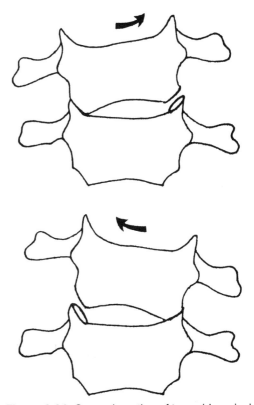

Figure 3.34. Coronal section of two midcervical vertebrae showing the motion of lateral flexion created by the planes of the uncovertebral joints (Courtesy ACAP).

DR. FAYE'S CLINICAL COMMENT #3.7

These restrictions of motion are often caused by covertebral articular fixation and spinous processes that refuse to separate during passive flexion. The doctor must be sure his technique not only affects the posterior intervertebral joints but also affects the joints of Luschka and the interspinous soft tissues.

are located on the anterolateral surfaces of the vertebral body and act as tracts that guide the motion of coupled rotation and lateral flexion and limit sidebending. These saddle-like joints, states Bergmann, begin development between the ages of 6 and 9 and are complete at 18 years. Whether they are true synovial joints is highly controversial. Gehweiler and associates feel that they represent functional adaptation by the cervical IVDs to the increased mobility of the cervical vertebrae at the time that the uncinate processes are reaching their full height. However, as these joints are not found in a large percentage of the population, some authorities feel that they are strictly an effect of degeneration.

Compensation in Lumbopelvic Scoliosis. During any type of lumbopelvic distortion where the sacral base has assumed an unnatural position, cervical accommodation normally occurs to maintain the eyes horizontally forward and near the midline. However, because the occipito-atlanto-axial complex allows only slight lateral bending, scoliotic compensation must occur *below* the axis. If this does not occur in habitually maintaining the axis on the horizontal plane, stress on the dura mater above will be produced. Thus, it can be acknowledged that any problem from above or below that interferes with the role of the axis will produce problems with considerable scope because of the extensive myofascial relationships. For this reason, Dove recommends that the function of the axis be checked in each case where problems manifest in the head, cervical area, upper thoracic area, and shoulder girdle.

Assessing Segmental Mobility Objectively

Physical Mensuration

Gillet's system of measurement has always recognized that there could be possibilities by which hypermobile segments could take up the motion that did not occur in hypomobile motion units. The actual occurrence of this in a particular patient may or may not be true. For those who desire to collect ob-

jective data, following are some techniques to show unequal ranges of motions:

1. *Lateral bending.* The head of a sitting patient is flexed to the side, taking care to prevent the shoulders from following this movement. With the patient in this position, a dot is placed on the tip of the C7 spinous process. A short plumb line is then dropped from the posterior-superior aspect of the ear, and the point where it strikes the shoulder is marked. The same is done during lateral bending to the other side. The distance from these two shoulder points to the midline dot over C7 are then compared to note discrepancies in the ROM of cervical lateral bending.

2. *Rotation.* Gillet prefers to measure rotation rather than lateral bending because it appears that the influence of hypermobile vertebrae shows up less in this movement. Rotate the head of the sitting patient to the maximum with one hand, taking care that the patient's shoulders do not move from the neutral position. With the patient in this position, drop a short plumb line from the tip of the patient's ipsilateral ear and mark where it strikes the shoulder on a level with the C7. Do the same after rotating the patient's head toward the other side. The distance from these two shoulder points to the midline dot over C7 are then compared to note discrepancies in the ROM of cervical rotation.

3. *Extension and flexion.* To measure cervical extension, stand to the side of the sitting patient. With your stabilizing hand on the patient's scalp, slowly tilt the patient's head into extension on the neck without disturbing the neutral position of the patient's shoulders. Drop a short plumb line from the back of the patient's ear to the patient's shoulder. Obviously, the greater the degree of backward flexibility, the farther posterior the line will strike the patient's shoulder girdle. In extremely flexible patients, the line may fall posterior to the patient's spine. This same process can be reversed to evaluate cervical flexion.

The above measurements evaluate only gross cervical motion. They do not show specific sites of segmental hypomobility and/or hypermobility. These must be determined by motion palpation and roentgenographic analyses. Such plumb line measurements, however, are helpful in judging the gross effects corrective therapy has on restricted and unstable conditions.

Applied Roentgenography

The Davis series (seven views of the cervical spine) is the standard for assessing the osseous architecture of the cervical spine and to rule out osseous pathology. On the lateral exposures during cervical flexion and extension, considerable information can be gained about intersegmental mobility. Once significant pathology has been ruled out and an evaluation of A-P and P-A function is the remaining objective, immobilization devices should not be used.

Pre- and post-therapy studies using overlays have much merit, and various authors have suggested several methods to gather helpful data. As each vertebra serves as the foundation for the one below, each vertebra becomes the established reference point for the movement of the segment above. Faye advises tracing the vertebral bodies and spinous processes. The neutral spine is traced on clear acetate in black as it appears on the standard Davis lateral view. Once this is done, it can be used to compare flexion and extension ROMs of each motion unit. Jackson's stress lines are another excellent method of demonstrating abnormal flexion and extension arcs.

Roentgenographic Analysis of Cervical Hypolordosis

Rehberger reports the typical radiographic findings to include loss of the normal lordotic curve by the straightened cervical spine (78% cases), anterior and posterior subluxation on flexion and extension views, narrowing of IVD spaces at C4—C6 in 46% cases, discopathy at the affected vertebral level as the injury progresses, and osteoarthritic changes that are often accompanied by foraminal spurring.

In his monograph, Bergmann mentions the radiographic studies of Jochumsen who measured the distance from the anterior body of C5 to a line running from the anterior arch of the atlas to the anterosuperior aspect of the body of C7. He then set up a classification of cervical curves as follows:

1. Hyperlordosis —   over +9 mm
2. Mean lordosis —   +3 to +8 mm
3. Hypolordosis —   +1 to +2 mm
4. Alordosis   —   +1 to -3 mm
5. Kyphosis   —   under -3 mm

Another approach used by some roentgenologists is to draw one line through the anterior and posterior tubercles of the atlas and another line through the inferior plate of C7. Secondary lines are then drawn at right angles from each of these base lines, and the angle created by the perpendicular lines is measured. From 35° to 40° is considered normal, less than 35° indicates hypolordosis, and an amount greater than 40° is classified as hyperlordosis.

Other methods can also be used. Pettibon states that mechanically the strongest and most resilient curve is an arc which has a radius of curvature equal to the chord across the arc, and he uses the Delmas index as described by Kapandji. As the radius increases, the curve increases (flattens, as in hypolordosis).

Differential Diagnosis

No where else in the spine are the bones, nerves, arteries, and veins so intimately associated as they are in the cervical region.

Tissue Sites of Pain Production

The neck contains an abundance of pain sensitive tissues within a relatively small and compact area of the body. Neck pain may be the result of trauma, irritation, prolonged tension, infection, or degenerative processes. The muscles, ligaments, glandular capsules, vessel walls, and skin of the anterior neck contain networks of nociceptors. Within the spinal complex, pain is primarily elicited from the perivertebral muscles and ligaments, sensory fibers of the nerve root and recurrent meningeal nerve root, dural sleeves and lining of the cord, vascular walls, and apophyseal capsules. Some investigators have traced a few sensory fibers to the posterior aspect of the IVD. Typical causes of posterior neck pain are shown in Table 3.5.

Table 3.5. Typical Causes of Posterior Neck Pain

Traumatic	Inflammatory	Neurologic Psychologic	Vascular	Endocrine Metabolic
Compression	Abscess	Brachial neuritis	Angina pectoris	
Contusion	Dental infection	Cervical subluxa-	Dissecting aor-	
Dislocation	Fibrositis	tion syndrome	tic aneurysm	
Fracture	Lymphadenitis	Multifidi trigger	Subarachnoid	
Hematoma	Meningitis	point	hemorrhage	
IVD syndrome	Myalgia	Postural subluxa-	Temporal ar-	
Subluxation	Rheumatoid	tion complex	teritis	
	arthritis	Psychoneurosis		
	Riedel's struma	Scalenus anticus		
	Trichinosis	syndrome		
	Tuberculosis	Sternocleidomas-		
		toid trigger point		
		TMJ dysfunction		
		Trapezius trigger		
		point		

Neoplastic	Degenerative Deficiency	Congenital	Allergic Autoimmune	Toxic
Carcinoma	Cervical spondylosis	Branchial cyst		
Cyst	Osteoarthritis	Cervical rib		
Hodgkin's disease	Pott's disease of	Congenital di-		
Metastasis	bone	verticulum		
Pancoast tumor		Platybasia		
Spinal cord tumor		Other anomalies		

Significant Neurologic and Orthopedic Tests

Evaluating vital signs and such proce-dures as inspection, static palpation, light touch/pain tests, muscle strength grading, and range of gross motion tests are so stan-dard within chiropractic physical examina-tion that there is no need to describe them here. This is also true for the evaluation of re-flexes pertinent to cervical syndromes such as the biceps, ciliospinal, deltoid, infraspina-tus, pectoral, radial, scapulohumeral, and triceps reflex. When suspicions arise of pos-sible cranial nerve deficits, facial (VII), glos-sopharyngeal (IX), hypoglossal (XII), tri-geminal (V), and vagus (X) nerve tests are especially pertinent. Besides these standard tests, the following orthopedic and neurolog-ic tests are helpful in the differential diag-nosis of cervical syndromes.

Cervical Compression Tests. Two tests are involved. First, with the patient sitting, stand behind the patient. The patient's head is laterally flexed and rotated about 45° to-ward the side being examined. Interlocked fingers are placed on the patient's scalp and gently pressed caudally. If an IVF is nar-rowed, this maneuver will further insult the foramen by compressing the disc and further narrowing the foramen, causing radiating pain and reduplication of other symptoms. In the second test, the patient's neck is pas-sively extended and your interlocked fingers are placed on the patient's scalp and gently pressed caudad. If an IVF is narrowed, this maneuver mechanically compromises the foraminal diameters bilaterally and causes radiating pain and reduplication of other symptoms. Pain at the spine only is proably facetal in origin.

Cervical Distraction Test. With the patient sitting, stand to the side of the patient and place one hand under the patient's chin and your other hand under the base of the patient's occiput (Fig. 3.35). Slowly and gradually the patient's head is lifted to remove weight from the cervical spine. This maneuver elongates the IVFs, decreases the pressure on the joint capsules around the facet joints, and stretches the perivertebral musculature. If the maneuver decreases pain and relieves other symptoms, it is a likely indication of narrowing of one or more IVFs or cervical facet syndrome. When stretched, spastic perivertebral muscles are painful.

Cervical Active Rotary Compression Test. With the patient sitting, observe while the patient voluntarily laterally flexes the head toward the side being examined. With the neck flexed, the patient is then instructed to rotate the chin toward the same side, which narrows the IVF diameters on the side of concavity. Pain or reduplication of other symptoms suggests a physiologic narrowing of one or more IVFs.

Shoulder Depression Test. With the patient sitting, stand behind the subject and bend the patient's neck laterally away from the side being examined. Stabilize the patient's shoulder with one hand and apply pressure alongside the patient's head with the palm of your other hand; stretching the dural root sleeves and nerve roots or aggravating radicular pain if the nerve roots adhere to the foramina. Extravasations, edema, encroachments, and the conversion of fibrinogen into fibrin may result in interfascicular, foraminal, and articular adhesions and inflammations that will restrict fascicular glide and the ingress and egress of the foraminal contents. Thus, radiating pain and reduplication of other symptoms during this test suggest adhesions between the nerve's dura sleeve and other structures around the IVF.

Swallowing Test. The sitting patient is asked to drink some water. If a pharyngeal lesion is ruled out (eg, tonsillitis), painfully difficult swallowing may suggest a space-occupying lesion at the anterior aspect of the cervical spine (eg, abscess, tumor, osteophytes, etc). See Figure 3.36.

Valsalva's Maneuver. The sitting patient is asked to bear down firmly (abdominal push), as if straining at the stool. This act increases intrathecal pressure, which tends to elicit localized pain in the presence of a space-occupying lesion (eg, IVD protrusion, cord tumor, bony encroachment) or of an acute inflammatory disorder of the cord (eg, arachnoiditis) or possibly the nerve root (radiculitis). Deep coughing will produce the same effect under like circumstances.

Cervical Percussion Test. The neck of the sitting patient is flexed to about 45° while you percuss each of the cervical spinous processes and adjacent superficial soft tissues with a rubber-tipped reflex hammer or the side of a closed fist. Evidence of point tenderness suggests a fractured or acutely subluxated vertebra or localized severe sprain or strain, while symptoms of radicular pain suggest IVF radiculitis or an IVD lesion.

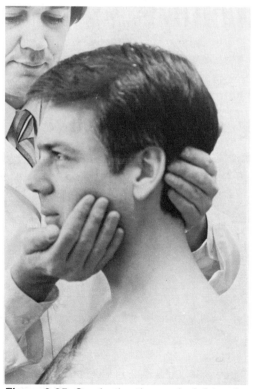

Figure 3.35. Conducting the cervical distraction test (Courtesy ACAP).

Following are some common tests that are helpful in the differentiation of a thoracic outlet syndrome.

Adson's Test. With the patient sitting or standing, palpate the patient's radial pulse and advise the patient to bend the head obliquely backward toward the side being examined, to take a deep breath, and then to tighten the neck and chest muscles on the side tested. This maneuver decreases the interscalene space and increases any existing compression of the subclavian artery and lower components (C8 and T1) of the brachial plexus against the 1st rib. Marked weakening of the pulse or increased paresthesias is a positive sign of pressure on the neurovascular bundle, particularly of the subclavian artery as it passes between or through the scaleni musculature (Fig. 3.37), thus suggesting a probable cervical rib or scalenus anticus syndrome. This test is sometimes called the *scalene maneuver*.

Allen's Test. The sitting patient elevates the arm and is instructed to make a tight fist to express blood from palm. You should then occlude the radial and ulnar arteries by finger pressure. The patient lowers the hand and relaxes the fist, while you release the arteries one at a time. Some examiners prefer to test the radial and ulnar arteries individually in two tests. The sign is negative if the pale skin of the palm flushes immediately when the artery is released. The patient should be instructed not to hyperextend the palm as this will constrict skin capillaries and render a false positive sign. The sign is positive if the skin of the palm remains blanched for more than 4 seconds. This test, which should be performed before *Wright's test*, is significant in vascular occlusion of the artery tested.

Eden's Test. With the patient seated, the examiner palpates the radial pulse and instructs the patient to pull the shoulders

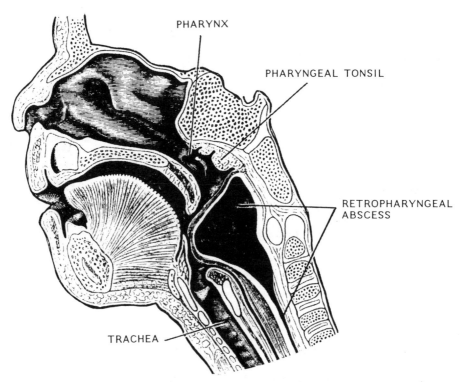

Figure 3.36. Schematic of a vertical section of the face and neck depicting how a retropharyngeal abscess or any other type of space-occupying lesion in this area would include dysphagia among the clinical features (Courtesy ACAP).

backward, throw the chest out in a "military posture," and hold a deep inspiration as the pulse is examined. The test is positive if weakening or loss of the pulse occurs, indicating pressure on the neurovascular bundle as it passes between the clavicle and the 1st rib, and thus a costoclavicular syndrome.

Wright's Test. With the patient sitting, palpate the radial pulse from the posterior in the downward position and as the patient's arm is passively moved through an 180° arc. If the pulse diminishes or disappears in this arc or if neurologic symptoms develop, it may indicate pressure on the axillary artery and vein under the pectoralis minor tendon and coracoid process or compression in the retroclavicular spaces between the clavicle and 1st rib, and thus be a hyperabduction syndrome.

Costoclavicular Maneuver. With the patient sitting, stand behind the patient and monitor the patient's radial pulse on the side being examined. Bring the patient's shoulder and arm posterior and then depresses the shoulder on the side being examined. This maneuver narrows the costoclavicular space by approximating the clavicle to the first rib, tending to compress the neurovascular structures between. When the shoulder is retracted, the clavicle moves backward on the sternoclavicular joint and rotates in a counterclockwise direction. An alteration or obliteration of the radial pulse or a reduplication of other symptoms suggests compression of the neurovascular bundle passing between the clavicle and the first rib (costoclavicular syndrome).

In addition to the tests described above, there are occasions when Bradburne's, Branham's, Brudzinski's cheek and neck, Klippel-Weil, and Rust's signs should be sought. This is also true for the application of Bakody's, Bikele's, Kernig's neck, Naffziger's, O'Donoghue's, Ruggeri's reflex, Soto-Hall's, and Spurling's tests. These tests are described in comprehensive texts on physical and differental diagnosis.

Vertebral Artery Deflection

The vertebral arteries are the major source of blood supply to the cervical spinal cord and brain stem, including the medulla oblongata, pons, and midbrain. They also supply the visual cortex of the cerebrum and cerebellum via the basilar artery. For an unexplained reason, one artery is usually smaller than its mate. In visualizing the course and distribution of the vertebral arteries, we should realize that they are captive vessels from C6 upward (Fig. 3.38). Severe deflection may be caused by any stretching or twisting of the artery during neck injury or cervical manipulation. In later years, chronic deflection is commonly associated with bony spurs from the covertebral joints or grossly hyperplastic apophyses from arthrosis.

The vertebral arteries are unique in their course through several bony foramina, and in this intermittently channeled course they must make four nearly right-angle turns (forming a half square) in just 20—30 mm between entering the C2 transverse and entering the foramen magnum. Adding to this tortuous course are the anomalous loops that occur in about one in every 5

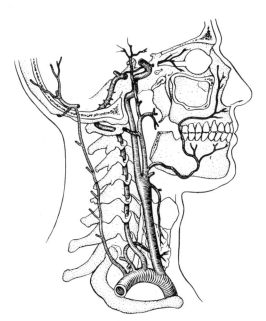

Figure 3.37. Diagram showing how the anterior and middle scalene muscles surround the brachial plexus and subclavian artery. Keep in mind that it is from the subclavian that the vertebral artery originates bilaterally. Right complex only is shown, as viewed from the anterior (Courtesy ACAP).

people. In addition, the C2 area is a common site for aneurysm.

With rotation, C1 moves forward from C2. On the side opposite to which the head is turned, the portion of the artery between the two segments is narrowed and stretched —first being affected near 30° rotation and markedly kinked at 45°.

Extension of the cervical spine allows the tip of the superior articular process of the motion unit to glide forward and upward. If sufficient, this motion may cause encroachment on the vertebral artery and/or the IVF. Deflection of the artery and any resulting symptoms are especially exaggerated by rotation plus extension of the neck. As a result of pressure against the artery, there may be temporary lessening in the volume of blood flow. Atheromatous changes may occur later within the vascular wall. The major symptoms include headache, vertigo, nausea, vomiting, nystagmus, and suboccipital tenderness, which may be exaggerated by cervical extension with or without added rotation. Sometimes the symptoms are aggravated by dorsal extension and relieved by forward flexion with cervical traction.

Vertebral-Basilar Artery Insufficiency Syndrome

The vertebral arteries also exhibit special features for particular sites of predilection for degeneration by the change of fixed and unfixed vessel parts, increased vulnerability to bone and muscle movements, and the occlusion of peripheral arteries in their circulation area by difficult to diagnose pathologic changes of the vascular walls. See Figure 3.39. These factors suggest the probability of advanced degenerative or inflammatory process. Trauma to the vertebral artery has even been reported after emergency resuscitation procedures where passive extension of the neck is necessary to insert an airtube.

Because cervical rotation may approach 47° or more, the vertebral artery can easily be stretched and twisted to the point of occlusion. Thus, the integrity of the vertebral arteries should always be evaluated before cervical manipulation or mobilization. Youth

is no exception to this rule. It is often young patients that experience transient ischemic attacks or a serious vascular accident after misapplied cervical manipulation.

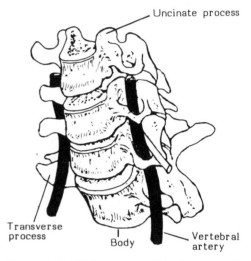

Figure 3.38. Oblique view of the lower cervical vertebrae (Courtesy ACAP).

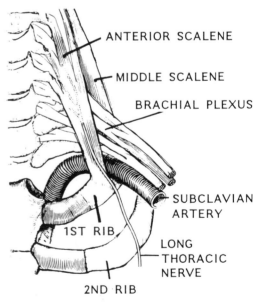

Figure 3.39. Lateral view of the course of the major arteries of the neck. Note the route of the vertebral artery through the transverse foramina of the cervical vertebrae (Courtesy ACAP).

Symptoms can usually be attributed to involvement of the plexus around the vertebral artery or intermittent disruption of the blood flow. Any compromise (eg, compression, atherosclerosis, thrombosis, vasospasm, kinking, longus colli and scalenus anticus spasm) producing an insufficiency of blood flow can lead to a singular symptom or a wide number of seemingly unrelated cranial manifestations such as occipital headaches, memory lapses, dizziness, tinnitus, nausea and vomiting, lightheadedness or syncope, intermittent blurred vision, suboccipital tenderness, and, sometimes, retrooccular pain (episodic), speech impairment, extremity paresthesia and weakness, drop attacks, and gait defects—all of which can be generally grouped under the title of *Barré-Lieou syndrome*, especially when cervical trauma and an underlying spondylosis are involved. These signs and symptoms, which sometimes fluctuate from side to side, can mimic a posttraumatic syndrome, multiple sclerosis, amyotrophic lateral sclerosis, or a tumor within the posterior fossa.

Severe interference (eg, advanced atherosclerosis, osteophytic kinking, spondylotic foraminal impingement, or extension effects of IVD degeneration) leads to involvement of the nucleus ambiguous of the vagus (eg, dysphagia, ipsilateral palatal weakness), descending root and nucleus of cranial V (ipsilateral facial hypesthesia, especially around the lips), descending sympathetic fibers (Horner's syndrome), vestibular nuclei (rotary nystagmus), midbrain and cerebellum (ipsilateral arm/leg malcoordination, intention tremor, ataxia), spinothalamic tract (contralateral hypesthesia), and the effects from impaired venous drainage and CSF flow, which is often referred to as *Wallenberg's syndrome*.

It can be projected that the many cranial-oriented symptoms that have been relieved by chiropractic adjustments to the cervical region can be attributed to normalization of vertebral artery blood flow. Here we have a clinical paradox in that the same treatment may cause possible distress if unusual precautions are not taken with some patients.

Several clinical tests that have only minor variations are portrayed in the literature. The six most commonly used are Barré-

Lieou's, George's, Hautant's, Maigne's, De-Kleyn's, and Unterberger's tests.

Barré-Lieou Test. The sitting patient is asked to slowly but firmly rotate the head first to one side and then to the other. Transient mechanical occlusion of the vertebral artery may be precipitated by this simple turning of the head, and this phenomenon is attributed to the compressive action of the longus colli and scalene muscles (Fig. 3.40) on the vertebral artery, just before coursing through the IVF of C6. A positive sign is exhibited if dizziness, faintness, nausea, nystagmus, vertigo, and/or visual blurring result—suggesting buckling, torsion, or compression of the vertebral artery. This mild test should be used before any others because if it is positive, there is no need to apply greater stress.

George's Tests. With the patient sitting, blood pressure and the radial pulse rate are taken bilaterally and recorded. Stenosis or occlusion of the subclavian artery is suggest-

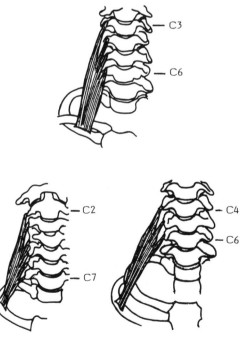

Figure 3.40. The scalene muscle group. The scalenus anterior is shown at the *top,* scalenus medius in the *bottom left,* and the scalenus posterior in the *bottom right* drawing (Courtesy ACAP).

ed when a difference of 10 mm Hg between the two systolic blood pressures and a feeble or absent pulse is found on the involved side. Even if these signs are absent, a subclavian deficit may be exhibited by finding auscultated bruits in the supraclavicular fossa.

Hautant's Test. Place the sitting patient's upper limbs so that they are abducted forward with the palms supinated. The patient is instructed to close the eyes while you extend and rotate the patient's head. This position is held between 20—30 seconds on each side. A positive sign is for one or both arms to drop into a pronated position.

Maigne's Test. Place the sitting patient's neck in extension and contralateral rotation. This position is held for about 30—60 seconds on each side. A positive sign is shown by nystagmus or symptoms of vertebrobasilar ischemia. In this and DeKleyn's test, unusual care must be exercised as each of these tests is designed to stress the vertebral arteries, which may be weakened.

DeKleyn's Test. Place the patient supine with the head rest lowered a few notches. Extend and rotate the patient's head, and hold this position for about 15—30 seconds on each side. A positive sign is the same as that in Maigne's test. Faye recommends that the position be held for 45—60 seconds and that it must be held long enough to cause brain ischemia owing to loss of patency of an arterial deficit (eg, compression, atherosclerosis, kink, etc).

Underburger's Test. Ask the patient to stand with the upper limbs outstretched, the eyes closed, and then to march in place with the head extended and rotated. The examiner should stand close to the patient during the test because a positive sign is a loss of balance. For this reason, it is not one of the most commonly used.

Other signs that help to determine a patient at risk include arteriosclerotic optic fundi changes, a subclavian or carotid bruit, positive Doppler ultrasound tracings, and positive roentgenographic changes.

Headaches of Cervical Origin: General Considerations

Markovich, the renowned neurologist, found that the most common headache is the type caused by neuromuscular skeletal imbalance. He points out that "the head in the human species has changed its position from the quadruped to the erect, thereby changing the basic relationship between the cervical spine and the head, with its important functional structures, and the rest of the body." He calls attention to the delicate interaction and highly sensitive biofeedback or servo-mechanisms that continually make adjustments in body balance, vision, and hearing with head and neck posture. "These regulatory, homeostatic mechanisms can be disturbed by a variety of conditions, originating at any level, including the inflammation and/or irritation of the cephalic projection of the upper cervical nerves (cervico-occipital neural-glias)."

Abnormal contraction of the muscles at the occipitocervical area appears to generate a type of "ischemic irritation" that includes the entrapment of the C2 nerves (greater and lesser occipital) as they pierce the thick muscle and ascend to the back of the head. Differentiation of various types of headaches is shown in Table 3.6, adapted from Markovich's findings. However, keep in mind that a patient may not exhibit such a clear picture. For example, vascular migraine may be superimposed on occipitocervical neuralgia or episodes may be interposed, depending on the causes involved.

Localized headaches may point to causative subluxations. Pioneer chiropractic was specific in relating certain types of headache with to specific spinal areas. Firth, then president of Lincoln Chiropractic College, taught that: "A headache located in the forehead or over the eyes (frontal or eye headache) is often caused by a local subluxation in the upper or middle cervical region. A headache located in the region of the temples (temporal headache) is usually caused by a subluxation in the region of T4. A headache in the back of the head (occipital headache) may be caused by an atlas or axis subluxation, but it is more frequently caused by a lumbar subluxation. A vertigo or sick headache may be the result and symptom of gastric indigestion that is frequently relieved by an adjustment in the T6—T8 region. A headache at the crown of the head is more rarely encountered than any of the others and frequently indicates kidney trouble. It can often be relieved by an adjustment to the T10—T12 region. Such subluxations may be primary subluxations or in compensation to a structural fault elsewhere in the spine or a reflex from a distant part."

Kraus states: "It has been my experience that the most common cause of headaches originates in the 'vicious circle' generated by the abnormal and painful contraction of the cervical-nuchal muscles, mainly the trapezius muscle. These contractions generate a type of 'ischemic irritation' that includes the entrapment of the second cervical nerves (greater occipital and lesser occipital) as they travel through the bulk of the muscle, ascending into the back of the head to innervate the posterior scalp region, temporal areas, and lobes of the ears, and sending terminal branches into the angle of the jaw, back of the eye, and vertex of the head. This creates a distinct clinical syndrome that is easily confused with atypical 'vascular migraine' because of the unilaterality of the symptoms and frequent complaints of pain in the back of the eye with or without visual disturbance."

Kraus goes on to say that the second common entity is the TMJ pain dysfunction syndrome that has been proven to be more common than many expect and has many protean manifestations—to the extent that it has become known as *The Great Imposter*. "The fact that a cervical nerve irritation can create a painful condition in the angle of the jaw or in the temple explains the possible common 'irritative' source of both syndromes." [See Clinical Comment 3.8]

True Migraine

With any type of vascular headache (migraine, cluster, hypertension), a patient will

---

DR. FAYE'S CLINICAL COMMENT #3.8

Cervicogenic headaches can usually be exacerbated by specific palpation of the muscle or joint fixation. The patient will tell you "that's it" when you find the "spot" or direction to challenge the joint that produces the chief complaint.

Table 3.6. Differentiation of Common Types of Headaches

Symptom/Sign	Occipito-cervical Neuralgia	Trigeminal Neuralgia	Vascular Migraine	Temporo-mandibular Traction
Pain	Throbbing, paroxysmal	Excruciating, paroxysmal	Severe, paroxysmal	Severe, dull
Quality	Muscle spasms	Stabbing	Throbbing	Dull ache
Location	Occipital	Facial	Unilateral	Facial
Aura	None	None	Visual	None
Duration	Days	Brief	Hours	Chronic
Associated symptoms and signs	Earache Eye pain Neck pain Paresthesias Anxiety Tinnitus Nausea	Trigger zones	Vomiting Photophobia Irritability	Bruxism Malocclusion Earache Joint clicks

feel more relief in the upright position. The recumbent position is more beneficial to patients with sinusitis and tension headaches. In addition, vascular headaches are commonly associated with a prodromal aura (usually visual) that is thought to be the result of an initial arterial spasm and local ischemia in the area affected. In females, attacks are more frequent just before the onset of menstruation.

In true migraine headaches, there is an initial vasoconstriction (amine release) that produces prodromal neurologic symptoms (eg, visual aura, motor or sensory perversions) in 10% of the cases from the ischemia, which initiates a period of vasodilation (vasoactive substance release) that, in turn, produces the headache. The initial site of pain is usually orbital, frontal, or temporal; unilateral and localized; and then radiates to the parietal and occipital areas. The side of the headache may at one time occur on the left and the next time on the right. Bilateral types, however, are not rare. An attack may last several days, but the typical attack lasts less than 24 hours. Bouts of a throbbing headache arise in late adolescence or early adult life. They are more common in females and frequently associated with a family tendency, but some type of stress usually precipitates an attack. They usually first occur before adulthood.

Prodromal neurologic manifestations (usually accentuated contralaterally) such as amblyopia, hemianopsia, hemiparesis, numbness, ophthalmoplegia, paresthesia, speech disturbances, and weakness may or may not be associated. Listlessness, social withdrawal, dejection, nausea and vomiting, and anorexia are frequently related. Scintilating scotomata are commonly associated with migraine but rarely with other types of chronic headaches. Birth control pills (attributed to the periodic withdrawal of exogenous progestogens) and excessive noise and/or light increase the pain and number of attacks. Attacks usually reduce in severity and rate during pregnancy. [See Clinical Comment 3.9]

Cervical Migraine

The generally accepted etiology of cervical migraine is upper-cervical angiospasm of the vertebral artery.

As with true migraine, cervical migraine may be preceded by an aura. Neurologic examination during a pain-free interval reveals nothing pertinent except a tender spot in the upper neck over the site where the occipital nerve pierces the aponeurosis of the upper neck muscles. See Figure 3.41.

According to Faye and associates, if the occipital nerve is cut, the pain of cervical migraine may be stopped. However, sometimes the pain may persist, suggesting that it can be elicited from any segmental level of the cervical spine. An even more puzzling observation is that cervical migraine is often relieved when a cervical rib producing brachialgia is removed. This might indicate a vertebral artery or sympathetic involvement.

Cervical migraine may be suspected if the headache is always localized on the same side during every attack. A history of cervical trauma is also important. Seek signs of cervical dysfunction. In cervical migraine, it has been Schafer's experience that the site of involvement will usually be in the C4—C6 area. Pressure over and around the spinous processes may elicit extreme tenderness. Cervical motions in various directions may start an attack, especially if the positions are held for 30—60 seconds.

Cluster Headaches

In cluster migraine (Horton's histamine cephalgia), the intense pain is unilateral. It may have an evening onset, but more commonly it awakens the patient after a few hours of sleep. The paroxysmal and localized pain begins initially in the temporal-supra-

---

DR. FAYE'S CLINICAL COMMENT #3.9

The atlanto-occipital lift is often very effective in clearing the migraine syndrome. There are often coexisting majors in the upper-thoracic spine and A-P lower-cervical fixations. The first rib and scalenius anticus syndromes can mimic migraine symptoms but usually have no teen-age history.

orbital area and progresses to the occipital area, or the opposite may appear: occiput to temple.

Attacks, which are invariably associated with adult males, are more common in the spring and fall, thus making an allergic or hormonal reaction a possible precipitating factor. A familial tendency is rarely involved. The pain may be so intense that suicide is contemplated. It usually lasts 30—90 minutes but may continue for several hours, reappearing in clusters that last from a day or two to several months, then it may remiss for several years. In both cluster and migraine headaches, severe bouts of pain are interspersed with pain-free episodes lasting several months. The reason for this pattern is not clear.

Nasal stuffiness, flush, injected conjunctiva, and other ipsilateral signs of vasodilation may be found. Rhinorrhea, profuse lacrimation, tenderness of the carotid arteries, and pupillary constriction commonly manifest. In addition, cluster headaches are frequently found associated with "silent" peptic ulcers, in which the duration of severe pain may be

extended to several hours. Such conditions are frequently aggravated by huge consumption of aspirin to relieve the pain but increase the gastritis that is producing the reflex mechanism. The patient will often report that everything is tried to gain relief, but nothing appears to help until the pain runs its course. Medication of any type, even morphine, has little effect; yet treatment to the hidden gastrointestinal fault will show immediate relief within a few days. It has been Schafer's experience that an occipitoatlantal fixation is usually involved in cluster headaches.

Occipital Neuralgia

Occipital neuralgia is caused by involvement of the greater and lesser occipital nerves, the greater nerve being affected with more frequency. These nerves are derived from the C2 and C3 segments of the spinal cord.

Typical occipital neuralgia displays paroxysms of pain provoked by movement of the head, suggesting that the nerve roots are under the influence of some type of mechanical pressure or irritation. The patient complains of pain in the back of the head and behind the ear. At the time, the pain is strictly occipital, unilateral or bilateral. Sometimes it radiates toward the mandible. The character of the pain varies from a dull aching soreness to a sharp shooting pain. Turning the head often increases the pain, and brushing the hair is annoying because of an hyperesthetic scalp. Attacks may arise with short-intervals of relief or the pain may be continuous.

Examination usually reveals a tender point, which aids the diagnosis, that is located: (1) midway between the tip of the mastoid and the atlas (greater occipital nerve), (2) at a point behind the mastoid, or (3) between the insertion of the sternocleidomastoideus muscle and that of the trapezius muscle.

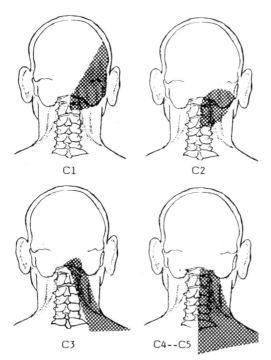

Figure 3.41. Areas of referred pain from C1—C5 nerve root irritation (Courtesy ACAP).

Vascular Tension Headache

Tension headaches, which frequently have an emotional base (eg, stress, anxiety, depression), are rarely present on arising but increase in severity as the day progresses and stress accumulates. The onset is typically gradual and may last from hours to months without relief. Attacks, which may be unilateral or bilateral, may occur daily or be constant for several days and then not recur for several weeks or months (similar to cluster headaches). Facial pain and cheek paresthesias and/or a sense of pressure behind an eyeball may be associated. Tension headaches must be differentiated from the referred pain of sinus disease, which may manifest in the occipital area, especially if the maxillary or sphenoid sinuses are involved.

Examination usually reveals suboccipital tenderness at a point midway between the tip of the mastoid and the midcervical vertebrae. Firm pressure on this tender point may sometimes ease the pain referred to the temple, face, or eyeball. Palpation or percussion of a temporal artery may reveal abnormal unilateral tenderness. This must be differentiated from arteritis.

Two types of tension headaches are reported: the "hat-band" type and the occipital type:

1. In the "hat-band" type with a history of a constriction feeling around the circumference of the scalp, the cause can usually be found in a history of emotional stress. Symptoms of chronic anxiety or depression and unusual fatigue may also be associated.

2. The occipital type exhibits severe contraction in the muscles of the neck and scalp that can be palpated and demonstrated in electromyography. The pain is typically bilateral or general, with radiation over the entire cranium and sometimes down the neck into a shoulder. Cervical stiffness, tension, and tingling in the occipitoparietal region are commonly associated. Trigger points can often be found in the suboccipital area and other cervical muscles. Anxiety symptoms and hyperactive deep reflexes are usually associated. The occipitoatlantal joint is inevitably hypomobile, suggesting a motion-unit fixation. During suboccipital spasm, the nerves in the area are vulnerable to irritation from C1 or C2 subluxations. Passive upper-cervical stretching reproduces the pain and possibly the paresthesia, and palpation of the area elicits deep tenderness.

Atypical Facial Neuralgia

Besides a pathologic intracranial lesion, facial pain may have its origin in a fixation-subluxation of the occiput or in the upper cervical spine. The pain may be referred to any or all distributions of the 5th cranial nerve so that, in some instances, it suggests tic douloureux. Some of the characteristic signs of trigeminal neuralgia, however, are absent. For example, the paroxysmal peripheral projection of pain is not present, and, in trigeminal neuralgia, the pain is described as being in the skin, gums, or tongue. In atypical facial neuralgia, the pain may be continuous.

The history may reveal that the attack was preceded by some type of physical or emotional stress. It may be associated with true migraine, and an associated tender point is often identical to that found in occipital neuralgia. Spinal examination usually elicits extreme tenderness over the articular processes of C2 and C3. An adjustment on this side is usually successful. Particularly seek signs of impaired flexion and A-P rotation motion, advises Faye.

Interscapulovertebral Pain Syndrome

Faye and associates have found that about 70% of common posterior upper thoracic pain is of lower cervical origin, is predominant in the interscapular region, and has a higher incidence in women. It is usually localized between the scapula and the spine, almost always unilateral, and radiates at times to the lateral (sometimes superior) border of the scapula. It may give the patient the impression of being deep seated, internal, or feel as a weighty, burning, or painful tension between the scapulae. Sharp pain may occur within 3—4 hours after working or it may arise a few minutes after the patient begins work. In other cases, it is episodic and elicited by faulty movement such as extremely abducting the arm backward.

The history will usually trace the cause to (1) occupations during which the hands are used at the level of where the elbows are not supported; (2) domestic activities such as ironing, cleaning, sewing, or carrying heavy packages; or (3) wearing a heavy overcoat, especially during prolonged standing, which may precipitate symptoms. Sometimes the pain occurs only at night, depending upon the position of the head on a pillow, the height and firmness of the pillow, and the side on which the patient habitually rests.

The presence of a positive anterior cervical "doorbell sign" (described later in this chapter) confirms the origin of the upper thoracic pain. A moderate pressure maintained for 2 or 3 seconds reproduces the pain of the patient's complaint. Palpation also reveals the presence of a fixed tender point that is invariably found about 2 cm lateral to the spinous processes of T5 or T6. This interscapular point is extremely tender. When pressure is applied, it also reproduces the pain that formed the basis of the patient's complaint. This tender point is over the site where the posterior branch of T2 emerges. The medial ramus becomes superficial at the T5 level, and from there it fans out horizontally to supply a large area of skin on the back. The fact that the posterior branch of T2 may be responsible for the pain does not explain why the cervical doorbell sign is positive. However, close study will show that there are anastomoses between the lower cervical and upper thoracic nerves. Also, T2 is an important segment as far as the cervical sympathetic nerves are concerned.

Posterior Nerve Branch Syndrome

The posterior rami of the spinal nerves innervate all the formations dependent on the posterior vertebral arch. Their motor distribution is in the muscles acting on the axial skeleton, and their segmental sensory distribution covers a large area of skin that extends without interruption from the vertex to the coccyx. Their role in the rich innervation of the posterior articulations of the spine is not well known. These nerve branches closely adhere to the articular structures, being fixed by fibrous attachments, and are affected by acute or chronic derangements of the posterior joints. In chronic fixations, there is pericapsular fibrosis of the posterior

apophyses and marginal osteophytosis that may irritate the nerve root. See Figure 3.42.

The posterior branches of a spinal nerve can be injured or inflamed near the IVF. When this occurs, the pain is limited to the perivertebral region and relatively localized. The pain may often be elicited by movements that especially slide the posterior articulations (eg, rotation). Perivertebral spasm, usually pronounced, is another consequence of irritation of a posterior ramus. When prolonged, such complications as torticollis or other deformities arise.

Lower Cervical Radicular Syndrome

This neuralgia features pain along the upper extremity from cervical nerve root compression or irritation (C5—C8). Either mechanical and/or inflammatory etiologies may be involved. See Figure 3.43. Pain constitutes almost the entire symptomatology. It may involve the entire dermatome supplied by the root or be isolated to a smaller area

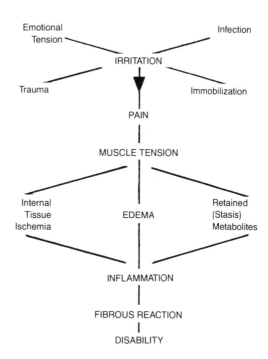

Figure 3.42. Basic mechanisms by which irritation can progress to functional impairment and end in pathologic disability (Courtesy ACAP).

such as the shoulder, elbow, or wrist. The patient almost always complains of simultaneous interscapular pain, which often precedes the radicular symptoms. It is usually increased when the patient is in bed and alleviated by certain movements such as placing a hand behind the head. In this position, the roots of the brachial plexus are relaxed.

An *anterior doorbell sign* is usually found. This sign contributes to the segmental localization and reveals the cervical origin of the symptoms. Keep in mind, however, the possibility that interspinal ligament pain and tenderness may alone be responsible for lower neck pain or pain referred to the posterior aspect of the shoulder or arm. In such cases, the anterior cervical doorbell will be absent.

After a thorough motion palpation examination, multidirectional pressure applied to the spinous process of the involved segment can help to analyze more precisely the level of the intervertebral block. When lateral pressure is applied, a counterpressure should be applied to the adjacent inferior spinous

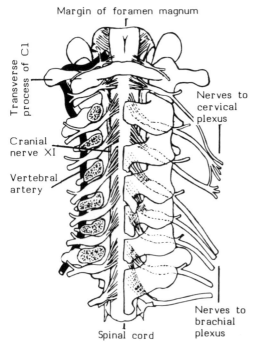

Figure 3.43. Posterior view of the cervical spine. Laminae have been removed on the left to show the vulnerable position of the IVF contents (Courtesy ACAP).

process. The related findings contribute to the determination of the most appropriate adjustive technic. Faye advises his students to remember that the major fixation is often above or below the level of radicular neuropathy. Other objective physical findings are present in only half the cases. For example, reflex changes are not often found, and motor changes are found in still fewer cases.

Anterior Doorbell Sign. The examiner faces the sitting patient. Mild pressure is applied over the emerging ventral roots of the cervical spine at the anterolateral aspect of the neck, under the sternocleidomastoideus muscle. Contact is made with the thumbs held horizontally. A positive sign is the reproduction or exaggeration of patient symptoms (eg, upper-extremity pain, paresthesia).

Adjustive Considerations. Manipulation is effective in many cases of cervical radiculitis. In the hyperalgesic forms in which neck movements are absent, one should not manipulate the cervical spine until palliative procedures have produced some substantial degree of pain-free motion. At times, adjustments are effective in the T3—T5 area when fixations, spontaneous pain, and point tenderness are located there. Pressure in this area may elicit brachial pain. In such cases, the pain does not show a typical radicular distribution; it resembles a sympathetic disturbance. Conversely, many interscapular neuralgias are improved by adjustments of the lower cervicals if fixated. After signs of inflammation and symptoms subside, reports Faye, gentle adjustments at the symptom level clears up the postinflammatory fixations.

Cervical IVD Syndrome

According to Grieve, the clinical picture of cervical disc disorders is typically a combination of "a hard osseocartilaginous spur, produced by the disc together with the adjacent margins of the vertebral bodies." Furthermore, "the mechanism by which pain and disability originate in the neck region," contends Cailliet, "can be considered broadly to result from encroachment of space or faulty movement in the region of the neck through which the nerves or blood vessels pass." This *encroachment of space* or *faulty movement* commonly comprise apophyseal subluxation with osteophyte formation, contributing to, or superimposed upon disc degeneration and/or protrusion. This occurs most frequently in the C4—C6 area. When a cervical disc protrusion is toward the posterior, *Lhermitte's test* will be positive.

Lhermitte's Test. With the patient seated, flexing the patient's neck and hips simultaneously with the patient's knees in full extension may produce sharp pain or shock-like sensations radiating down the spine and/or into the upper extremities. When this is elicited, it is a sign of cervical pathology suggesting spinal cord myelopathy by a protruded cervical disc, tumor, fracture, or multiple sclerosis.

The discs below C3 exhibit a higher incidence and the greatest severity of herniation. The C5 disc is the most frequently involved, followed by the C6 disc. The C2 disc is the least frequently involved of any in the neck. The specific neurovascular manifestations of acute cervical disc herniation are:

• *C2 disc protrusion (C3 nerve root level):* posterior neck numbness and pain radiating to the mastoid and ear. The reflexes test normal.

• *C3 disc protrusion (C4 nerve root level):* posterior neck numbness and pain radiating along the levator scapulae muscle and sometimes to the pectorals. The reflexes test normal.

• *C4 disc protrusion (C5 nerve root level):* lateral neck, shoulder, and arm pain and paresthesia, deltoid weakness and possible atrophy, hypesthesia of C5 root distribution over middle deltoid area (axillary nerve distribution). The reflexes test normal.

• *C5 disc protrusion (C6 nerve root level):* pain radiating down the lateral arm and forearm into the thumb and index finger, hypesthesia of the lateral forearm and thumb, decreased biceps reflex, biceps and supinator weakness.

• *C6 disc protrusion (C7 nerve root level):* pain radiating down the middle forearm to the middle fingers, hypesthesia of the middle fingers, decreased triceps and radial reflexes, triceps and grip weakness.

• *C7 disc protrusion (C8 nerve root level):* possible pain radiating down the medial forearm and hand, ulnar hypesthesia, intrinsic muscle weakness of the hand. However, these symptoms are uncommon. The reflexes test normal.

The above symptoms vary depending on the direction of the disc bulge; eg, on the nerve root, IVF vessels, spinal cord, or combinations of involvement. In some acute and many chronic cases, peripheral numbness may manifest without pain. In some cervical disc herniations, the features may be confused with those of shoulder or elbow bursitis, epicondylitis, or subluxation, especially when no local cervical symptoms exist.

Vague autonomic symptoms may also be exhibited such as dizziness, blurred vision, and hearing difficulties. These can usually be attributed to a complicating involvement of the sympathetic plexus around the vertebral artery or intermittent disruption of the blood flow of the vertebral artery. *Horner's syndrome* (ptosis, meiosis, hypohidrosis) often occurs in diseases affecting the cervical cord. According to Faye, autonomic symptoms also occur when flexion and A-P cervical rotation fixations stress the sympathetic ganglion chain.

Shoulder-Hand Syndrome

This reflex dystrophy is often referred to as *Steinbrocker's syndrome*. It is a condition that simulates many of the common lesions about the shoulder joint and often erroneously diagnosed as periarthritis, bursitis, tendinitis, or frozen shoulder.

The signs and symptoms that involve the shoulder and hand include pain, swelling, stiffness, restricted motion, trophic changes of the soft tissues, and osteoporosis in some cases. It may start with a burning causalgic-type pain in the shoulder joint, followed by joint stiffness and trophic changes. The first sign in the hand may be stiffness and swelling of the fingers, with an inability to close the fist. The palmar fascia may contract. In its early stages, it resembles bursitis, neuritis, or any of the so-called rheumatic conditions that affect the shoulder.

Steinbrocker's syndrome is usually an aftermath of trauma or disease involving the upper-extremity, neck, or cranium. Symptoms may not appear for days, weeks, or even months following the cause. It is also common following myocardial vascular damage. Regardless, the condition is regarded as a motor and neurovascular symptom complex that primarily affects the upper extremity. Various etiologic theories have been proposed, but none have been widely confirmed. One again, advises Faye, pay close attention to the flexion and A-P rotation cervical fixations.

One widely held theory states that the reflex starts from an area of local tissue disturbance. Impulses from these areas travel centrally along the usual afferent pathways and enter the internuncial system of spinal cord neurons, which is an interconnected and widely ramified network of CNS nerve fibers. In shoulder-hand syndrome, the noxious impulses apparently set up a central disturbance in the nature of a widespread continuous agitation of the internuncial pool. Impulses spread steadily to fire the anterior and lateral horn cells, which are not ordinarily affected by afferent impulses from the periphery. This incessant stimulation is expressed peripherally by motor and neurovascular symptoms. Spasm and vasomotor imbalance result and produce the characteristic clinical features of the shoulder-hand syndrome.

A variety of seemingly unrelated clinical disturbances have been described for many years as separate entities. These disorders include causalgia, Sudeck's atrophy, posttraumatic osteoporosis, painful shoulder disability following coronary occlusion, postinfarctional sclerodactylia, palmar and digital contractures, the swollen atrophic hands associated with cervical osteoarthritis, and certain changes in the limbs of hemiplegics. Increasing evidence suggests that, although the etiology of these various syndromes may be different, many of their clinical characteristics, and probably the neurophysiologic mechanisms underlying their development, are extremely similar if not identical.

THERAPEUTIC APPROACH

To repeat for emphasis, no where else in the spine are the structures as vulnerable to the effects of a poorly controlled adjustment than in the cervical region. Because of the possibility of a subclinical vertebral artery lesion, an adjustment with a shallow depth is a must in the cervical spine. We need only to open a joint less than an eighth of an inch to obtain an audible release of a fixation.

Before making a proper adjustment, the doctor must be well armed with a sound knowledge of anatomy, pathophysiology, and be able to visualize the tissues involved and the plane of articulation of the segment(s) to be mobilized. This is true for all articulations to assure that the correction is made most efficiently and with the least discomfort to the patient. Faye recommends that the DC administer an impulse at the point of lock, into the fixation, assures adequate velocity with minimal amplitude.

Adaptability to Partial Mobility

For reasons not fully explained, Gillet only adjusts *total fixations* in the upper cervical area. He rarely adjusts partial fixations. One reason he gives is because they are so easily relieved spontaneously by the correction of more caudad total fixations. When it is deemed beneficial to adjust an upper-cervical partial fixation, a rotary-type adjustment is preferred by Schafer because he believes that a recoil-type thrust is usually too traumatic on muscular fixations in this area, tending to enhance the fixed state at a later date because of the superimposed irritation. Gillet mentions that the rotary technic in such cases is one of his favorites. Faye states that it is important to adjust into the direction of each restricted direction of motion.

It is rarely possible to produce an *immediate* complete correction in a chronic upper-cervical total fixation because (1) the chronic state of the articular and periarticular soft tissues requires time to adapt to the renewed mobility, and (2) the six occipitoatlantal muscles are especially affected by conditions more caudad in the spine. The fixation will either normalize itself after release, little by little, as the articulations are used or be encouraged to do so when the remainder of spinal fixations are mobilized.

In rare occurrences, it may be found that the amount of correction achieved during the initial adjustment was so slight that the fixation returned to its state of total fixation within a few days. If this occurs, consideration should be given to using a more efficient technic. On this point, Faye states that the technic should utilize more than one adjustive thrust into a motion unit. "Often three or more specific thrusts are necessary to release a total fixation in all its directions of fixation."

Adjusting Occipitoatlantal Articular Fixations

The most important total fixation found in the spine appears to be at the occipitoatlantal articulations. In adjusting a total occipitoatlantal fixation, Gillet applies a forward thrust (P—A) on the readily palpable posterior arch of the atlas while holding a firm contact just posterior to the lateral masses. This places the contact point on the largest and strongest aspect of the atlas.

An occipital lift, taught by Faye, is also an extremely effective technic for releasing total occipitoatlantal fixations and jammed facets (Fig. 3.44).

Occipital Lift

Patient Supine. Place the patient supine on an adjusting table with the head-piece level with the floor. Stand at the head of the table, facing the patient. Turn the patient's head so that the fixation is upward and the contralateral side of the occiput can be cradled within your stabilizing hand. The middle

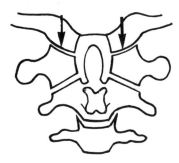

Figure 3.44. Suboccipital jamming often resulting in distention fixation (Courtesy ACAP).

finger of this hand should firmly contact the rim of the patient's occiput. Shift your position slightly so that it will be more lateral to the patient. With your active hand, apply a pisiform contact on the rim of the occiput on the side of fixation, fingers pointing toward the patient's vertex. Widen your stance for stability, raise the patient's head to slightly laterally bend the occipitoatlantal area, shift your body weight slightly forward from the patient to apply axial traction, and then deliver a quick shallow distracting impulse to just separate the locked occipitoatlantal joint. See Figure 3.45. This same procedure can be adapted to the patient in the prone position (Fig. 3.46).

Patient Sitting. Stand directly behind the sitting patient. The patient should be sitting erect, with the feet flat against the floor, and exhibiting the normal sitting lumbar lordosis. Take a moderately wide stance for stability. Rotate the patient's head away from the side of fixation. Reach around in front of the patient with your active hand, and apply a contact with your middle finger under the rim of the occiput, posterior to the mastoid process. Your index finger and thumb should avoid contact with the patient's ear. Reach around the other side of the patient with your stabilizing hand, and place it over your active hand for reinforcement. Bend over slightly and flex your knees so that the patient's skull can be firmed against your sternum. Your shoulders should be parallel with the patient's shoulders. With these contacts held firm, lean forward slightly more to produce a few degrees of lateral flexion of the patient's upper cervical spine and straighten your knees slightly to apply a slight vertical lift (distraction). At the end of resistance, apply a short dynamic impulse directed upward to separate the occipital condyle from the atlas. The thrust is delivered simultaneously with your contact hands and torso, assisted by quickly extending your knees (Fig. 3.47). Take care not to apply any pressure against the patient's mandible. If a bilateral fixation has been found, reverse the procedure for the contralateral side.

Patient Prone. Place the patient prone on an adjusting table with the head-piece lowered about 15°. Rotate the patient's head away from you so that the side of fixation is upward. Apply a knife edge contact with the medial edge of your active hand on the rim of the occiput, and grasp your active wrist with your stabilizing hand. Slowly apply pressure to the point of firm resistance, and deliver an impulse thrust directed forward against the occiput.

Another common technic applied with the patient in the prone position and the head turned so that the site of fixation is upward is to take a double knife-edge contact: one under the patient's occipital rim and the other just above the patient's vertebra prominens (viz, C7 or T1 spinous process). Your fingers will be entwined, and your hands will be placed in somewhat of a pyramidal design. In this position, apply opposing forces for long-axis cervical elongation (by opening the pyramidal base of your hands), then add a short distracting impulse (by dropping body weight slightly) at the end of resistance.

Occipital Posterior Rotation on Atlas Fixation

Patient Supine. Although active rotation of the occiput on the atlas is usually slight in degree, there should be distinct end play. If not, all other motions of the condyles will be affected. To correct this restriction, place the patient supine with the head level (Fig. 3.48). Turn the patient's head so that the fixated side is upward. Stand at the head of the table facing the patient, and place your stabilizing hand under the patient's head. Apply a light thumb contact anteriorly against the patient's zygomatic arch and a firm index finger contact posteriorly against the rim of the occiput. Avoid pressure against the patient's ear. Slowly rotate the patient's head a little farther with your stabilizing hand until firm resistance is felt, then deliver a short quick dynamic impulse to further this rotation.

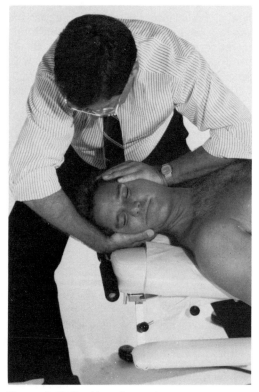
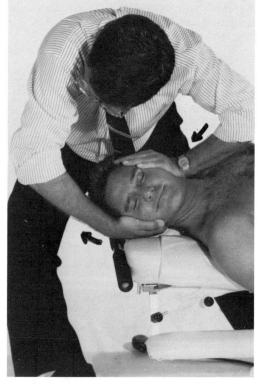

Figure 3.45. Positions for applying a left occipital lift with the patient supine; contact *(left)*, thrust *(right)*.

With slight modification, an occipital anterior rotation on the atlas fixation can be corrected by applying the technic described above on the contralateral side.

Adjusting Atlantoaxial Fixations

Atlantal Posterior Rotation on Axis Fixation

Patient Supine. Place the patient supine with the head-piece of the adjusting table level with the floor. Stand at the head of the table, obliquely facing the patient on the side of fixation. Rotate the patient's head so that the side of fixation is upward. Reach under the patient's head, and cup the patient's ear with your stabilizing hand. Bend forward over the patient, and with your active hand, apply an index finger or pisiform contact on the posterior arch of the atlas. Slowly rotate the patient's head farther with your stabilizing hand until firm resistance is felt, then add a short dynamic rotatory impulse with your active hand. This adjustment is delivered with the whole body, not just the contact point.

Patient Sitting. If a posterior rotation fixation between the atlas and axis is found on the right, for example, stand behind the patient and turn the patient's head away from the side of fixation. The patient should be sitting erect, with the feet flat on the floor. Take contact on the right posterior arch of the patient's atlas with your supinated right index finger, other fingers pointing slightly downward and your palm cupping the patient's right ear. Cup your stabilizing hand over the patient's left ear, and just slightly extend the patient's neck. Avoid lateral flexion. Slowly rotate the patient's head a little farther, and shift your position so that it

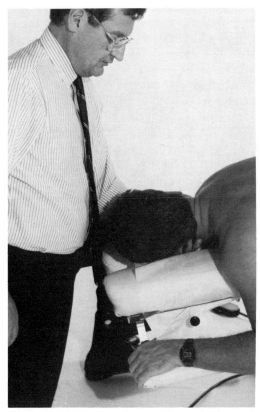 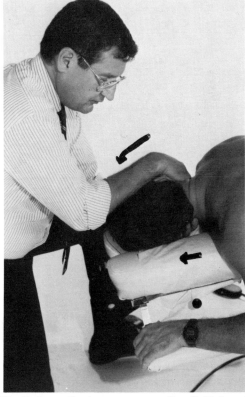

Figure 3.46. Positions for applying a right occipital lift with the patient prone; preparation *(left)*, thrust *(right)*.

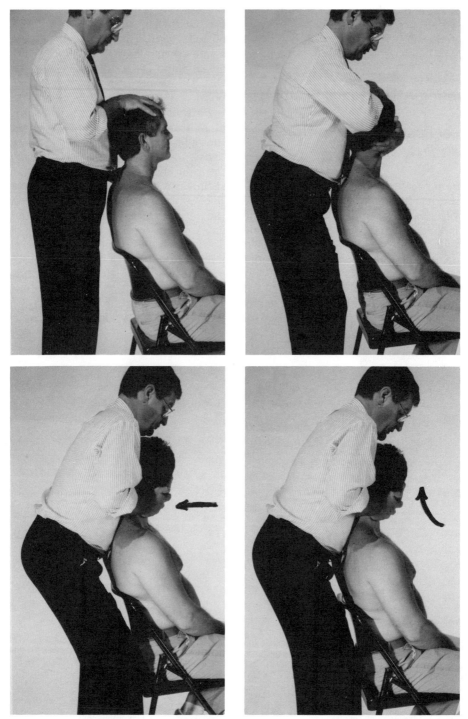

Figure 3.47. Occipital lift with the patient sitting; starting position *(upper left)*, contact *(upper right)*, thrust *(lower left and right)*.

follows the back of the patient's head. Once firm resistance is felt, add a short dynamic impulse to continue the rotation.

Atlantal Lateral Flexion on Axis Fixation

Patient Supine. If a lateral bending fixation is found between the atlas and axis, place the patient supine, stand at the head of the table and face the patient, turn the patient's head away from the side of fixation, and place your stabilizing hand under the patient's head. With your active hand, apply a pisiform contact on either the tip of the transverse process or the posterior arch, with your little finger extended along the ramus of the patient's jaw. Lift upward with your stabilizing hand to slightly laterally flex the upper cervical area. Apply counterpressure with your contact hand, and, when firm resistance is felt, add a short dynamic impulse to increase the lateral flexion (Fig. 3.49).

Patient Prone. With the patient positioned face down on the adjusting table, stand on the side of involvement. Bend down so that you can apply a thumb contact against the posterior arch of the atlas. Reinforce this contact with the thumb of your stabilizing hand. Apply pressure horizontally. Your fingers will be extended over the back of the patient's neck, and your arms should be almost parallel to the floor. Increased contact pressure until firm resistance is felt, then add a short dynamic recoil-type of impulse by extending your elbows. This is an excellent technic to use with the elderly when a lateral fixation exists and there is mild suspicion of but no overt signs of vertebral artery insufficiency.

Atlantal Anterior Rotation on Axis Fixation

Patient Supine. Stand at the head of the table facing the patient. Turn the patient's head toward the side of fixation. With your

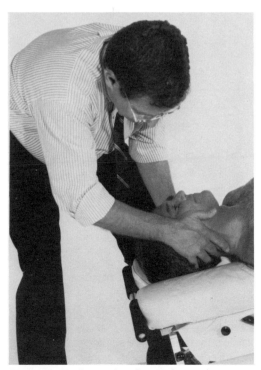

Figure 3.48. Preparing the supine patient to receive an occipital adjustment.

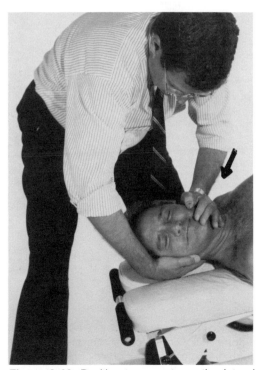

Figure 3.49. Position to correct an atlas lateral flexion on axis fixation with the patient supine.

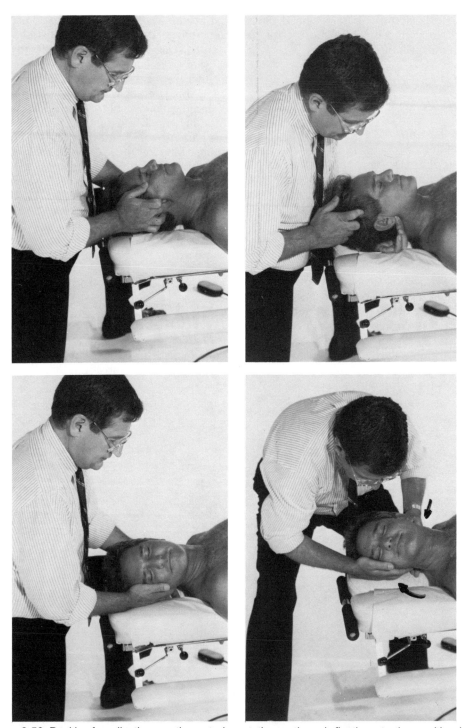

Figure 3.50. Position for adjusting an atlas anterior rotation on the axis fixation; starting position *(upper left)*, taking contact *(upper right)*, preparing the patient *(lower left)*, thrust *(lower right)*.

contact hand, cup the patient's atlas in the web of your active hand so that the tip of your index finger can contact the anterior aspect of the transverse process of the patient's atlas on the side of fixation. The patient's occiput will be supported by your palm. Cup the patient's uppermost ear with your stabilizing hand. Increase the rotation of the patient's head against the fixation with your stabilizing hand. Once firm resistance is obtained, apply traction with your stabilizing hand and deliver an impulse against the fixation by rotating the atlas posteriorly on the side of fixation with your contact fingers (Fig. 3.50). It should be noted that during this adjustment the active hand also laterally flexes toward the stabilizing hand.

Patient Sitting. This fixation is usually attended by a degree of flexion fixation. Stand facing the sitting patient, oblique to the side of fixation. The stabilizing hand cradles the patient's head firmly enough to apply a slight degree of distraction. Slide the pisiform of your active hand up the angle of the scalenus anticus attachments until it contacts the anterior aspect of the transverse process of the patient's atlas. Slightly lift, rotate, and tilt the patient's upper cervical area with both hands to produce tension of the scaleni attachments. When firm resistance is felt, add a quick dynamic impulse with your pisiform that will produce a short anterior-to-posterior movement of the atlas on the axis. A variation of this technic is to use a thumb contact rather than a pisiform contact.

Adjusting Middle and Lower Cervical Fixations

Posterior Rotation Fixations: C3—C7

Patient Supine. The patient is placed face up on the adjusting table, with the head-

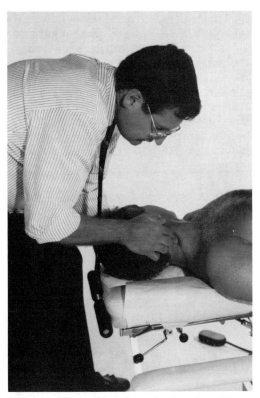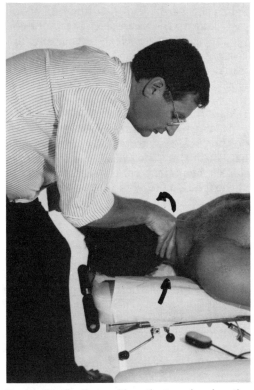

Figure 3.51. Positions for adjusting C3—C7 posterior rotation fixations with patient supine; locating contact site *(left),* thrust *(right).*

piece of the table level or up a notch. Stand at the head of the table facing the patient. Your stabilizing hand should support the patient's head and turn it away from the side of fixation. With your contact hand, push the trapezius laterally and take contact on the lamina or articular process of the involved segment, using either an index finger contact (straight or crooked) or a pisiform contact. Shift your weight slightly to the side of fixation, increase the rotation of the patient's neck to firm resistance, and deliver a short quick impulse directed along the plane of articulation to mobilize the blocked P-A motion (Fig. 3.51).

Patient Sitting. Stand directly behind the sitting patient. Locate the fixed processes with the thumb of your contact hand by sliding the trapezius laterally, then take contact with your index finger, palm supinated. Your stabilizing hand should be supporting the contralateral side of the patient's neck at the same level as your active contact. Rotate the patient's head away from the side of fixation, let the neck extend slightly, and shift your weight slightly to the side of contact. Take up the tissue slack with your contact, rotate the neck a little farther until firm resistance is felt, and deliver a short quick impulse against the blocked articulation (Fig. 3.52). Your line of drive should be along the plane of the articulation, designed to release the blocked P-A motion.

An alternative technic is a slight variation on the classic rotatory adjustment with the patient in the sitting position. Stand at the side of the patient, contralateral to the side of the fixation. Reach around in front of the patient with your contact hand so that your middle finger can firmly grip the lamina of the involved segment on the side of fixation. Pronate the palm of your stabilizing hand, and raise the elbow high so that you can grasp your fingers around the rim of the patient's occiput on the contralateral side of the fixation. Rotate the patient's face away from the side of fixation, take up any tissue slack under your contact finger, increase the rotation to firm resistance, and give a short quick impulse with your contact hand along the plane of articulation to release the blocked P-A motion (Fig. 3.53). It often helps if both the contact hand and the stabilizing hand

simultaneously apply a slight vertical distraction pull during the adjustment.

Patient Prone. Place the patient face down on the adjusting table with the head-piece level. Stand on the side of fixation, facing perpendicular to the patient. Take contact on the involved articular process with your thumb, fingers relaxed horizontally over the back of the patient's neck. Place your stabilizing thumb over your contact thumb in a like manner for reinforcement. Shift your weight so that it is centered over the patient, relax your elbows, take up the tissue slack under your contact thumb, and deliver a short quick recoil-type impulse by quickly adducting your elbows. The line of drive should be towards the floor and slightly headward to be in line with the plane of articulation.

An alternative technic is the classic cervical rotatory adjustment with the patient in the prone position. Stand on the same side as the fixation, turn the patient's face away from the side of fixation, so that the involved side will be facing the floor. Take contact on the lamina of the involved segment with the side of your index finger, elbow almost perpendicular to the patient's neck, and stabilize the patient's occiput by placing the heel of your stabilizing hand on the patient's temporal area above the ear. Remove any tissue slack under your contact finger, apply slight traction with your stabilizing hand, and deliver a short quick impulse with your contact hand against the blocked P-A motion of the segment.

Lateral Bending Fixations: C3—C7

The suggested technics used for releasing lateral bending fixations are similar to those described above for posterior rotation fixations with the major exception that the line of drive is directed perpendicularly against the block processes rather than directed to rotate the superior segment of the involved motion unit anteriorly (Fig. 3.54).

Extension Fixations: C3—C7

Patient Supine. With the patient facing the ceiling and the head-piece of the table

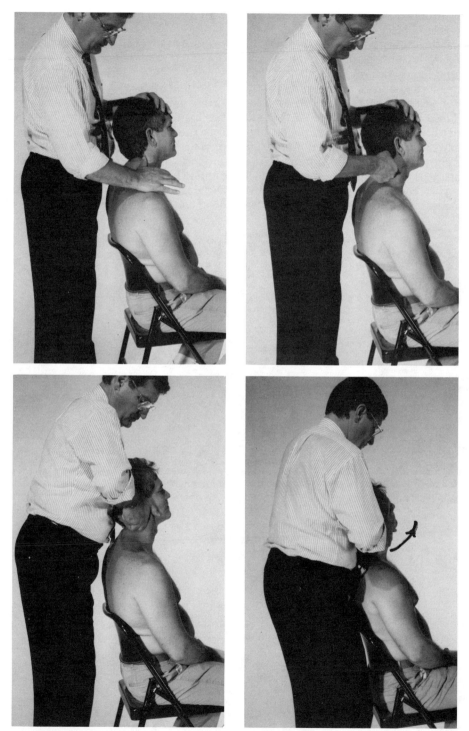

Figure 3.52. Positions for adjusting C3—C7 posterior rotation fixations with patient sitting; seeking contact site *(upper left)*, localizing contact site *(upper right)*, applying contact *(lower left)*, thrust *(lower right)*.

136

level or dropped a notch, stand at the head of the table and face the patient. Support the patient's head on the opposite side of the fixation with the fingers and palm of your stabilizing hand. With your active hand, place an index finger contact on the lamina of the superior segment of the involved motion unit. Raise both hands a little so that the patient's head will roll backward slightly and the cervical spine will be placed into extension. Your elbows will be low and pointing obliquely to the floor. Take up any tissue slack under your contact finger, and when firm resistance is felt, apply a short quick impulse

with your contact finger that is directed anteriorly (upward) and slightly medial to release the extension block. The slight medial direction is added only to avoid contact slippage.

Patient Sitting. Stand directly behind the sitting patient, supinate the palm of your active hand and place an index finger contact over the inferior articulating process of the fixated process. Your stabilizing hand should support the patient's neck in a similar manner and be positioned at the same level. Keep the patient's head near your sternum for good control. Shift your body weight slightly

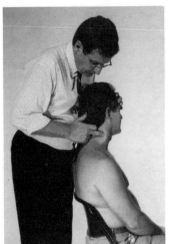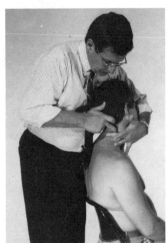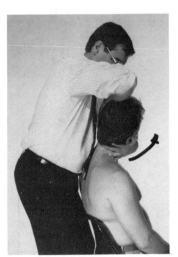

Figure 3.53. Positions for applying alternative technic for adjusting C3—C7 posterior rotation fixations with patient sitting; localizing contact site *(left),* applying contact *(middle),* thrust *(right).*

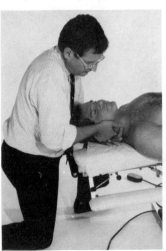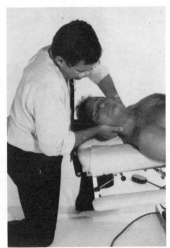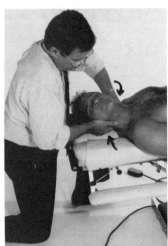

Figure 3.54. Positions for adjusting C3—C7 lateral flexion fixations with patient supine; applying contact *(left),* preparing patient for adjustment *(middle),* thrust *(right).*

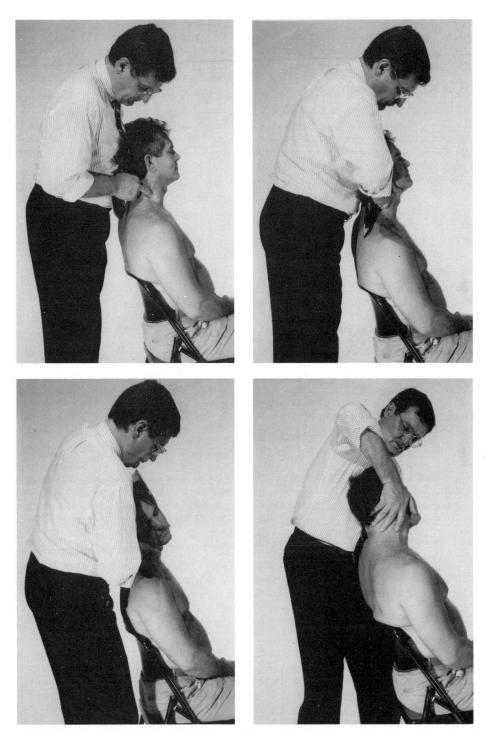

Figure 3.55. Positions for adjusting C3—C7 anterior rotation fixations with patient sitting; localizing contact site *(upper left)*, applying contact *(upper right)*, thrust *(lower left)*, view of stabilizing hand during thrust *(lower right)*.

to the side of fixation, extend and slightly distract the patient's neck with both hands to a point of firm resistance, and administer a short quick impulse directed anterosuperiorly against the extension block (Fig. 3.55).

Patient Prone. Position the patient face down. The head-piece can be either level or raised a notch or two. Stand at the head of the table, obliquely facing the patient, on the side opposite the fixation. With your active hand, make contact on the lamina of the superior segment of the involved motion unit with your index finger so that the thumb of this hand can be placed on the contralateral lamina. Place your stabilizing hand upon your active hand for reinforcement. Shift your torso over your hands, relax your elbows, but increase pressure until firm resistance is felt. The adjustment is made by delivering a short recoil-type of impulse by quickly adducting your elbows. The line of drive is downward (anteriorly) and slightly cephalad to mobilize the extension block.

Anterior Rotation Fixations: C3—C7

Patient Supine. Position the patient face up on an adjusting table with the head-piece level. Stand at the head of the table and face the patient. Lift the patient's occiput with your stabilizing hand so that you can reach under the back of the patient's neck and apply a web contact with your active hand around the posterior aspect of the superior segment of the involved motion unit. The tip of your active index or middle finger should be on the anterolateral aspect of the segment's transverse process. Once firm contact is made, place the palm or heel of your stabilizing hand against the patient's ipsilateral temporal area, and rotate the patient's face away from the side of fixation. Remove all tissue slack under your active finger by adding mild counterpressure with your stabilizing hand. The adjustment is made by simultaneously pulling your active contact so that the segment will rotate from the anterior to the posterior while your stabilizing hand applies some tensile force.

An alternative technic with the patient supine is to apply contact on the anterolateral aspect of the involved transverse process

with the side of the index finger of your active *ipsilalateral* hand. Turn the patient's face *away* from the side of fixation, and countersupport the patient's head or neck with your stabilizing hand. The correction is made by delivering an anterior-to-posterior impulse with your contact finger.

Patient Sitting. With the patient sitting, stand directly behind. Support the patient's neck contralaterally with your stabilizing hand and make contact with the side of your active hand's supinated index finger on the anterolateral aspect of the transverse process of the superior segment of the involved motion unit. Shift your weight slightly toward the side of fixation, laterally bend the patient's head toward the side of fixation (over your active contact finger), and apply slight extension of the patient's neck with both hands. Apply A-P motion until firm resistance is felt, and then administer a short quick rotatory anterior-to-posterior impulse with your active finger against the anterior rotation block, while lifting upward with your stabilizing hand to add some traction to open the facets.

Long-Axis Elongation Fixations: C3—C7

After all cervical flexion-extension, rotation, and lateral bending fixations have been mobilized, check the integrity of motion-unit distraction. Restriction here sometimes remains after all other corrections have been made. To make this correction, assume the same doctor-patient positions as used during long-axis elongation palpation (Fig. 3.56). If no or distinctly subnormal separation is felt between certain segments during traction, hold the traction and apply a short quick mild additional long-axis pull (a faint release should be palpable or heard), and sustain mild traction for several seconds to allow for tissue adaptation. Release the tension slowly. The prior traction before the correcting stretch is important to avoid tearing some tissue. Never "snap" the spine. This is often an extremely effective maneuver, but gentleness, the utmost of control, and sound clinical judgment are necessary in its application.

Table 3.7. Selected Effects of Cervical Area Hypertonicity

Muscle	Effect of Prolonged Hypertonicity
Interspinales	Excessive muscle tone between the spinous processes tends to hyperextend the motion unit.
Obliquus capitis inferior	Increased tone tends to produce a rotary torque of the atlas-axis motion unit.
Obliquus capitis superior	Contraction tends to roll the occiput anterior and inferior and pull the atlas posterior and superior to produce a lateral occiput tilt and condyle jamming.
Rectus capitis posterior major	Hypertonicity tends to pull the occiput posterior, inferior, and medial and the spinous of the axis superior, lateral, and anterior. Strong hypertonicity will lock the occiput and axis together so that they appear to act as one unit even though they are not contiguous.
Scalenus anterior	Contraction tends to pull the C3—C6 transverse processes inferior, lateral, and anterior and the 1st rib superior and medial.
Scalenus medius	Excessive tone tends to pull the C1—C7 transverse processes inferior, lateral, and anterior and the 1st rib superior and medial.
Scalenus posterior	Hypertonicity tends to pull the C4—C6 transverse processes inferior, lateral, and anterior and the 2nd rib superior and medial.
Splenius capitis	Increased tone tends to pull the C5—T3 spinous processes lateral, superior, and anterior and to subluxate the occiput inferior, medial, and posterior.
Sternocleidomastoideus	Contraction tends to pull the sternum and clavicle posterior and superior and the occiput inferior and anterior.
Upper trapezius	Hypertonicity tends to pull the occiput posteroinferior, the C7—T5 spinous processes lateral, and the shoulder girdle medial and superior.

Adjusting Muscular Fixations in the Cervical Spine

Some major biomechanical effects of cervical hypertonicity are shown in Table 3.7. Should the practitioner wish to adjust muscle fixations in the cervical spine rather than allowing them to correct themselves spontaneously by relieving primary fixations found elsewhere, Gillet offers the following comments.

Intertransversarii, multifidi, and rotatores respond well to a rotatory adjustment designed to pull one end of the shortened muscle away from the other end; ie, to produce a stretch. The transverse process is the best contact point to accomplish this. On the other hand, interspinous fixations tend to relax more when a thumb contact is used against the spinous process of the superior segment of the fixed motion unit when the patient's head is held in lateral flexion. A fixation of an obliquus muscle may be stretched at the atlas transverse when it is in rotation with the occiput, or the spinous of the axis may be stretched from the atlas on the opposite side.

140

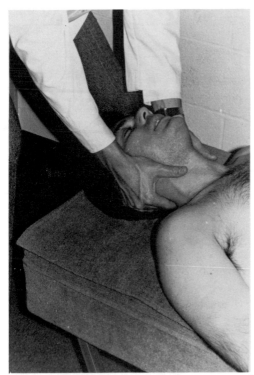

Figure 3.56. Position for evaluating segmental cervical distraction (Courtesy ACAP).

One transverse process of the atlas may palpate more prominently than the other. If this is not a structural anomaly, it is likely from hypertonicity of the ipsilateral rectus capitis minor posterior or the contralateral rectus capitis minor anterior. In either case, an occipital adjustment will "reposition" the atlas if the adjustment is designed to stretch the shortened muscles involved. A favorite method of Gillet is a rotary adjustment in which the head of the sitting patient is turned and the lateral aspect of the temporal bone (just above the ear) is nested against the lower part of his sternum. Contact is made on the contralateral transverse process of the atlas with the middle phalanx of the 2nd finger. Your other hand can be placed over this finger for reinforcement. Without moving the patient's head, remove the tissue slack and direct a short brisk rotation of the atlas anteriorly. With the patient's cranium firmed against your sternum, this technic is quite specific.

The technics that have been described with the patient in the sitting position can also be modified to be conducted with the patient supine or prone. In recumbent positions, special care must be taken in most instances to move only the contact hand and not the stabilizing hand unless it is being used for reinforcement.

Bibliography

Bailey RW: *The Cervical Spine.* Philadelphia, Lea & Febiger, 1974, pp 91-97.
Bard G, and Jones M: Cineradiographic recording of traction of the cervical spine. *Archives of Physical Medicine and Rehabilitation,* August 1964.
Bergmann T: Integrated chiropractic methods. Oklahoma seminar, April 23, 1983, NWCC, pp 8—12.
Bovee ML: *The Essentials of the Orthopedic & Neurological Examination.* Place of publication not shown, published by author, 1977, p 7.
Brodin H: Cervical pain and mobilization. *Manuelle Medizin,* 20:90-94, 1982.
Cailliet R: *Neck and Arm Pain.* Philadelphia, F.A. Davis, 1974, p 37.
Cailliet R: *Soft Tissue Pain and Disability.* Philadelphia, F.A. Davis, 1980, pp 61, 107-124, 128-130, 135-140, 142-148.
Chusid JG: *Correlative Neuroanatomy & Functional Neurology,* ed 19. Los Altos, CA, Lange Medical, pp 68, 297.
Craton EF: Cranial vertebral junction autopsy. *Today's Chiropractic,* pp 29-30. September-October 1985.
De Rusha JL: Upper cervical technic correlated with neurodiagnosis. *ACA Journal of Chiropractic,* September 1961.
Dimnet J, Pasquet A, Krag MH, Panjabi MM: Cervical spine motion in the sagittal plane: Kinematic and geometric parameters. *Journal of Biomechanics,* 15:959-969, 1982.
Dove CI: The occipito-atlanto-axial complex. *Manuelle Medizin,* 20:11-15, 1982.
Duckworth JAW: Dissection seminar conducted at the Canadian Chiropractic Memorial College. Toronto, CMCC, 1983.
Dvorak J, Orelli FV: How dangerous is manipulation of the cervical spine? Case report and results of an inquiry. *Manuelle Medizin,* 20:44-48, 1982.
Epstein BS: *The Spine: A Radiological Text and Atlas.* Philadelphia, Lea & Febiger, 1962, pp 268-269.
Faye LJ, et al: Spine II: *Motion Palpation and Clinical Considerations of the Cervical and Thoracic Spine.* Huntington Beach, CA, Motion Palpation Institute, 1986, pp 1-2, 4-9, 12-15, 18-21, 24-41.
Faye LJ: Motion Palpation and Manipulation of the Lower Cervicals [Videotape]. Dynaspine, Inc, 10780 Santa Monica Blvd, Suite 400, Los Angeles, CA 90025.
Faye LJ: Motion Palpation and Manipulation of the Upper Cervicals [Videotape]. Dynaspine, Inc, 10780 Santa Monica Blvd, Suite 400, Los Angeles, CA 90025.
Faye LJ: Motion Palpation: Spine 2, Cervicals and Thoracics [Cassette tape program]. Huntington Beach,

CA, Motion Palpation Institute, 1986, 6 tapes.

Felding JW, Francis WR, Hawkins RJ: The upper cervical spine. In Feldman F (ed): *Radiology, Pathology, and Immunology of Bones and Joints: A Review of Current Concepts*, New York, Appleton-Century-Crofts, 1978, pp 303-312.

Fisk JW: *The Painful Neck and Back*. Springfield, IL, Charles C. Thomas, 1977, pp 28-37.

Gehweiler JA Jr, Osborne RL Jr, Becker RF: *The Radiology of Vertebrae Trauma*. Philadelphia, W.B. Saunders, 1980, p 74.

Gemmell HA: Biomechanics and function examination of the cervical spine. *Journal of the Chiropractic Association of Oklahoma*, 6(2):12-13, Spring 1988.

George AW: A method for more accurate study of injuries to the atlas and axis. *ACA Journal of Chiropractic*, pp 41-51, December 1983.

George PE: New techniques to identify the potential stroke victim. *International Review of Chiropractic*, p 23, January/March 1981.

Gillet H, Liekens M: *Belgian Chiropractic Research Notes*. Huntington Beach, CA, Motion Palpation Institute, 1984, pp 5-7, 19-20, 27-28, 38-43, 70-71, 107-108, 142-144.

Gillet H: Normal and abnormal cervical mobility. *Bulletin of the European Chiropractic Union*, 28(4):47-49, 1980.

Gillet H: Occiput-atlas-axis fixation. *Journal of Clinical Chiropractic*, 1(12): 30-33, 1976.

Glerak RA: Vertebral artery compression and vascular insufficiency of the brain. *Archives of California Chiropractic Association*, 2:28-39, 1972.

Goodheart GL: *Collected Published Articles and Reprints*. Montpellier, OH, Williams County Publishing, 1969, pp 15, 59-60, 65.

Gregory R: Biomechanics of the upper cervical spine. *The Digest of Chiropractic Economics*, September/October 1983.

Grice AS: A biomechanical approach to cervical and dorsal adjusting. In Haldeman S (ed): *Modern Developments in the Principles and Practice of Chiropractic*. New York, Appleton-Century-Crofts, 1980, pp 331-349.

Grieve GP: *Common Vertebral Joint Problems*. London, Churchill Livingstone, 1981, pp 41, 125-134, 312-314, 319-324.

Grove AB: *Chiropractic Technique—A Procedure of Adjusting*. Madison, WI, Straus Printing & Publishing, 1979, p 40.

Hadler NM: *Medical Management of the Regional Musculoskeletal Diseases*. New York, Grune & Stratton, 1984, pp 123-126.

Hadley LA: *Anatomico-Roentgenographic Studies of the Spine*. Springfield, IL, Charles C. Thomas, 1981, pp 160-162.

Henderson DJ: Significance of vertebral dyskinesia in relation to the cervical syndrome. *Journal of Manipulative and Physiological Therapeutics*, 2:1, 1979.

Herbst RW: *Gonstead Chiropractic Science and Art*. Sci-Chi Publishers. Other publication data not shown.

Hohl M, Baker HR: The atlantoaxial joint, roentgenographic and anatomical study of normal and abnormal motion. *Journal of Bone & Joint Surgery*, 46A:

1739, 1964.

Jackson R: *The Cervical Syndrome*, ed 4. Springfield, IL, Charles C. Thomas, 1978.

Jeffreys E: *Disorders of the Cervical Spine*. Boston, Butterworths, 1980, pp 2-14.

Jirout J: Changes in the atlas-axis relations on lateral flexion of the head and neck. *Neuroradiology*, 6:215, 1973.

Johnston WL, Hill JL: Spinal segmental dysfunction: incidence in the cervicothoracic region. *Journal of the American Osteopathic Association*, 81:67-76, September 1981.

Johnston WL, Vorro J, Hubbard RP: Clinical/biomechanic correlates for cervical function: part I, a kinematic study. *Journal of the American Osteopathic Association*, 85(7):429-436, July 1985.

Kapandji IA: *Physiology of the Joints: The Trunk and Vertebral Column*, ed 2. New York, Churchill Livingstone, 1980, vol three, pp 20-21, 154, 172-244.

Kale M: The upper cervical specific. *Today's Chiropractic*, part 1, pp 28-29, July/August 1984; part 2, pp 27-30, September/October 1984.

Keggi, Granger, Southwick: Vertebral artery insufficiency secondary to trauma and osteoarthritis of the cervical spine. *Yale Journal of Biology and Medicine*, 38:471-478, 1966.

Kos J: The cervical spine. Toronto, Canadian Memorial Chiropractic College, CMCC continuing education program.

Kraus H: Muscular aspects of oral dysfunction. In Gelb H (ed): *Clinical Management of Head, Neck and TMJ Pain and Dysfunction*. Philadelphia, W.B. Saunders, 1977, pp 117-124.

Lommbardi G: The occipital vertebra. *American Journal of Roentgenology*, 86:260, 1961.

Lysell E: Motion in the cervical spine. *Acta Orthopaedia Scandinavia* (Supplement), 123:1, 1969,

Macnab I: Symptoms in cervical disc degeneration. In The Cervical Spine Research Society: *The Cervical Spine*. Philadelphia, Lippincott, 1983, pp 388-394.

Mapstone T, Spetzler RF: Vertebrobasilar insufficiency secondary to vertebral artery occlusion. *Journal of Neurosurgery*, 56:581-583, 1982.

Markovich SE: Painful neuro-muscular dysfunction syndromes in the head: a neurologist's view. Paper presented to the American Academy of Cranio-Mandibular Orthopedics Meeting, New Orleans, September 1976.

Markovich SE: Pain in the head: A neurological appraisal. In Gelb H (ed): *Clinical Management of Head, Neck and TMJ Pain and Dysfunction*. Philadelphia, W.B. Saunders, 1977, pp 125-139.

McRae DL: The significance of abnormalities of the cervical spine. *American Journal of Roentgenology*, 84:3, 1960.

Mertz JA: Videofluoroscopy of the cervical and lumbar spine. *ACA Journal of Chiropractic*, pp 74-75, August 1981.

Meyermann R: Possibilities of injury to the artery vertebralis. *Manuelle Medizin*, 20:105-114, 1982.

Mumenthaler M: *Neurology*, ed 2. Translated by EH Burrows. New York, Thieme-Stratton, 1983, pp 157-158.

Murphy C, Rankin I, Jones BE, Jayson MIV: Continuous recording of neck rotation: preliminary observations. *Spine*, 9:657-658, 1984.

Nash CL, Moe JH: A study of vertebral rotation. *Journal of Bone & Joint Surgery*, 51:223, 1969.

Nelson JM: Conservative approaches to the management of thoracic outlet syndrome. In Coyle BA, Martinez DP (eds): *Proceedings of the Second Conference on Current Topics in Chiropractic: Reviews of the Literature;* May 4-5, 1985. Sunnyvale, CA, Palmer College of Chiropractic—West, 1985, section B1.

Ng SY: The relationship between atlas deposition and cervical curvature. *ACA Journal of Chiropractic*, 13:79-83, September 1979.

Ng SY: Upper cervical vertebrae and occipital headache. *Journal of Manipulative and Physiological Therapeutics*, 3(3):137-141, September 1980.

Pettibon Bio-Mechanics Institute: *Pettibon Spinal Bio-Mechanics: Theory and Implications*, ed 2. Vancouver, WA, Pettibon BioMechanics, 1976, pp 44-46, 94-99.

Phillips RB: Upper cervical biomechanics. *ACA Journal of Chiropractic*, October 1976.

Rehberger LP: Reversal of the normal cervical curve. *Roentgenological Briefs*, Council on Roentgenology of the American Chiropractic Association, Des Moines, IA, date not shown.

Reid JD: Effects of flexion-extension movements of the head and spine upon the spinal cord and nerve roots. *Journal of Neurology, Neurosurgery and Psychiatry* (British), 23:214. 1960.

Reinert OC: Anatomical characteristics of subluxation: C2 through C7. *ACA Journal of Chiropractic*, pp 62-69, May 1984.

Rude J: Morphology of the occipital condyles and movement of the atlanto-occipital joint. *Manuelle Medizin*, 22:101-106, 1984.

Sandoz R: A classification of luxation, subluxation and fixation of the cervical spine. *Annals of the Swiss Chiropractors Association*, 6:219-276, 1976.

Saternus KS, Fuchs V: Is the artery vertebralis endangered in resuscitation. *Manuelle Medizin*, 20:101-104, 1982.

Schafer RC: *Chiropractic Management of Sports and Recreational Injuries*. Baltimore, Williams & Wilkins, 1982, pp 331, 340-341, 357.

Schafer RC: *Chiropractic Physical and Spinal Diagnosis*. Oklahoma City, American Chiropractic Academic Press, 1980, pp VI:24-26, VIII:9-32.

Schafer RC: *Clinical Biomechanics: Musculoskeletal Actions and Reactions*. Baltimore, Williams & Wilkins, 1983, pp 175, 177, 183, 184-186, 194, 264-271, 279-285.

Schafer RC: Physical examination of the TMJ, posterior neck, and cervical spine. In Schafer RC: *Physical Diagnosis: Procedures and Methodology in Chiropractic Practice*. Arlington, VA, American Chiropractic Association. Scheduled to be released in 1989. Chapter 15.

Schafer RC: *Symptomatology and Differential Diagnosis*. Arlington, VA, American Chiropractic Association, 1986, pp 228, 455, 552-555, 569-570.

Schmorl G, Junghanns H: *The Human Spine in Health and Disease*. New York, Grune & Stratton, 1971.

Sheehan S, Bauer RB, Meyer JS: Vertebral artery compression in cervical spondylosis, arteriographic demonstration during life of vertebral artery insufficiency due to rotation and extension of the neck. *Neurology*, 10:968-986, 1960.

Smith DM: Vertebral artery. *Roentgenological Briefs*. Council on Roentgenology of the American Chiropractic Association, date and number not shown.

Snijders CJ, Timmerman P: Motions and forces in the atlanto-occipital joint during flexion of the cervical spine. *Manuelle Medizin*, 20:51-58, 1982.

Stonebrink RD: Palpation for vertebral motoricity. *ACA Journal of Chiropractic*, III:S11-14, February 1969.

Sutherland S: Anatomical perivertebral influences on the intervertebral foramen. In Goldstein M (ed): *The Research Status of Spinal Manipulative Therapy*, NINCDS Monograph No. 15, DHEW Publication No. (NIH) 76-998, Stock No. 017-049-0-0060-7, Washington, DC, U.S. Government Printing Office, 1975.

Sweat RW: Scanning palpation: cervical spine. *Today's Chiropractic*, pp 23-24, January/February 1985.

Sweat RW, Sievert T: Chiropractic and the vertebral arteries. *Today's Chiropractic*, part 1, pp 45-48, September/October 1984; part 2, pp 23-24, November/December 1984.

Telford ED, Mottershead S: Pressure at the cervical brachial junction: an operative and anatomical study. *Journal of Bone & Joint Surgery*, 30B:249-250, 1948.

Toole J, Tucker SH: Influence of head position upon cerebral circulation. *Archives of Neurology* (AMA), 2:616-623, 1960.

Von Torklus D, Gehle W: *The Upper Cervical Spine*. New York, Grune & Stratton, 1972, p 22.

West HG: Vertebral artery considerations in cervical trauma. *ACA Journal of Chiropractic*, pp 18-19, December 1968.

White AA, Panjabi MM: *Clinical Biomechanics of the Spine*. Philadelphia, J.B. Lippincott, 1978, pp 65-74, 82-87, 123-166, 183-184, 196-218, 235, 271, 294-296.

Chapter 4

The Thoracic Spine

This chapter describes the *dynamic chiropractic* approach to the correction of fixations of the thoracic spine and related tissues. Diagnostic and therapeutic considerations are described, as well as some significant points in differential diagnosis.

BASIC CONSIDERATIONS

It is common knowledge that the thoracic spine is the most often manipulated region of the spine; yet, its fixations are frequently the least efficiently corrected. This chapter has been designed to resolve common points of confusion and offer the practitioner a rational approach relative to thoracic fixations.

Applied Anatomical Considerations

Some unique factors should be considered about the stability of the thoracic spine. Fifteen important points are, in comparison to the cervical and lumbar regions of the spine, that the thoracic spine:
• Has an anatomic curvature directed posteriorly
• Is biomechanically stiffer
• Is less mobile
• Has restricting costal articulations
• Has a great resistance to extension
• Possesses coupling variants from top to bottom
• Is the major source of supply of sympathetic fibers
• Has thin discs

• Has IVD nuclei almost centered within the anuli
• Has thicker yellow ligaments
• Has thinner and looser apophyseal capsules
• Has thinner and weaker interspinous ligaments
• Has a smaller vertebral canal
• Has less vascularity for the cord
• Tends to be clinically unstable during flexion.

Planes of Articulation

The direction of the superior articulations in the thoracic spine is slightly posterolateral, and the inferior processes face slightly anteromedially. This slant comes closer to the vertical axis as one progresses caudally downward. The facets are inclined 60° or more to the vertical plane in the midthoracic spine. These articular planes allow greater rotation but less flexion and extension than that seen in the more horizontal articular planes of the lumbar vertebra.

Vertebrae normally move in the planes of their articulations, and it is at the level of the posterior intervertebral articulations that most fixations occur and influence the IVFs. Exception for bony outgrowths near IVFs, structural changes in the diameter of IVFs result from an abnormal joint position, which predisposes to further subluxation or kinetic disturbances as well as being a direct factor in altering the curves of the particular region of the spine in which this structural/functional defect is found. This, of course, is in addition of any affect placed on the IVF contents.

The Intervertebral Foramina

An IVF is bounded above by the inferior pedicle notch of the superior vertebra, anteriorly by the centrum of the superior segment and slightly by the IVD, and posteriorly by the superior and inferior articular processes. The pedicle notch of the typical thoracic vertebra above is quite deep, and the result is a pear-shaped canal with sharp bony edges that predispose to fibrotic changes from chronic irritation. The vertebral body and disc of the superior vertebra form most of the IVF's anterior boundary. See Figure 4.1.

When viewed laterally, an IVF is generally elliptical in shape, with the diameter of its vertical axis about double its lateral dimension. Because of this, there is usually adequate space for changes in vertical dimension (eg, axial traction or compression and disc flattening) without injury to the IVF contents as long as there is adequate fat and fluid present. However, reduction of an already short transverse diameter can produce many noxious effects. Thus, complete disc collapse vertically is often asymptomatic, while a slight posterolateral herniation may protrude on the IVF and produce overt symptoms.

The Spinocostal Joints

The Costovertebral Joints. Posteriorly, the convex-shaped head of a rib articulates (slides and pivots) on two adjacent thoracic vertebral bodies at the concave demifacets, above and below disc level, within a single richly innervated synovial joint. Exceptions to this are the 1st rib and floating ribs whose heads articulate with only one vertebra. Typically, the capsule of a costovertebral joint is thin and weak by itself but stronger anteriorly than posteriorly. It is attached to the anulus via the intermediate intra-articular ligament that divides the cavity and attaches to the rib head between the facets. Interosseous fibers also extend from the rib head superiorly to the vertebral body above and inferiorly to the vertebral body below. These intermediate, superior, and inferior fibers greatly strengthen the inherently weak capsule proper. Posteriorly, capsule fibers merge with the lateral extensions of the posterior longitudinal ligament. During inspiration, the rib heads undergo a slight rotatory and gliding movement, much like a bucket handle being lifted away from the side of the pail.

The Costotransverse Joints. As a rib is directed posteriorly from the attachment of its head, a convex posterior tubercle on the rib articulates with a concave facet on the anterior tip of the transverse process of the same vertebra (Fig. 4.2). This is also a richly innervated synovial joint that allows lubricated movement. The T1—T7 joints are concave to allow rotation, while the T8—T10 joints are flat and situated more superiorly and horizontal to allow gliding. Strength is provided to the thin capsule via medial and lateral costotransverse ligaments. A strong superior costotransverse ligament connects an adjacent rib neck below to the transverse process above, but it offers only slight protection to the costotransverse capsule. Dur-

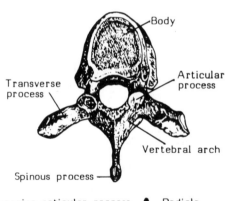

Body

Transverse process

Articular process

Vertebral arch

Spinous process

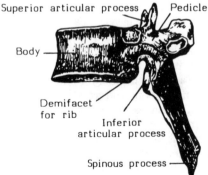

Superior articular process

Pedicle

Body

Demifacet for rib

Inferior articular process

Spinous process

Figure 4.1. Diagrams of a typical thoracic vertebra (T6) from above (*top*) and left lateral (*bottom*) (Courtesy ACAP).

ing inspiration, the tubercle glides superiorly and posteriorly. The lower two or three ribs have neither articular tubercles nor costotransverse joints.

Biomechanical Considerations

As in the lumbar spine, all thoracic movements are somewhat three-dimensional with rotation and lateral flexion being the most evident. Gillet points out that within

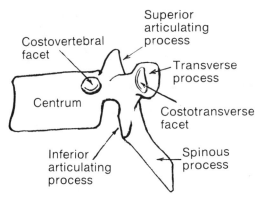

Figure 4.2. Schematic of a typical T5 vertebra.

oversimplified teachings, the thoracic spine is "often singled out as a string of bones" with the existence and movements of the attached ribs left out of the functional picture. Yet, the thoracic vertebrae normally move by carrying their attached ribs, and vice versa. See Figure 4.3.

The Righting Reflexes and Their Effect on the Spine

To maintain an erect posture with whatever postural abnormality may be present, the righting reflexes (if intact) attempt to distribute the weight of the body over the area occupied by the feet. To some extent, this accommodation process is limited by the gravitational forces involved that direct the postural variations which are possible. The components that are distinguishable in the majority of postural defects when viewing the body from the lateral plane are: (1) an increase or decrease in the angle of the sacral base, (2) the presence or absence of a fixed thoracolumbar tendency toward kyphosis, (3) the presence or absence of a mid-

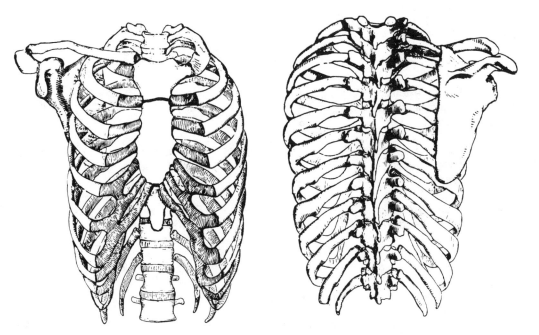

Figure 4.3. The thorax and shoulder girdle, as viewed from the front (*left*) and rear (*right*) (Courtesy ACAP).

thoracic hyperkyphosis, (4) the presence or absence of a flattening of the thoracic spine (with Pottenger's saucering), and/or (5) an increase or decrease in the cervical curve. Some of these distortions will be readily apparent on visual analysis, especially when a grid or plumb line is used. However, the determination of the cause(s) of the distortion must be based on detailed physical (eg, motion palpation) and roentgenographic analyses.

Kinematics

Gravitational forces fall upon the articular surfaces in such a manner as to force each vertebra more inferior, posterior, and medial until gravity brings the curve back toward the centered balance point.

Flexion and Extension. Flexion and extension of the thoracic spine are comparatively limited; ranges are shown in Table 4.1. As in other spinal areas, excessive A-P and P-A motions are restricted by the check ligaments, but the thoracic cage adds a strong additional mechanical barrier to flexion and intercostal and intervertebral straps to restrict extension.

Thoracic extension from full flexion is described in the literature of spinal biomechanics as taking place in two phases:

1. The articular surfaces glide posteriorly and inferiorly, the interspinous spaces close, and the stretched posterior anulus of the disc returns to its normal shape as the individual achieves the erect position. There is no appreciable change in the anterior aspect of the disc's anulus or its nucleus.

Table 4.1. Normal Ranges of Thoracic Motion

Motion Unit	Movement	Degrees*	Motion Unit	Movement	Degrees*
T1—2	Flexion/extension	4	7—8	Flexion/extension	6
	Lateral bending	6		Lateral bending	6
	Rotation	10		Rotation	7
2—3	Flexion/extension	4	8—9	Flexion/extension	6
	Lateral bending	6		Lateral bending	6
	Rotation	9		Rotation	6
3—4	Flexion/extension	4	9—10	Flexion/extension	6
	Lateral bending	6		Lateral bending	6
	Rotation	8		Rotation	4
4—5	Flexion/extension	4	10—11	Flexion/extension	10
	Lateral bending	6		Lateral bending	7
	Rotation	8		Rotation	3
5—6	Flexion/extension	4	11—12	Flexion/extension	12
	Lateral bending	6		Lateral bending	9
	Rotation	8		Rotation	2
6—7	Flexion/extension	6	12—L1	Flexion/extension	12
	Lateral bending	6		Lateral bending	8
	Rotation	7		Rotation	2

*These ranges are approximate. Authorities differ in several degrees in their reported findings. The above is a composite of findings.

2. It is not until the shingle-like facets, transverse processes, and spinous processes reach their limit as the spine is extended posterior to the midline that the anterior discs and anterior intercostal spaces begin to widen. On forced extension, the articular processes impact. The vertebrae then push between their ribs, and the rib heads and their angles are moved slightly aside by the transverse processes.

Thoracic A-P and P-A mobility from the neutral position includes a good amount of facet gliding, but it is far less than that of the cervical region where the facets almost separate on forward flexion. Because of the rather limited normal movement of individual segments of the thoracic spine, the gross idiopathic type scolioses in this area are difficult to comprehend when little structural damage is present.

As in other spinal areas, the anulus and nucleus bulge in opposite directions during A-P, P-A, and lateral bending moments to stabilize each other. During forced extension, the anulus thins and bulges posteriorly, and it stretches and contracts anteriorly. The nucleus bulges anteriorly without appreciable shifting. The anterior ligaments are put under tension while the posterior ligaments relax. At the end of forced extension, the inferior facets tend to pivot open as their inferior aspect jams on their neighbors below. These actions are quite minimal when the normal kyphosis is present, but they may be exaggerated in the flat "military-type" spine. During flexion, the mechanisms described above for extension are opposite.

From a slightly different perspective, Gillet also describes thoracic A-P and P-A motions as normally taking place in two parts:

1. If the patient is brought back from full forward flexion, the *first* movement that takes place is not an opening of the motion unit's disk space anteriorly or of the respective anterior costocostal space but a closing of the posterior spaces. The articulating surfaces glide backward and downward (posteroinferiorly), and the interspinous space closes before any appreciable change take place in the movement of the vertebrae at their anterior aspect. It is only when these structures and their ribs arrive at their extension end point and continued further

will the anterior portion of the IVD and anterior intercostal spaces widen. Thus, in the everyday movements of the average human, thoracic motion primarily takes place in the posterior half of the involved motion units. It appears that Gillet is describing the changes occurring at the anterior aspect of the motion unit during extension to be the result of the superior facets acting as pivot points for the inferior facets.

2. Thoracic forward flexion and backward extension at any starting position also includes a certain amount of gliding but less so than found with the cervical spine. At the end of this movement, a small degree of supplementary movement also occurs between the involved vertebrae and attached ribs.

Lateral Bending. Although lateral flexion is hampered by the rib cage, the average person should be able to touch the ipsilateral knee with the fingertips. Of course, this could be accomplished in a fixated thoracic spine compensated by an extremely flexible lumbar spine and hip joints. During lateral flexion in either the neutral or forward flexed position, there is generally thought to be some coupled rotation where the upper vertebral bodies swing toward the concave side of the curve and the spinous processes rotate toward the convexity as in the cervical spine. This sidebending-rotation requires transverse process movement anteriorly, pushing against the rib on the convex side and posterior transverse process movement pulling away from a rib on the concave side. This appears to be the primary restricting mechanism, with the ligaments playing a lesser role except in traumatic forces.

According to various papers on the subject, the vertebral bodies in the lower thoracic segments swing toward the convex side and the spinous processes rotate toward the concavity as in the lumbar spine. Grieve states that an opposite effect occurs during lateral flexion when the spine is in the extended position, where vertebral body rotation is towards the convexity in the upper thorax and toward the concavity in the lower thoracic region. This fact tends to explain how various primary fixation-subluxations influence the direction a scoliosis will take; ie, a focal vertebral motion unit locked in either neutral, flexion, or extension.

If the ligament attachments are supple (eg, as those of a healthy child), the ribs react to this movement of the transverse processes and enhance rotation. The rib spaces on the convex side will not open until the ribs on the concave side have reached their limit of apposition. In the adult thoracic spine, however, there is generally thought to be little rotation accompanying lateral bending except in the lower thoracic region where the ribs float. On forced lateral bending where the ribs appose on the concave side and their limit is reached, the involved vertebrae are capable of slight additional lateral gliding. The function of a thoracic vertebra locked in lateral flexion is identical to that of the static subluxation description in the neutral position where one facet has glided inferoposteriorly while its counterpart has glided upward and forward (superoanteriorly).

In the classical description of thoracic lateral bending in which the mechanism is described as lateral flexion coupled with rotation (in which the centra rotate posteriorly on the side of the convexity of the curve and the spinouses rotate toward posteriorly of the side of the concavity), it is generally explained that one transverse process and its attached rib are pushed anteriorly on the concave side of the curve while the other transverse process and its attached rib are pulled posteriorly on the convex side of the curve. However, Gillet points out that while this does occur in the young child in which the thorax is normally supple, it is rare in the adult except in the lower thoracic spine (in the area of the floating ribs). He reports that, in the typical adult, the transverse processes on the convex side do separate (but only to a small degree), while the opposite transverse process rarely, if ever, succeeds in pushing its attached rib forward. Therefore, for all practical purposes, lateral bending in the thoracic spine is normally a pure sideways flexion except in the lower thoracic area where the floating ribs are able to follow vertebrae rotation with much less restriction. This lateral bending motion is accompanied by a gliding action; ie, a lateral tilting of the centra and the articulations toward from the side of the concavity.

Rotation. Rotation of the thoracic spine, possibly coupled with some vertebral body tilting, is somewhat greater than flexion and extension that are about equal in range. According to Grice, there are also a few degrees of coupled flexion during upper-thoracic rotation and a few degrees of coupled extension during lower-thoracic rotation. This becomes a significant point in analyzing scolioses.

A study of thoracic rotation, states Gillet, must also take into consideration the attached ribs, "for he who has looked closely at a patient in this position (thoracic rotation) will have immediately noticed that the spine does not turn *between* the ribs, but *with* them." It is his belief that the *normal* center of rotation is not in the spine but at the *sternum.* "In fact, the movement at the vertebrae is also a lateral gliding. This can readily be ascertained, as Illi has done, by measuring the plane lines of the surfaces of the articulation. It is evident, therefore, that the involved vertebrae rotate and flex *with* their attached ribs, which also glide laterally on their neighbor below. It is only when this movement is forced a little beyond the elastic limit that a new movement takes place, and this new movement can be described as flexion, extension, lateral bending, or rotation of the vertebrae to a degree that is further than the ribs can move."

Disc Changes During Rotation. During axial rotation, the oblique fibers of the anulus that course in the direction of rotation become tensed while those running in the opposite direction relax. This puts a twist on the anulus, but there are no appreciable shear forces involved in the thoracic spine during pure axial rotation.

Rib Changes During Rotation. It can be readily noted during thoracic rotation that the spine does not rotate between the ribs but with the ribs, and this is accompanied by a degree of lateral gliding of the vertebrae involved. However, when rotation is forced beyond the limit of rib motion, there is a slight push by the transverse process against the rib head on the side moving anteriorly and a slight pull by the transverse process complex on the rib head on the side moving posteriorly. This motion is often revealed by palpation, rarely by roentgenography. It is recognized easier in the upper thoracic region where rotation is greater and the ribs are firmly attached to the sternum than in the lower thoracic area where the floating ribs more readily follow vertebral movement. According to its design, the thoracic spine would have a considerable range of rotary motion if it were not for the restricting thoracic cage. This is exhibited in scoliosis, where every movement of the spine is registered by a corresponding movement in the attached ribs.

The gliding action of each involved vertebra as a whole is accompanied by a similar movement of the pair of ribs attached to the vertebra being studied. This gliding is, by itself, perceptible—both at the motion unit's spinous processes and the lateral angles of the attached ribs.

On forced *extension*, each involved vertebra is pushed forward a little between its pair of attached ribs. The ribs heads and rib angles are pushed aside by the vertebrae centra and transverse processes from 1—2 mm, according to Gillet's studies. The posterior aspects of the ribs appose first, and then the anterior costocostal spaces open after the ribs contact. In forced *lateral* flexion, the vertebrae flex slightly more *between* their attached ribs than the ribs bend laterally. Apart from the lateral gliding that accompanies the vertebrae, the external spaces open on the convex side and close on the concave aspect of the curve.

On this subject, Faye states: "This subtle movement of the upper thoracic vertebrae translating anterior between the ribs is essential for normal cervical extension. Adjusting to restore this motion is important in a large percentage of patients. See Figure 4.29, and adapt by lowering the head piece and raising contact to T1, T2, T3, or T4."

During *rotation*, as with lateral bending, the same action occurs as the upper ribs rotate progressively more than the lower ribs. In the lower thoracic region, because there the ribs are attached relative loosely at the sternum, they will have a much greater tendency to follow their respective vertebrae in their different movements. In fact, in many ways, the lower thoracic spine behaves more like the lumbars than the mid- and upper-thoracic vertebrae. In forced rotation, a similar small amount of mobility is possible that is characterized by the rib on the active side going forward and inward (anteromedially) and the one on the passive side, moving backward and outward (posterolaterally). While these three movements (forced extension, lateral bending, rotation) are small, and almost imperceptible to most roentgenographic mensuration systems, they are important because of the sympathetic ganglia in the vicinity of spinocostal motion.

The ribs have one more movement that is characteristic of them and which has been adequately described in standard anatomy and physical diagnosis texts: lateral tilting of each rib during respiration. This movement, as all others, will be influenced by fixations owing to hypertonus of the intercostal muscles.

The ribs attach bilaterally to the thoracic spine at the centrum (costovertebral joint) and at the transverse process (costotransverse joint) of the same segment. If one of these joints is structurally fixed, the other is functionally fixed. Thus, these two joints are often referred to collectively as the *spinocostal* articulations.

Costovertebral and Costotransverse Coupling. Kapandji points out that the costotranverse joint and the costovertebral joint serve as a mechanical couple that restricts normal movement to only rotation about an axis that passes through the center of each of these joints. These joints, along with the elasticity of the sternocostal articulations, produce pivot points from which the ribs elevate and depress laterally. Because the axis running through the costotransverse and costovertebral joints lies close to the frontal plane in the upper ribs and nearly parallel to the sagittal plane in the lower ribs, elevation of the ribs during inspiration appreciably increases only the lateral diameter of the upper thorax, increases both the lateral and transverse diameters in the midthorax, and increases only the transverse diameter of the lower thorax. He notes that all these changes in thoracic diameters can be accomplished by the diaphragm itself.

Concepts of Coupled Spinal Rotation and Lateral Bending

A search of the literature regarding coupled rotation and lateral bending in the thoracic spine reveals a mass of conflicting data. Although the subject of coupled rotation during thoracic lateral bending appears on the surface to be readily definable, this is not the case. Several authorities appear to disagree on what occurs, especially when flexion or extension is introduced. About the cervical and upper thoracic spine, White/Panjabi state that the direction of coupling of axial rotation with lateral bending is directed in such a manner "that axial rotation of the vertebral body causes its anterior aspect to point toward the concavity of the lateral bending curve. In other words, the spinous processes point more to the convexity of the physiologic curve." These investigators also report that the same pattern occurs in the mid- and lower-thoracic spine, but to a lesser extent, inconsistently present, and with possibly the reverse motion occurring in the upper thoracic and cervical regions.

Grice is in general agreement with this when he reports: "In the upper thoracic spine, rotation during lateral flexion is similar to that in the cervical spine; ie, the rotation of the spinous process is toward the convexity." He is more specific, however, when it comes to the lower thoracic spine during lateral flexion: "...the upper thoracic vertebrae behave similar to a cervical motion segment while the lower thoracic vertebrae behave similar to a lumbar segment." On the other hand, in writing of the T3—T10 area, Grieve states: "In neutral and extension, sidebending and rotation occur to opposite sides. In flexion, they occur to the same side, as in the cervical spine." Shrader appears to initially agree with White/Panjabi and Grice: "When the spine is in a neutral position (easy normal) and side bending is introduced, the bodies of the vertebrae will rotate toward the concavity." However, he goes on to report that "When the spine is either forward or backward bent and side bending is introduced, the vertebrae will rotate toward the concavity."

In clinical application, however, the moot question of such "normal" movements may not be that important as pathologic changes readily alter normal dynamics. Although Jirout was referring to the cervical spine, his thoughts would be applicable here: "Any manipulation philosophy based on the supposed 'correctness' of this or that set movement 'logically' based on the plane of the facets may be fallacious." Grieve underscores this point by stating that it may seem wise to "...allow the joints of individual patterns to speak for themselves, in the prime matter of the nature and direction of the most effective therapeutic movement" and "...clinical assessment of individual responses takes precedence over theories of biomechanics and theories of 'correct' techniques."

Features of the Thoracic Spine Under Stress

Three points should be kept in mind when listening to the history of thoracic strain/sprain:

1. During axial rotation, the thoracic cage is biomechanically stressed so that the ribs are pushed posteriorly on the side of movement and pulled anteriorly on the other side. This subjects the sternum to shear forces, and the sternum minutely tips obliquely toward the direction of rotation.

2. Segmental motion is generally greater in the direction of loading in the thoracic spine than in other directions. The one exception is axial compression, which exhibits almost 50% more translation horizontally than axially.

3. The costovertebral joints exhibit their highest stiffness property in the lateral direction and their lowest stiffness against superior or inferior loading. The sternocostal joints act just the opposite. They exhibit higher resistance against vertical forces and lower resistance against A-P and P-A forces.

DIAGNOSTIC CONSIDERATIONS

Evaluating vital signs and such procedures as cardiac signs, thoracic auscultation and percussion, light touch/pain tests, muscle strength grading, range of gross motion tests, inspection, and static palpation are so standard within chiropractic physical examination that there is no need to describe them here. This is also true for the evaluation of reflexes pertinent to thoracic syndromes such as the pectoral reflex and scapular reflex and often the meridian alarm points. Besides these standard tests, the following orthopedic and neurologic tests are helpful in the differential diagnosis of thoracic syndromes.

Significant Neurologic and Orthopedic Tests

Abdominal Reflexes. These superficial reflexes are tested by light stroking with a blunt instrument such as a tongue blade toward the middle of the abdomen from the lateral border, at the level of the umbilicus, and above and below it. Some authorities recommend that a pinwheel be used. The upper abdominals are supplied by T8—T10; lower, T10—T12 segments of the spinal cord. Contraction of the abdominal muscles on the same side causes a pulling of the umbilicus toward the stimulus. This test of superficial abdominal reflexes is unreliable in the obese, pregnant, or those with lax abdominal walls. Similar contractions elicited by tapping neighboring bony structures are called *deep abdominal reflexes.*

Adams' Sign. If the patient has an S or a C scoliosis, note if the scoliosis straightens when the spine is flexed forward. If it does, it is a negative sign and evidence of a functional scoliosis. A positive sign is noted when the scoliosis is not improved, thus evidence of a structural scoliosis.

Bainbridge Reaction. Any condition that produces increased venous pressure in or distention of the great vessels results in a sympathetic reflex with a resultant increase in heart rate.

Barkman's Reflex. This normal sign features ipsilateral contraction of the rectus abdominis muscle when the skin just below the nipple is stimulated. It is often used to test the integrity of the T4—T5 (approximately) segmental levels.

Beevor's Sign. Note the position of the umbilicus when the patient tenses the abdominal muscles as in trying to rise from a recumbent position with the hands behind the head. Movement of the umbilicus upward signifies paralysis or weakness of the lower abdominal muscles. If the umbilicus

moves toward the right, weakness of left abdominal muscles is indicated. If the umbilicus moves toward the left, weakness of the right abdominal muscles is indicated. A positive sign points to segments T6—T10 such as in spinal cord or vertebral injury, disease, or tumor such as vertebral or cord tumor, anterior poliomyelitis, transverse myelitis, compression fracture, multiple sclerosis, and disc protrusions.

Cataneo's Sign. When heavy percussion over the spinous processes of the thoracic vertebrae causes red spots to develop directly over the processes, tracheobronchial adenopathy should be suspected.

Chapman's Test. With the patient in the supine position, stabilize the patient's legs and ask the patient to attempt to flex the trunk to the sitting position without using the hands. This test, which requires strong contraction of the abdominals, is positive for abdominal weakness if the patient is unable to sit upright but abdominal pain is not produced. If abdominal pain is produced during the attempt, an inflammatory abdominal lesion should be suspected.

Chest Expansion Test. With the patient standing, chest measurements are taken around the circumference of the thorax near the nipple level: first after the patient inhales and then after the patient exhales completely. A 2-inch difference (possibly less in females) is a negative sign. A positive sign is indicated by no or little difference in measurements and suspect of osteoarthritic ankylosis or ankylosing spondylitis. Roentgenography should offer confirmatory evidence.

Comolli's Sign. Shortly after trauma to the upper posterior thorax, a triangular swelling may develop in the region of the involved scapula owing to an accumulation of blood anteriorly and posteriorly to the scapula. For anatomical reasons, the blood cannot escape; hence, a cushion-like swelling develops more or less corresponding to the outline of the scapula that may persist for several days. This sign, which can be confused with an intramuscular hematoma (eg, of the rhomboideus major, infraspinatus, trapezius) is helpful in the physical diagnosis of fracture of the surgical neck and body of the scapula.

Forestier's Sign. The patient in the upright position is asked to bend laterally, first to one side and then to the other. Normally, the contralateral perivertebral muscles will bulge because of the normal coupling rotation of the lumbar spine (exhibited by the spinous processes pointing to the ipsilateral side of lateral flexion). However, in ankylosing spondylitis (Marie-Strümpell's disease) or a state of extensive spinal fixation, the muscles will appear to bulge greater on the side of the curve's concavity.

Grocco's Sign. This sign is a manifestation of an area of percussion dullness at the base of the chest alongside the spinal column, on the side opposite a pleural effusion.

Kernig's Neck Test. Biomechanically, this test is the cephalad representation of Lasegue's straight-leg-raising test. The supine patient is asked to place both hands behind the head and forcibly flex the head toward the chest. Pain in either the neck, lower back, or down the lower extremities suggests meningeal irritation, nerve root involvement, or irritation of the dural coverings of the nerve root. That is, some hypersensitive tissue is being aggravated by the tensile forces (Fig. 4.4). When the examiner passively flexes the patient's neck and trunk, it is called the *Soto-Hall test* or *Lindner's test*, depending on the examiner's or patient's position.

Kernig's Sign. This sign constitutes a reflex hypertension of the hamstring muscles when a patient's thigh is flexed on the trunk at a right angle in the supine position, and an attempt is made to extend the lower leg, and motion is arrested about half way between the right angle and full extension. This reaction is of value in the diagnosis of spinal meningitis, though allowance must be made for the stiffness of old age. The sign is by no means pathognomonic but is of some confirmatory value. It is generally held that if pain or resistance is encountered as the leg extends, the sign is positive for a spinal cord lesion provided there is no hip or knee stiffness or sacroiliac disorder. The precise opposite of Kernig's sign (ie, a great slackness, hypotonus, of the hamstrings) is often a valuable confirmatory sign in tabes dorsalis.

Leser-Trelat Sign. When warts, pigmented foci, and senile angiomata of fairly recent origin appear on the skin, carcinoma should be suspected.

Lewin's Supine Test. This test is identical to Chapman's test, except that Lewin believes a positive sign is indicative of an ankylosing dorsolumbar lesion.

Lindner's Test. The patient is placed supine, and the examiner slowly flexes the patient's head forward so that the neck and thoracic spine curve forward. This test often helps to localize diffuse spinal pain. Essentially, it is the passive form of *Kernig's neck test* and quite similar to the *Soto-Hall test* except for the examiner's position.

Lombardi's Sign. This sign refers to the presence of varicosities in the region of the spinous processes of C7—T3. This "varicose zone of warning" strongly suggests early degenerative pulmonary disease such as tuberculosis.

Naffziger's Test. This test, when positive, offers a suspicion of an abnormal space-occupying mass such as a spinal tumor or disc protrusion. It is performed by having the patient sit or recline while the examiner

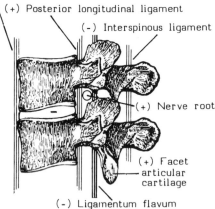

(+) Anterior longitudinal ligament
(+) Posterior longitudinal ligament
(-) Interspinous ligament
(+) Nerve root
(+) Facet articular cartilage
(-) Ligamentum flavum

Figure 4.4. The posterior and anterior longitudinal ligaments, nerve root, apophyseal articular cartilage and capsule, perivertebral muscles and fascia, walls of the arteries and veins, and periosteum of the centrum are pain-sensitive tissues (+). The deep and anterolateral aspects of the IVD, ligamentum flavum, and interspinous ligament are generally considered to be nonsensitive (—) because they are devoid of sensory fibers (their external surfaces, however, are usually innervated (Courtesy ACAP).

holds digital pressure over the jugular veins for 30—45 seconds. The patient is then instructed to cough deeply. Pain following the distribution of a nerve may indicate nerve root compression. Though more commonly used for low back involvements, thoracic and cervical root compression may also be aggravated. Local pain in the spine does not positively indicate nerve compression; it may point to the site of a strain, sprain, or another lesion. The sign is almost always positive in the presence of cord tumors, particularly spinal meningiomas. The resulting increased intrathecal pressure above the tumor or disc protrusion causes the mass to compress or pull on sensory structures to produce radicular pain. The test is contraindicated in geriatrics and extreme care should be taken with anyone suspected of having atherosclerosis. The patient should always be alerted that jugular pressure may result in dizziness.

Pectoralis Flexibility Test. With the patient placed supine and the hands clasped behind the head, the elbows are allowed to slowly lower laterally toward the table. If the elbows do not approximate the tabletop, shortening (eg, spasm, inflexibility, contracture) of the pectoralis group is indicated.

Sargent's Sign. This sign is produced by a light stroke drawn in the median line from above downward over the abdominal wall. When a distinct white line appears, it is an indication of increased sympathetic tonus or hyperadrenia.

Soto-Hall Test. This test is primarily employed when fracture of a vertebra is suspected. The patient is placed supine without pillows. One hand of the examiner is placed on the sternum of the patient, and a slight pressure is exerted to prevent flexion at either the lumbar or thoracic regions of the spine. The other hand of the examiner is placed under the patient's occiput, and the head is slowly flexed toward the chest. Flexion of the head and neck on the chest progressively produces a pull on the posterior spinous ligaments from above, and when the spinous process of the injured vertebra become involved, an acute local pain is experienced by the patient.

Spinal Percussion Test. With the patient prone or in a sitting forward-flexed position, percuss the spinous process of the

involved area. Induced pain suggests intervertebral sprain, fracture, acute subluxation, IVD lesion, or dislocation. If negative, the perivertebral soft tissues (about 1—2 inches lateral) are percussed. Induced pain suggests strain, radiculitis, transverse process fracture, or a costovertebral lesion. A variation of this test is to place a c-128 tuning fork on suspected segments to see if symptoms are aggravated. A positive sign often manifests during the acute phase.

Sternal Compression Test. Floorward pressure is slowly applied against the sternum of a supine patient. Sharp, localized pain arising laterally suggests a fractured rib.

Trousseau's Line Sign. This refers to the production of a bright red line where the finger is drawn across the trunk or forehead. It commonly occurs in meningitis.

Dynamic Palpation of the Thoracic Spine: General Considerations

As with the cervical spine, the motions that must be evaluated in the thoracic spine are flexion, extension, and right and left rotation and lateral bending. In addition to these, we must also consider the action of the costotransverse and costovertebral joints. The most common fixations in the thoracic spine, thus the priority consideration, are posterior intervertebral fixations, interspinous fixations, costotransverse fixations, anterior ligament fixations, intercostal fixations, and anterior thorax fixations.

Motion palpation of the thoracic spine must of necessity include the apophyseal joints, the costovertebral joints, and the sternocostal joints. Areas of total fixation are found most commonly at the upper and middle thoracic segments and the thoracolumbar junction. Joint play is more difficult to assess because of the increased stiffness of the thorax as compared to that of the cervical and lumbar spine.

Spinocostal Kinematics from Gillet's Perspective

As described earlier, Gillet views thoracic motion as taking place in two phases. As the spine moves from full flexion toward extension, there is first an inferior gliding of the prezygapophyses and closing of the interspinous spaces. This motion is readily palpable by placing a palpating thumb or finger pad in the interspinous space being evaluated and sensing the changes that occur as the patient is moved from flexion into extension. A wide range of change should be noted; thus, this is an excellent maneuver for student's to begin their motion palpation training. From here, sites of more subtle motion can be mastered. Second, when the facets and spinous processes closely appose each other at their extreme range of motion, there is still a certain amount of further motion possible. If extension is forced at this point, the spinous processes will be felt to move forward, with the superior segment of the motion unit gliding slightly anterior on its subjacent neighbor. During such motion, it appears obvious that the interfacial space must open anteriorly and the anterior aspect of the IVD must widen.

Two other important movements also take place:

1. The thoracic vertebrae tend to move forward between the ribs. This anterior motion occurs as the vertebrae spring the ribs laterally. One might think that such a motion would be impossible because of the ligamentous complex existing between the ribs and the thoracic vertebrae, but motion palpation will reveal that these tissues are normally much more pliable than generally thought. In fact, this motion can be perceived at the bulky T1 level. With experience, it is possible to palpate the vertebra's laminae, transverse processes, and also the heads of the first ribs as they articulate with it.

2. As the spinous processes appose and separate, so do the posterior portions of the ribs. Thus, there is also an intercostal motion (felt between the ribs): an opening during flexion and closing during extension of the intercostal spaces.

These movements require the action, or at least a good degree of flexibility, of the intercostal muscles anteriorly, posteriorly, and laterally if a total range of motion is to be achieved. At the extreme ranges of motion, there is a gliding motion in the lateral intercostal spaces, similar to that described of the occipital condyles on the superior surfaces of the lateral masses of the atlas.

Recognizing these factors this gives us several possible causes of motion restriction in the thoracic spine: (1) total articular fixations, (2) interspinous muscular fixations, (3) interspinous ligamentous fixations, (4) anterior body ligamentous fixations, (5) spinocostal articular fixations, and (6) costocostal muscular fixations. Gillet discloses that the latter may be found individually or allied with another type of local fixation.

Thoracic Fixations

The entire thoracic region is prone to many muscle, ligament, and spinocostal fixations. In addition, Gillet observes that primary thoracic fixations tend to produce secondary areas of fixation in the cervical spine. Jirout and others have also reported similar observations.

Most fixations found in the thoracic area are muscular in type. This is fortunate, states Gillet, because difficult to manage fibrous ankylosis can readily develop in the thoracic spine. "While fibrous ankylosis does not contraindicate manipulation, the tissues adapt slowly and correction takes frequent care

DR. FAYE'S CLINICAL COMMENT #4.1

I have found over the years that a successful treatment schedule for patients over 50 years of age with reversible kyphotic thoracic spines has been twice a week for a minimum of 6 months. Full mobility and a postural change takes a year or more in the more elderly. After age 65, mobility improves but not enough to allow postural changes.

A major biomechanical insult in the lower cervical region is the loss of upper-thoracic mobility. C5—C6 becomes hypermobile and hyperlordotic, and degenerative changes occur. For the cervical spine to fully extend, the upper thoracics must move anteriorly between the ribs. Thus, this action is extremely significant clinically in cervical brachial syndromes.

utilizing a wide scope of therapy over many months, if not years, to obtain an appreciable change because of the poor vascularity of the tissues involved." [See Clinical Comment 4.1]

The Longitudinal Ligaments of the Spine

Apart from possible shortening of the anterior longitudinal ligament, Gillet believes that the only other common ligamentous fixations in the thoracic spine and posterior thoracic cage are found between the vertebrae and the ribs (eg, at the costotransverse and costovertebral articulations), between the transverse processes, and/or of the intercostal ligaments at the angles of the ribs. See Figure 4.5.

The Anterior Longitudinal Ligament. Shortening of the anterior longitudinal ligament is a common site of fixation in the thoracic spine, but it is rare in the lumbar region. It is manifested by an increased kyphosis and a decreased anterior disc space on a lateral roentgenograph and may be confused with anulus degeneration that may or may not be present. The normal IVF space will appear elongated. Gillet feels that this traction appears to have considerable effect on the sympathetic nerves (visceral symptoms), be a source of noxious reflex activity, but have little or no effect on the somatic nerves. Some authorities believe that this condition is encouraged in compensation to hyperlordotic lumbar and/or cervical curves or in women with large heavy breasts.

According to the studies of Gillet and associates, the "anterior ligament" fixation that is due to shortening of the anterior longitudinal ligament is rarely found in the lumbars, frequently found in the thoracic spine, and especially so as we palpate upwards toward T1. This shortening tends to pull the anterior aspects of the involved motion units together, "pinching" the anterior aspect of the IVDs. This type of fixation tends to force the involved IVFs open, but, in spite of this, it seems to be pathogenic according to Gillet. "It rarely produces any irritation of the cerebrospinal nerves (eg, intercostal neuritis), but it does seem to be very irritable

to the sympathetic fibers—producing a large variety of visceral signs and symptoms. It also produces a typical reflex fixation."

The Posterior Longitudinal Ligament. For some unexplained reason, shortening of this ligament is rarely seen. This could possibly be explained by the greater flexion exercise required in normal activity, keeping in mind that A-P and P-A thoracic motion is minimal at best. While this may explain the thoracic state, one would think that these ligaments would be shortened in chronic cervical or lumbar lordosis, but Gillet believes that this is rarely demonstrated.

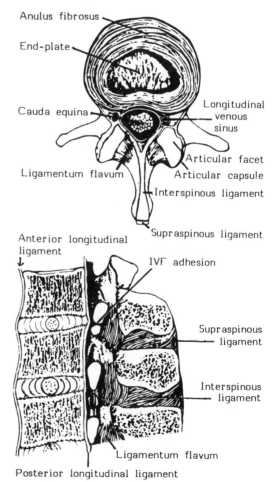

Figure 4.5. *Top,* the major spinal ligaments of the thoracic spine as viewed from above; *bottom,* lateral view of a midsagittal section (Courtesy ACAP).

It has been stated previously that, for some unknown reason, some articulations, ligaments, and muscles are far more often the seat of fixations than others. Normally, we should find the posterior longitudinal ligament also in a state of shortening in certain areas, but Gillet has not found this to be true in the research conducted to this point. When it occurs, ossification of the posterior longitudinal ligament in the cervical region is often associated with signs of radiculomyelopathy. However, when this ligament ossifies in the thoracic spine, it is typically, but not always, asymptomatic. For an unknown reason, the disorder occurs predominantly in females when the thoracic region is involved and almost always in Japanese males when the cervical region is affected.

Special Considerations in the Lower Thoracic Spine

The lower thoracic region (T9—T12) is probably more prone to fixation development than any other area of the thoracic spine. This is likely because of the abrupt change in facet planes between the superior and inferior processes of the transitional vertebra, the altered stiffness between thoracic and lumbar vertebrae, the lack of strong supporting muscles enjoyed by the lumbar region, the lack of firm anterior support of the floating ribs, and the large compressive forces concentrated at this area. According to mechanical laws, a sudden change in the stiffness properties of a structure at a given point will subject the structure to stress concentration at that point. This can lead to eventual mechanical failure.

It is here, in the lower thoracic spine, that we meet with (1) vertebra/rib fixation caused by hypertonic serratus muscles that tend to pull the floating ribs downward and inward (inferomedially); (2) shortened intertransverse muscles, which are common here but not in the more superior thoracic spine; and (3) diaphragmatic fixation. In the latter, we have an unusual type of fixation that does not bind two osseous structures together but can be likened to a "knot" within a broad muscle. It can be palpated quite close to the spine, just under the floating ribs.

We are indebted to Illi for bringing this fixation to our attention. Gillet states that Illi puts some emphasis on the diaphragmatic fixation, finding in it one cause of lumbago that he attributes to an abnormal diet. The three types of lower-thoracic fixations enumerated above are common. Although it is not yet known if they are pathogenic or not, they are corrected just as all other fixations that are found in routine analyses.

Special Considerations in the Midthoracic Spine

In the midthoracic spine, it is common to find (1) anterior body fixations; (2) fixations between the head of the ribs and the bodies of the respective vertebra; (3) fixations between the transverse processes and the angles of the ribs; (4) costospinal fixations as the result of local serratus or levator costorum muscle shortening; (5) vertebrovertebra fixations caused by local rotatores, multifidus, or spinalis shortening, of which the latter tend to reproduce the interspinous fixations found in the lumbars and cervicals; and (6) costocostal fixations found in the anterior, lateral, and/or posterior aspects of the ribs. All these fixations can be found almost anywhere in the thoracic spine, but they are prevalent in the midthoracic region and thus must always be searched for and corrected if found. Gillet has found that these fixations produce, in turn, specific secondary fixations in the cervical spine. He also believes that it is possible to differentiate one fixation from another by searching for the reflex fixation it provokes.

Local fixations of the midthoracic vertebrae can be palpated when the patient is in the neutral resting position as sometimes being rotated or laterally flexed. Theoretically, all fixations occurring between ribs or vertebrae from hypertonus of the serratus or levator costorum muscles will restrict rotation of one segment over another. Fixation between a vertebra and its attached rib is observed easier when the spine is put in lateral flexion or rotation (Fig. 4.6). All these fixations tend to fix the structures in one position without completely restricting all spinocostal motion.

Sternal fixations as well as anterior-body fixations tend to force the local spine into exaggerated kyphosis. With the ribs, hypertonic anterior muscles of the thorax also tend to pull the segments into hyperkyphosis. On the other hand, hypertonic posterior muscles tend to flatten the thoracic curve and possibly produce local segmental lordosis. Lateral costocostal fixations tend to pull the ribs together at their widest aspects, in which case a relative *lateral* flattening of the normal rib bulging can be felt.

Palpation of the intercostal spaces, on the anterior and lateral aspects of the thorax, will show where these are abnormally narrow—suggesting areas in which the intercostal muscles are pulling the ribs toward each other. In each of these cases, a relative hypermobility of the area of the ribs opposite the seat of shortening can be felt. This is also true in the spine, for example, when a sternal fixation forces a relative hypermobility on the interspinous spaces during full forward flexion. Thus, all forward flexion movements that normally take place in the thorax are forced to occur at the posterior aspects of the intervertebral and costocostal spaces.

Gillet describes an unusual type of midthoracic fixation that can be seen when the patient is moved into a position of full rotation. In this position, the chain of spinous processes is followed with the fingerpads. In certain cases, the spinous processes of T5—T7 do not follow those above or below; they may appear to counterrotate. This phenomenon may be unilateral or bilateral, and Gillet reports that a double transverse adjustment will usually correct this unusual motion anomaly.

It has been Gillet's experience that the midthoracic spine seems to be the meeting place of all thoracic-type fixations so far found. It is a region that can give much trouble in analysis and correction because it is the seat of continual recurrent fixations until the focal cause is found and eliminated. [See Clinical Comment 4.2]

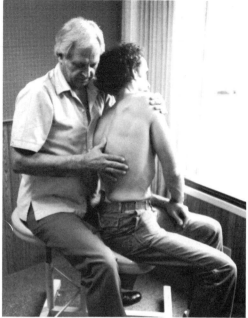

Figure 4.6. Motion palpation of a midthoracic motion unit during left lateral flexion.

Consumption of Brewed Coffee. A common cause of recurrent fixations in the midthoracic spine has been linked to coffee drinking. This linkage, states Gillet, was first reported by Illi whose investigation found that (1) each patient had a personal threshold (1—10 cups/day) over which any additional cups consumed would bring on a hypertonic state and fixation in the T4—T8 region, including the attached ribs. (2) It was also discovered that it was not the caffeine content of the coffee that was responsible, but the oil of the coffee bean that was "burnt in" during the roasting process. Certain brands of coffee appear to be especially dangerous because oils are added to the coffee before roasting to enhance the flavor.

Extensive Rotatore Shortening. The rotatore muscles of the spine may become extensively hypertonic. When they do so unilaterally, or more so on one side, they tend to pull the spinouses of the vertebrae to which

---

DR. FAYE'S CLINICAL COMMENT #4.2

The need to be able to palpate and apply specific adjustments is demonstrated often clinically. It is not uncommon to produce three or four audible releases with three or four separate manipulations in one thoracic region or as specific as one motion unit.

they are attached into a degree of flexion-rotation. If they become involved bilaterally, they can effectively halt the rotation of each vertebra on its subjacent neighbor. They can also hinder the lateral gliding that normally occurs during lateral bending. However, a small amount of local lateral flexion can be felt, in which one transverse moves superiorly and the other inferiorly. Hypertonic rotatores are usually hidden except in the upper-thoracic region where they are visible, usually protruding from the vertebral groove. They are often accompanied by bulging levator costorum muscles.

A unilateral hypertonic rotatores, which courses in the groove between the spinous and transverse processes, will pull the corresponding spinous process into rotation and the transverse process below into counterrotation, similar in effect to that of intertransverse hypertonicity. This unilateral state, usually acute, commonly extends over several thoracic segments. Bilateral rotatores hypertonicity, often a generalized reflex condition in the thoracic spine, tends to initiate the interspinous syndrome. Rotation is restricted and lateral bending is inhibited slightly less. This condition is more readily palpable in the upper dorsal area and usually accompanied by bulging levator costarum muscles. Reflex muscular fixations palpate as being springy and should not be confused with those fixations exhibiting a hard end-feel that we adjust. Gillet believes that this disorder is frequently secondary to a primary fixation in one or both feet.

The Interspinous and Intertransverse Muscles. Bilateral interspinous and/or intertransverse muscle hypertonicity produces a fixation that resists flexion. In unilateral intertransverse hypertonicity, the transverse processes appose, the disc thins ipsilaterally, and the height of the IVF is reduced. The subjacent superior articulation is pulled into a stressed position away from the inferior process. The interarticular space exhibits an abnormal V-shaped appearance. The IVD space increases at the anterior and decreases at the posterior. The acute stage is produced by muscular spasm; but in prolonged conditions, the ipsilateral muscles become fibrotic and the perivertebral ligaments shorten. Stretching occurs on the contralateral side.

Special Considerations in the Upper-Thoracic Spine

The upper-thoracic spine, especially in the T1—T3 area, is the site of two common fixations. One of them is felt in local lateral flexion, with the palpating fingerpad placed deep along the side of the spinous process. The spinous processes should move laterally when the head and neck are laterally flexed. If they do not, and this resistance is springy, Gillet believes that this suggests a primary fixation in the pelvis due to shortening of the sacrotuberous ligaments. These pelvic ligaments are readily palpable and the technique will be described in a subsequent chapter. Gillet states, however, that the upper-thoracic sign is even more accurate than direct palpation of the sacrotuberous ligaments. He also reports that correction of the pelvic fixation will be immediately evident by demonstrable release of the upper-thoracic fixation, if indeed a muscular fixation exists.

Another common type of fixation found in the upper-thoracic spine is that of the "anterior-body," described previously, which usually concerns shortening of the anterior longitudinal ligament. This type of fixation, states Gillet, is often associated with a secondary muscular fixation between the occiput and the axis. He also reports that it requires a spinous contact for the adjustment, but he offers no explanation as to why. [Refer to adjustment of thoracic interspinous fixation with patient prone, described later in this chapter.]

Upper-Thoracic Rotatore Shortening. Unilateral hypertonic rotatores are usually acute. In contrast, bilateral hypertonic rotatores are often reflexively related to remote primary fixations. This, states Gillet, is especially true for fixations within the upper thoracic spine, which may be caused by fixations in the feet. "This can be easily proved by noting the effect of foot adjusting on these fixations. The effect has been shown to be total and immediate by a two-man team: one palpating the reflex fixation while the other adjusts the primary fixation in the foot."

Rhomboid Shortening. The rhomboid group, which is innervated by the dorsal scapular nerve, is often involved in shortening that is associated with upper-thoracic fixations. See Figure 4.7. This is especially true of the rhomboideus major. The *rhomboideus major* (greater) arises from the spinous processes of T2—T5 and inserts at the vertebral margin of the scapula. The *rhomboideus minor* (smaller), arises from the spinous processes of C7, T1, and the lower portion of the nuchal ligament and inserts at the vertebral margin of the scapula at the root of the scapular spine. The action of the rhomboids (greater and smaller) is to retract and stabilize the scapula. During a state of fixed hypertonicity, these muscles tend to pull the scapula backward and upward. During unilateral shortening, one shoulder will appear to be held higher than the other. In this context, Gillet states, "Here we are again at the limit of the long and short muscles, and those which are attached to the spine or not. Logically, hypertonus of these muscles should be secondary to some other fixation but it (the site of fixation) can be adjusted locally. We are also uncertain whether this fixation is pathogenic or not."

The Upper-Thoracic Mensuration

Gillet reports that it is not practical to use the vertical line technique described in Chapter 2 for the cervical spine to measure the lateral flexion mobility of T1—T6

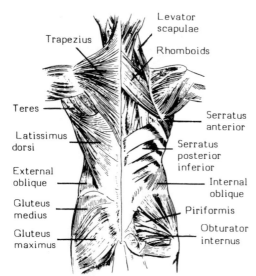

Figure 4.7. Some major muscles of the back. Superficial muscles are shown on the left, deeper muscles on the right (Courtesy ACAP).

because this technique is too easily influenced by the suppleness of the spine below it. Thus, we must revert to the measurement of rotation to calculate the degree of mobility in this region of the spine.

Unfortunately, here we encounter another difficulty; viz, that of eliminating the effects of rotatory restriction caused by scapular fixations, where one or both scapulae fail to properly revolve around the rib cage during rotation of the shoulders on the thorax, or due to a fixation existing at one or both sternoclavicular joints. In addition, scapular rotation causes confusing movement of the skin overlying the spinous processes if we draw a vertical dotted line upward from T7. It is therefore imperative that the patient be rotated before dotting the spinous processes and to repeat this process during rotation to the posterior on the other side. Granted, it is also possible to palpate for and correct the possible fixations of the sternoclavicular joints beforehand.

Another difficulty in producing an accurate measurement line over the upper thoracic spine is the necessity of drawing it perpendicular to a line that cuts the shoulders at equal points. To do this, the examiner must reach around the patient anteriorly, take hold of the patient's knees and legs, and rotate them around to the side while the examiner's stabilizing hand keeps the shoulders from turning. At the end of this maneuver, the patient will be fully rotated but the examiner will be looking at the patient's shoulders. The T7 spinous can now be marked and a vertical line extended upward to connect with the shoulder line. Do the same thing when the patient is rotated posteriorly on the other side. Return the patient to the neutral resting position, and you should see two lines on the patient's back that portray the actual degree of movement taken by this region of the patient's spine. Ideally, the lines will appear as a V, but this is rarely the case. If one of them curves sharply inward, somewhat resembling a C, a significant sign has been discovered (Fig. 4.8).

Determining Flexion-Extension Fixations

The characteristic movement of the spinous processes in the thoracic spine can be

160

felt during passive flexion and extension. The pads of the index and middle fingers (or thumb and index finger) are placed within the interspinous spaces of adjacent verte-

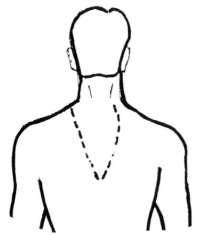

Figure 4.8. A significant sign of upper-thoracic fixation as the result of upper-thoracic mensuration.

brae while the patient is brought up from full flexion to full extension. If a spinous process is felt to move slightly laterally, rather than arcing posteroinferiorly, a unilateral muscle or ligament fixation is suggested. If no motion is perceived during this A-P maneuver, a total fixation is indicated if no springy end-feel exists.

During examination, slowly and completely flex and extend the patient's spine while you evaluate the corresponding segmental kyphotic and lordotic motions (Fig. 4.9). Incomplete symmetrical motion, complete fixation, or excessive motion (hyperkinesia) is easily noted; the latter being particularly evident owing to the usually associated palpable instability of the supraspinal ligament. Keep in mind that when the thoracic spine is normally extended from a forward flexion position, there is first an inferior gliding of the inferior facets on the superior facets below and the interspinous spaces close. This can sometimes be best determined by placing a horizontal palpating thumb within

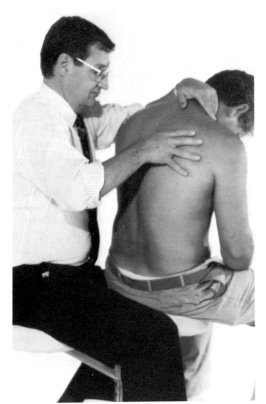
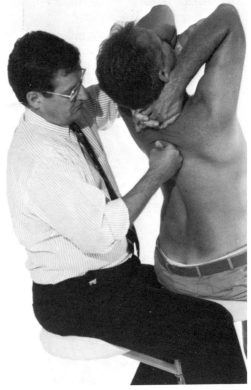

Figure 4.9. Determining thoracic flexion-extension fixation.

the interspinous space being examined. During forward flexion, the spinous processes will open unless there is an interspinous fixation.

According to Gillet, the first partial fixation to occur is usually that which resists forced extension. The involved segment will be kyphotic. When hyperextension is forced, the spinous process will normally be felt to move slightly anterior as the inferior facets of the vertebra above pivot (open anteriorly) on the superior facets of the vertebra below. This paradoxical anterior shift is a normal action that can be restricted by shortening at the anterior motion unit (eg, anterior longitudinal ligament).

Asymmetrical movement from underlying spinal fixations feature certain gross characteristic kinematic signs: (1) a motion unit fixed in extension shows a lesser degree of kyphotic movement on flexion and a much greater degree of hyperextension motion. (2) With segments fixed in flexion, the sign is opposite; ie, flexion of the area shows a great-er tendency of segmental kyphotic movement and hyperextension of the spine causes less segmental lordosis.

Determining Lateral-Flexion Fixations

Because of the relative rigidity of the thoracic spine, lateral flexion of the neck of only 30° will yield palpable motion in the lumbar spine. With the patient seated, palpation for vertebral motion is conducted with the thumbpad placed over the inferolateral aspect of the spinous process of the segment being examined and the fingers extending over the perivertebral musculature (Fig. 4.10). The side of the thumb may be placed over the corresponding zygapophysis for further kinesthetic awareness. Some examiners prefer to use one hand for the contact with the index finger placed on the tip of the spinous process and the thumb and middle finger placed over the transverse processes

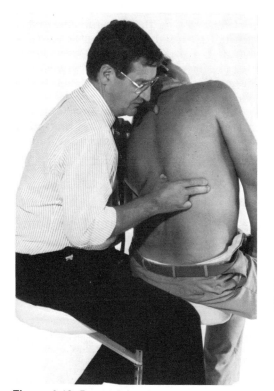
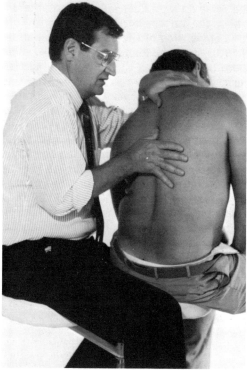

Figure 4.10. Determining thoracic lateral flexion fixation.

of the vertebra below the segment being examined. Thus, comparative movement of the superior segment on its base may be appraised. The other arm and forearm of the examiner may be placed anteriorly around the patient's shoulders to guide the patient through the various spinal movements.

Gillet feels that a lateral muscular fixation at C7—T2 is a secondary manifestation that is commonly linked to shortening of the pelvic sacrotuberous ligament. He reports that stretching the ligament in the knee-chest position immediately corrects this secondary fixation. If the thoracic fixation is primary, this effect cannot be confirmed.

During lateral bending, the movements felt will be (1) vertebral lateral gliding, (2) vertebral lateral tipping, and (3) rib tipping as the vertebra carries the rib with it. You will find that rotational coupling during lateral flexion is much stronger in children than adults.

Although Lovett states the theory, which is widely held, that pure lateral flexion is abnormal in the spine, this premise must be amended in light of findings elicited by motion palpation. In the child, lateral bending of the spine does produce a flexion-rotation in which the vertebrae rotate posteriorly on the convex side of the curve. By palpating the ribs, it will be found that they also slide more posteriorly on the convex side of the curve. In the adult, however, this is rarely the case because the thoracic cage has lost most of the suppleness (flexibility, plasticity, elasticity) that is so characteristic of the young. Thus, in adulthood, the flexion-rotation motion observed during lateral bending of children is replaced by a flexion-gliding action in which each vertebra moves laterally in toto, taking with it its attached ribs. This can easily be felt at the exterior angles of the ribs. The ribs not only separate during lateral bending of the spine, they glide outward to a perceptible degree.

This same motion can be felt with the method previously described for the cervicals. Two finger pads can be placed close together on either side of the spinous process while the patient's spine is laterally flexed by the examiner's free hand on the patient's shoulder. The shoulder is curved laterally downward. As always, care should be taken to try to localize, as much as is possible, movement at the area of the spine being palpated. [See Clinical Comment 4.3]

Liekens teaches that interspinous motion can be felt with even greater precision by placing the palpating fingerpad against the lateral aspects of two adjacent spinous processes, first on one side and then on the other. It is then possible to perceive slight fixations that still permit a partial movement.

The lateral glide of the vertebrae is obviously not the only movement that occurs here. During segmental motion palpation, a local lateral flexion can be perceived that takes place in two phases. First, the vertebra tips laterally from its subjacent neighbor. It also tips between its attached ribs. Second, as the motion becomes greater, the attached ribs follow the tilting of the vertebra. To feel this lateral tipping, the palpating fingerpads must be separated about a half an inch so that they are over the costotransverse joints Fig. 4.11). Because of the tissues between the fingerpads and the osseous structures, a good degree of sensitivity must be developed to fully appreciate this movement on the anterior aspect of the transverse process. It is also possible to use a thumb contact on the transverse process of the vertebra being examined, either on the concave or convex side of the curve, or even on the related ribs.

Determining Rotational Fixations

In the standard palpating position, rotate the patient to the right and left. A rotational

---

DR. FAYE'S CLINICAL COMMENT #4.3

Motion palpation will detect the loss of movement, but it is necessary to spring the end resistance to see if the elastic barrier is limited. My clinical experience has convinced me that adjusting those joints which have lost their elastic end-feel and palpate as a hard end-feel is advantageous. These fixations also often need to be adjusted in more than one direction and over a series of visits before complete range of motion is normal.

fixation, by being further accentuated, may be confirmed by palpating just lateral to the spinous process (Fig. 4.12). Assisted lateral flexion to the right or left helps to confirm the analysis of a fixation. Further confirmation of ankylosis, fixation, or segmental hyperkinesia may also be made during these range of motion studies.

Normal vertebral rotation can be greatly impaired by a rib fixation because the ribs must move with the rotating transverse processes. Similarly, hypertonicity of the rotatores, multifidi, and levator costorum will restrict rotation. These conditions are often found in the upper thoracic area. The intertransverse muscles may be a cause of fixation in the mid-to-lower thoracic area and can be best determined by intertransverse palpation during lateral flexion.

Thoracic vertebrae do not just turn around their vertical axes in a semicircle during rotation. There is always an additional (and far more prominent) anterosuperior and posteroinferior gliding action of the inferior facets on the subjacent superior facets. This upward-forward motion on one side and downward-backward movement on the other side is also exhibited by the attached ribs, with the center of motion being located near the sternum. This action can be observed simply by moving a patient into total thoracic rotation and noting the relative positions of the vertebrae and ribs.

This means that (1) total fixations will render normal rotation impossible, with the fixed motion unit turning as one solid mass; (2) any partial fixation involving a motion unit's attached ribs will also impede rotation; and (3) while a fixation at the costovertebral or costotransverse interface will *not* completely halt thoracic rotation, it will impede it enough that trained fingers will readily sense the difference from normal. This latter motion at the spinocostal joints will also be restricted by shortening of the rotatory, multifidus, and levatores costarum muscles of the ribs.

The rotatores, which course vertically be-

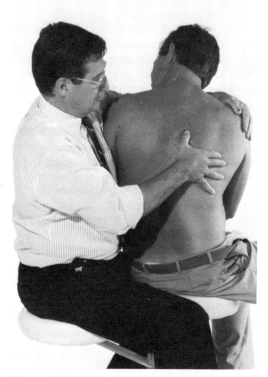

Figure 4.11. Determining costotransverse joint fixation.

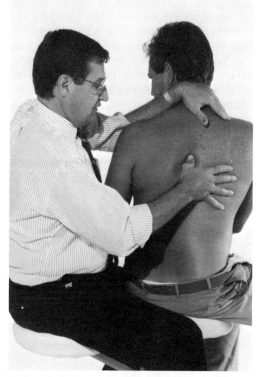

Figure 4.12. Determining zygapophyseal rotation fixation.

tween spinous processes of subjacent vertebrae to transverse processes of the unit above, take an active part in the rotation of the vertebrocostal complex, and it is evident that rotatore hypertonicity will impede the action they are meant to produce. In comparison, fibers of the levatores costarum of the ribs arise from the transverse processes of C7—T11 and insert at the medial angle of the rib below. They aid in elevation of the ribs during respiration. When hypertonic, they tend to pull the attached rib upward, producing a intervertebral fixation. These two muscles, the rotatores and levatores costarum, are often found to be contractured in the upper-thoracic region of the spine. Fortunately, they are easily released with a spinous or transverse process contract that is directed to stretch the involved shortened muscle(s).

Contrary to other thoracic vertebrae, the lower thoracic vertebrae have distinct intertransverse muscles. Similar muscles have been described in the previous chapter concerning the cervical spine. Higher in the thoracic spine, these muscles blend with the intercostals which assume their function. Intertransversarii shortening in the lower thoracic spine, as well as in the lumbar region, does not appear to be strong enough to pull the attached transverse processes together to any significant degree. However, their hypertonicity does seem to restrict opening of the intertransverse space on the contralateral side of lateral bending, even though the involved IVDs narrow on the concave side of the curve. Thus, again, we will have partial movement occur, which can be felt at the spinous process or within the intertransverse space.

Gillet's Spinous Process Contact

In palpation of the thoracic spine, the doctor-patient position is similar to that described for the scanning examination except that it is usually best for the examiner to grasp the patient's shoulder from the anterior. The forearm of your stabilizing hand should be held high enough that the patient's cheek can rest on it during maximum rotation.

It is possible to feel the movement of a spinous process with the same contact during lateral bending and rotation. A definite restriction of motion will be felt, which Gillet describes as a "holding back of the spinous," preventing it from following its neighbors. This is especially evident in the thoracic spine where, at times, one fixation will cause a restriction in several consecutive vertebrae.

To apply this technique, the examiner's thumbpad is placed against T12, for example, and the examiner's free arm is passed around in front of the patient to grasp the opposite shoulder. This permits the examiner to force the spine easily into full rotation or lateral bending. With the patient in the same position, and by decreasing and increasing thoracic lateral bending or rotation in a series of small movements, it is possible to feel, with a probing thrust applied just lateral to the spinous process, a little additional end play.

It is also possible to keep the patient in this position and to observe the alignment of spinouses during passive movements. The spinous process(es) that "hold back" become visible immediately.

It appears that apart from the wide rotation of a vertebra and its attached ribs around a point centered near the sternum, there is a small "counterrotation" action that takes place between the vertebrae and their attached ribs. This occurs near the end point of forced rotation. In this movement, the ribs seem to try to move just a little farther than the spine. This forces the proximal portion of the rib slightly forward (anteromedially from the vertebra) ipsilaterally and backward (posterolaterally from the vertebra) contralaterally. If a costovertebral fixation exists, the lack of motion should be perceived. Although a large variety of fixations can exist in the thoracic spine, the entire area can be examined rapidly once the art of motion palpation has been mastered.

Faye's Method

This is a slight modification of Gillet's technique. The thumbpad of the palpating hand is placed just lateral to the spinous process. This will be over the articular pillar. Keep in mind that there will typically be from ½ to 1½ an inch of fat and muscle tissue between your palpating finger and the transverse process. In muscular patients, it is often necessary to place your palpating thumb just lateral to the erectors, and then slide it medially under the muscle bulk. Holding a firm contact while the patient is rotated, check end play at the extreme range of motion by adding a mild push. With this same contact and the same doctor-patient position, the examiner will be able to check rotation, extension, and lateral flexion by moving the patient into and out of these movements passively.

Determining Anterior Ligament Fixations

While in the standard doctor-patient palpating position, extend the patient's thorax at the level of palpation until the normal range of motion is reached and then hyperextend the thoracic spine to see if a normal "springy end-feel" exists as the anterior ligament stretches, allowing the anterior aspect of the IVD space to open.

Anterior Rib and Sternal Fixations

These fixations of the anterior thorax will be described in Chapter 8.

Total and Related Fixations in the Thoracic Spine

Total fixations may be determined with a thumb contact, one after the other, during flexion, extension, lateral bending, and rotation maneuvers. However, it is far easier and more rapid to elicit them by using the back of the fingers as explained for the scanning examination in Chapter 2. As there is no movement at all in total fixations, fixated areas are readily localized in this manner.

True total fixations are always of the articular type; ie, the fixative element is in the articulation. However, multimuscular and ligamentous fixations may feel just as hard under the palpating fingers. See Figure 4.13. Total fixations are commonly found in the mid- and upper-thoracic spine. The upper thoracics are sometimes difficult to palpate, and it is often necessary to extend the patient's neck. [See Clinical Comment 4.4]

For the specific localization of articular fixations, it is possibly better to change the contact from the back of the fingers to the

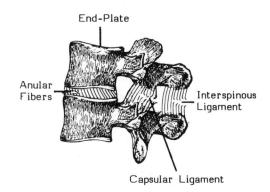

Figure 4.13 Common sites of vertebral motion sprain than can result in severe posttraumatic fixation. T11 and T12 are shown in the example (Courtesy ACAP).

DR. FAYE'S CLINICAL COMMENT #4.4

More recently Dr. Leander Eckard has described from x-ray image intensification of thoracic spine movement, as shown on a video monitor, the motion of y-axis translation during mechanical distraction. This long-axis extension is viewed as the parallel separation of the vertebral body end plates. In other words, the disc spaces are distracted and remain parallel. Eckard also observed that narrowed disc spaces widened during treatment. The motorized flexion traction table has now become a practical aid in palpating this fixation. This method has not been previously recorded in the literature.

This fixation exists when the interspinous space fails to separate during the distractiom phase of the motorized mechanical distraction. Normally, the interspinous spaces separate dramatically and close again with each distraction cycle.

Eckard was also able to demonstrate that an interspinous knife-edge contact and a short, sharp thrust directed anterosuperiorly would restore y-axis distraction capability.

thumbpad, moving from right and left from the spinous process to the articular pillars, the transverse process, the levatores costarum muscle, and then the rib. As with the scanning examination, a series of short P-A pushes can be used with the contact not leaving the skin. Your free hand can be used to stabilize the patient's shoulders.

During middle and late life, it is frequently found that the midthoracic area is full of total fixations as the result of fibrous degeneration. The lower cervical spine may express a similar state. It appears that no amount of "cracking" will be effective in correcting such an area, even when bony ankylosis is absent. Gillet believes that it is useless to try to correct this state with one or two adjustments as is often possible in many other types of total fixation. He feels that the area needs comprehensive care over many months or possibly years to achieve even a slight degree of mobility. Fortunately, this area of fixation is rarely the site of acute irritation. On the other hand, as long as it remains stiff, other vertebra of the spine will have great difficulty in achieving a high degree of correction.

As soon as all total (major) fixations are released, it is necessary to find and correct any remaining partial fixations—going from the greater to the lesser. Gillet suggests that the priority partial fixations to correct are those that restrict extension (flexion fixations). These are usually exhibited by palpatory and visual signs of segmental or short regional areas of hyperkyphosis during full flexion or kyphosis during full extension.

It is also easy to move the patient into full thoracic extension and to push forward on one spinous after another, marking those that resist the passive P-A push. From 2—5 vertebrae will typically offer resistance, and it is invariably a segment at the superior aspect of the kyphosis that offers the greatest resistance.

Special attention should be given to the upper thoracic spine. Once the "kyphotic" fixations described above are mobilized, the next priority are interspinous fixations. These are exhibited by palpatory and visual signs of segmental or short regional areas of flattening or lordosis during full flexion. Such fixations are commonly found among the cervicals and of the T4 and L5 segments.

They will also be revealed by motion palpation during lateral bending when the contact fingers straddle the spinous processes. If fixated, the vertebrae will not glide laterally, but they do tilt to various degrees.

The Costotransverse Joints

Gillet and associates have found that fixations found between the ribs and the vertebrae, either between the head of the rib and the vertebral body or between the angle of the rib and the transverse process, are probably produced by some type of shortening of the local capsular ligaments for they are undoubtedly articular in nature but still permit a certain torsion motion of the ribs during respiration. See Figure 4.14. Extremely chronic fixations in these areas have been found to cause soft-tissue degeneration that may extend to the sympathetic ganglia themselves. This degeneration, states Gillet, is nearly always found related to degenerative cardiovascular disease.

Dynamic Palpation

In palpating the costotransverse joints, a position is taken similar to that described for evaluating thoracic rotation. The palpating thumbpad contact is applied about 1½ inches lateral to the spinous process so that contact is made over the tip of the transverse process. Hold a firm contact during rotation, check end play at the extreme range of mo-

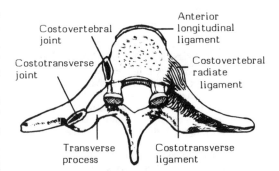

Figure 4.14. Highlights of the costovertebral and costotransverse joints of the midthoracic spine as viewed from above (Courtesy ACAP).

tion, and then release the thorax. A fixated rib will feel more prominent than usual.

The costotransverse joint articulates on the anterior surface of the lateral aspect of the transverse process in the upper-thoracic area and most of the midthoracic area, thus it is directly unpalpable. From T7 downward, the articulation moves more superiorly until it is almost on top of the transverse process in the area of the false ribs. In this area, the joint can be palpated in some extremely lean patients. However, the spring end-feel of the joint is always palpable due to this leverage on the angle of the rib.

Posterior rib fixations resulting in decreased chest excursion can be determined by motion palpation of the thoracic cage during deep inspiration with the patient either standing or prone. First, traction the skin of the lateral thorax towards the spine with broad bilateral palmar contacts and place your thumbs near the dorsal midline on the rib being examined. As the patient inhales deeply, note if both thumbs move equally. If the rib rises and the interspace opens, it is considered normal; if it remains

down to some extent compared to the opposite side, it is considered "locked." Thumb motion restricted unilaterally suggests the side of fixation.

The Costovertebral Joints

The unpalpable costovertebral joints are located on the superoposterior aspect of the centrum (Fig. 4.15). In the lower portion of the thoracic spine, the facet tends to move progressively inferior to a more central position on the posterior aspect of the vertebral body.

It is unlikely that a costovertebral fixation would exist independently from a costotransverse fixation. Any force efficient enough to free a costotransverse fixation will also release a costovertebral fixation. Gillet describes rare cases in which an extremely deep thoracic ache persisted after all other thoracic fixations were corrected. In these cases, which he attributed to a costovertebral fixation, they were released with a firm but shallow thrust on the rib. Symptomatic relief followed. Even such a shallow adjustment, however, would usually be contraindicated in the elderly unless extreme precautions are taken.

Characteristics of Thoracic IVD Lesions

The position of the protrusion determines the clinical picture. A midline protrusion usually produces intermittent pain, sensory impairment, pyramidal signs, and possibly bowel and bladder symptoms. Protrusion laterally causes more pain, is radicular in distribution, and is associated with fewer cord signs.

• *The upper thoracic spine.* Pain radiates anteriorly along the affected intercostal nerve. If the T1 root is involved, pain usually radiates down the medial aspect of the arm to the little finger. Sensory loss may be found on the medial side of the forearm, hand, little finger, and half of the ring finger. Weakness is typically exhibited in the intrinsic muscles of the hand. If the T2 root is involved, pain will be referred to the axilla and the medial aspect of the arm.

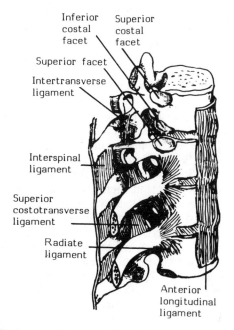

Figure 4.15. Highlights of the costovertebral joints and spinal ligaments of the midthoracic area as viewed from the oblique lateral. Normal kyphosis is not depicted (Courtesy ACAP).

• *The midthoracic spine.* Pain and sensory impairment are typically intercostal (dermatomal) in nature.

• *The lower thoracic spine.* Pain is referred anteriorly to the abdomen, pelvic organs, or groin, depending on the level of involvement. Segmental sensory impairment will help to isolate the lesion.

Centra Lipping

Vertebral body lipping is a sign of osseous hypertrophy and disc degeneration. In addition, it can be a sign of covert visceral pathology. A high incidence of osteophytic lipping in the thoracic region has been described in patients with gastrointestinal disorders, diabetes mellitus, and coronary heart disease. Bergfeldt and associates have shown a strong correlation between asymptomatic ankylosing spondylitis and sacroiliitis with disturbances of the cardiac conduction system.

Spondylitis

The ankylosed osteoporotic spines of patients with chronic spondylitis are prone to fracture from what may appear to be trivial forces. These injuries, which have a higher incidence in the cervical region than the thoracic region, can easily be overlooked when neurologic signs are absent.

Fixations of Chemical Origin

Illi's and Gillet's observations that certain thoracic fixations can be caused or perpetuated by the use and abuse of certain brands of coffee has been previously described in this chapter. This syndrome does not appear to be related to the caffeine content of coffee as it has not been found to be associated with the consumption of caffeine-rich tea. It is assumed to be related to oils within or added to the coffee beans during the roasting process, which some authorities have claimed to be carcinogenic. With this statement, the reader may reply, "and what substance commonly consumed has not been classified as being carcinogenic by some authority somewhere at sometime." Regardless, if the specific fixation in question is corrected by any number of different technics, there will still be a strong tendency of recurrence until the use of the offending brand of coffee is eliminated. Until such elimination is made and sustained for a while, you can expect the patient's back muscles to react abnormally to the reflex hammer; viz, a rapid contraction followed by relaxation. Headaches, heartburn, etc, are also reported to be commonly associated in the clinical picture that will disappear once the offending chemical is removed from the patient's diet.

The site of the fixation in question can be palpated as a vertical ridge of contracted muscle over the transverse processes in the T4—T6 region. It is assumed that this mass is the result of erector hypertonicity. This contracture-like mass is readily palpable by gliding the fingers down the thoracic transverse processes in a wide band. If in doubt, the thumbpads can be glided from the root of the spinous processes laterally.

Faye states that it can take multiple thrusts directed specifically into the sites of fixation before the complete thoracic fixation is mobilized in all directions. Obviously, if after the first or second adjustment there is still palpable loss of end-spring, one would thrust into the direction of the resistance to increase the lost motion.

Gillet points out that the oil in certain brands of coffee is not the only allergen that can be responsible for such a fixation. He also believes that the use of tobacco may have a similar effect in producing muscular fixations in the *midthoracic* area, especially at the T5—T6 level. Here, it is not the nicotine within tobacco that seems to be the culprit but the coal tar, which when burnt, is also attributed to be a cancer-causing agent in many people. As the fumes of burning animal fat, as experienced in fast frying or charcoal broiling a steak, has been classified as being thousands of times more carcinogenic than cigarette smoke, such a custom also brought out in the patient's history may be significant.

It is reported by Gillet that similar fixations are often found lower at the T6—T7 segments. However, the specific cause has not been determined. In rare instances, the

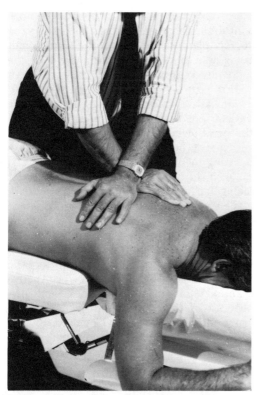

Figure 4.16. Applying a double-transverse contact on a midthoracic vertebra.

overuse of white sugar, white flour, or alcohol has been tentatively assumed to be the cause. A sophisticated food elimination diet would likely pinpoint the specific food substance containing the allergen, and it can be initially assumed from Gillet's observations that it will not be the substance as a whole being the cause as much as it is some associated compound.

THERAPEUTIC APPROACH

Unlike upper-cervical articular fixations, total fixations in the middle and lower thoracic spine may be corrected with one adjustment. Once upper cervical and sacroiliac fixations have been mobilized, it often appears that thoracic and lumbar fixations "invite" correction.

In Gillet's practice, all total fixations in the thoracic and lumbar spine are corrected with a firm double transverse contact (Fig. 4.16) followed by a rapid, short dynamic thrust directed at right angles to the spine (Fig. 4.17)—with the objective of separating the fixed intra-articular space. Many authorities in this country, however, recommend that the thrust be delivered in a line that is parallel to the plane of articulation of the particular segment adjusted.

The use of a particular technique is not important in regards to releasing the fixation. For example, adjusting a vertebrae to produce lateral rotation on the right will undoubtedly release a lateral rotation on the left fixation. Because the segment is a whole, motion induced on one side must produce motion on the contralateral side. However, the more efficient the technique is biomechanically, the less patient discomfort and the less iatrogenically produced injury (eg, "retracing").

It cannot be overemphasized that the examination must be thorough. The reason for this, as far as motion palpation is concerned, is that fixation at the posterior facet joints, the IVD interfaces, the costotransverse joint, or the costovertebral joint can cause aberrant motion at any or all of the other joints.

Specificity of palpation can also uncover the one direction of fixation that may not have been adjusted and needs further attention so the patient is not left with a partial fixation.

Thoracic Spine Fixations

Described below is a summary of the more common adjustments to release fixations associated with the thoracic spine and posterior aspect of the ribs. After each adjustment, the patient should be repalpated to assure that a *correction* has been made at the joints, and not just a mobile joint gapped for an audible release of no therapeutic significance.

Interspinous Fixations

Thoracic Interspinous Fixation: Patient Prone. Place the patient face down on the adjusting table, with the head-piece level.

Stand at the side of the table, obliquely facing the patient, and apply a knife-edge contact (medial edge of hand) with your active (cephalad) hand just below the spinous process of the superior segment of the locked motion unit. Your fingers will be horizontal. Place your caudad stabilizing hand over your active hand for reinforcement. Shift your body weight over the patient, keep your elbows locked, take up any tissue slack under your active hand, and, with a quick body drop, deliver a short impulse cephalad and slightly downward (superoanteriorly) against the spinous process. See Figure 4.18.

During this adjustment, the level of your arms relative to the patient's thoracic kyphosis must be changed. That is, your arms will be almost parallel to the patient's spine for fixations in the lower-thoracic region, slightly more oblique when treating the mid-thoracic area, and slightly further oblique when treating the upper-thoracic spine. The correct angle of thrust will be determined by the perception of the most resistance. If the plane of your arms is too upright or too horizontal, the force will not be centered at the correct plane of resistance. The result of not being able to feel this resistance will be the tendency to apply too much force.

Mid- and Lower-Thoracic Interspinous Fixation: Patient Supine. Place the patient face up on the adjusting table, with the head-piece level. Have the patient grip the back of the neck with both hands, elbows pointing forward. Stand at the side of the table on the opposite side of fixation, at first facing fairly perpendicular to the patient. Place your cephalad stabilizing hand under the hands of the patient (clasped behind the neck), curl the patient upward about 30°, and then roll him/her toward you slightly so that you can apply your contact. Insert the flexed middle or index finger of your active (caudad) hand between the locked spinous processes. Using your flexed finger as a fulcrum and pry, roll the patient back over toward your active hand to a considerable degree but without applying excessive pressure

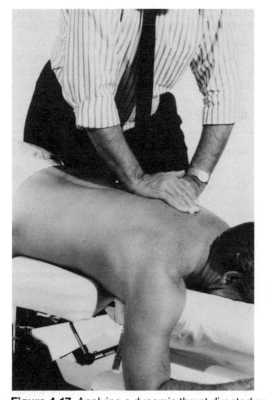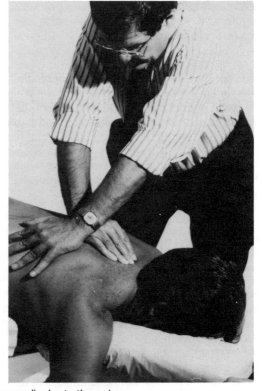

Figure 4.17. Applying a dynamic thrust directed perpendicular to the spine.

against your active hand. Lean over the patient so that your chest firmly contacts the patient's elbows, remove any slack, and quickly impulse downward to flex the patient's spine primarily at your contact finger. See Figure 4.19.

Note: the patient's spine must be flexed for proper release, not extended. The line of drive of your chest against the patient's elbows is towards the patient's navel and into the maximum resistance that you may feel.

Lateral-Flexion Fixations

Upper-Thoracic Lateral-Flexion Fixation: Patient Sitting. Our example here will be a T2-T3 motion unit in which the superior segment is fixed in lateral flexion on the right. Have the patient sit erect on a low stool. Stand behind the patient perpendicular to the site of involvement. If the stool is wide enough, lift your flexed left knee and place your left foot on the stool near the

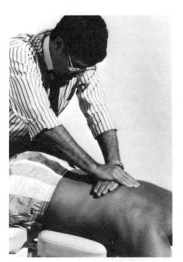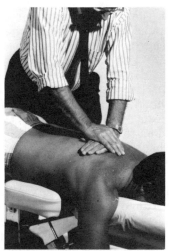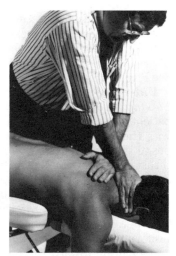

Figure 4.18. Applying a knife-edge contact against an interspinous fixation. *Left,* lower thoracic spine; *center,* midthoracic spine; *right,* upper thoracic spine.

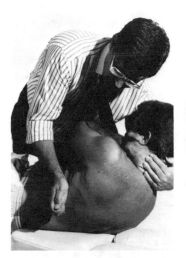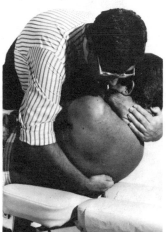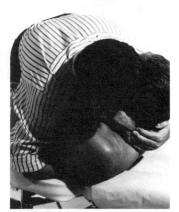

Figure 4.19. Correcting a lower-thoracic interspinous fixation with the patient supine. *Left,* preparing the patient for the adjustment; *center,* applying contact with the active hand; *right,* making the correction.

patient and drape the patient's left arm over your left thigh. With your active (left) hand, apply a thumb contact on the spinous process of the involved segment, and allow your fingers to curl forward over the patient's shoulder. Your flexed left elbow will be near the horizontal plane. Place the palm of your stabilizing hand (right) on the right side of the patient's head, just above the ear. Shift your weight slightly over the patient, laterally flex the patient's head and neck toward the side of your contact, and simultaneously deliver a corrective impulse by creating segmental lateral flexion to the left. The line of drive will be toward a point slightly above the patient's right shoulder, directed into the site of greatest resistance between T2 and T3. See Figure 4.20.

Mid- and Lower-Thoracic Lateral-Flexion Fixation: Patient Prone. Place the patient face down on the adjusting table, with the head-piece level. Stand on the opposite side of involvement, so that you can thrust into the lateral-flexion fixation, facing perpendicular to the patient. Your contact will be on the nearside of the spinous process of the superior segment of the fixated motion unit. Apply a specific contact with the pisiform of your active (caudad) hand, fingers pointing toward the patient's occiput. Place the heel of your stabilizing hand (cephalad) on the contralateral side of the pa-

tient's spine, fingers pointing horizontally across the patient's back. Shift your weight over the patient, lock your elbows, take up any tissue slack under your hands, and with a body drop, deliver a short quick impulse directed towards the floor and forward (anterolaterally) to produce segmental lateral flexion. To clarify: If the patient cannot laterally flex toward the left, stand on the left side because the joints on the right side are failing to open. See Figure 4.21.

Upper-Thoracic Lateral Flexion: Patient Prone. Similar to above except that a thumb contact is applied against the spinous process and the stabilizing hand lifts the patient's head and laterally flexes the head and neck toward the thumb contact and away from the side of fixation just before the thrust is made. See Figure 4.22.

Mid- and Lower-Thoracic Lateral-Flexion Fixation: Patient Laterally Recumbent. Place the patient in a sidelying position on a low adjusting table, with the head-piece level or slightly raised. The side of fixation should be facing downward. Stand on the ventral side of the patient, reach over the patient, and apply a thumb contact deep against the upper side of the spinous process of the superior segment of the involved motion unit. Place the thumb of your stabilizing hand over your active thumb for reinforcement. Shift your weight over the pa-

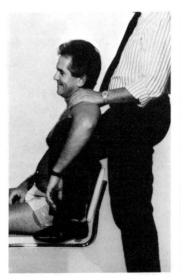 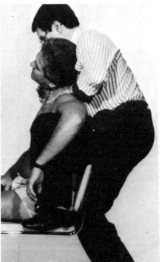 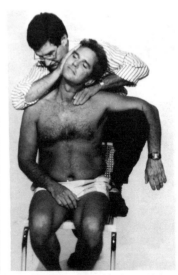

Figure 4.20. Adjusting an upper thoracic lateral-flexion fixation with the patient sitting. *Left,* applying the thumb contact; *center,* side view of the adjustment; *right,* frontal view of the adjustment.

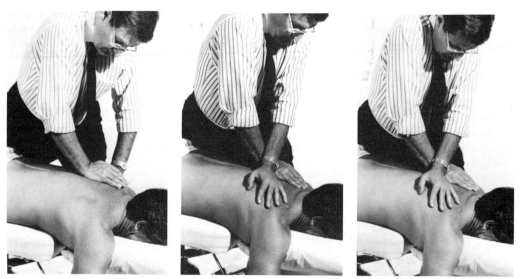

Figure 4.21. Correcting a midthoracic lateral-flexion fixation with the patient prone. *Left,* apply the contact; *center,* preparing to deliver the adjustment; *right,* adding body drop.

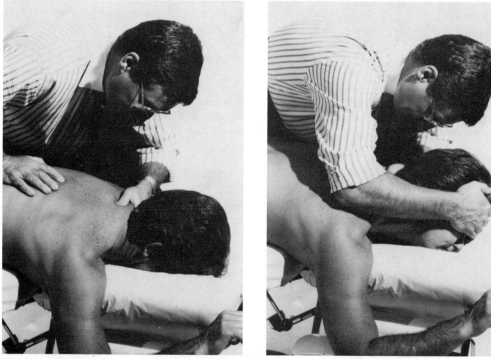

Figure 4.22. Adjusting an upper-thoracic lateral-flexion fixation with the patient prone. *Left,* applying the contact; *right,* making the correction.

tient, lock your elbows, take up any tissue slack under your contact thumb, and with a body drop, deliver a short recoil impulse directed toward the floor, perpendicular to the fixation, to produce segmental lateral flexion. See Figure 4.23.

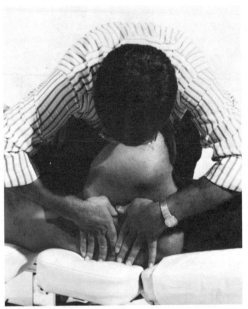

Figure 4.23. Position for correcting a midthoracic lateral-flexion fixation with the patient laterally recumbent.

Rotational Fixations

Mid- and Lower-Thoracic Rotational Fixation: Patient Sitting. Have the patient seated on a palpation stool, facing forward and arms crossed over the chest. Sit obliquely behind the patient, facing toward the site of fixation. Place your outer-positioned leg against the patient's leg to prevent the patient's pelvis from turning toward you during the maneuver ahead. With your stabilizing hand cupped over the patient's elbows, rotate the patient's thorax toward the side of fixation in a manner similar to that you would do during motion palpation. With your active hand, take a pisiform contact against the nearside of the spinous process of the superior segment of the involved motion unit. Turn the patient into maximum rotation with your stabilizing hand, and then, when all slack is removed, deliver a dynamic impulse with your active hand to further rotate the motion unit and mobilize the rotational block. The direction of drive is lateral and slightly upward into the plane of greatest resistance. Do not thrust if you cannot feel the resistance of the fixation that was palpated. See Figure 4.24.

Mid- and Lower-Thoracic Rotation Fixation: Patient Prone. Place the patient face down on the adjusting table, with the

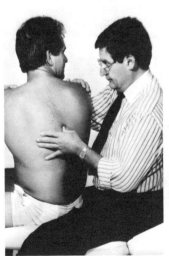
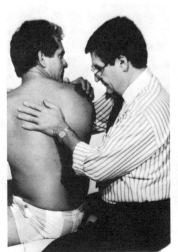
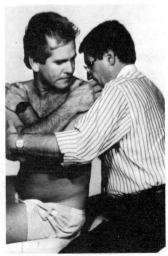

Figure 4.24. Correcting a lower-thoracic rotational fixation with the patient sitting. *Left,* locating the fixation; *center,* applying a pisiform contact; *right,* frontal-oblique view showing position of the stabilizing hand.

head-piece level. Stand on the side of involvement, oblique to the patient. Apply a pisiform contact on the nearside of the spinous process of the superior segment of the involved motion unit, fingers pointing toward the patient's occiput. Place your stabilizing hand over your active hand for reinforcement. Lock your elbows, raise up slightly on your toes and flex your knees, take up any tissue slack under your active hand, and with a body drop, impulse, or recoil, deliver a short quick thrust that is directed into the resistance—downward, lateral, and slightly toward the patient's contralateral shoulder to produce segmental rotation. See Figure 4.25.

Upper-Thoracic Rotation Fixation: Patient Prone. Place the patient face down on the adjusting table, with the head-piece level. Stand on the side of involvement, obliquely facing the patient. Apply a pisiform contact against the nearside of the spinous process of the superior segment of the involved motion unit. Place your stabilizing hand against the ipsilateral side of the patient's head above the ear, and rotate the patient's head and neck toward the side of fixation. Lock the elbow of your active hand, and take up any tissue slack underneath your contact. Raise up, and with a body drop or recoil, deliver a short quick thrust that is directed downward and laterally into the resistance to produce segmental rotation ipsilaterally from the posterior to the anterior. See Figure 4.26.

If you prefer, the same result can be achieved by standing on the other side and setting your contact over the contralateral articular or transverse process. See Figure 4.27.

Mid- and Lower-Thoracic Rotation Fixation: Patient Supine. For this adjustment, the doctor-patient positions are the same as those described for releasing an interspinous fixation with the patient supine except that flexed fingers are placed under the locked facets and the body drop against the patient's elbows is directed to rotate the patient's spine over your contact finger(s) to mobilize the blocked rotation of the motion unit. If you choose, you may use a pisiform contact on the contralateral side of the spinous process of the superior segment of the

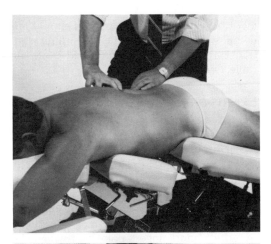

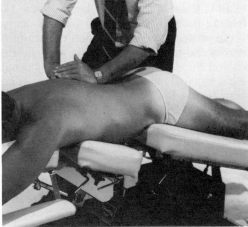

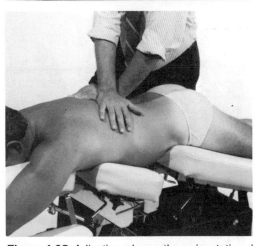

Figure 4.25. Adjusting a lower-thoracic rotational fixation with the patient prone. *Top,* localizing the involved spinous process; *middle,* applying a pisiform contact; *bottom,* positioned to deliver the corrective thrust.

involved motion unit. The patient should not be allowed to return to the full supine position; only the side being adjusted is on the table. See Figure 4.28.

Extension Fixations

Mid- and Lower-Thoracic Extension Fixation: Patient Prone. Place the patient face down on the adjusting table, with the head-piece level. Stand on the side of involvement, obliquely facing the patient. Apply contact over the involved inferior articular process with the pisiform of your active (caudad) hand, fingers pointing toward the head of the table. Place the heel of your stabilizing hand over the contralateral transverse process, fingers extended horizontally across the patient's back. Shift your weight so that it is slightly over the patient, lock your elbows, and take up any tissue slack under your hands. Raise up, and with a body drop or recoil, deliver a short quick thrust that is directed downward (anteriorly) and cephalad to produce segmental extension.

A vertebra locked in extension (which restricts flexion), sometimes called a posterior vertebra, can also be adjusted with a crossed-hand bilateral contact with the pisiforms on the laminae. This is similar to but

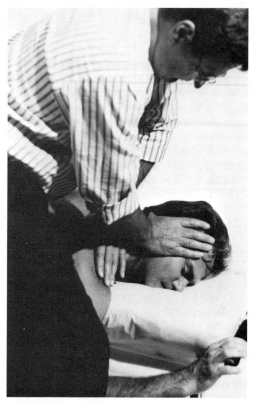

Figure 4.27. Correcting an upper-thoracic rotational fixation from the contralateral side of the table.

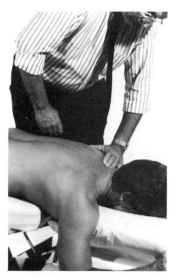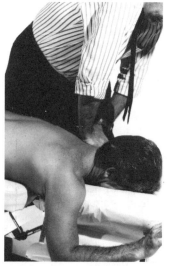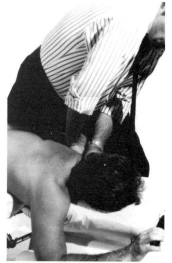

Figure 4.26. Correcting an upper-thoracic rotational fixation with the patient prone. *Left,* applying a pisiform contact; *center,* securing the contact; *right,* releasing the fixation.

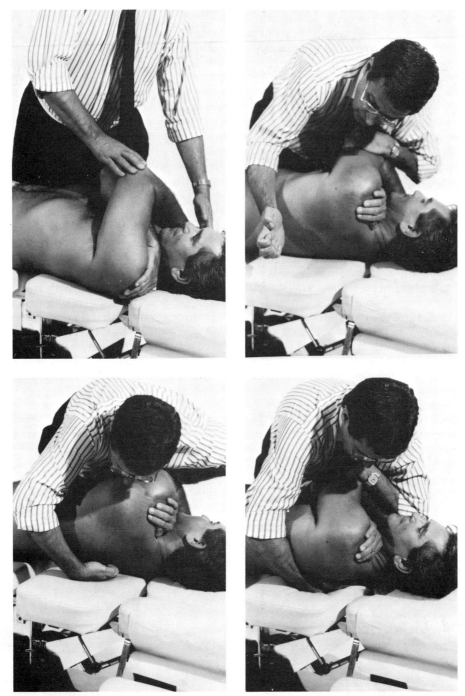

Figure 4.28. Adjusting a midthoracic rotational fixation with the patient supine. *Top left,* positioning the patient; *top right,* preparing to apply the contact hand; *bottom left,* securing the contact hand; *bottom right,* delivering the corrective thrust.

safer than a double transverse contact because the laminae are stronger than the transverse processes. The impulse is directed downward and headward, in line with the plane of facet articulation. [See Clinical Comment 4.5]

Mid- and Lower-Thoracic Extension Fixation: Patient Supine. For this adjustment, the doctor-patient positions are similar to those described for releasing an interspinous fixation with the patient supine with a few important modifications: (1) the spinous process of the superior segment of the involved motion unit is inserted between your flexed fingers on one side and the thenar eminence on the other side. This contact will serve as a fulcrum during the adjustment. (2) As you desire the spine to extend in this adjustment, your stabilizing hand is not placed at the back of the patient's neck; rather, the forearm of your stabilizing limb is placed horizontally across the patient's folded arms. (3) The body drop of your chest against your forearm is directed to extend the patient's spine over your contact fingers to mobilize the blocked extension of the

motion unit. Thus, the line of drive is directed toward the patient's sternal notch. (4) Lowering the head-piece a few notches is also helpful. See Figure 4.29.

Some practitioners always prefer to use a broad palm contact anteriorly on the patient's crossed arms rather than a chest contact during thoracic adjustments with the patient in the supine position.

Anterior Longitudinal Ligament Fixations

Mid- and Lower Thoracic Anterior Longitudinal Ligament Fixation: Patient Prone. Place the patient face down, head-piece level or slightly lowered. Stand on either side and face the patient obliquely. Apply a knife-edge contact with your active hand just below the spinous process of the superior segment of the involved motion unit (ie, within the interspinous space). Place your stabilizing hand over your contact hand for reinforcement. Keep your arms low so that they will be appropriate for the ar-

---

DR. FAYE'S CLINICAL COMMENT #4.5

Remember that the facet angles on a dry spine (model) or those seen in the shadows of a radiograph do not exhibit the actual shape of the articular surfaces. In vivo, the hyaline-coated articular surfaces provide a convexoconcave congruence. Preceding a thrust, I always feel the resistance in the direction palpated. The line of drive for the thrust is into the resistance.

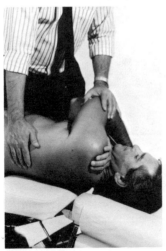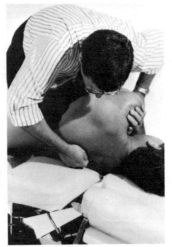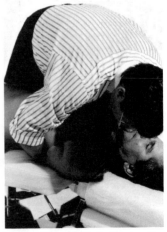

Figure 4.29. Correcting a midthoracic extension fixation with the patient supine. *Left,* positioning the patient; *center,* securing the contact; *right,* applying the thrust.

ticular plane of the facets. Lock your elbows, take up any tissue slack under your contact hand, and deliver a short quick impulse that is directed downward and cephalad. This will be in a "scooping" manner, "down and through" (against) the fixation. See Figure 4.30.

Upper-Thoracic Anterior Longitudinal Ligament Fixation: Patient Prone. This adjustment is similar to that above except that the adjustive force is directed more towards the floor to create segmental extension designed to stretch the anterior longitudinal ligament. It is frequently held that this adjustment is often the key to successful recovery in chronic radiculitis of this area. Another exception to the above technic is that rather than placing your stabilizing hand over your active hand, it is usually best used to cup the patient's occiput to stabilize the cervical spine. While stabilizing, exert moderate traction while the active hand impulses against the fixation. Added body drop during delivery of the impulse is often helpful.

Costotransverse Fixations

Mid- and Lower Thoracic Costotransverse Fixations

Costotransverse Fixation: Patient Prone. Place the patient face down on the adjusting table, with the head-piece level or dropped a notch. Stand at the side of the table, obliquely facing the patient. Apply a pisiform contact under the edge of the angle of the involved rib, just lateral to the tip of the transverse process, fingers pointing toward the head of the table. Place the heel of your stabilizing hand over the contralateral transverse process, fingers pointing horizontally over the patient's back. Shift your weight so that it is over the patient, lock your elbows, take up any tissue slack under your contact hand, and deliver a short quick impulse that is directed to release a left lateral-flexion fixation of the involved costotransverse joint. If a release is not felt, rotate your body and hands so that a similar thrust will release a right lateral-flexion fixation of the involved costotransverse joint. See Figure 4.31.

Costotransverse and costovertebral fixations may also be released with the standard double-transverse contact applying a dynamic thrust, keeping in mind that the depth of the thrust is much less than that applied to a muscular type of fixation. Costotransverse and costovertebral fixations are often bilateral and rarely associated with isolated overt malalignment in the resting position.

Costotransverse Fixation: Patient Supine. For this adjustment, the doctor-patient positions are identical to those described for releasing a thoracic rotational fixation with the patient in the supine position except that the contact is made on the

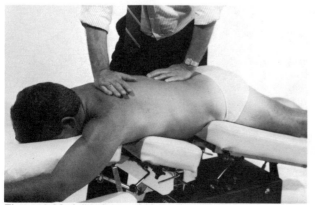
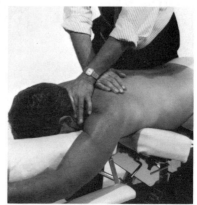

Figure 4.30. Adjusting a midthoracic anterior longitudinal ligament fixation with the patient prone. *Left,* applying a knife-edge contact; *right,* preparing to deliver the corrective thrust.

angle of the rib, just lateral to the tip of the transverse process. See Figure 4.32.

Costotransverse Fixation: Patient Standing. Stand behind the standing patient who has the arms crossed over the chest. Reach around the patient and cup the patient's adducted elbows in both hands. It sometimes helps to interlace your fingers. Lean closer so that chest pressure can be directly against the angle of the involved rib. Apply traction to remove any tissue slack, and then quickly lift the patient upward and slightly backward into extension (by curving backward yourself), using your chest as a fulcrum. This adjustment is identical to the classic osteopathic maneuver for distracting the thoracic spine except that the sternal contact is against the angle of the rib rather than against the apex of the patient's kyphosis.

First Rib Costotransverse Fixations

Place a palpating finger on the angle of the 1st rib, which can be found just in front of the trapezius in the fossa at the base of the neck. Hold this contact while your other hand extends the patient's neck, rotates the head away from the side of palpation, and laterally bends the neck toward your palpating finger. Normally, the 1st rib should then have dropped away from the palpating finger and

no longer be perceptible. If it can still be felt, it can be considered locked, having failed to move inferiorly.

Patient Supine. With the patient supine, stand on the ipsilateral side of the involved rib, facing caudad. With your lateral hand, take an open-web contact on the involved rib's crest that is high on your lateral hand's index finger, with the thumb anterior and your fingers posterior to the patient's chest. The point of contact is about 4 inches lateral to the T1 spinous. The stabilizing palm is cupped over the patient's contralateral ear, with your fingers supporting the patient's occiput (Fig. 4.33). To relax the ipsilateral neck muscles, raise the patient's neck several inches with your stabilizing fingers and let the occiput extend into your palm. Rotate the patient's head 20°—30° away from the fixation, laterally bend the neck toward your contact hand, and deliver a moderate thrust that is directed caudad and slightly posteromedially toward T4 into the resistance of the first rib to move it inferiorly.

Patient Prone. Some DCs prefer the following alternative approach: With the patient prone, stand on the ipsilateral side of the involved rib facing the patient's contralateral shoulder. With your lateral hand, take an open-web contact on the rib's crest that is high on your lateral hand's index finger as above. The elbow of your active limb will be

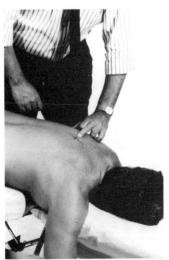
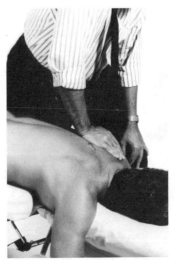
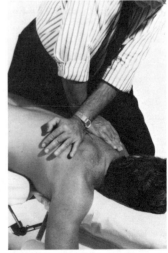

Figure 4.31. Correcting a left midthoracic costotransverse fixation with the patient prone. *Left,* localizing the contact; *center,* applying a pisiform contact; *right,* applying the corrective impulse.

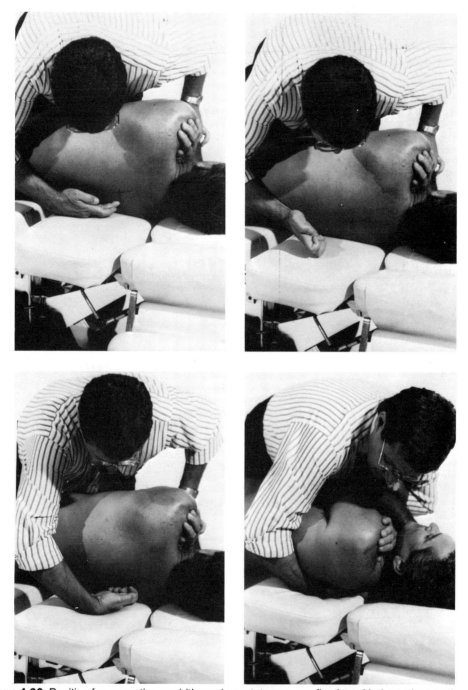

Figure 4.32. Position for correcting a midthoracic costotransverse fixation with the patient supine. *Top left,* localizing the site of fixation; *top right,* preparing the contact hand; *lower left,* securing the contact hand; *lower right,* releasing the fixation.

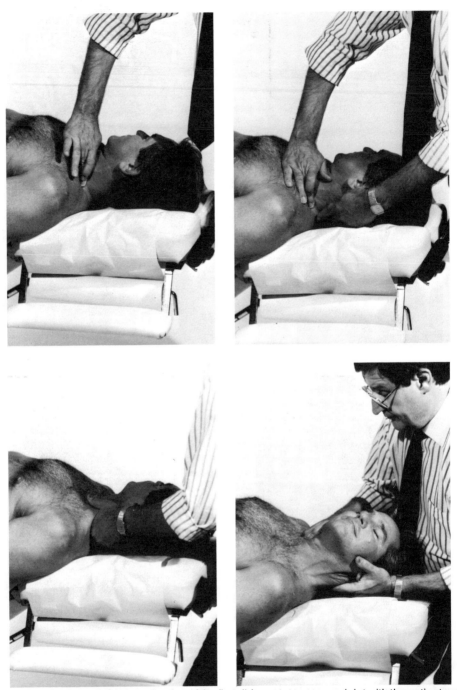

Figure 4.33. Position for adjusting a fixation of the first rib's costotransverse joint with the patient supine. *Top left,* localizing the site of fixation; *top right,* applying the contact; *lower left,* preparing for the adjustment; *lower right,* adjustment position shown from the contralateral side.

flexed and pointing superolaterally as you lean over the patient. A palm contact is made with your stabilizing hand on the patient's forehead. With your stabilizing hand, lift the patient's head slightly, rotate the head away from the involved rib, and apply mild lateral flexion to relax the ipsilateral muscles. Then deliver a thrust with your contact hand that is directed caudad and medial toward T4 into the resistance of the 1st rib. See Figure 4.34.

Costovertebral Fixations

Gillet's early studies of the thoracic spine encountered great difficulty because of the existence on the strong rib attachments in this area of the spine. He comments that "In chiropractic, these structures are practically ignored, contrary to our osteopathic colleagues who teach the existence of rib 'lesions' and the 'springing' of ribs."

Unfortunately, research related to the movements of the thoracic spine relative to their attached ribs is extremely meager except for studies of costal motion during the respiratory process. It can be easily understood that the study of fixations between (1) the vertebrae, (2) the vertebrae and ribs, and (3) the ribs themselves are still perplexing problems worthy of our special attention.

Adjusting Costovertebral Fixation: Patient Prone. Place the patient's face down on the adjusting table, head-piece level or dropped a notch. Stand at the side of the table on the side of involvement, and obliquely face the patient. Lean over the patient, and apply a knife-edge contact at the inferior edge of the involved rib's angle. Place your stabilizing hand over your active hand for reinforcement. Lower the angle of your arms so that they are almost parallel to the patient's spine, lock your elbows, take up any soft-tissue and rib slack under your contact hand, and deliver a short quick impulse that is directed cephalad and slightly downward (superoanteriorly), along the long axis of the rib (Fig. 4.35).

The articulations between the rib head and vertebral body or between the rib tubercle and the transverse are common sites of fixation and often due to serratus and/or levator costarum hypertonicity. Gillet believes this type of fixation is contributed to by capsular shortening that allows enough torsion for unrestricted breathing during nondemanding activities. Associated adhesion-type bands could easily irritate an entrapped sympathetic ganglia during normal motion. Posterior rib fixations are rarely complete. They usually tend to restrict mobility in one or more directions but not in all directions.

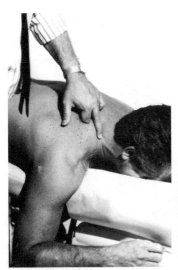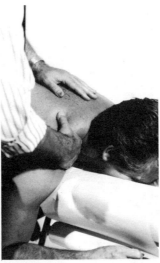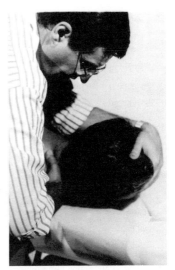

Figure 4.34. Position for adjusting a fixation of the first rib's costotransverse joint with the patient prone. *Left,* localizing the site of fixation; *center,* securing the contact hand; *right,* making the correction.

Intertransverse Fixations

Both muscles and ligaments connect adjacent transverse processes. Fixation can be palpated by contacting each intertransverse space with a thumb contact and forcing the spine into lateral flexion. If a fixation exists, it will be felt as a slight resistance of one or two vertebrae. It will usually be bilateral. Gillet recommends a local rotatory thrust, on both sides, to release such fixations. Correction occurs with only moderate force if it is not attempted too early in the course of case management.

Costocostal Fixations

Costocostal fixations are often classified as ligamentous fixations although they are probably of muscular origin; ie, intercostal muscles that have degenerated into a toughened state of fibrosis. If they are found somewhere far into the phases of Gillet's

therapeutic routine, a degenerative state is likely because costal muscular fixations would have long since disappeared spontaneously. Resistance to light preadjustive thrusts will often suggest the site of major fixation (Fig. 4.36).

Adjusting Posterior Costocostal Fixations

The adjustive thrust in a posterior rib—rib fixation is commonly made with the heel of the hand, with the patient placed in the prone position. Care must be taken to direct the thrust cephalad, never toward the sternum, to separate a rib from its inferior partner. A slight but distinct "release" is often felt and/or heard even though there is no articulation at this point.

Note: This adjustment must be delivered with extreme caution. Many patients nearing and over the age of 40 tend to have

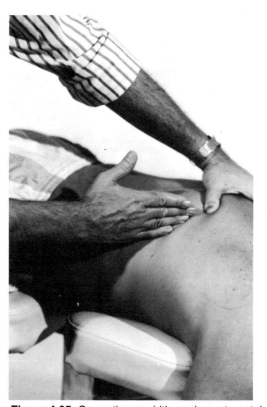
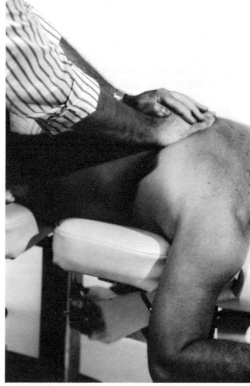

Figure 4.35. Correcting a midthoracic costovertebral fixation with the patient prone.

brittle ribs, and this would be especially true if the intercostals are in a state of degeneration. This is true in spite of the absence of roentgenographic signs of osteoporosis. A localized force directed at right angles to fixated ribs can easily produce a fracture. The possibility of this occurring can be greatly minimized by directing the thrust cephalad and keeping the thrust light and shallow. Some practitioners prefer to use one thumb contact against the inferior edge of the superior rib and another thumb contact against the superior edge of the inferior rib. This double-thumb contact may cause more patient discomfort momentarily, but it is far more specific than a palm heel contact.

Once identified and released, a general rib-mobilization technique with and without tracion on the ipsilateral iliac crest or shoulder can then be applied on the angles of the ribs involved to further loosen restrictions. This is frequently best followed by a regimen

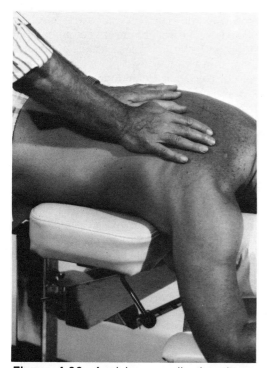

Figure 4.36. Applying preadjustive thrusts against the midthoracic rib angles to screen the presence of costocostal fixations.

of heat, muscle stimulation, and graduated stretching exercises.

Integrated Treatment Approach

Trigger Points

Because trigger-point development has been shown to interfere with homeostasis, Hitchcock points out that a patient's condition can usually be improved by modifying or deleting an excessive reaction on the musculoskeletal system, especially when such a reaction is related to the same levels of the CNS that innervate the area of pathophysiologic disturbance.

Some refer to a trigger point as a myofascitis. They state that trigger points are specific and sclerotomal in distribution and can be treated effectively with spray and stretch methods, acupressure or Nimmo techniques, electrotherapy, and other methods. Travell, on the other hand, describes a trigger point as a site of localized myodysneuria within muscle tissue, not an overlying fascial inflammation, and that the course of the pain frequently does not follow any known anatomical path of distribution (ie, dermatome, myotome, or sclerotome). Some professional papers conclude that the course of referred trigger-point pain often follows meridian paths described in Chinese literature.

Postural Realignment

In postural alignment of a scoliotic thoracic spine and shoulder girdle, the primary muscles requiring strengthening are (1) the quadratus lumborum on the side of concavity, (2) the upper and lower trapezius and the major and minor rhomboids to improve scapular adduction and rotation, and (3) the infraspinatus and teres minor to improve lateral rotation of the shoulder. In addition, it is unusual in thoracic distortions that certain muscles do not need stretching. Typical examples are (1) the quadratus lumborum on the side of lower thoracic convexity, (2) the latissimus dorsi, teres major, and subscapularis to improve shoulder adduction and medial rotation, and (3) the pectoral group to improve shoulder adduction and medial rotation. Invariably, stretching of the intercostals on the side of thoracic concavity is necessary.

McGall and associates have shown that long-term immobilization in plaster casts for scoliosis, including the duration of the adolescent growth spurt, leads to an increase in height of the vertebral bodies and a decrease of their height-to-width ratio. These changes appear to be at the expense of the disc, which is *reduced* in thickness. It is thought that this stimulating effect on vertebral body growth is due to the alteration of mechanical forces. The counterrotation exercises described by Michele are extremely helpful, as is the walking traction used by Illi and Betge.

Schafer's Basic Adjustive Concepts: Articular Fixations

Schafer states that he applies four cardinal rules in the application of any adjustive technic. They are primarily based on his training at Lincoln Chiropractic College in diversified technic courses and early training by his father (a DC). He makes no claim that their application is any better than any other generally taught procedures but feels that they have served him well and can be justified according to the established principles of applied anatomy and articular biomechanics. They concern (1) preadjustment patient positioning, (2) directing the impulse drive carefully in line with the segment's plane of articulation, (3) applying the active contact on the strongest logical point of the segment, and (4) applying segmental distraction before the thrust. A brief explanation of these points and their rationale are listed below for the reader's consideration:

1. *Patient positioning.* Ideal patient positioning is that position which best encourages spontaneous release if such were possible. This often requires the use of padded wedge-shaped cushions and/or various alterations in treatment table adjustment. The objective is to enlist the forces of gravity and reduce compressive forces on the involved facets. With such positioning, half the adjustment is accomplished and only a minimal additional applied force by the physician is necessary to complete the release. For example:

a. If a thoracic vertebra is fixed in extension, the patient is placed prone, the head-piece of the table is lowered, the thoracic-abdominal support is raised and tension is increased, and the front end of the pelvic-thigh support is raised—all of which will add gravitation force that encourages thoracic flexion (hyperkyphosis).

b. If a thoracic vertebra is fixed in flexion, the patient is placed prone, the head-piece of the table is raised, tension is released from the thoracic-abdominal support, and the front aspect of the pelvic-thigh support is lowered—all of which will add gravitation force that encourages thoracic extension (flattening). Care must be taken, however, not to induce a degree of extension that would cause overt jamming of the facets to be released. Thus, specific positioning will be a matter of compromise and clinical judgment of the situation (primarily, the degree of habitual thoracic kyphosis).

c. If a thoracic vertebra is fixed in lateral flexion to the right, the patient is carefully placed in the right lateral recumbent position, with the contralateral side of involvement upward. The head-piece of the table is raised, the thoracic-abdominal support is lowered and its tension is reduced, and the front aspect of the pelvic-thigh support is raised—all of which will add gravitational force that encourages the area involved to laterally flex to the left (curve toward the floor).

d. If a thoracic vertebra is fixed in posterior rotation on the right, the patient is placed prone with a wedge-shaped cushion inserted under the patient's left shoulder girdle and upper thorax to encourage thoracic rotation toward the posterior on the left. If the patient's thoracic spine as a whole presents with a distinct kyphosis, the thoracic-abdominal support is made level. If the patient's thoracic spine as a whole is unusually flat, the thoracic-abdominal support and pelvic-thigh supports are adjusted to induce a moderate kyphosis. Various other positioning modifications and a hip wedge may be helpful depending on the individual design of the patient's thoracic scoliosis, if one exists.

2. *Plane of articulation.* A line of drive that is directed exactly parallel to the plane of articulation is the most mechanically efficient and induces the least amount of articular injury (and related patient discomfort). See Figure 4.37. As postapophyseal midthoracic facets face almost straight toward the anterior, the adjustive impulse must be directed as parallel to the spine as is possible; ie, headward, minimally downward. Granted, this appears to be an awkward position, but the more downward impulse, the

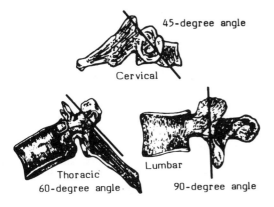

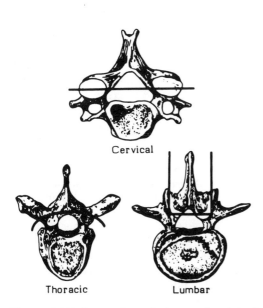

Figure 4.37. Comparison of planes of vertebral facets shown from the side and from above. These planes should be considered during the application of any articular adjustment (Courtesy ACAP).

more articular jamming will be induced, encouraging articular bruise and the subsequent development of an inflammatory reaction leading to adhesion development in the weeks or months ahead. It should also be remembered that the superior articular processes of the subjacent segment extend somewhat upward as "rabbit ears." They could easily be fractured by a sharp force directed anteriorly if not for the stability provided by the rib cage. Refer to Figure 4.1.

It would appear to be of little far-reaching clinical value to the patient to release a fixation only to set the stage for another in the future. Thus, for instance, while Gillet recommends that an anterior body fixation be released by a force directed perpendicular to the plane of articulation to stretch the anterior longitudinal ligament and widen the IVD space anteriorly, Schafer usually prefers to accomplish this by patient positioning and to release the fixed facets with a force that is parallel to their plane of articulation. "In this era of increasing malpractice claims, I believe it best to give patient safety an extraordinary priority over a loss of a few ounces of mechanical efficiency."

The plane of articulation of an individual patient's particular involved thoracic segment must be considered. Textbook descriptions are based on population averages and do not consider the factors of individual genetic design or the effects of unique trauma and osseous erosion from long-term postural imbalance.

Faye states: "The last word in line of drive is determined by the direction of the loss of motion and the greatest point of resistance into that direction is the prethrust, lockpoint one has to 'feel' before one thrusts. This lock-point is that point in the load separation graph where the elastic barrier is met and one is just short of the physiological space. A short, sharp, high-velocity low-amplitude thrust, impulse causes the joint space to separate sufficiently to create cavitation ('crack') and greatly increase the postmanipulative range of motion. This new motion stimulates the previously dormant mechanoreceptors and pain relief is experienced. This mechanostimulation also causes muscles that move the joint to relax due to the normalized articular neurostimulation."

3. *Point of contact.* Most classic adjustive technics apply contact on the spinous process or transverse process for greater leverage. Whenever possible, a laminal contact would allow the force to be directed against the strongest aspect of the posterior portion of the vertebra. Some leverage is lost with a laminal contact, but added safety is gained. Unless cautiously applied, a transverse process contact holds the inherent danger of the contact slipping laterally, which can easily result in rib injury. A transverse or laminal contact is less painful to the patient than a spinous contact because of the padding afforded by the intervening musculature). A broad contact (eg, knife-edge, hand heel), although less specific, is less painful to the patient than a contact applied with a smaller surface area (eg, thumb, pisiform, adjusting gun).

4. *Segmental distraction.* Because of the reduction of interarticular friction, articular distraction applied an instant before delivering the corrective impulse will enhance mechanical efficiency of the induced movement. This is especially important in extension and rotational fixations that almost always are complicated by a degree of articular jamming; unimportant in flexion fixations that normally present with widened interarticular spaces. A mild vertical axial traction force can be applied by the stabilizing hand, patient positioning, an assistant, a traction apparatus, or a combination of these methods.

Faye recommends the motorized mechanical distraction table. "Leander has published data showing a 40%—50% less thrust is needed if thoracic distraction is occurring."

The use of segmental distraction (prethrust traction) was considered a fundamental factor in chiropractic adjustive therapy from the early part of the century through the 1950s. It was emphasized in the writings of Willard Carver, J. S. Riley, and Oakley Smith (1900—1920), especially. Michael Grecco, of the Chiropractic Institute of New York, incorporates it in his 1953 text *Chiropractic Technic Illustrated;* Homer Beatty, then president of the University of Natural Healing Arts (Denver), emphasized it in his 1939 text *Anatomical Adjustive Technic,* and it was found consistently within the technic notes of Lincoln College. A photograph in *Chiropractic Health Care* shows an automated "traction couch" being demonstrated on the campus of Palmer Chiropractic College in Davenport in 1914 by inventor D.W. Risland.

Background: Underlying Biomechanical Principles

The application of a chiropractic adjustment is an art, an art that must be well-founded on an understanding of the underlying pathophysiologic processes involved with an particular patient and an understanding of the basic principles of biomechanics. These factors should never be taken lightly.

The Intervertebral Interface. The faces of the articular facets are covered by tough hyaline cartilage and separated by meniscus-like tabs of synovium that originate from the synovial lining. These tabs glide in and out of the joint during motion but are rarely nipped during joint jamming (eg, extension). The tabs appear to allow a degree of extra shock-absorbing and pressure-absorbing protection for the articular cartilage.

Biomechanical Viscoelasticity. Although widely variant in degree, all neuromusculoskeletal tissues are organic viscoelastic substances. The critical factor in *viscoelastic stability* involves both load and a *time element.* That is, a viscoelastic substance can resist a certain load for a period of time and then fail without the load being altered. Thus, *all musculoskeletal structures have a time-dependent stability factor.* This factor is usually structurally adapted to in living tissue if the time element is prolonged (eg, redesign of trabeculae). It is emphasized that the combined components of viscosity and elasticity allow for relaxation and creep, and both relaxation and creep are a function of time.

Biomechanical Fatigue and Hysteresis. The viscoelastic nature of IVDs and other joint connective tissues therefore offers time-dependent properties such as *fatigue* and *hysteresis,* which vary in reaction whether the load is applied quickly with high amplitude (jerk) or slowly with a low magnitude (pressure fatigue failure). As the repair and regeneration capabilities of discs and cartilages are low, their fatigue life is comparatively low when subjected to repetitive loading. On failure, the result is tissue tearing.

During cyclic loading and unloading, a viscoelastic substance shows a loss of energy in the form of heat. This phenomenon is *hysteresis.* When an IVD, for instance, is subjected to reptitive cycles of loading and unloading (eg, hopping), the shock waves directed from the feet to the head are substantially dissipated by disc hysteresis. This effect is minimal in the T9 L2 area. It decreases when the load-unload cycle is prolonged (eg, constant bumping) and during old age when viscoelasticity is low.

The process of developing structure cracks when subjected to cyclic loading is called *fatigue* in engineering. The magnitude of the load is usually far below that of the ultimate load of the particular structure, and thus well within the elastic range. The result is a summation effect in which a fatigue crack reaches a size that causes the remainder of the structure to become so weakened that the entire structure fails. In biomechanics, this factor is popularly called the *time* or *aging factor* of a body structure, and the time of failure decreases as the magnitude of the load increases.

The term *endurance limit* refers to the least load that produces a failure from structural fatigue. If healing processes are inhibited or impaired, if the body's reserves are depleted, or if the healing processes do not have adequate time to repair structural cracks in bone or cartilage, for example, a *fatigue fracture* occurs. Such "cracks" commonly occur microscopically in articular cartilage except in the menisci of the knee where they are frequently gross.

Biomechanical Creep and Relaxation. The *viscoelastic* properties of a fibrocartilage such as an IVD and somewhat of articular cartilage offer it *creep* and *relaxation* behavior. The greater the load, the greater the deformation and the faster the rate of creep. A degenerated disc, for example, exhibits less viscoelasticity, less creep, and less capability of attenuating shocks and

vibrations uniformly over the full surfaces of the end plates. Thus, stress relaxation is the viscoelastic property of a tissue of retaining a constant deformation after a load is removed. Relaxation, popularly called "give," is a steady deformation that occurs with less force over a period of time. This is demonstrated in a tissue being stressed at a constant magnitude where the force necessary to maintain the deformation decreases with time.

Creep is the viscoelastic property of slowly increasing deformation under a constant load. That is, there is an initial deformation followed by a slowly increasing degree of deformation. Unlike plastic behavior, creep begins even with a minimal force and the recovery is slow. Creep is exhibited in the loss of an individual's height from many hours in the upright position owing to the phenomenon occurring in the intervertebral discs where a constant weight has been borne over a period of time. When a constant force is applied to viscoelastic substances such as bones, muscles, tendons, cartilage, and ligaments, the property of creep becomes apparent. When a deformation is fixed, stress relaxation becomes apparent.

Loading Considerations. When articular cartilage is subjected to weight bearing, deformation develops instantaneously according to the tissue's stiffness property. This initial rapid deformation stage has a negligible matrix fluid flow, and the contour of the tissue changes but not its volume. This stage is followed by a slower *time-dependent creep* that is related to the flow of water through the matrix according to the magnitude of the load, the fiber elasticity, the quantity of surface area loaded, the uniformity of force distribution, the matrix permeability (which is low even when unloaded), the osmotic pressure of the matrix colloid, and the length of the flow path.

When load is removed during rest, the stressed cartilage begins to return to its original thickness—quickly at first (90%) because of the elastic recoil of the collagen fibers and then slowly thereafter from the absorption of water that is governed by the Donnan osmotic pressure of the proteoglycans in the matrix gel. This recovery by absorption is enhanced by oscillation of the unloaded joint and limited by the collagen fiber's stiffness and strength that are subjected to increasing tensile forces as the swelling develops.

Because fluid flow within a connective tissue's matrix is time dependent, cartilage response to compression depends on the magnitude of the load, the length of time the load is applied, and if the load is applied statically or cyclically. A small amount of water is expressed through the matrix even during a briefly applied load, and its absorption is *time dependent.* If a second load is applied before the matrix is fully reimbibed, as during cyclic loading, the result is incomplete recovery that summates as the cyclic loading continues. In addition, all cartilage can be considered prone to biomechanical fatigue.

Joint Lubrication. Joint lubrication is another factor to consider. The complex lubrication system of human joints far exceeds that of similarly designed man-made bearings. Much of this is due to (1) the renewable coating of glycoprotein molecules that blanket the surface of articular cartilage, (2) the ingress and egress of fluid from the cartilage's matrix, (3) the porosity and elasticity of cartilage that also affords fluid imbibement and expulsion during load compression and relief, and (4) the unique folding and sliding action of interarticular synovial folds during movement.

Position of Fixation. A segment's position in fixation, besides its affect on the contents of the IVF, is another important factor. See Figure 4.38. Vertebral tilting in the neutral position as seen in disorders with disc wedging alters the relationship of apposing articular surfaces to produce a change in the direction of compressive forces on these joints. In contrast, severe fixed rotation produces a jamming compression on ipsilateral facets and contralateral facet opening. When continuous compression is applied to any active mobile joint, cartilaginous erosion followed by arthritis and its sequelae can be expected.

Clinical Application. The properties of tissue relaxation, creep, and fatigue should be considered whenever articular correction, traction, lifts, or braces are used. For example, the soft tissues involved in spinal distortion will retain a degree of relaxation

for some time after adverse forces have been relieved. Thus, some means of rest and support are often necessary until the deformed tissues can adapt to new conditions. When certain adjustive forces, a pressure brace, or a shoe lift is applied, they should be done slowly in increments so that the degree of creep reversal obtained and the residual relaxation present can be evaluated. This would not be apparent with rapid maneuvers.

In most circumstances that contribute to abnormal soft-tissue stiffness where true ankylosis has not occurred, a large degree of functional shortening is superimposed on structural changes. When adjusting a vertebral or extraspinal motion unit that is obviously fibrotic, Schafer has found that mild traction and a broad contact with mild transverse pressure held in the direction of correction for 30—60 seconds just before the corrective adjustment helps to "reverse" the established creep and elastic fiber shortening produced by gravity, hypertonicity, etc. This is usually on the side of disc or cartilage thinning or musculotendinous shortening. When the adjustment is delivered, it appears to be with further palpable movement and with far less discomfort to the patient than would otherwise be achieved. The same mild contact following specific adjustment appears to enhance "holding" of the correction achieved. Facilities for postadjustment rest offer an excellent means of providing the time factor for the soft-tissue fibers to adapt without fighting gravity and for some corrective disc imbibition. However, this approach of applying biomechanical principles within articular therapy is an empirical observation on his part that he feels needs further study to be confirmed.

Personal Approach

Schafer approaches the subject of chiropractic articular correction as "a noninvasive surgical procedure, a *chiurgical art.*" "This takes time, and it takes time to assure proper patient positioning, assure that the impulse drive is exactly parallel to a particular patient's facet design, assure that the safest and most efficient point of contact is

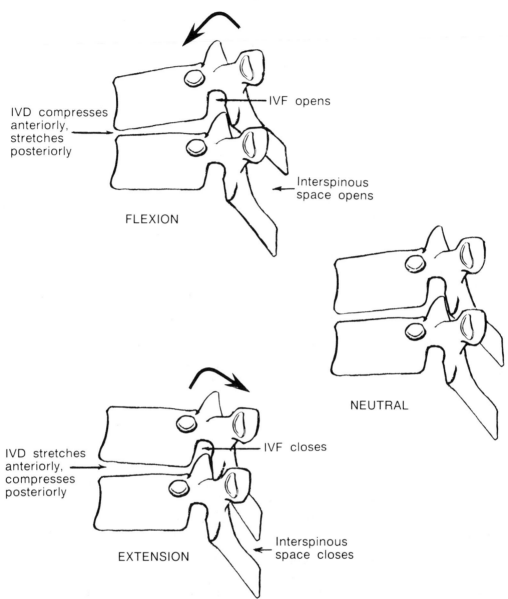

IVD compresses anteriorly, stretches posteriorly

IVF opens

Interspinous space opens

FLEXION

NEUTRAL

IVD stretches anteriorly, compresses posteriorly

IVF closes

Interspinous space closes

EXTENSION

Figure 4.38. *Top,* schematic of a typical midthoracic motion unit in full flexion; *middle,* in the neutral position; *bottom,* in full extension. Note that during flexion, the IVF opens vertically. This would have little effect on IVF contents unless the dural sleeve is firmly attached to both of the apposing processes. However, during extension, compression of the IVF contents can be severe, depending on the extension range of motion. Because compression thins the posterior aspect of the IVD, a weakened anulus would tend to protrude further into the vertebral canal. Thus, in most instances, it can be projected that fixations in extension would be more symptomatic than fixations in flexion. It can also be projected that in rotation to the posterior on the left, for example, where the left inferior facet of the superior segment glides down the left superior facet of the subjacent vertebra and the right inferior facet of the superior segment glides up the right superior facet of the subjacent vertebra, symptoms would be expected to be greater on the left. In rotation to the posterior on the right, opposite conditions occur.

selected, and assure that the proper impulse velocity and depth have been predetermined according to the circumstances at hand (eg, patient age, size, development, individual pain threshold, underlying pathophysiologic status, etc).

"When determined to be necessary or helpful, time is taken to assure that adequate *preadjustive* therapy is applied to render the tissues involved to be more receptive to the adjustment (eg, tissue plasticity, elasticity, and flexibility) and that adequate *postadjustive* therapy is applied to enhance the healing process (eg, neurocirculatory processes, pain control)." Schafer also feels that it is important that the patient be allowed to rest undisturbed in a comfortable position (and draped with a sheet and light blanket to avoid chilling) for 20—30 minutes or more following an adjustment because "The encouragement of physiologic *normalization* within viscoelastic substances takes time. I believe that it is imperative that this period of postadjustive rest be allowed before the physiologic and structural demands of weightbearing and cyclic loading are applied. Traumatized and pathologic tissues characteristically have low endurance and high biomechanical fatigue properties."

CLOSING REMARKS

Faye believes that the adjustment is an imposed demand for motion and if repeated at proper intervals stimulates a specific adaptation. "The thrust must be in sufficient directions to increase the lost ranges of motion of the motion unit and just forceful enough to cause cavitation and its audible release. The new demands of motion cause a specific response of increased lubrication, viscoelasticity, normalization of the neurophysiology and muscular changes necessary to accommodate the increased intersegmental range of motion. Just like weight training the adjustment by being repeated every other day at first becomes an imposed demand."

Bibliography

Agostoni E, et al: Forces deforming the rib cage. *Respiratory Physiology*, 2:105, 1966.

Albrand OW, Corkill G: Thoracic disc herniation: treatment and prognosis. *Spine*, 4:41-46, 1979.

Andriacchi T, et al: A model for studies of mechanical interactions between the human spine and rib cage. *Journal of Biomechanics*, 7:497-507, 1974.

Baltzell LG, Mackey RH (eds): *Firth's Technic Notes (Revised)*. Place of publication not shown, 1967, pp 45-48.

Barge FH: *Scoliosis*. Davenport, IA, published by author, 1981, vol III, pp 147-149.

Beatty HG: *Anatomical Adjustive Technic*, ed 2. Denver, CO, published by author, 1939.

Benson DR: The back: thoracic and lumbar spine. In D'Ambrosia RD: *Musculoskeletal Disorders: Regional Examination and Differential Diagnosis*. Philadelphia, J.B. Lippincott, 1977, pp 247-253, 308-309.

Bergfeldt L, Edhag O, Vedin L, Vallin H: Ankylosing spondylitis: an important cause of severe disturbances of the cardiac conduction system. *American Journal of Medicine*, 73:187-191, 1982.

Bernick S, Cailliet R: Vertebral end-plate changes with aging of human vertebrae. *Spine*, 7:97-102, 1982.

Blits J: Thoracic disk herniation. *Ortho Briefs*, ACA Council on Chiropractic Orthopedics, Spring 1982, pp 8-9.

Bowerman JW: *Radiology and Injury in Sport*. New York, Appleton-Century-Crofts, 1977, pp 87-92, 189.

Branton P: Behavior, body mechanics, and discomfort. *Ergonomics*, 12:316-327, 1969.

Cailliet R: *Low Back Pain Syndrome*, ed 2, Philadelphia, F.A. Davis, 1968, p 25.

Carver FJ: Postural adjusting. *Journal of the National Chiropractic Association*, April 1940.

Carver W: *Carver's Chiropractic Analysis*, ed 4. Oklahoma City, published by author, vol one, 1921.

Carver W: *Carver's Chiropractic Analysis*, ed 4. Oklahoma City, published by author, vol two, 1922.

Chin WS, Oon CL: Ossification of the posterior longitudinal ligament of the spine. *British Journal of Radiology*, 52:865-869, 1979.

Cox J, Gideon D, Rogers F: Incidence of osteophytic lipping of the thoracic spine in coronary heart disease: results of a pilot study. *Journal of the American Osteopathic Association*, 82:837-838, 1983.

Craig AS: Elements of kinesiology for the clinician. *Physical Therapy*, 44:470-473, 1964.

Daniels L, Worthingham C: *Therapeutic Exercise for Body Alignment and Function*, ed 2. Philadelphia, W.B. Saunders, 1977, pp 73-74, 66-71.

Evans DC: Biomechanics of spinal injury. In Gonza ER, Harrington IJ: *Biomechanics of Musculoskeletal Injury*. Baltimore, Williams & Wilkins, 1982, pp 200-204.

Faye LJ: Chiropractic Manipulation of the Thoracic Spine [Videotape]. Dynaspine, Inc, 10780 Santa Monica Blvd, Suite 400, Los Angeles, CA 90025.

Faye LJ, et al: *Spine II: Motion Palpation and Clinical Considerations of the Cervical and Thoracic Spine*. Huntington Beach, CA, Motion Palpation Institute, 1986, pp 10-15, 21-23.

Faye LJ: Motion Palpation: Spine 2, Cervicals and Thoracics [Cassette tape program]. Huntington Beach, CA, Motion Palpation Institute, 1986, 6 tapes.

Faye LJ, Weary B, Hooper P: *Motion Palpation and Clinical Considerations of the Upper Extremi-*

ties. Huntington Beach, CA, Motion Palpation Institute, 1986, p 30.

Gehweiler JA Jr, Osborne RL Jr, Becker RF: *The Radiology of Vertebrae Trauma.* Philadelphia, W.B. Saunders, 1980, pp 76-78, 259-373.

Gillet H, Liekens M: *Belgian Chiropractic Research Notes.* Huntington Beach, CA, Motion Palpation Institute, 1984, pp 7-8, 15, 18-19, 27-28, 43-46, 69, 78-81, 92, 106-107, 139-141.

Gonza ER, Harrington IJ: *Biomechanics of Musculoskeletal Injury.* Baltimore, Williams & Wilkins, 1982, p 202.

Grecco MA: *Chiropractic Technic Illustrated.* New York, Jarl, 1953.

Gregerson GG, Lucas DB: An in vivo study of axial rotation of the human thoracic-lumbar spine. *Journal of Bone and Joint Surgery,* 49A:247, 1967.

Grice AS: A biomechanical approach to cervical and dorsal adjusting. In Haldeman, S (ed): *Modern Developments in the Principles and Practice of Chiropractic.* New York, Appleton-Century-Crofts, 1980, pp 339-340, 351-352.

Grice AS, Fligg DB: Class notes. Department of Biomechanics/Kinesiology, BK202. Toronto, Canadian Memorial Chiropractic College, date not shown, pp 81-82.

Grice AS: Radiographic biomechanical and clinical factors in lumbar lateral flexion: part I. *Journal of Manipulative and Physiological Therapeutics,* 2(1): 26-34, March 1979.

Grieve GP: *Common Vertebral Joint Problems.* New York, Churchill-Livingstone, 1981, pp 10, 33, 47-48, 134, 235.

Hadley LA: *Anatomico-Roentgenographic Studies of the Spine,* ed 5. Springfield, IL, Charles C. Thomas, 1981, pp 36-37, 42-45.

Hilton RC, Bail J: A systematic pathological study of the dorsolumbar spine. *Journal of Rheumatology,* 9:95-96, 1983.

Hitchcock ME: Myofascial considerations in the thoracic area. *Osteopathic Medicine,* 85, December 1978.

Holmes GW, Robbins LL: *Roentgen Interpretation.* Philadelphia, Lea & Febiger, 1947, pp 111, 170.

Janse J: *Principles and Practice of Chiropractic.* Lombard, IL, National College of Chiropractic, 1976, pp 99, 105-109

Jirout J: Pattern of changes in the cervical spine in lateroflexion. *Neuroradiology,* 2:164, 1971.

Johnston WL: The role of static and motion palpation in structural diagnosis. In Goldstein M (ed), *The Research Status of Spinal Manipulative Therapy.* NINCDS Monograph No. 15, DHEW Publication No. (NIH) 76-998, Stock No. 017-049-00060-7, Washington, DC, U.S. Government Printing Office, 1975, pp 249-252.

Kapandji IA: *The Physiology of the Joints: The Trunk and the Vertebral Column,* ed 2. New York, Churchill Livingstone, 1974, vol III, pp 138, 146-150.

Krupp MA, Tierney LM Jr, Jawetz E, Roe RL, Camargo CA: *Physician's Handbook,* ed 21. Los Altos, CA, Lange Medical, 1985, pp 16-17.

Maurer EL: The thoraco-costal facet syndrome with introduction of the marginal line and the rib sign. *ACA Journal of Chiropractic,* X:S-158-159, December 1976.

McAndrews JF: Spinal motion examination. *ACA Journal of Chiropractic,* III:S-38, 39, May 1969.

McGall IW, Galvin E, O'Brien JP, Park WM: Alterations in vertebral growth following prolonged plaster immobilisation. *Acta Orthopaedica Scandinavica,* 52: 327-330, 1981.

McGee DJ: *Orthopedic Physical Assessment.* Philadelphia, W.B. Saunders, 1987, pp 142-169.

Miyasaka K, Kaneda K, Ito T: Ossification of spinal ligaments causing thoracic radiculomyelopathy. *Radiology,* 143:463-468, 1982.

Moore KL: *Clinically Oriented Anatomy.* Baltimore, Williams & Wilkins, 1980, pp 1, 4-12, 15-16, 18-28.

Morris JM: Biomechanics of the spine. *Archives of Surgery,* 107:418-423, 1973.

Ono M, Russell WJ, Kudo S, Yoshigoro K: Ossification of the thoracic posterior longitudinal ligament in a fixed population. *Radiology,* 143:469-474, 1982.

Orne D, Liu YK: A mathematical model of spinal response to impact. *Journal of Biomechanics,* 4:49-71, 1971.

Panjabi MM, et al: Mechanical properties of the human thoracic spine. *Journal of Bone and Joint Surgery,* 58A:642-651, 1976.

Panjabi MM, et al: Three dimensional flexibility and stiffness properties of the human thoracic spine. *Journal of Biomechanics,* 9:185-192, 1976.

Ponsetti IV, et al: Biomechanical analysis of intervertebral discs in idiopathic scoliosis. *Journal of Bone and Joint Surgery,* 54:1993, 1972; 56A, 1973.

Reinert OC: *Fundamentals of Chiropractic Techniques and Practice Procedures.* Chesterfield, MO, Marian Press, 1983, pp 84-87.

Riley JS: *Science and Practice of Chiropractic with Allied Sciences.* Place of publication not shown, published by author, 1925.

Roaf R: A study of the mechanics of spinal injuries. *Journal of Bone and Joint Surgery,* 42B:810-823, 1960.

Roaf R: Rotation movements of the spine with special reference to scoliosis. *Journal of Bone and Joint Surgery,* 40-B:312-332, 1958.

Rosse C, Clawson DK: *The Musculoskeletal System in Health and Disease.* New York, Harper & Row, 1980, pp 122-124, 129.

Salter RB: *Textbook of Disorders and Injuries of the Musculoskeletal System.* Baltimore, Williams & Wilkins, 1981, pp 117, 119-123, 279-281, 489, 496-498.

Schafer RC: *Chiropractic Health Care.* Des Moines, IA, Foundation for Chiropractic Education and Research, 1976, p 30.

Schafer RC: *Chiropractic Management of Sports and Recreational Injuries.* Baltimore, Williams & Wilkins, 1982, pp 271, 272, 420-425, 427.

Schafer RC: *Chiropractic Physical and Spinal Diagnosis.* Oklahoma City, Associated Chiropractic Academic Press, 1980, p X-26, 27, 29; XIII-25.

Schafer RC: *Clinical Biomechanics: Musculoskeletal Actions and Reactions.* Baltimore, Williams & Wilkins, 1983, pp 80, 193-194, 331, 334-335, 337-338, 367-370, 372-373, 397.

Schafer RC (ed): *Basic Chiropractic Procedural Manual,* ed 4. Des Moines, IA, American Chiropractic Association, 1984, pp 85, 92-93.

Schoenholtz F: Conservative management of costovertebral subluxation. *ACA Journal of Chiropractic,*

14:S-77-78, July 1980.

Shrader TL: Council on technic (column). *ACA Journal of Chiropractic*, p 90, December 1985.

Stierwalt DD: *Fundamentals of Motion Palpation.* Place of publication not shown, published by author, 1977, pp 18-24.

Stonebrink, RD: Palpation for vertebral motoricity. *ACA Journal of Chiropractic*, III:S-11-14, February 1969.

Sweere JJ: Type II round back deformity. *Orthopedic Brief*, ACA Council on Chiropractic Orthopedics, August 1985.

Teranel JA: *Chiropractic Orthopedics and Roentgenology.* Newark, NJ, Medusa Press, 1953, pp 107-108.

Turek SL: *Orthopaedics: Principles and Their Application*, ed 3. Philadelphia, J.B. Lippincott, 1977, pp 1358-1359, 1380-1381.

Van Dusen LG: *Chiropractic Relationship to Gravitational Force.* Sodus, NY, published by author, 1968, pp 71, 93, 105, 107.

Walters RL, Morris JM: An in vitro study of normal and scoliotic interspinous ligaments. *Journal of Biomechanics*, 6:343, 1973.

Weis EB Jr: Spinal geometry: Normal and abnormal. In Goldstein M (ed): *The Research Status of Spinal Manipulative Therapy.* NINCDS Monograph No. 15, DHEW Publication No. (NIH) 76-998, Stock No. 017-049-00060-7, Washington, DC, U.S. Government Printing Office, 1975.

Weitz EM: The lateral bending sign. *Spine*, 6:4, July-August, 1981.

White AA, Panjabi MM: Basic kinematics of the human spine. *Spine*, 3:1, March 1978.

White AA, Panjabi MM: *Clinical Biomechanics of the Spine.* Philadelphia, J.B. Lippincott, 1978, pp 74-78, 93, 166-179, 236-244, 250-251.

White AA, Panjabi MM: Spinal kinematics. In Goldstein M (ed): *The Research Status of Spinal Manipulative Therapy.* NINCDS Monograph No. 15, DHEW Publication No. (NIH) 76-998, Stock No. 017-049-00060-7, Washington, DC, U.S. Government Printing Office, 1975.

Winsberg F: Roentgenographic aspects of aging. In Rossman, I (ed): *Clinical Geriatrics.* Philadelphia, J.B. Lippincott, 1971, p 267.

Zuidema GD, et al: *The Management of Trauma*, ed 3. Philadelphia, W.B. Saunders, 1979, pp 12-13, 379-384, 610-616.

Chapter 5

The Lumbar Spine

This chapter describes the *dynamic chiropractic* approach to the correction of fixations of the lumbar spine and related tissues. Emphasis is on biomechanical, fixation, and therapeutic considerations. Some significant points in differential diagnosis are also described.

BASIC CONSIDERATIONS

Gillet's investigations found that the lumbar region is the only area of the spine (along with the lower thoracics) in which Lovett's principles are true. However, this will depend on the initial position of the vertebrae. If the region is in a lordosis (patient standing), lateral flexion produces maximum accompanying rotation. With the patient sitting and the lumbars in a "balanced medium" or even in kyphosis, the amount of rotation will be reduced to a minimum. This is an important point to remember in this chapter.

The Interview

Information gathering about the nature of patients' problems may begin as early as when they call for an appointment and attempt to describe their pain and its onset to the receptionist. Faye poses the following questions as the patient navigates around the office and he observes their ease of movement and posture: Is there difficulty straightening when rising from a chair? Can the patient sit down at all? Is he or she bent laterally to either side or to the anterior? Is there a limp or shuffle during gait? Does the patient's facial expression reflect pain? Is the patient's attitude cheerful or does it suggest obvious distress?

The interview should be conducted as quickly and efficiently as possible while still making sure that important details are covered. Listen to the patient's uninterrupted description of the chief complaints. Then, during the systems review, interview the patient in a manner designed to confirm or rule out probable diagnoses. Pertinent questions to be asked may be derived from the lists of characteristic findings of each of the syndromes discussed here and within standard differential diagnosis texts. The nerve function of the lumbosacral plexus is shown in Table 5.1.

According to Faye, the three most common types of low back pain are (1) the lumbar facet syndrome, (2) the sacroiliac syndrome, and (3) the lumbar radicular syndrome, which may be discogenic or biomechanical in origin. Each of these types can be acute or chronic, traumatic or nontraumatic, and have varying degrees of concomitant pathomechanics. The syndromes are named according to the level of inflammation or pain-producing structures and more than likely not the area in need of adjustments. Their typical cause may be due to sprain/strain, overuse, poor posture, disuse, joint dysfunction (fixation/hypermobility), development abnormality, degenerative changes, or various combinations of these origins. In addition, the possibility of viscerosomatic and somatosomatic reflexes should not be overlooked.

Applied Anatomical Considerations

Many of the abnormal orientations found in the lower spine can be because the facet

Table 5.1. Nerve Function of the Lumbosacral Plexus

Nerve	Function
Femoral	*Sensory* to skin over anterior and medial thigh, knee, leg, dorsum of foot to base of 1st metatarsal. *Motor* to iliacus, pectineus, sartorius, quadriceps femoris.
Genitofemoral	*Sensory* to skin over scrotum, upper anterior thigh area. *Motor* to the cremaster.
Iliohypogastric	*Sensory* to skin over hypogastric and lateral gluteal areas.
Ilioinguinal	*Sensory* to skin over genitalia and upper medial thigh area.
Inferior gluteal	*Motor* to gluteus maximus.
Lateral femoral cutaneous	*Sensory* to skin over lateral thigh.
Muscular branches	*Motor* to major and minor psoas, quadratus femoris, gemellus inferior and superior, piriformis, obturator internus.
Obturator	*Motor* to adductor longus, brevis, magnus; obturator externis; gracilis.
Posterior femoral cutaneous	*Sensory* to skin over inferior buttock, posterior thigh, popliteal space, perineum, external genitalia.
Pudendal	*Sensory* to skin of genitalia, anus, scrotum, labium major, penis, clitoris. *Motor* to levator ani, coccygeus, sphincter ani externus, transversus perinei superficialis, profundus, bulbocavernosus, ischiocavernosus, sphincter urethrae membranacae.
Sciatic	*Sensory* to skin over posterolateral aspect of leg and lateral foot; heel; over upper third of lateral aspect of leg below knee; over anterolateral aspect of leg and dorsum of foot and toes; medial aspect of sole, great toe, 2nd to 4th toes; lateral aspect of sole, 4th and 5th toes; on dorsum of foot between great toe and 2nd toe. *Motor* to hamstrings, adductor magnus, gastrocnemius, plantaris, soleus, popliteus, tibialis anterior and posterior, flexor and extensor digitorum longus and brevis; peroneus longus, brevis, and tertius; abductor and adductor hallucis, flexor hallucis brevis, extensor hallucis longus, quadratus plantae, abductor digiti quinti brevis, all interossei, and 1st through 4th lumbricals.
Superior gluteal	*Motor* to gluteus minimus and medius, tensor fascia lata.

joints of the lumbar spine are not determined until the secondary curves are firmly developed in the erect position. The stresses imposed during the development stage can easily lead to the high incidence of asymmetry.

The Lumbar Vertebrae

Because vertebral segments increase in size and strength progressing caudally to sustain increasing weight load, the lumbar vertebra are relatively large (Fig. 5.1). The centra are kidney shaped, larger in width than from front to back, and thicker anteriorly (except L2). A line crossing horizontally at the uppermost aspect of the iliac crests normally cuts the body of L4.

Each lumbar vertebra exhibits strong stout laminae, pedicles, and spinous processes that project directly backward on a horizontal plane (Fig. 5.2). The transverse processes, which arise at the junction of the pedicles and laminae, project laterally and slightly backwards and increase in length progressing caudally. The neural ring is triangular, and the vertebral canal is larger than that of the thoracic spine but smaller than that of the cervical spine.

Lumbar articular processes are especially strong. Because the inferior articular processes face laterally and slightly anteriorly and the superior processes face medially and

slightly posteriorly, rotatory ROM is somewhat restricted. Mamillary processes (rounded tubercles) project from the posterosuperior border of each superior articular process (Fig. 5.3).

L5 differs from its neighbors above in that its centrum has the largest circumference and is thinner in height, its superior facets face more posteriorly, its inferior facets face more anteriorly, and it has a short rounded spinous process. While the entire lumbar spine is encased in strong ligaments that may shorten, the iliolumbar ligaments are especially vulnerable to the stress of daily living and degenerative changes, sometimes to the point of firmly anchoring L5 to the ilium and/or sacrum, unilaterally or bilaterally.

Lumbar Intervertebral Foramina

All vertebrae normally move in the planes of their articulations, and it is at the zygapophyses that most fixations and subluxation complexes seem to originate to influence the integrity of the related IVFs. Changes in the diameter of normal IVFs are both the result and the cause of abnormal joint function that predisposes further kinetic disturbances. These disturbances tend to alter the curves of the particular region of the spine in which the structural-functional defect is found. The lumbar region is no exception.

In the lumbar region, the IVFs are shaped like a kidney bean. It requires considerable posterolateral disc protrusion to encroach the nerve exiting at the same level because

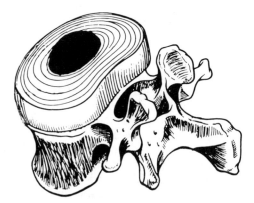

Figure 5.1. Drawing of a lumbar vertebra (superior oblique view) showing its superior disc. The nucleus pulposus is shown in black, surrounded by the rings of the anulus (Courtesy ACAP).

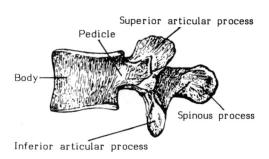

Figure 5.2. Lateral view of an L2 vertebra (Courtesy ACAP).

the lumbar IVFs are comparatively large in this area of the spine. When disc protrusion does cause trouble, it is usually from encroachment on the laterally placed nerve root on the vertebra above.

Sunderland emphasizes that the passage of the medial branch of the lumbar dorsal ramus and its accompanying vessels through the osseofibrous tunnel and the intimate relationship of the neurovascular bundle to the capsule of the apophyseal joint represents a potential site of fixation and entrapment following pathologic changes involving the joint.

The Nerve Roots

The segmental innervation of the lumbosacral spine supplying the major associated muscles and the related skin and tendon reflexes are shown in Table 5.2.

There are about twice as many sensory fibers than motor fibers in the lumbar roots.

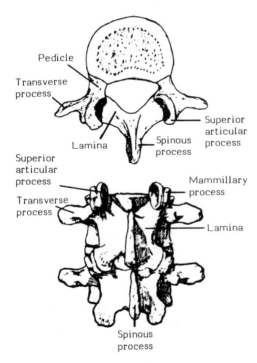

Figure 5.3. A midlumbar vertebra as viewed from above, top drawing, and behind, bottom drawing (Courtesy ACAP).

When the anterior nerve root is irritated, pain is felt in the peripheral distribution of the fibers affected and the pain often becomes self-perpetuating from the focal spasm produced. When the posterior root is irritated, the pain can be perceived to be in the dermatome, myotome, sclerotome, or possibly the viscerotome.

Planes of Articulation in the Lumbar Spine (Normal and Abnormal)

Lumbar facets have moderately sloped surfaces rather than a single-plane angle as seen in the cervical and thoracic area, and they are near parallel to the vertical plane. The convex inferior facets mate with concave superior facets. From L1 to L5, the plane of the articular facets generally change from mediolateral to anteroposterior and lie in the sagittal plane.

The lumbosacral facet planes are slightly more horizontal than those above and allow greater A-P, P-A, and lateral motion but less joint locking as compared to the vertebrae above. This horizontal and anterior inclination of L5, spreading out toward the coronal plane, becomes progressively more vertical upward from L4 to L1.

An important influence on interspinal posture is that of the facet facing of each posterior intervertebral joint, with alterations of the facings most commonly occurring in the lumbar and lower cervical regions. These facings are more frequently altered between L4 and L5 than at any other level in the vertebral column.

Symmetric facets glide with little friction produced. If the facets deviate in their direction of movement, however, the unparallel articulating surfaces "scrub" upon one another, which leads to degenerative changes. Variances of the articular structures often occur even in the absence of injury at the level of abnormality. They are characterized by thickening of the covering of the facet and marginal sclerosis. This hardening process is usually followed by hypertrophy or exostosis that produces an irregular articular surface when the facet is viewed in profile in roentgenography. Coexistent with this finding, the interarticular spaces gradually become narrowed, hazy, obscured, and even obliterated on x-ray films.

Because these various facet and interarticular manifestations are from either chronic abnormal weight-bearing or specific trauma, the term *arthrosis* is often used today rather than the phrase *posterior intervertebral osteoarthritis.* Arthrosis is a more reasonable descriptor because of the implications of the suffix "itis." Although there may not be evidence of direct bony encroachment from the process of arthrosis directly into the IVFs, one must consider that the process of arthrosis *does* produce a general narrowing of the diameters of the IVFs and hence can predispose interference with the normal expression of nerve impulse and axoplasmic flow transmission.

When the spine is in good postural balance, facet articulation offers minimal friction. In scoliosis, the articular surfaces are no longer parallel and the result is articular friction leading to erosion, arthrosis, and impingement. This is the result of normally reciprocal articulating surfaces operating in an abnormal relationship.

Biomechanical Considerations

From the middle of the anterior surface of T12, the body's gravity line extends downward to the anterior aspect of the sacral base. Weight distribution in the lumbar region is governed chiefly by the inclination of each vertebral body. The lumbosacral articulations are slightly more horizontal than those above them, allowing for greater P-A and lateral motion and offering less joint locking during extension as compared to the vertebrae above.

The horizontal inclination of L5, spreading out toward the coronal plane, becomes progressively more vertical from L4 to L1 as the dorsolumbar articulation is approached. These changes in articular planes allow the

Table 5.2. Segmental Innervation of the Lumbosacral Spine

Segment	Major Muscles Supplied
L1—L2	Cremaster
L1—L5	Iliopsoas
L2—L3	Sartorius, pectineus, abductor longus
L2—L4	Quadriceps, gracilis, adductor brevis
L3—L4	Obturator externus, adductor magnus and minimus
L4—L5	Tibialis anticus
L4—S1	Semimembranosus, semitendinosus, extensor hallucis longus, popliteus, plantaris, extensor digitorum longus, extensor hallucis brevis, gluteus medius and minimus, quadratus
L5—S1	Peroneus longus and brevis, tibialis posticus, flexor digiti brevis, abductor hallucis
L5—S2	Gluteus maximus, obturator internus, biceps femoris, soleus, gastrocnemius, flexor hallucis longus
S1—S2	Lumbricales, piriformis, abductor digiti, flexor digiti, opponens, quadratus plantae, interossei
S2—S4	Levator ani, bulbocavernosus, ischiocavernosus
S4—S5	Sphincter vesicae
S5—Cx1	Sphincter ani, coccygeus

Segment	Skin Reflexes	Segment	Tendon Reflexes
L1—L2	Cremasteric	L2—L4	Patellar
L4—S1	Gluteal	S1—S2	Achilles
S1—S2	Plantar		
S5—Cx1	Anal		

lower back to bend and twist to accommodate gravitational force during movement. The upper lumbar joints are J-shaped when viewed from the lateral, thus their anterior aspect resists forward displacement.

The lateral center line of gravity falls on different points in the lumbar spine because of gradual changes in the angles of the inclined planes of the various articular surfaces. This tends to force each lumbar segment more inferior, medial, and anterior or posterior until gravity brings the apex of the curve back toward the balancing point. The lateral line of gravity in the pelvic area passes just anteriorly to the S2 segment.

Except for the lesser role of the pelvic basin, superimposed body weight is carried in the lower back essentially by the L5 disc and then dispersed to the sacral base, sacroiliac joints, and acetabulae. This burden on the L5 disc is forced slightly forward on the load-bearing surfaces. Defective weight bearing is usually caused by some impairment in the anterior portion of the vertebral motion unit (eg, disc deficit, anterior ligament fixation). In contrast, faults in the direction of distortions can usually be attributed to the posterior aspect of the motion unit; eg, total or partial fixations involving the apophyseal joints, pillar erosion and distortion, osseous pathology, etc. The anterior portion of the motion unit is mechanically designed for weight bearing, the posterior pillars are not. Thus, when the pillars are forced to assume the constant role of weight bearing because of some biomechanical fault altering spinal equilibrium and the distribution of load (intrinsic or extrinsic), structural failure and compensatory remodeling of the posterior elements is likely to occur eventually.

Kinematics of the Lumbar Spine

In the absence of fixation, the range of gross lumbar motion is primarily determined by the sum of individual IVD resistance to distortion, the thickness of the discs, and the angle and size of the articular surfaces.

As in other regions of the spine, the movements of the lumbar spine are flexion, extension, lateral bending, and rotation. While lumbar motion is potentially greater than

that of the thoracic spine because of the lack of rib restriction, facet facing and heavy ligaments check the range of rotatory motion.

A patient may be observed who replaces normal lumbar motion with exaggerated hip motion, or vice versa. If so, the ranges of motions of the restricted lumbar or hip joints should be tested. Any disorder of the hip joint itself (eg, fracture, tuberculosis, osteoarthritis, fixation) or of the hip flexor, adductor, abductor, or extensor muscles may result in limited hip motion. Compensation of hip deficits will be attempted at the nearest movable segment(s) such as the sacroiliacs, lumbars, knees, and/or ankles.

Muscle Weakness That May Affect Lumbar Function

The trunk is held erect by the flexors and extensors of the spine and the extensors of the hip. The muscles and ligaments that hold the trunk erect are much stronger as a whole

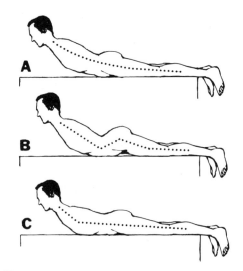

Figure 5.4. A, if both the back extensors and the hip extensors are strong, the patient will smoothly coordinate hip extension with spinal extension. B, if the spinal extensors are strong but the hip extensors are weak, the patient will hyperextend the trunk but the pelvis will fail to rotate posteriorly. C, if the spinal extensors are weak but the hip extensors are strong, the trunk will fail to arch but the pelvis will rotate posteriorly (Courtesy ACAP).

than those of the pelvis. After a long illness, for example, a patient can sit erect long before he can stand.

Extension. Because P-A trunk motions are the most common movements used in daily living and as flexion is assisted by gravity, the spinal extensors are the most important muscles of the trunk from a biomechanical viewpoint. Muscles of the back are rarely weak unless paralysis is present. Kendall places the incidence of weak spinal erectors at less than 1% in the nonparalytic. When signs of extension weakness are evident, differentiation must be made between weak spinal extensors and weak hip extensors. A screening test can easily be done with the patient prone (Fig. 5.4).

Lateral Flexion. Trunk raising from the lateral recumbent position exhibits the strength of trunk lateral flexors and hip abductors. A simple screening test to differentiate weakness in these groups is shown in Figure 5.5.

Flexion. Leg raising from the supine position is a two-phase combination between strong abdominals and strong hip flexors. A screen test to differentiate weakness of the two groups is shown in Figure 5.6.

Muscle Shortening That May Affect Lumbar Function

The postural patterns exhibited in forward flexion from the supine position can offer distinct clues to shortening of specific muscles and muscle combinations. Six typ-

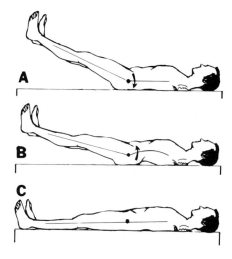

Figure 5.6. Slow leg raising and lowering in the supine position evaluates the strength of the abdominals and hip flexors. A, if the abdominals and hip flexors are both strong, leg raising and lowering can be accomplished by the patient consciously rotating the pelvis backward so that the lumbar spine is kept flat on the table. B, if the abdominals are weak but the hip flexors are strong, the lumbar spine will arch acutely into hyperlordosis at the higher degrees, the pelvis will rotate anteriorly, and the abdominals will stretch, increasing the sternal-pubic distance. C, if the abdominals are strong but the hip flexors are weak, the patient will be unable to lift the extremities from the table but there will be strong abdominal contraction that tends to decrease the sternal-pubic distance (Courtesy ACAP).

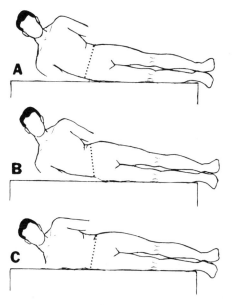

Figure 5.5. A, if both the flank muscles and the hip abductors are strong, the patient will smoothly coordinate trunk and hip lateral flexion. B, if the flank muscles are strong but the hip abductors are weak, the upper shoulder will flex and the upper pelvis not fixed by body weight will tend to move cephalad, reducing the rib-ilium distance. C, if the flank muscles are weak but the hip abductors are strong, the upper shoulder will fail to move much but the pelvis will tend to move caudad, increasing the rib-ilium distance (Courtesy ACAP).

ical patterns are shown in Figures 5.7 and 5.8.

Motion at the Thoracolumbar Transitional Area

Descriptions of normal articular angles in any text are approximations. There is considerable variation from one person to another and of the transitional segment between one region of the spine and another. For example, the transitional vertebra between the thoracic and lumbar regions is usually given as T12, but it might be any vertebra from T9—L1 according to White/ Panjabi.

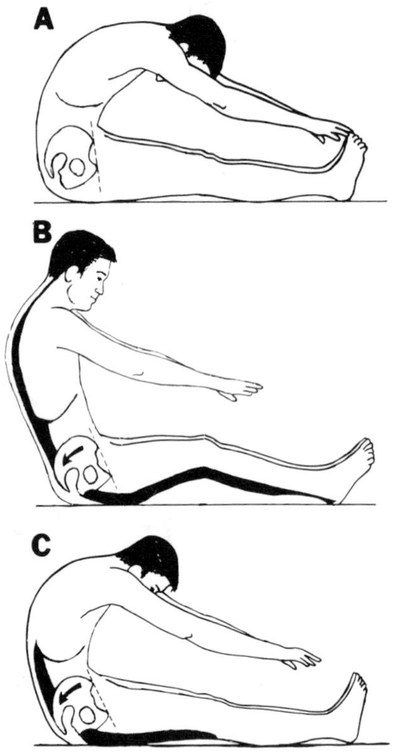

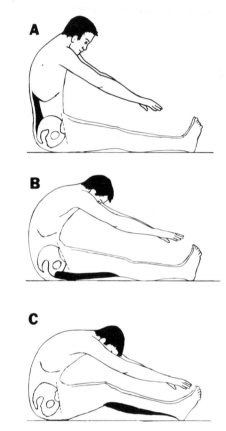

Figure 5.7. Testing length of some posterior muscle combinations. A, if the posterior spinal, thigh, and calf muscles have not shortened, forward flexion from the sitting position will produce a smoothly curve spine with little if any movement of the pelvis or knees. B, if the posterior muscles of the spine, thigh, and calf muscles have all shortened, forward flexion will be extremely limited, the pelvis will rotate posteriorly, and the knees will flex. C, if the lower back and hamstrings are moderately tight but the upper spinal and calf muscles are not shortened, flexion will be restricted with the upper thoracic region arching smoothly, the lumbar region flattening, and the pelvis rotating posteriorly, but the knees will remain flat on the table (Courtesy ACAP).

Figure 5.8. More tests for posterior muscle shortening combinations. A, if the posterior lower back muscles are severely shortened but the upper thoracic, hamstrings, and calf muscles are flexible, flexion will be restricted with the lumbar region holding some lordosis but the pelvis and knees remaining stable. B, if the hamstrings are shortened but the spinal and calf muscles are flexible, flexion will be restricted with the pelvis rotating posteriorly. The spine will curve smoothly and the knees will remain extended. C, if the calf muscles have shortened but the spinal and posterior thigh muscles are flexible, the spine will curve smoothly, the pelvis will remain stable, but the knees will flex (Courtesy ACAP).

Owing to the restricted movements in the thoracic spine as the result of the attached thoracic cage and the mobile lumbar spine in flexion below, the intervening thoracolumbar area must achieve a degree of hypermobility in all three body planes. Because of this, as is true to some extent in all spinal transitional areas, the thoracolumbar junction is more prone to overstress from both above and below because of its unusual role.

The superior facets of the transitional vertebra resemble thoracic facets and are designed primarily for rotation and lateral flexion, even though these motions are restricted somewhat by the free ribs. While the stiff thoracic spine tends to move as a whole, most rotation takes place in the lower segments that are not restricted by the rib cage. The inferior facets of the transitional vertebra are of the lumbar type; ie, designed more for flexion and extension. Although great curves can be observed in the lumbar area, most of the apparent rotation seen is from distortion of the lumbar spine's base, vertebral and pelvic tipping, and the lumbar lordosis viewed out of its normal plane (planar displacement or malposition).

Lumbar Lateral Bending

In the lumbar spine as a whole, lateral flexion is relatively free, followed in order of mobility by extension, flexion, and minimal rotation. Significant to gross movements in the lumbar spine is the fact that all movements are to some degree three dimensional; ie, when the lumbar spine bends laterally, it tends to also rotate posteriorly on the side of convexity and assume a hyperlordotic tendency. Thus, *fixation effects are also coupled.*

During lateral bending in the erect position, considerable rotation accompanies the abduction of the trunk if there is a significant degree of lordosis. However, if the lumbar spine is flattened or if the lateral bending is performed in the sitting position, the amount of associated rotation is minimal but enough to be determined by Grice on kinematic stress films.

The intertransverse spaces of the normal spine open on the convex side and close on the concave side during lateral bending. In

normal extension and distinct lordosis, however, the facets jam and lateral flexion is so restricted that the vertebrae must severely rotate to allow lateral flexion.

Lumbar Flexion

During lumbar flexion and extension, there is considerably less facet gliding than seen in other areas of the spine during such motions. Widening of the anterior disc space

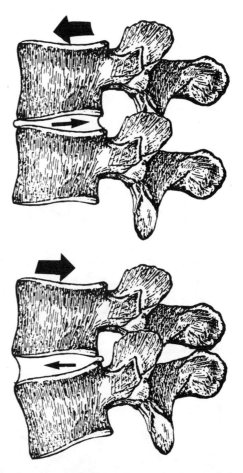

Figure 5.9. The hydraulic mechanisms of the IVD. During normal flexion (top), the anterior anulus bulges anteriorly from compression and the posterior aspect of the anulus stretches from the tensile load. The nucleus follows the linear action by shifting slightly posteriorly but bulges and contracts in opposite directions to those of the anulus. During normal extension (bottom), the opposite mechanisms occur (Courtesy ACAP).

on extension or of the posterior disc space on flexion does not occur until movement *nears its full range of motion*. Even then, it is far less than that seen in other areas of the spine. See Figure 5.9.

The anterior longitudinal ligaments relax during flexion, and the supraspinal and interspinal ligaments stretch. Opposite effects occur during extension. Although many disorders result in decreased flexion, paraspinal muscle spasm and total fixations are the primary suspects. [See Clinical Comment 5.1]

Lumbar Extension

Gillet's studies found that lumbar flexion-extension movements are similar to those of other regions of the spine but with less forward or backward gliding. Extension is, states Gillet, also a movement that takes place in two parts with the anterior inter-

body space opening only after backward bending has reached its limit. This opening anteriorly is, however, a smaller movement than that which occurs in other regions of the spine.

The extent of lumbar extension is primarily controlled by the tautness of the anterior longitudinal ligament, the elasticity of the posterior ligaments, and the tonicity of rectus abdominis anteriorly and the spinal extensor muscles posteriorly. See Figure 5.10. In IVD herniation posteriorly, facet inflammation, or spondylolisthesis, pain will be increased during extension but not on flexion. This is a helpful point in differential diagnosis.

According to McKenzie, reduced lumbar extension is frequently the result of poor sitting posture and/or inadequate extension mobilization following injury in which scar tissue prevents a full range of extension. Reduced extension (1) causes chronic stress on the soft tissues of the posterior motion unit

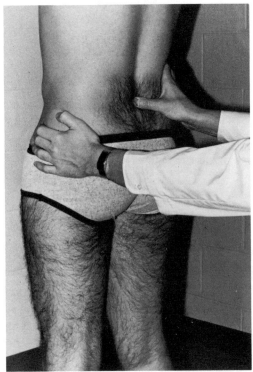 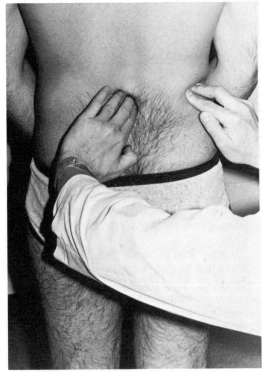

Figure 5.10. *Left,* locating the L4—L5 interspinous space, which normally lies on the same level as a line drawn across the tops of the iliac crests. *Right,* static palpation of the integrity of the midlumbar supraspinous and interspinous ligaments (Courtesy ACAP).

and an increased intradiscal pressure during sitting; (2) restricts a fully upright posture during relaxed standing, leading to a stooped appearance in stance and gait; and (3) produces a *premature* fully stretched lumbar posture when arising from a forward flexed posture.

Keep in mind that the fibers of the posterior anulus are the weakest. The anterior and lateral aspects of the anulus are almost twice as thick as the posterior aspect. The anular fibers at the posterior aspect of the disc are less numerous, narrower, and more parallel to each other than at any other portion of a disc.

If a person must work habitually in a prolonged forward flexed position, periodic lumbar extension will relieve the stress of the posterior anulus and tend to shift a loose nucleus pulposus anteriorly; ie, away from the spinal cord and IVF. Many manual laborers do this stretching maneuver instinctively.

Lumbar Rotation

Only slight rotational fixation is necessary to affect P-A, A-P, and lateral bending motions. Because the facial planes are no longer reciprocal when a fixation exists, normal motion is restricted and sets up dyskinesia.

If the axis of rotation of lumbar vertebrae were at the tips of the spinous processes, as sometimes is taught, the spinous process of L1 would be directly in line with the spinous process of L5 during rotation while the vertebral bodies rotate to a greater degree towards the direction of movement. But because the center of rotation of T12 is distinctly anterior, it must pull L1 with it during rotation. This pulls the lumbars into rotation and flexion, jamming the facets on the side moving posteriorly and opening the facets on the side swinging anteriorly. This effect in the lumbar spine continues caudally to the sacrum, which also flexes and rotates with the lumbars.

Segmental Stability and Instability

It is obvious that each spinal segment rests on the one beneath it and that the interposed joint surfaces serve as the support base of the separate segments. The force of gravity acting on each segment must be individually neutralized if the body as a whole is to be in complete gravitational balance.

Joint stability normally depends on (1) the size of the joint surfaces, (2) the height of the segmental centers of gravity above the joint surface, (3) the horizontal distance of the common gravity line to the joint's center, and (4) the integrity of the supporting ligaments. While these facts are true in all areas of the spine, their importance are increased in the lumbar spine because of the increased weight load.

In the adult lumbar spine, the interspinous and supraspinous ligaments play a lesser role in segmental stability than they do in upper regions. White/Panjabi report that these ligaments are frequently absent, degenerated, or ruptured.

The lumbars normally tend to remain stable during gait, according to Illi, Gowitzke, and LeVeau. See Figure 5.11.

The Role of Ligaments in Static Balance

When standing upright, the normal tendency is to rest on the axial joints and ligaments. There is only light and intermittent muscular activity. As ligament support does

---

DR. FAYE'S CLINICAL COMMENT #5.1

In chronic low-back pain cases, it is important to take a series of lateral lumbar radiographs: neutral, forward flexion, and backward flexion positions. An unstable motion unit will appear to be normal in the neutral view but demonstrate antero- or postero-listhesis in stress films. This sign makes for a worse prognosis and the possible necessity for spinal fusion if disc degeneration is advanced or if correcting the etiological dysfunction does not cause a tightening of the ligaments involved. I x-ray again after 4—6 months of symptom relief. Continual severely painful episodes should suggest an orthopedic consultation.

not consume much energy, it does not contribute to fatigue. Chronic ligament tension, however, must be intermittently relieved by muscle activity and position changes to avoid chronic sprain leading to ligamentous fixation.

The primary ligaments involved in static balance are the lumbar anterior longitudinal ligament, which restricts lumbar "sinking"; the iliofemoral Y ligaments at the anterior hip, which guard hip hyperextension; the tensor fasciae latae of the thigh, which assist the Y ligaments, restrict lateral sway, and help the knees to lock; and the posterior knee ligaments, which lock the knees in extension. The ankles cannot be locked, thus they require slight intermittent contraction of the leg muscles.

Several authorities report that the key to lumbar ligament stability is the angle of the pelvis. Lateral pelvic tilting from a unilateral short leg, for example, is accompanied by load shifting to the lowered hip and pelvic rotation that unlocks the weight-bearing joints of the lower extremities. The lumbar spine will not bend laterally without some rotation. This change in equilibrium forces imposes increased muscular effort to maintain balance that, in turn, leads to chronic fatigue and eventual articular degeneration and fixation.

DIAGNOSTIC CONSIDERATIONS

Significant Neurologic and Orthopedic Tests

Evaluating vital signs and such procedures as light touch/pain tests, muscle

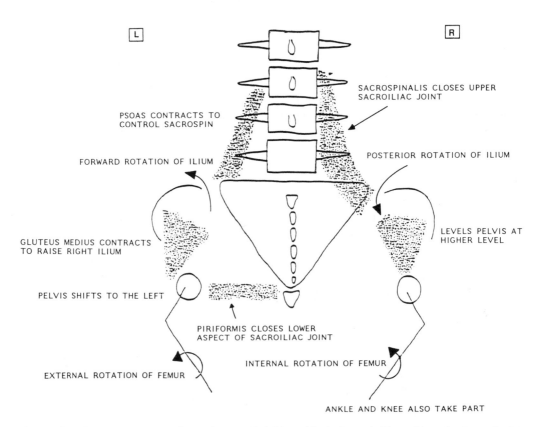

Figure 5.11. The lumbars normally tend to remain fairly stable during gait. The schematic above depicts some primary lumbopelvic actions when the right foot steps forward.

strength grading, range of gross motion tests, inspection, and static palpation are so standard within chiropractic physical examinations that there is no need to describe them here. This is also true for the evaluation of reflexes pertinent to low-back syndromes such as Achilles, adductor, anal, ankle clonus, Babinski's plantar, cremasteric, Giegel's, hamstring, patella, patella clonus, and quadriceps reflexes, as well as Jendrassik's maneuver, Valsalva's maneuver, and Adams' sign. Besides these standard procedures, the following orthopedic and neurologic tests are helpful in the differential diagnosis of lumbar syndromes.

Beery's Sign. This sign is positive if a patient with a history of lower trunk discomfort and fatigue is fairly comfortable when sitting with the knees flexed but experiences discomfort in the standing position. It is typically seen in spasticity or contractures of the posterior thigh and/or leg muscles.

Bragard's Test. If Lasegue's SLR test is positive at a given point, the leg is lowered below this point and dorsiflexion of the foot is induced. The sign is negative if pain is not increased. A positive sign is a finding in sciatic neuritis, spinal cord tumors, IVD lesions, and spinal nerve irritations. A negative sign points to muscular involvement such as tight hamstrings. Bragard's test does not stress the sacroiliac or lumbosacral articulations and is therefore negative in facet and sacroiliac syndromes.

Dejerine's Sign. This sign constitutes aggravated symptoms of radiculitis, resulting from a space-occupying lesion within the spinal cord, during any Valsalva maneuver (eg, coughing, sneezing, abdominal straining) that would increase intrathecal pressure.

Demianoff's Test. This is a variant of Lasegue's SLR test used by many in lumbago and IVF funiculitis with the intent of differentiating between lumbago and sciatica. When the affected limb is first extended and then flexed at the hip, the corresponding half of the body becomes lowered and with it the muscle fibers fixed to the lumbosacral segment. This act, which stretches the muscles, can induce sharp lumbar pain. Lasegue's sign is thus negative as the pain is caused by stretching the affected muscles at the posterior portion of the pelvis rather than stretching the sciatic nerve. To accomplish this test with the patient supine, the pelvis is fixed by the examiner's hand firmly placed on the ASIS, and the other hand elevates the leg on the same side. No pain results when the leg is raised to an 80° angle. When lumbago and sciatica are coexistent, Demianoff's sign is negative on the affected side but positive on the opposite side unless the pelvis is fixed. The sign is also negative in bilateral sciatica with lumbago. The fixation of the pelvis prevents stretching the sciatic nerve, and any undue pain experienced is usually associated with ischiotrochanteric groove adhesions or soft-tissue shortening.

Deyelle-May Test. This test may be helpful in differentiating the various etiologies of sciatic pain and is particularly designed to differentiate between pain from pressure on the nerve or its roots and pain produced by other mechanisms in the lower back. Compression or tractional pressure on muscles, ligaments, tendons, or bursae may cause reflex pain that often mimics true direct nerve irritation. Reflex pain does not usually follow the pattern of a specific nerve root, is more vague, does not cause sensory disturbances in the skin, comes and goes, but may be an extremely intense ache. The procedure in the sitting position is to instruct the patient to sit still and braced by the hands in a chair. The painful leg is passively extended until it causes pain, then lowered just below this point. The leg is then held by the examiner's knees and deep palpation is applied to the sciatic nerve high in the popliteal space that has been made taut (bow string) by the maneuver. Severe pain on palpation suggests a definite sciatic syndrome as opposed to other causes of back and leg pain such as the stretching of strained muscles and tendons or the movements of sprained sublumbar articulations.

Double-Leg Raise Test. This is a two-phase test: (1) The patient is placed supine, and a straight-leg-raising test is performed on each limb: first on one side, and then on the other. (2) The SLR test is then performed on both limbs simultaneously; ie, a bilateral SLR test. If pain occurs at a lower angle when both legs are raised together than when performing the monolateral SLR maneuver, the test is considered positive for a lumbo-sacral area lesion.

Ely's Test. To support iliopsoas spasm suspicions, the patient is placed prone with the toes hanging over the edge of the table, legs relaxed. Either heel is approximated to the opposite buttock. After flexion of the knee, hip pain makes it impossible to perform the test if there is inflammation of the psoas muscle or its sheath. The buttock will tend to rise on the involved side. However, a positive Ely's test can also suggest rectus femoris contraction, a lumbar lesion, a contracture of the tensor fascia lata, or an osseous hip lesion.

Fajersztajn's Test. When straight-leg raising and dorsiflexion of the foot are performed on the asymptomatic side of a sciatic patient and this produces pain on the symptomatic side, there is a positive Fajersztajn's sign, which strongly suggests a sciatic nerve root involvement such as a disc syndrome, dural root sleeve adhesions, or some other space-occupying lesion. This is sometimes called the *well-leg* or *cross-leg straight-leg-raising* test. From a biomechanical viewpoint, this test would be suggestive but not indicative.

Gaenslen's Test. In this test, the patient is placed supine with knees, thighs, and legs acutely flexed by the patient who clasps his knees with both hands and pulls them toward the abdomen. This brings the lumbar spine firmly in contact with the table and fixes both the pelvis and lumbar spine. With the examiner standing at right angles to the patient, the patient is brought well to the side of the table and the examiner slowly hyperextends the opposite thigh by gradually increasing force by pressure of one hand on top of the patient's knee while the examiner's other hand is on the patient's flexed knee for support in fixing the lumbar spine and pelvis. Some examiners allow the hyperextended limb to fall from the table edge. The hyperextension of the hip exerts a rotating force on the corresponding half of the pelvis. The pull is made on the ilium through the Y ligament and the muscles attached to the AIISs. The test is positive if the thigh is hyperextended and pain is felt in the area of the sacroiliac joint or referred down the thigh, providing that the opposite sacroiliac

joint is normal and the sacrum moves as a unit with the side of the pelvis opposite to that being tested. The test should be conducted bilaterally. A positive sign may be elicited in a sacroiliac, hip, or lower lumbar nerve root lesion. If the L4 nerve is involved, pain is usually referred anteriorly to the groin or upper thigh. If the sign is negative, a lumbosacral lesion should be first suspected. This test is usually contraindicated in the elderly.

Goldthwait's Test. The patient is placed supine. The examiner places one hand under the lumbar spine with each fingerpad pressed firmly against the interspinous spaces. The other hand of the examiner slowly performs an SLR test. If pain occurs or is aggravated before the lumbar processes open (0°—30°), a disc or sacroiliac lesion should be suspected. Goldthwait believed that if pain occurred while the processes were opening at 30°—60°, a lumbosacral lesion was suggested; at 60°—90°, an L1—L4 disc lesion. If pain is brought on before the lumbar spine begins to move, a lesion, either arthritic or a sprain involving the sacroiliac joint, is probably present. If pain does not come on until after the lumbar spine begins to move, the disorder is more likely to have its site in the lumbosacral area or less commonly in the sacroiliac areas. The test should be repeated with the unaffected limb. A positive sign of a lumbosacral lesion is elicited if pain occurs near the same height as it did with the first limb. If the unaffected limb can be raised higher than the affected limb, it is thought to be significant of sacroiliac involvement of the affected side. White/Panjabi, however, dispute such specific indications in orthopedic maneuvers as this. There are too many variables.

Kemp's Test. While in a seated position, the patient is supported by the examiner who reaches around the patient's shoulders and upper chest from behind. The patient is directed to lean forward to one side and then around to eventually bend obliquely backward by placing the palm on the buttock and sliding it down the back of the thigh and leg as far as possible. The maneuver is similar to that used in oblique cervical compression tests. If this compression causes or aggravates a pattern of radicular pain in the thigh and leg, the sign is positive and suggests nerve root compression. It may also suggest a strain or sprain and thus be present when the patient leans obliquely forward or at any point in motion. Not to be dismissed lightly would be the possibility of shortened contralateral paraspinal ligaments and tendons that would force erratic motion on the side of lateral flexion. [See Clinical Comment 5.2]

Lasegue's Rebound Test. At the conclusion of a positive sign during Lasegue's supine SLR test, the examiner allows the limb to drop to a pillow without warning. If this rebound test causes a marked increase in pain and muscle spasm, then a disc involvement is said to be suspect. However, it would appear that any site of irritation in the lower back and pelvis would be aggravated by such a maneuver.

Lasegue's Standing Test. The patient attempts to touch the floor with the fingers while the knees are held in extension during the standing position. Under these conditions, the knee of the affected side will flex, the heel will slightly elevate, and the body will elevate more or less to the painful side. It should be noted that this would also be true with shortened posterior thigh and calf muscles.

Lasegue's Straight-Leg-Raising (SLR) Test. The patient lies supine with legs extended. The examiner places one hand under the heel of the affected side and the other hand is placed on the knee to prevent the knee from bending. With the limb extended, the examiner most cautiously flexes the thigh on the pelvis to the point of pain, keeping the knee straight. The patient will normally be able to have the limb extended to almost 90° without pain. If this maneuver is markedly limited by pain, the test is positive and suggests sciatica from a disc lesion, lumbosacral or sacroiliac lesion, subluxation syndrome, tight hamstring, spondylolisthetic adhesion, IVF occlusion, or a similar disorder.

Lewin-Gaenslen Test. The patient is placed in the lateral recumbent position with the underneath lower limb flexed acutely at the hip and knee. The examiner stabilizes the uppermost hip with one hand. With the other hand, the uppermost leg is grasped near the knee and the thigh is extended on the hip. Initiated or aggravated pain suggests a sacroiliac lesion. [See Clinical Comment 5.3]

Lewin's Standing Test. With the patient standing with the back to the examiner, the examiner cautiously forces first the right and then the left knee into complete extension. Then both knees are straightened at the same time. In lumbosacral, lower lumbar, sacroiliac, and gluteal disturbances, these movements will be accompanied by increased pain and the knee will snap back into flexion.

Lewin's Supine Test. Lewin believes a positive sign in this test indicates an ankylosing dorsolumbar lesion. With the patient supine, the examiner places his arms or a strap across the patient's thighs just above the knees. The patient is directed to sit up straight without using the hands. The sign is positive if the patient is unable to do this maneuver, and during the attempt, the patient is frequently able to localize the site of pain. It is frequently associated with lumbar arthritis, lumbar fibrosis, degenerative disc

DR. FAYE'S CLINICAL COMMENT #5.2

Mennell teaches a modified Kemp's maneuver that is helpful: The sitting patient leans backward against the doctor and rotates his trunk posteriorly to the point of low-back pain and/or radiation of pain to a buttock and leg. The doctor then reaches around to the opposite side and pulls the patient's ASIS posteriorly to ease the contralateral pressure on the sacroiliac joint. Pain relief confirms a sacroiliac lesion. If no relief occurs, suspicion of a lumbar facet lesion is confirmed.

DR. FAYE'S CLINICAL COMMENT #5.3

Grice teaches that if the hip is flexed as far as possible and the leg is not held straight, one can test for iliopsoas and quadriceps shortening. If the iliopsoas is shortened, the patient's thigh will raise and the heel will not raise from the table. If the quadricep group has shortened, the patient's lower leg will raise from the table. This test plus hamstring tests are important in assessing causes of low-back pathodynamics.

thinning with protrusion, sacroiliac or lumbosacral arthritis, or sciatica.

Lindner's Test. The patient is placed supine, and the examiner slowly flexes the patient's head forward so that the neck and thoracic spine curve forward. This test often helps to localize diffuse spinal pain. This is the passive form of *Kernig's neck test* and similar to the *Soto-Hall test* except for the examiner's position. [See Clinical Comment 5.4]

Minor's Sign. Sciatic radiculitis is suggested by the manner the patient with this condition rises from a sitting position. The weight is supported on the uninvolved side by holding on to the chair for firm support in arising or the patient places the hands on the knees or thighs while working into the upright position, balances on the healthy leg, places one hand on the back, and flexes the leg and extends the thigh of the affected limb. The sign is often positive in sacroiliac lesions, lumbosacral strains and sprains, fractures, disc syndromes, dystrophies and myotonias.

Milgram's Test. The supine patient is asked to keep the knees straight and lift both legs off the table a few inches and to hold this position for as long as possible (Fig. 5.12). The test stretches the anterior abdominal and iliopsoas muscles and increases intrathecal pressure. Abnormal intrathecal pressure can be ruled out if the patient can hold this position for 20 seconds without pain. If this position cannot be held or if pain is experienced early during the test, a positive sign is offered that indicates pressure on the cord from some source (eg, cord pathology, IVD lesion).

Naffziger's Test. This test offers a suspicion of an abnormal spaceoccupying mass such as a spinal tumor or disc protrusion. It is performed by having the patient sit or recline while the examiner holds digital pressure over the jugular veins for 30—45 sec-

onds (Fig. 5.13). The patient is then instructed to cough deeply. Pain following the distribution of a nerve may suggest nerve root compression. Though more commonly used for low back involvements, thoracic and cervical root compression may also be aggravated. Local pain in the spine does not positively prove nerve compression; it may suggest the site of a strain, sprain, or another lesion. The sign is almost always positive in the presence of cord tumors, particularly spinal meningiomas. The resulting increased intrathecal pressure above the tumor or disc protrusion causes the mass to compress or pull sensory structures to produce radicular pain. The test is contraindicated in geriatrics and extreme care should be taken with anyone sus-

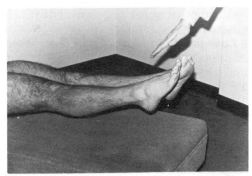

Figure 5.12. Milgram's test (Courtesy ACAP).

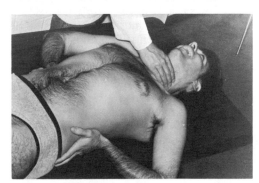

Figure 5.13. Naffziger's test (Courtesy ACAP).

DR. FAYE'S CLINICAL COMMENT #5.4

When a thoracolumbar adhesion tends to pull a lumbar nerve root cephalad and produce radicular symptoms, this test will be positiive and produce great patient apprehension during the maneuver. Some disc cases are the effect of incomplete ruptures (anular bulges). Cephalad traction on the root changes its normal angle as it exits the IVF, producing an abnormal tensile stress on the root involved. See Breig for full explanation. Manipulation of the thoracolumbar fixation will greatly reduce the patient's discomfort within 24 hours when this pseudo disc syndrome is present.

pected of having atherosclerosis. The patient should always be alerted that jugular pressure may result in vertigo.

Neri's Bowing Sign. This sign is positive when a standing patient can flex the trunk further without low back discomfort when the ipsilateral leg is flexed than when both knees are held in extension. A positive sign suggests hamstring spasm, contractures of the posterior thigh and/or leg muscles, sciatic neuritis, a lumbar IVD lesion, or a sacroiliac subluxation syndrome.

Skin Rolling Test. This test, according to Faye, will cause increased pain over a facilitated segment in the midline. He reports that, for a reason he is not aware of, this test can be positive unilaterally in a mechanical dysfunction segment (eg, a unilateral fixation).

Yeoman's Test. The patient is placed prone. With one hand, firm pressure is applied by the examiner over the suspected sacroiliac joint, fixing the patient's anterior pelvis to the table. With the other hand, the patient's leg is flexed on the affected side to the limit, and the thigh is hyperextended by the examiner lifting the knee off the examining table. If pain is increased in the sacroiliac area, it is significant of an anterior sacroiliac or hip lesion because of the stress on the anterior sacroiliac ligaments. Normally, no pain should be felt on this maneuver.

In addition to the tests described above, there are occasions when Babinski's sciatic, Baron's, Barre's pyramidal, Bonnet's, buckling, Duchenne's, Gower's, iliopsoas spasm, Kernig's, Lloyd's, Murphy's kidney, Pitres', Shober's, Sicard's, toe-in, Turyn's, Vanzetti's, and Westphal's signs should be sought. This is also true for the application of Astrom's, Bechterew's, belt, bent-knee pull, heel walk, iliopsoas contracture, Nachlas', O'Connell's, quadriceps flexion, Romberg's station, Smith-Peterson's, thigh hyperextension, and toe walk tests. These tests are described in comprehensive texts on physical and differential diagnosis.

Practical Sequence

As with any clinical examination procedure, the examination of the lumbar spine should be performed in an orderly and efficient manner designed to gain the maximum amount of information while provoking the patient's condition as little as possible. One helpful method uses a tape recorder for the doctor to dictate findings as the examination is performed. This speeds up the examination and eliminates the need for the doctor or other personnel to record findings by hand. An efficient sequence of examination, states Faye, might be as follows:

1. Patient vital statistics are taken and recorded while the patient is seated on the motion palpation stool.

2. Full spine motion palpation.

3. Low-back orthopedic testing with patient sitting.

4. Low-back orthopedic testing with patient standing, including postural analysis, sacroiliac palpation, observation of gait, heel and toe walk, etc.

5. Low-back orthopedics and neurologic testing with the patient supine (eg, reflexes, pin-wheel testing, motor strength testing, etc).

6. Low-back orthopedic testing with the patient prone.

7. When the examination is complete, the doctor decides what x-ray films are necessary. When acute spasm and antalgia exist, motion studies may not reveal significant information and it may be prudent to take standard views while delaying motion studies until muscular function has normalized enough to allow intersegmental motion to occur.

It then becomes the chiropractor's task to combine the information of the patient's history, orthopedics and neurologic examination, motion palpation examination, and x-ray findings to form a diagnosis, prognosis, and treatment regimen. These routines, when practiced to proficiency and coupled with compassion and integrity, will result in great success in the understanding and management/treatment of most low-back pain syndromes.

Lumbar Fixations

Iliolumbar Ligament Fixations

In the Belgium group's studies of fixation, they found that the 5th lumbar vertebra acts as part of the pelvis and at that level the most common ligament at fault is the ilio-lumbar. When these ligaments are shortened, they pull the crests of the ilia towards each other during standing, thereby forcing the ischia outward, the base of the sacrum forward, and the sacral apex backwards in the typical position that these structures assume during sitting. Gillet reports that this fixation is difficult to differentiate from that caused by the contracture and degeneration of the lower part of the quadratus lumborum. Fortunately, from a therapeutic viewpoint, the adjustment is the same, except that if the muscle is not degenerated, its hypertonicity may be reflexively produced by an articular fixation of the proximal fibulotibial articulation.

Quadratus Lumborum Fixations

The quadratus lumborum is a large muscle that has considerable importance by itself in producing both local and reflex fixations. Physiologically, it acts as one muscle, on either side, but individual bundles of its fibers, going from the iliac crest to a vertebra, can become "contractured" and pull the spine into distortion and fixation. This muscle, states Gillet, normally produces a flexion-rotation of the lumbar spine towards the side of the contraction. This movement takes place around a normal center of flexion-rotation in such a way that the superior and inferior articular surfaces remain in contact with each other. When in fixation, however, this normal gliding does not take place. On the contrary, the movement turns around an abnormal center of rotation that is at the opposite articulation. The articulations on the side of fixation are then forced open, with the inferior articulation being pushed into the IVF and against the nerve. This, states Gillet, is the "pressure on nerves" concept in all its simplicity and is one mechanism by which sciatica on the convex side of the lumbar curve is produced.

One special type of muscular fixation occasionally found seems to be of the vertical branch of the quadratus lumborum. It is often found to be hypertonic but quickly relaxes as other specific fixations are corrected.

Interspinous Muscle Fixations

Gillet reports that the next "ligamentous" fixation to be found as palpation moves cephalad is "that which can be considered as being pathognomonic of chronic lower back pain; ie, the lower lumbar lordosis that will not disappear when the patient is flexed forward. In its acute form, this fixation is produced by hypertonus of the interspinous muscles, but when it becomes chronic, either the muscular tissue changes into fibrous tissue, or the interspinous, supraspinous, or sacrolumbar ligaments take over and shorten. The muscular degeneration may even spread laterally over an area from 1 inch to 1½ inches in width on both sides. It then must be taken care of in a special manner."

This fixation, states Gillet, forces the vertebral articulations in a position that is not physiologic; ie, the pre- and post-zygapophyses are pulled apart at their superior edges and the interarticular spaces deform into a V shape. This, according to Gillet, forms what is usually called the facet syndrome, in which the vertebrae can be said to be "displaced." In the lateral x-ray view, this fixation gives the characteristic shape of the IVD, which is wedge shaped with the anterior part widened.

Rotatore Muscle Fixation

This muscle, states Gillet, is often found to be unilaterally hypertonic: it pulls the corresponding spinous into rotation and pulls the transverse of the vertebra below into counterrotation (Fig. 5.14). The fixation resem-

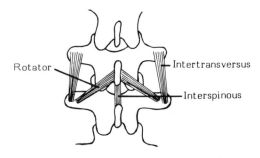

Figure 5.14. Schematic of the deep spinal extensor muscles (Courtesy ACAP).

bles that caused by the intertransverse muscle (flexion-rotation in one case and rotation-flexion in the other). Fortunately, the muscle responsible can easily be palpated. It is often important to be able to pin-point the offending muscle accurately because the contact site for the adjustment will vary accordingly. Some authorities recommend adjusting along the long axis of the contracted muscle.

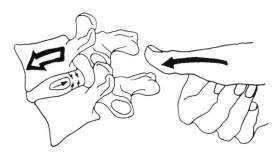

Figure 5.15. Evaluating intersegmental flexion.

Intertransverse Fixations

It was described in the previous chapter that thoracic interspinous fixations are often found associated with chronic low-back pain. The intertransverse muscles in the lumbar region have a similar role in the production of sciatic pain. "Contrary to the subluxation produced by the quadratus lumborum muscle," states Gillet, "[shortening of] this muscle is responsible for the pain on the side of concavity. It pulls the two transverse processes of the vertebrae together and pinches the disc and the contents of the intervertebral foramen on that side."

Erector Spinae Fixations

Gillet's studies found that lumbar erector spinae contractures pull the region into lordosis. In rare cases, this muscle is found, bilaterally, in a type of fibrous shortening that stops the region from moving into complete kyphosis. These cases are not frequent and sometimes difficult to manage.

Motion Palpation of the Lumbar Spine

Faye recommends that the lumbar spine be routinely palpated to determine which, if any, motion units are fixated; ie, which indicate the lack of a springy end feel at the end of all ranges of motion. The patient (sitting) and the doctor (sitting obliquely behind) should assume their standard positions for spinal motion palpation.

Flexion

Flexion is determined by interspinous separation (positive theta x). When testing for flexion freedom of the *posterior aspect* of the motion unit, the examiner's thumb is placed between the spinous processes while the patient's spine is passively flexed forward (Fig. 5.15). Try to center this flexion at the level of the motion unit being evaluated,

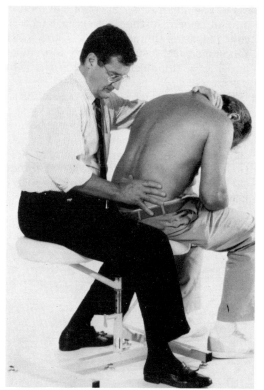

Figure 5.16. Seeking a sign of interspinous lumbar flexion fixation.

and then push anterosuperiorly on the superior spinous to see if a springy end feel exists (Fig. 5.16). The degree of intersegmental flexion motion varies considerably from patient to patient, but a distinct opening of the interspinous space should be perceived between segments that are not fixated.

This test evaluates only the *posterior aspect* of the motion unit; ie, the perception of motion may be normal even though the anterior ligaments have degenerated and tightened considerably.

Extension

During motion palpation for the integrity of segmental extension, two factors should be checked; ie, facetal extension and elasticity of the anterior longitudinal ligament.

1. *Extension of the zygapophyses (negative theta x)*. Extension freedom of the posterior aspect of the motion unit is indirectly tested by extending the patient's spine a few degrees and then pushing the articular process of the superior segment of the motion unit anteriorly (further into extension) with your palpating thumb (Figs. 5.17 and 5.18). You should feel a subtle springy movement under your thumb signifying that the joint has closed.

This motion, which evaluates the integrity of the *posterior aspect* of the superior segment of the motion unit, may appear normal even though an anterior fixation exists. Although fibers of degenerated ligaments lose their elasticity and plasticity to tensile forces, they still retain a large degree of their flexibility and are able to twirl to some degree.

2. *Extension, as determined by anterior longitudinal ligament testing in hyperextension*. The examiner's thumb is placed over the spinous process of the superior segment of the motion unit being evaluated. The patient's lumbar region is slightly hyperextended by the examiner's stabilizing arm, and then a forward push is made with the examiner's palpating hand (Fig. 5.19). Once the end of the ROM is reached, check for the normal springy end feel. If the anterior ligaments have degenerated, this springy end feel will be absent and the patient will report feeling quite uncomfortable.

Lateral Flexion

Right and left lateral flexion (positive and negative theta z). To check lumbar lateral bending to the left, the examiner's thumb is placed against the left side of the spinous process of the superior segment of the mo-

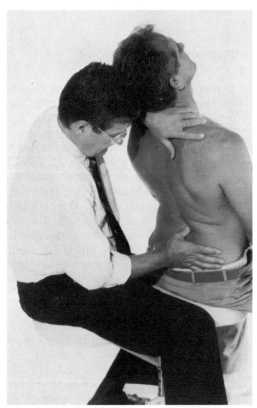

Figure 5.18. Seeking a sign of interspinous lumbar extension fixation.

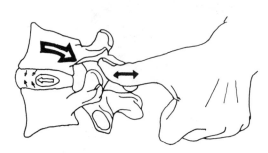

Figure 5.17. Evaluating intersegmental extension.

tion unit being evaluated (Fig. 5.20). As the patient is passively laterally flexed to the left with your stabilizing arm, your right thumb should push against the left aspect of the spinous process to produce a greater opening between the contralateral facets (ie, on the right, the side of convexity). See Figure 5.21. This slight movement should be perceived. Reverse your oblique position and these procedures for testing opening of the left articulation during lateral bending to the right. Again, a springy end-feel is normally sensed. A blocked resistance with a nonlingering painful discomfort indicates a fixation of significance.

Rotation

Left (clockwise) and right (counterclockwise) rotation, as determined by P-A motion of the zygapophyses (positive and

negative theta y). The examiner and patient should attain the basic starting (neutral) position. In testing the capability of the inferior facet of the superior segment of the motion unit to rotate counterclockwise on the right

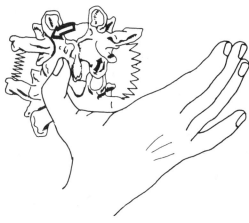

Figure 5.20. Schematic close-up view of thumb position when testing lateral flexion mobility.

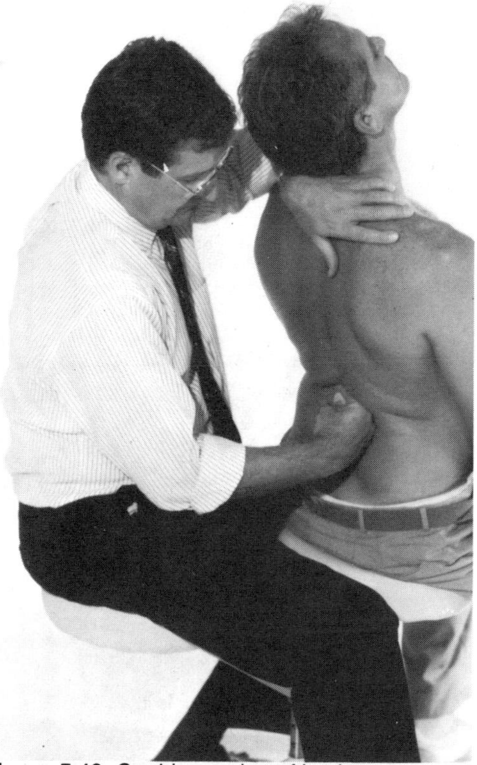

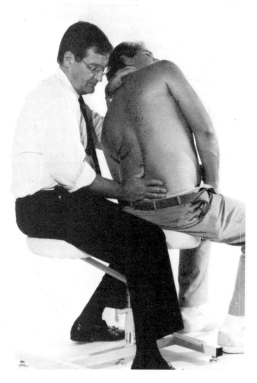

Figure 5.19. Seeking a sign of lumbar extension fixation resulting from anterior longitudinal ligament shortening.

Figure 5.21. Evaluating mobility of lumbar lateral flexion to the left.

(slightly superiorly, anteriorly, and medially on the superior facet of the segment below), the examiner's right thumb is placed against the right inferior process of the superior segment of the motion unit (Fig. 5.22). Rotate the patient's trunk counterclockwise (anteriorly on the right, posteriorly on the left) with your stabilizing arm, and, at the end of the ROM, check for a springy end feel by pushing forward with your thumb (Fig. 5.23). It is important during this maneuver to maintain constant contact against the inferior articular process being evaluated. Reverse your oblique position and these procedures for testing the contralateral articulation.

It should be noted that intersegmental rotatory motion may appear normal (but inhibited) even though extensive anterior and/or posterior partial fixations exist. As previously explained, this is because degenerated connective-tissue fibers retain some freedom to spiral and may be flexible. However, if a unilateral total (articular) fixation exists, rotatory motion will be absent on either side of the segment, according to Gillet and Schafer. Faye states that the fixation must be bilateral.

Applied Roentgenography

Lumbar studies, states Faye, should be conducted with a 72-inch tube-film distance, 100 KVP, 12:1 ratio grid with 103 lines, rare earth screens, and fast film. Considerable roentgenographic research has been done with patients sitting on a stool, but many clinicians use a standing A-P or P-A view quite successfully. Gonadal shields should always be employed. To read these functional films accurately, the examiner must be sure the pelvis did not side slip in lateral flexion.

Flexion-extension views are becoming more significant as investigations discover the significance of segmental instability. Motion studies with nonionizing radiation (eg, ultrasonic, magnetic) appears to be the standard of the future. The high KVP and rare earth screen combination is the best x-radiation reducer so far. The diagnosis of pathology is not the aim of a *function study* in dynamic chiropractic; therefore, stabilization is not used to immobilize the region.

The radiograph can show hypo- and hyper-mobility, but this finding will not rec-

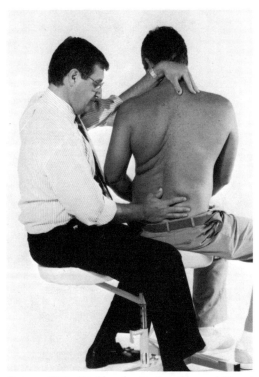

Figure 5.23. Position for testing the mobility of lumbar rotation posteriorly on the left.

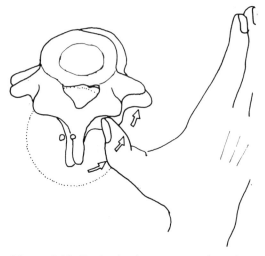

Figure 5.22. Evaluating intersegmental rotation.

ommend an articular adjusting procedure. Chronic hypermobilities seem to respond to stabilization if associated hypomobilities are corrected. More research is necessary in this area of our work. Personal observation of occasional cases such as those shown in MPI slides portray the return of hypermobile segments to a normal range of motion with time and correction of associated hypomobile articulations.

Flexion/extension overlay studies are extremely helpful for recording pre- and post-treatment changes. There are many methods recommended by different authors. Faye advises tracing the body and spinous process as it seems a more accurate method. Three colors of pointed pens that write on clear acetate sheets are also preferred. Each vertebra becomes the established reference point for the movement of the vertebra above. The neutral spine is traced first as it appears on the neutral lateral film. The clear acetate with the neutral spine traced on it in black is then used to compare flexion and extension ROMs of each motion unit.

In combined lumbar-sacroiliac disorders, the sacroiliac joints can be radiographed for pathology and anomalies. Faye uses a P-A view, stating that it gives a better picture of both sacroiliac joints. However, the professional standard is to use an A-P view. Most authorities agree that an oblique view is best for analyzing a particular sacroiliac joint.

Differential Diagnosis

Differential diagnosis is an art, not a pure science. The significance of the diagnosis depends on the perspective when the problem is approached. In our case as doctors of chiropractic, states Faye, "we need a double diagnosis. The classic diagnosis of allopathic medicine enables us to communicate with other professionals, insurance companies, etc. The chiropractic diagnosis is essentially a working knowledge of the five components of the subluxation complex."

To differentiate low-back pain, the chiropractic physician attempts to systematize, and hopefully simplify, the chiropractic diagnosis of low-back syndromes through a better understanding of the major types of low-

back pain and accurate significant examination. This is not an exhaustive approach to low-back diagnosis as it is assumed that at the postgraduate level the doctor is already versed in the mechanisms of referred pain, the clinical implications of x-ray findings, recognizing pain of organic pathology, and that occasionally patients problems don't always follow a classic pattern and are subject to variation in their clinical presentation. Kirkaldy-Willis and Cassidy state: "Moreover the many different causes of back pain are not always readily apparent. With the exception of back pain from entrapment of the spinal nerve root by degenerative changes or by disc herniation, most causes of low-back pain lack objective signs and overt pathological changes. Nevertheless, these obscure causes are responsible for most of the back pain seen in clinical practice." This further emphasizes the need for an ever-increasing understanding of biochemical mechanisms, pathologic joint movement, and consequential nervous system dysfunction.

Lumbar or Lumbosacral Facet Syndrome

The pain of lower lumbar facet syndrome is usually in the midline, presenting with an achy (sometimes sharp) pain that improves in the morning after rest and becomes worse in the evening after prolonged weight bearing. The patient's discomfort is aggravated by any maneuver causing extension of the lumbar spine such as with Kemp's, Lewin-Gaenslen's, or Ely's tests, and often relieved by forward flexion or when in the fetal position.

Faye reports that associated referred pain, usually mild to moderate, can refer to the (1) ipsilateral iliac crest; (2) ipsilateral buttock; (3) ipsilateral groin, scrotum, labium occasionally; or (4) leg, usually above the knee. There are no conclusive neurologic signs (reflexes +2, sensory negative, motor negative). There is usually no pain on coughing or sneezing, but the skin rolling test may be positive over the level of inflammation. Faye also states that the most common sites of causation fixation are at the (1) sacroiliac joints, (2) thoracolumbar or lumbar joints, or (3) the hip joints.

Lumbar Disc and Radiculitis Syndromes: General Considerations

One early clinical concern is to differentiate inflammatory conditions from noninflammatory joint dysfunction syndromes. If a patient can point specifically to an exact joint as the source of the pain, it is likely the pain arises from that joint. If the patient moves the whole hand over a general area, then a specific joint is not usually the correct diagnosis.

Percussing the area of pain causes a sharp pain in dysfunction: an "ouch" reaction. However, more serious pathology is suggested if percussion produces a deep, throbbing, aching pain that lingers after the springing test. Differentiating signs of lumbar disc protrusion, sprain, and strain are shown in Table 5.3.

With either IVD lesions or lumbar radiculitis, Faye describes that the patient usually presents with an acute antalgic posture, bent either laterally or anteriorly. There may or may not have been a traumatic onset. There is pain on coughing or sneezing, and it may radiate down either leg. The leg pain extends from below the knee to the foot. There may be neurologic signs such as paresthesia, weakness of the big toe, weak foot and ankle dorsiflexion, and/or weak plantar flexion eversion. Atrophy of the affected limb is possible.

Table 5.3. Typical Signs of Lumbar Disc Protrusion, Sprain, and Strain

Feature	Disc Protrusion	Sprain	Strain
Area of pain	Concave side of pain	Convex side of curve	Over muscle
Curve pattern	Segmental distortion	Segmental distortion	Antalgic, if any
Deep pressure pain	Often bilateral, localized, usually one joint	Unilateral pain, localized, often one joint	Usually bilateral, large area, in muscle
Effect of rest	Relieves pain	Relieves pain	Stiffens area
Iliac position	Low on pain side	High on pain side	High on pain side
Initial feeling	Lock	Snap	Tearing
Location of pain	Segment	Lumbosacral or sacroiliac area	Involved muscle
Major cause of pain	Root/cord irritation	Synovitis	Myositis
Most painful action	Hyperextension with torsion	Hyperextension	Flexion
Onset of pain	Minor trauma	Unprepared joint	During lifting
Percussion	Sharp pain that radiates	Sharp local pain	Little increased discomfort
Position of rest	Still position	Still position	Moves frequently

SLR, leg-lowering, and Kemp's tests will be positive. Bragard's, Minor's, and Neri's bowing tests may be positive or negative. The patient's discomfort becomes worse with activity, improves with rest; is worst in the evening; and improves in morning. The most common causative fixations are at the (1) thoracolumbar junction, (2) sacroiliac joints, (3) hip joints.

Intervertebral Disc Lesions in the Lumbar Spine

The firm diagnosis of IVD rupture can only be made during surgical intervention; myelography is no exception. Thus, only a tentative diagnosis of disc protrusion can be made when the conclusions are drawn from clinical signs and symptoms. A classification of IVD syndromes is shown in Table 5.4.

In the abscence of severe trauma, disc height is a reflection of disc hydration. As dehydration increases with age and late degeneration, the nucleus tends to lose its turgor, and disc height can be used as a sign of these two factors. But this is not to say that advanced degeneration cannot be found in a disc of normal height. During roentgenographic analysis, the tip of the superior articular facet should not reach a line extending backward from the undersurface of the vertebral body above (Macnab's joint body line) if disc degeneration is absent (Fig. 5.24).

Most exacerbating and remitting spinal pain cannot be attributed to the disc itself. Rather, involvement of the sensitive articular facets and IVF contents is much more likely.

Types of Intervertebral Disc Pathology. One method of classifying the various types of IVD pathology is Charnley's method:

Type I: acute sprain, usually from unexpected loading. There typically are severe pain and muscle spasm. Nonsciatic referred pain is usually associated. Rupture of some of the peripheral or central anular fibers, slight end plate fracture, and stress to the capsular or interspinous ligaments and posterior arch muscle fibers occur. Lasegue's straight-leg raising test is negative.

Type II: a nontraumatic, idiopathic, sudden intake of fluid by the nucleus pulposus, causing irritation of the peripheral anular fibers because of the nuclear pressure being transmitted horizontally. There are back pain and muscle spasm without referred pain or sciatica. Lasegue's test is negative.

Type III: slight abnormal bulging of some of the posterolateral fibers with slight IVF encroachment. In addition to local back pain, pain may be referred into the sacroiliac area, buttocks, hip, and posterior thigh. There is no neuromuscular deficit, and Lasegue's sign is negative.

Table 5.4. Classes of Intervertebral Disc Syndromes

Grade	Description
Grade I	The patient has intermittent pain and spasm with local tenderness. There is very little or no root compression. Paresthesia and/or radiculitis may extend to the ischial area.
Grade II	Some nerve root compression exists along with pain, sensory disturbance, and occasionally some atrophy. Paresthesia and/or radiculitis may extend to the knee.
Grade III	Marked demonstrable muscle weakness, pronounced atrophy, and intractable radicular pain. Paresthesia and/or radiculitis may extend to the ankle or foot.
Frank herniation	Complete extrusion of the nucleus through the anulus into the canal or IVF. All above symptoms are found in herniation, and, in addition, pain is worse at night and not generally relieved by most conservative therapies.

Type IV: herniation of part of the nucleus into the peripheral anulus that, in turn, bulges into the vertebral canal (Fig. 5.25). Local back pain increased with Valsalva's straining maneuvers, true sciatica, and a positive Lasegue's test occurs. These are signs of irritation of a nerve root.

Type V: floating nuclear fragment. This chronic condition is sometimes associated with disc degeneration. There are episodes of back pain, with or without sciatica, depending on the position of the fragment and the magnitude of stress.

Type VI: anchored nuclear fragment. This disorder is often the aftermath of Type V where the nucleus is fixed within the peripheral anulus or vertebral canal with probable IVF encroachment. The nerve root becomes chronically irritated from mechanical pres-sure, chemical irritation, autoimmune response, or a combination of these factors. True sciatica with a positive Lasegue's sign occurs. A narrowing of the IVD space is usually associated.

Type VII: advanced disc degeneration. When a disc is not well hydrated and nourished, it is unable to serve its hydraulic function. Disc narrowing and arthrotic processes of the vertebral bodies are invariably associated. Symptoms vary from severe to none and may be chronic or intermittent.

Lumbar Radiculitis

Signs and symptoms of lumbar radiculopathy vary somewhat depending on which root(s) are involved. See Table 5.5. In general, it can be said that painful lumbar attacks of radiculogenic erector splinting, often with brief episodes of paresis and paresthesiae, are sudden in onset and frequently bilateral as opposed to the invariably unilateral pain of a posterolateral disc protrusion. In this syndrome, the paravertebral ligaments are extremely tender, and pain is increased by rotation. Neurologic signs and Lasegue's SLR test are usually negative or unconclusive. The acute attacks of instability are often quickly relieved by rest and support. See Figure 5.26.

Several authorities suggest and clinical observation concurs that radicular inflammation can often be produced by hypermobility and consequential nerve root stress at the level involved. If the patient improves to any substantial degree with bed rest, physiotherapy, and gentle manipulation in 3—5 days, disc herniation is unlikely to be the etiologic factor. When disc tissue is compromised and produces nerve root compression, a much slower progress occurs (1—3 months) and the prognosis should be guarded. If no progress occurs within 2—4 weeks, referral to an orthopedist or neurosurgeon should be considered, especially if progressing muscle weakness and atrophy or an enlarging area of paresthesia/anesthesia is witnessed. If a cauda equina syndrome develops, the need for surgery may be urgent.

The practitioner who has been recently introduced to the precepts of *dynamic chiro-*

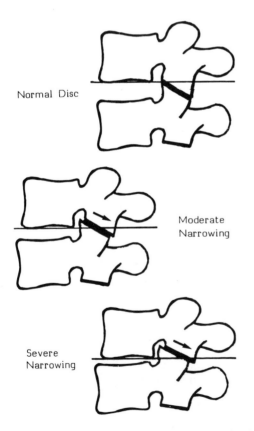

Normal Disc

Moderate Narrowing

Severe Narrowing

Figure 5.24. Effects of various degrees of IVD thinning on the IVFs and facets (Courtesy ACAP).

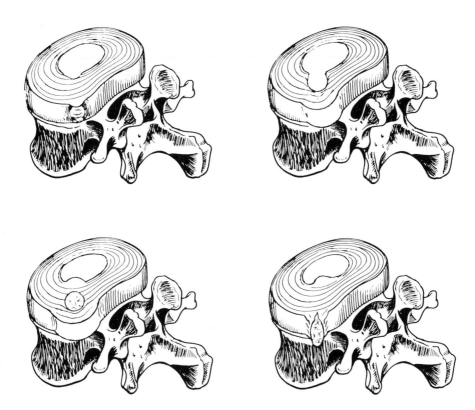

Figure 5.25. *Top left,* Type III IVD protrusion, exhibiting a slight protrusion at the posterolateral aspect of the disc; referred hip and thigh pain is common with this type of lesion. *Top right,* Type IV IVD anular bulge, in which nerve root irritation frequently exhibits sciatica. *Lower left,* Type V IVD disruption with a floating isolated nuclear fragment; pain usually exacerbates with an increase in intra-abdominal pressure or certain movements. *Lower right,* Type VI IVD rupture with a protruding sequestration; the nuclear fragment may or may not be anchored at some point (Courtesy ACAP).

practic will soon realize that almost all IVD lesions and local inflammatory nerve lesions (radiculitis) occur at the level of *hypermobile* segments. It is at such sites that overstress is concentrated. Thus, primary sites of fixation must be sought and corrected. Manipulating or adjusting a hypermobile segment would only aggravate the patient's problem.

Most lumbar disc lesions occur at the L5-S1 and L4-L5 levels, and it will be found that the majority of associated (and often responsible) primary fixations will be at or near the thoracolumbar transitional segments (eg, between T10 and L2). Faye believes that this is also true for cases of well-adapted chronic lower lumbar spondylolisthesis.

Malingering-Oriented Tests

Although there are many tests for differentiating malingering from a somatic, visceral, or psychic cause, Faye emphasizes Hoovers' and Mannkopf's tests.

Hoover's Test. This is a test for malingering associated with an active straight-leg-raising test. When the patient attempts to raise his leg, the examiner cups one hand under the heel of the opposite foot. When the typical patient tries to raise his affected limb, he normally applies pressure on the heel of the opposite limb for leverage and a downward pressure can be felt. If this pressure is not felt, the patient is probably not really trying.

Mannkopf's Test. This is an old, but reliable, objective test for pain, and it is not restricted to musculoskeletal complaints. The patient is placed in a relaxed position and the pulse is taken. The examiner then precipitates the pain (eg, by probing, applying heat or electrostimulation, etc). The pulse rate is then re-evaluated. In situations of true pain, the pulse rate will increase a *minimum* of 10%.

THERAPEUTIC APPROACH

Adjusting Lumbar Fixations

Flexion: Interspinous Separation Fixation

Place the patient in the lateral recumbent position with both knees and hips flexed, arms crossed, and adjust the head-piece of the adjusting table to patient comfort. This is a modification of the classic side posture adjustment position. The patient may lie on either side during the adjustment, for here we are dealing with a midline fixation.

Avoid rotating the patient's lumbars during patient placement. The patient's knees are stabilized by the doctor's thigh as he or she stands over the patient's flexed lower limbs. Once the patient is properly positioned, apply a pisiform contact on the tip of the spinous of the superior segment of the involved motion unit and direct an impulse cephalad and slightly forward to produce further flexion (kyphosis) of the superior segment on the inferior segment. See Figure 5.27.

Once lumbar interspinous soft-tissue fixations become chronic and degenerative processes are well established, they respond less to adjustments. See Figure. 5.28. Some type of stretching exercise is usually necessary to facilitate the effects of a mobilizing adjustment. One frequently used technique is to place the patient supine and flex both of the patient's knees toward the patient's chest, adding your own body weight if necessary, in an attempt to curl the patient's lumbar spine into flexion and place a slow stretch on the posterior elements. The sacral apex should be raised from the supporting surface (eg, a low therapy table). Try to direct the greatest force at the apex of the patient's lumbar lordosis. It may be necessary to place one hand under the patient's sacral apex and lift upward and cephalad to enhance this curling motion. See Figure 5.29.

With slight modifications, this stretching maneuver can be used as the primary adjustment with large patients that are difficult to manage in the lateral recumbent position. The modifications are to apply a knuckle contact with your active hand be-

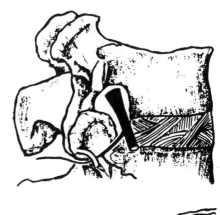

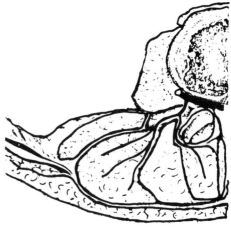

Figure 5.26. *Top,* the lumbar nerve root descends obliquely through the upper aspect of the IVF. The posterior ramus runs laterally across the superior articular process and through a ligamentous tunnel. Only a small portion of this channel is shown in the drawing. *Bottom,* the posterior division of the nerve root as view from above. Only the main branches are shown (Courtesy ACAP).

Table 5.5. Major Neurogenic Signs in the Lumbosacral Radiculopathies

Feature	L3 Root L2—L3 IVD	L4 Root L3—L4 IVD	L5 Root L4—L5 IVD	S1 Root L5—S1 IVD
Ankle reflex	Normal	Normal	Normal	Diminished
Back pain radiates to:	Buttocks, dorsal thigh, anterior knee	Buttocks, dorsal thigh, medial calf	Buttocks, lateral calf, dorsal foot, great toe	Buttocks, mid calf, plantar foot, heel
Lasegue's supine sign (SLR)	Usually negative	+ at 80° or more	+ at 50°—60° or more	+ at 30°—40° or more
Muscle weakness	Quadriceps femoris group	Quadriceps, iliopsoas	Gluteus med., ant. tibialis, hallucis ext.	Gluteus max., hamstrings, gastrocnemius, soleus.
Patellar reflex	Normal	Diminished	Normal	Normal
Sensory sign	Knee numbness	Lower medial leg numbness	Numbness at cleft between 1st and 2nd toe, dorsal foot	Numbness inferoposterior to lateral maleolus, heel, dorsal calf, lateral foot

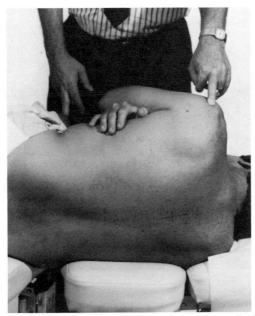 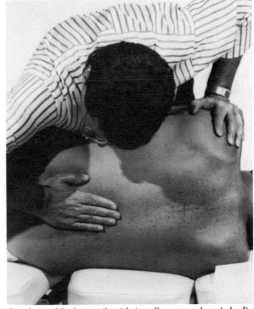

Figure 5.27. Adjusting a lumbar interspinous flexion fixation with the patient laterally recumbent. *Left,* positioning the patient; *right,* making the correction.

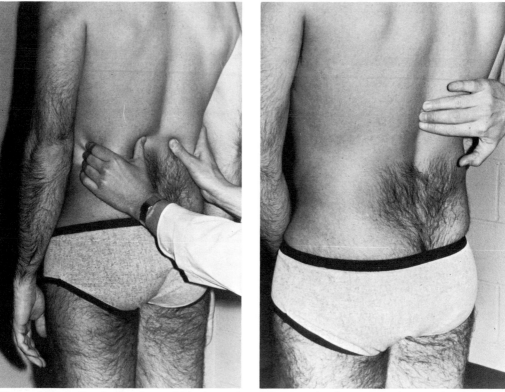

Figure 5.28. *Left,* palpating the perispinal muscles of the upper lumbar area and comparing their tone bilaterally. *Right,* static palpating of the upper lumbar spinous processes (Courtesy ACAP).

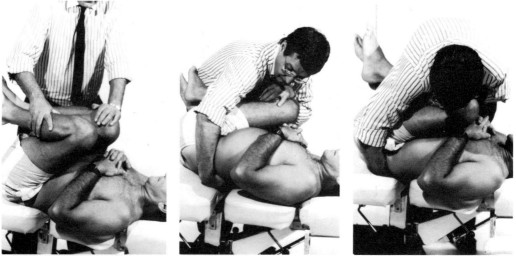

Figure 5.29. Stretching lumbar interspinous flexion fixations. *Left,* positioning the patient; *center,* curling the patient's lumbar spine; *right,* applying the stretch.

tween the fixed spinous processes, lean well over the patient with your stabilizing arm across the patient's uppermost thigh, and then deliver a body drop directed against your contact finger that serves as a fulcrum.

Extension: Zygapophyseal Fixation

Place the patient in the classic lateral recumbent position, involved side upward, with the uppermost hip and knee flexed over the underneath extended limb resting on the surface of the adjusting table. Position the patient so that the lumbar spine is lordotic (curved in moderate extension); ie, the patient's hips and shoulders are further from you than the patient's abdomen. Apply a pisiform contact on the involved articular process and direct an impulse anteriorly and slightly cephalad to produce extension (lordosis) of the superior segment on the inferior segment (Fig. 5.30). An added body drop during this adjustment is usually beneficial.

Extension: Shortened Anterior Longitudinal Ligament, Patient Prone

Place the patient prone, raise the pelvic support of the adjusting table slightly, lower the head-piece a few notches, and relax the tension from the chest-abdomen support of the adjusting table to place the patient's lumbar spine in extension (Fig. 5.31). With the patient in this "swayback" position and pressure is applied to achieve maximum extension, it only takes a slight impulse delivered obliquely anteriorly and cephalad (using a crossed-hand double-pisiform contact against the laminae bilaterally) to stretch the anterior longitudinal ligament. See Figure 5.32.

Extension: Shortened Anterior Longitudinal Ligament, Patient Sitting

Place the patient in the sitting neutral position, and stabilize the patient's shoulders as during motion palpation. Slightly flex the patient's lumbars to open the interspinous space so that you can obtain a firm thumb contact between the spinous processes of the involved motion unit. Return the patient's spine to the neutral and then into extension while continuously maintaining a firm contact with your thumb. Once the maximum ROM of extension is achieved, deliver an impulse with your thumb that is directed anteriorly and slightly cephalad (Fig. 5.33). Faye recommends this technic

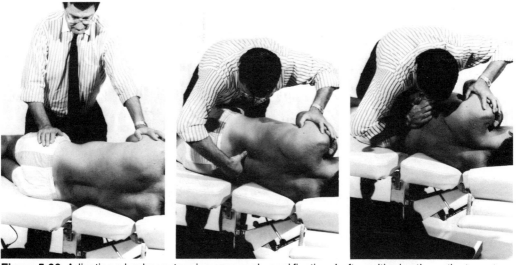

Figure 5.30. Adjusting a lumbar extension zygapophyseal fixation. *Left,* positioning the patient; *center,* producing lumbar lordosis; *right,* apply the corrective thrust.

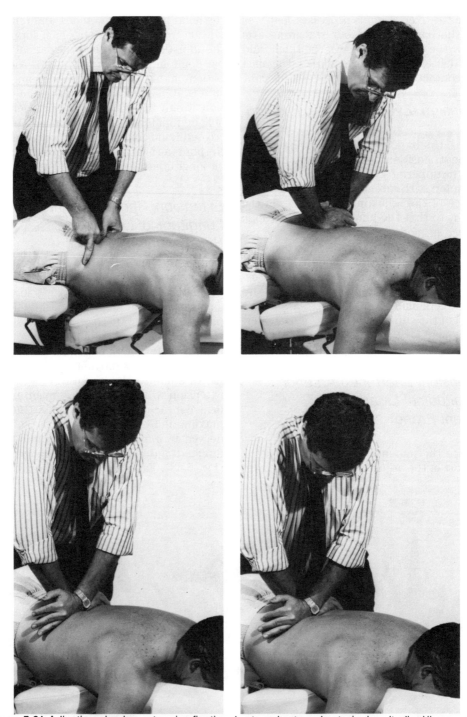

Figure 5.31. Adjusting a lumbar extension fixation due to a shortened anterior longitudinal ligament with the patient prone. *Top left,* localizing the site of fixation; *top right,* securing the right hand; *bottom left,* securing the left hand; *bottom right,* applying the corrective impulse.

when a shortened anterior ligament fixation is found during a housecall.

Gillet and Faye report that shortening of the lumbar anterior longitudinal ligament frequently occurs at one or two motion units, tending to push one or both of the involved

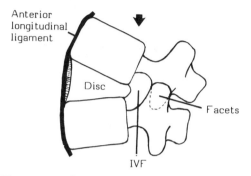

Figure 5.32. Side view of a healthy motion unit in extension. Note the movement required at the anterior longitudinal ligament, disc, and posterior facets. As the IVD contracts anteriorly during extension, the fibers of the anterior longitudinal ligament that attach to the disc are stressed (Courtesy ACAP).

segments into a state of local kyphosis (Fig. 5.34). The same condition may also be found in the thoracic and cervical spine. At times, such kyphotic segments in the lumbar spine will not be the effect of a shortened anterior longitudinal ligament; rather, they may be the result of iliopsoas spasm or hypertonicity. This point should be underscored for the iliopsoas has been shown to play a major role in many low-back pain complaints.

Schafer points out that the term "shortened anterior longitudinal ligament" should not be taken literally. It is a term that has been carried over from Gillet's writings, and it is likely that something became misinterpreted during translation. Shortened *ventral spinal tissues* would probably be a more correct general phrase. Although the anterior longitudinal ligament may degenerate, it is such a thin structure in the lumbar spine that tightening of this ligament in itself would unlikely interfere greatly with lumbar movements. Observation during surgery reveals that more important to restricting lumbar extension would be degeneration of the strong tendons and fascia of the iliopsoas

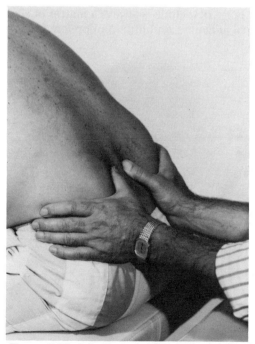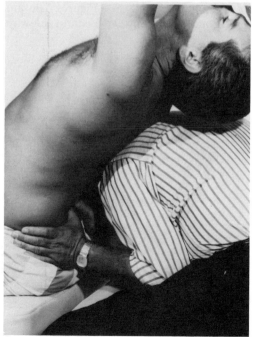

Figure 5.33. Adjusting a lumbar extension fixation, due to a shortened anterior longitudinal ligament with the patient sitting. *Left,* obtaining a firm thumb contact between the fixated spinous processes; *right,* delivering the corrective impulse with the patient's spine extended.

muscle (and some fibers of the retroperitoneal fascia) that firmly attach anteriorly to the vertebral bodies, IVDs, and transverse processes along with fibers from the anterior longitudinal ligament (Fig. 5.35). This ligamentous and tendinous complex should be considered clinically as a whole. It would be an unusual circumstance if degenerative processes would attack fibers of the anterior longitudinal ligament in this area of the spine and leave adjacent ligament, fascia, and tendon fibers unaffected.

Extension: Shortened Anterior Longitudinal Ligament, Patient Standing

This adjustment can be performed in several ways. One method is similar to that described for a shortened anterior longitudinal ligament in the thoracic spine. For the lumbar region, Faye stands backwards to the patient so that his buttocks fits into the patient's lumbar lordosis, reaches backward to grip the patient's crossed arms, and flexes forward to induce distraction and extension of the patient's spine. See Figures 5.36 and 5.37. Some doctors prefer to stand sideways

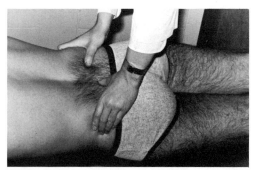

Figure 5.34. Locating the spinous process of L5 with the left thumb, patient prone (Courtesy ACAP).

to the patient and place their hip against the patient's lordosis just before the lifting maneuver is performed.

As an alternative to these technics with the doctor and patient in the standing position that are designed to stretch the anterior longitudinal ligament and induce intersegmental traction, Schafer achieves the same objective with the patient supine by applying intermittent mechanical spinal traction to the patient while a small Dutchman's roll is been placed under the patient's lumbars. Choice of technic is always a matter of clinical judgment and physician preference.

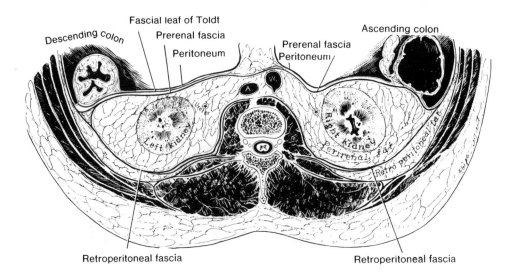

Figure 5.35. Transverse section of body at L2 level showing the relationship of the musculature and fascia at this level (Courtesy ACAP).

Zygapophyseal Rotatory Fixation, Patient Laterally Recumbent

Place the patient in the classic lateral recumbent position, involved side either upward or downward. Maneuver the patient's spine to apply a passive rotatory force against the site of fixation. The objective here is to induce a torque between the facets that exhibit restricted rotatory motion. With the patient positioned as described above, this can be accomplished in either of two ways depending on if the superior segment is restricted in its clockwise or counterclockwise motion (from a bird's-eye view with the patient sitting). If restricted in counterclockwise motion, the superior segment is moved in this direction against the fixation while the inferior segment is moved in the opposite (clockwise) direction. The adjustment is achieved by finger or thumb contact under the lateral aspect of the spinous process of the superior segment lifting obliquely upward and the contact over the lateral aspect of the spinous process of the inferior segment simultaneously pushing obliquely downward in line with the plane of articula-

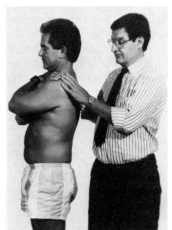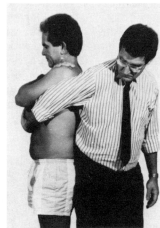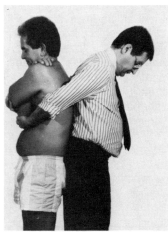

Figure 5.36. Preparing to adjust a lumbar extension fixation due to anterior longitudinal ligament shortening. *Left,* preparing the patient in the initial position; *center* and *right,* assuming the initial adjusting position.

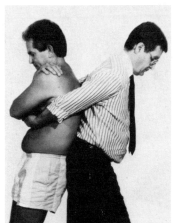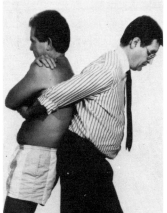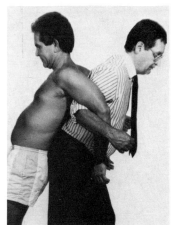

Figure 5.37. Adjusting a lumbar extension fixation due to anterior longitudinal ligament shortening. *Left* and *center,* doctor flexing forward to induce extension and distraction of the patient's lumbar spine; *right,* an alternative method of supporting the patient.

tion (Fig. 5.38). These counterrotations are centered at the fixated facet, and a mild added body drop will enhance this adjustment. The same effect can be achieved by stabilizing one segment and rotating the other. This latter method is the technic taught by Faye.

If the superior segment is restricted in clockwise motion, either the contacts and direction of force can be reversed or the patient can be placed on the other side. Keep in mind that restricted clockwise motion of the superior process is the same as restricted counterclockwise motion of the motion unit's inferior process, and vice versa, for facetal motion is relative to the gliding positions of the articulating surfaces.

This reciprocity of facetal motion is readily recognized in gross motions of the spine: if a patient's shoulders are stabilized and the patient's pelvis is rotated clockwise, the motions induced in the movable articulations of the patient's spine are no different than those that occur when the patient's pelvis is stabilized and the patient's shoulders are rotated counterclockwise. The same principle is true at the segmental level, for gross motions are only the sum of the actions taking place at segmental levels. For this reason, a large variety of technics can be applied in different fashions and yet achieve the same objective (the release of restricted joint motion or, conversely, the increase in joint motion freedom).

Zygapophyseal Rotatory Fixation, Patient Sitting

If necessary for the circumstances at hand, correction of restricted rotatory motion can be achieved with the patient in the sitting position. The doctor and patient positions are the same as those used for motion palpation of segmental rotation except that a pisiform contact is used rather than a thumb contact. If counterclockwise rotation is restricted on the right, the patient is ro-

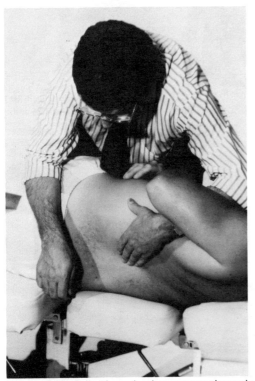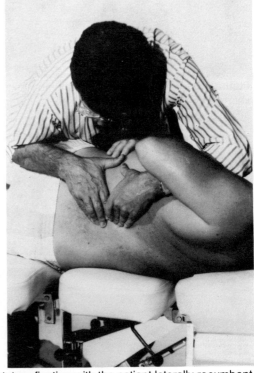

Figure 5.38. Adjusting a lumbar zygapophyseal rotatory fixation with the patient laterally recumbent. *Left,* localizing the site of fixation; *right,* applying the contacts.

tated into maximum counterclockwise ROM by the doctor's stabilizing arm. With the doctor's contact hand, an impulse is then directed anteriorly, slightly cephalad, and medially against the medial aspect of the right transverse process of the superior segment of the fixed motion unit.

Zygapophyseal Rotatory Fixation, Patient Prone

The patient is placed prone, the headpiece of the adjusting table is lowered, the abdominal support is raised slightly, and the front aspect of the pelvic support is raised slightly to place the patient's spine in mild flexion to slightly open the posterior elements of the lumbar vertebrae. If the superior unit of a motion unit exhibits restricted counterclockwise motion on the right, for example, Schafer recommends applying a crossed-hand double-pisiform contact, with

one contact applied against the right lamina of the superior segment and the other contact applied against the left lamina of the inferior segment of the motion unit. With elbows almost locked, the adjustment is delivered bilaterally anteriorly and cephalad (in line with the plane of articulation) with equal force to produce an intersegmental torque within the restricted articulations. See Figure 5.39.

Restricted Lateral Lumbar Flexion, Patient Laterally Recumbent

The patient is placed in the classic lateral recumbent position, and care should be made to avoid any degree of lumbar rotation. If lateral bending is restricted on the right, the patient is positioned so that side is upward, and vice versa. Release the tension on the abdominal support, and slightly raise the front aspect of the pelvic support. Stand

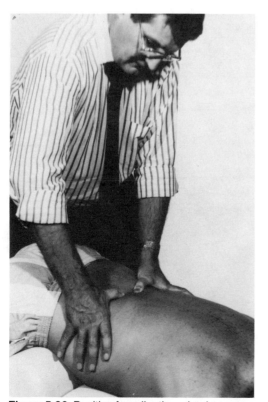 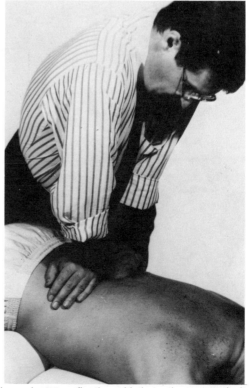

Figure 5.39. Position for adjusting a lumbar zygapophyseal rotatory fixation with the patient prone. *Left,* localizing the site of fixation; *right,* applying the adjustive impulse.

in front of the patient, perpendicular to the site of involvement. Reach over the patient and apply a pisiform contact deep against the lateral aspect of the spinous process of the superior segment of the involved motion unit. Apply firm pressure downward (and slightly anteriorly to avoid slipping) to produce lateral flexion under your contact, and, at the maximum ROM, deliver an impulse and mild body drop directed obliquely downward, cephalad, and anterior (in line with the place of articulation). See Figure 5.40.

Note: It should be realized that this adjustment can only be effective if the tension on the abdominal support is released to allow free lateral flexion. If the adjustment is delivered with the patient on a firm table, as sometimes must be demonstrated, the pressure contact and downward impulse on the spinous process (the most posterior lever on the motion unit) will not produce lateral flexion, it will produce clockwise rotation of the segment; ie, as the spinous process is forced downward, the centrum will rotate in

the opposite direction. The unyielding table surface will inhibit lateral flexion. The ideal contact to release a lateral flexion block would be on the lateral aspect of the contralateral articulating processes. As this is impossible without producing injury to the overlying tissues, patient and table positioning to achieve passive preadjustment lateral flexion against the fixation is almost mandatory.

Iliolumbar Ligament Fixations

Shortening of the iliolumbar ligaments, which extend from the transverse processes of L5 to the iliac crests bilaterally, tend to pull the pelvis in the standing position into the shape it normally takes in the sitting position. This produces a low lordosis in the standing position but of a different type than that caused by lumbar interspinous ligament fixations.

Iliolumbar shortening can be relieved by

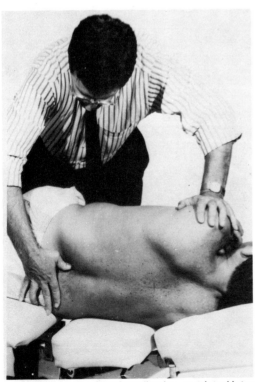
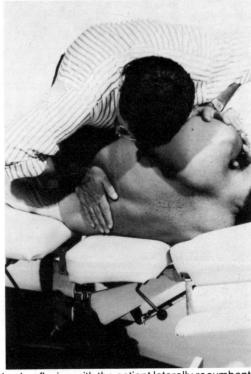

Figure 5.40. Position for adjusting restricted lateral lumbar flexion with the patient laterally recumbent. *Left,* localizing the site of fixation; *right,* applying the adjustive thrust.

placing the patient in the lateral recumbent position and applying a roll-type adjustment with contact held on the iliac crest on the side of the shortest iliolumbar ligament (Fig. 5.41). The objective is to increase the distance between ligament's origin and insertion. With the patient in the prone position and the tension on the abdominal support eased, an alternative technic can be applied by giving a short, stiff thrust against the midpoint of the shortened ligament.

Integrated Treatment Approach

Once the diagnosis is first established, it is best to consider it as the *working diagnosis*. This temporary diagnosis is usually confirmed or replaced in 2—3 weeks.

"The first concern therapeutically is the reduction of any inflammation and pain," states Faye. "The most effective methods of reducing inflammation, also reduces pain. I found electrotherapy and ice were more effective than ultra sonar. Restoring joint mobility also had a great pain relieving effect. In acute cases, the trauma has to be differentiated as invasive or a biomechanical insult. Thrust adjusting is contraindicated in invasive trauma. Manipulation of the area of dysfunction is indicated in trauma caused by biomechanical insult. The area of manipulation is more often not at the level of the inflammation treatment. The flow chart (refer to Fig. 2.5) helps in scheduling."

In developing an integrated treatment approach for low-back pain complaints, Faye emphasizes the inclusion of muscle testing, locating and treating associated trigger points, using a lumbar spine PNF stretching procedure, and physical therapy.

Lumbar trigger points are commonly found within each belly of the quadratus lumborum muscle; the multifidus, rotatores, and intertransversarii muscles; and the erector spinal muscles. Faye mentions that gluteus and piriformis trigger points are also commonly concomitant.

In PNF stretch of the lumbar spine, the patient sits for these stretches with arms crossed, hands on shoulders, and each range of motion is resisted for 8 seconds and than actively stretched to tolerance by the antagonist with gentle help from the doctor.

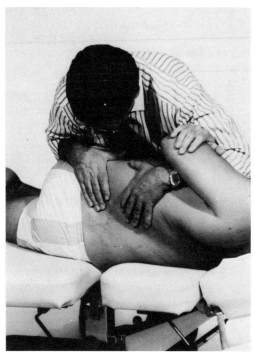

Figure 5.41. Stretching a shortened iliolumbar ligament with the patient laterally recumbent.

Muscles can be tested by judging the power of a contraction against resistance or by using a dynamometer such as a Cybex™ unit. A weak muscle or muscle group should be tested to see if it contracts when faradic current is applied. If it does, states Faye, it will recover in a few weeks. If no contraction occurs but galvanic current can cause a contraction, then from 8 to 12 months can be expected for a recovery. Faye reports that no response to galvanism means no recovery can be expected.

If physical therapy is employed in your practice, the doctor should use a modality to achieve a specific predetermined physiologic effect. The following considerations are recommended by Faye:

1. Reduce swelling and inflammation of acute condition—ice, electrotherapy, compression, elevation.

2. Reduce pain and thus anxiety caused by pain—electrotherapy, ice.

3. Promote healing by increasing metabolism and circulation—heat (eg, diathermy, infrared, etc).

4. Promote healing by changing polarity of

pathology area—electrotherapy, electromagnetic field therapy.

5. Promote muscle strengthening by electrical stimulation—faradic, galvanic, Russian stimulation, tetanizing currents with proper rest phases.

6. Extinguish active or latent trigger points —electrotherapy, ischemic compression, percussion vibration, spray-and-stretch.

7. Promote a positive feeling of getting well, which is so essential to the patient's psychology of getting well.

These notes provide a foundation for a chiropractic approach to many pelvic and lumbar spine complaints. Faye recommends that the involved segmental areas be adjusted often even though no low back pain syndrome is present. "The biomechanical model of joint function and the locomotor system as an integral unit of harmony of joints, muscles and neurobiological mechanisms is the chiropractic model of health and disease. We hope this approach stimulates your thinking and practical expertise in practicing rational chiropractic."

Motion Palpation Recumbent on a Mobile Adjusting Table

With the introduction of chiropractic adjusting tables that produce both y-axis distraction and lateral flexion, new methods of motion palpation are now possible. These innovations have been shown by Martin and associates to be as accurate in interreliability studies as our traditional methods conducted in the sitting posture.

A motorized table leaves both hands of the examiner free for palpation. Y-axis distraction can be palpated in the lumbar, thoracic, and cervical spine. In the lumbar spine, all ranges of motion can be examined while the patient is prone.

For the methods described below, the table needs to swing laterally between its abdominal and pelvic sections.

Lumbar Rotation: Patient Prone

With this type of motion palpation, do not drop the center abdominal section because a flattened lumbar spine is easier to palpate

than one that is lordotic. Unlock the lateral flexion mechanism. Position yourself on that side of the table which allows your nondominant hand to laterally flex the table. This will leave your dominant hand free to palpate.

The first step is to place your palpating thumb against the spinous process of L5 and push it away as you simultaneously pull the upper half of the table toward you. During the first few degrees of table motion, spring the L5 spinous to see if it can rotate a degree or so. The second step is to push the table back toward neutral, and hook your index and third finger over the contralateral side of

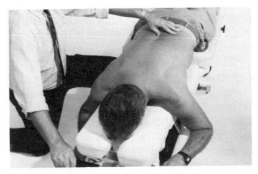

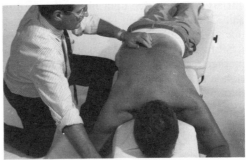

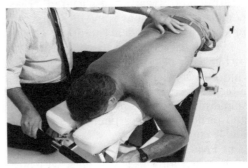

Figure 5.42. Evaluating lumbar rotation mobility on a mobile adjusting table with patient prone. *Top,* step one; *middle,* step two; *bottom,* step three. Refer to text for explanation of each step.

L5's spinous process. Then the third step is to pull and spring the L5 spinous process toward you as you push the table a few degrees laterally away. See Figure 5.42. Repeat this process up through the thoracolumbar junction to above the T11 level.

It is important to note that the spinous processes move in the opposite direction when the spine is in the prone position; ie, the spinous processes rotate to the convexity during lateral flexion. This rotation is only a degree or so. The significant feature to evaluate is the springy elastic barrier of the joint being examined. The lack of this rotation often releases during the testing procedure. [See Clinical Comment 5.5]

Lumbar Lateral Flexion: Patient Prone

Using the same method described above, pull the upper half of the table into full lateral flexion and continue to push the spinous process being tested toward the spinal convexity. The spinous process will serve as a lever to help you determine if a springy motion is palpable at full lateral flexion. Loss of joint motion on the convex side of the lumbar curve will restrict lateral flexion. Once again, (1) pull the table toward yourself and push the spine away by using your thumb against the spinous process of the segment being tested; then (2) push the table away and pull the spinous process with your index and 3rd finger to see if the ipsilateral joints are opening during lateral flexion (Fig. 5.43).

Y-Axis Translation

Palpate a potential y-axis fixation with the abdominal piece of the motorized table dropped. The superior edge of the patient's iliac crests should be positioned in line with the top edge

of the pelvic cushion. As the position of the pelvic section of the table descends at the caudad end, palpate the degree of separation within the interspinous spaces. In addition, push gently with the heel of your hand to determine if slight z-axis translation occurs (Fig. 5.44). The spinous processes should separate, and the lumbar joints should have a springy end point. You will likely find that gentle thrusts on the spine during the downward stroke of the pelvic section will often release both y-axis and z-axis restrictions.

Flexion/Extension of Lumbar Spine: Patient Laterally Recumbent

With the patient placed on their side and the downward iliac crest on the pelvic por-

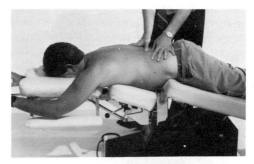
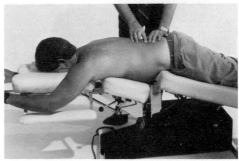

Figure 5.43. Evaluating lumbar y-axis translation on a mobile adjusting table. *Top,* step one; *bottom,* step two. Refer to text for explanation of each step.

DR. FAYE'S CLINICAL COMMENT #5.5

Spinal adjusting during motorized motion is a fairly new method of restoring fixated joints to normal function. With a motorized y-axis distraction table, less physically endowed doctors can now much more easily restore specific ranges of spinal motion. It has been shown by Eckard in a personal demonstration that up to 50% less force is necessary for some forms of lumbar and thoracic manipulation when using motorized mechanical traction. The test equipment used by Eckard contained computerized pressure gauges located underneath the sections of the table.

tion of the table: (1) Position the table's abdominal and head sections to produce lumbar flexion of the patient's spine. The patient's interspinous spaces should separate and approximate as the table is pushed back into neutral. (2) Continue pushing the table back until extension of the patient's spine occurs. The spinous processes should then close farther. Spring the joints at the end of each range of motion to see if normal zygapophyseal end play exists. See Figure 5.45.

Closing Remarks

Experience with motion palpation will greatly improve the chiropractor's efficiency in the diagnosis and treatment of patients with low-back pain complaints. Prior to training in motion palpation, it is not uncommon for the physician to wonder why one case responds well and another is a failure. When you are able to monitor the spinal corrections you achieve with dynamic chiropractic, you will soon learn from past successes and temporary failures. In this way,

you will improve with each spine placed in your care.

The large bonus, states Faye, is that your patients will also respect your ability to examine a spine. They will want you to conduct the same examination on the members of their families, their friends, and acquaintances. The need for your services in your community will grow with your increasing ability to change spinal mobility and improve subluxation complexes. And you will know why!

It is important to note that motion palpation is a method of analyzing the movement component of a subluxation complex. It does not matter what particular technique you use in practice. If you desire, you can see objectively just how effective your method is in a particular patient. Your successes will demonstrate improvement in spinal mobility and your failures will not. The alert doctor will determine the cause of why these fixations are not responding and change his or her therapeutic approach or find the source of the cause (Fig. 5.46).

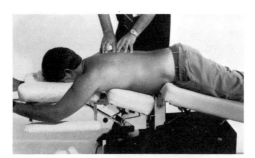

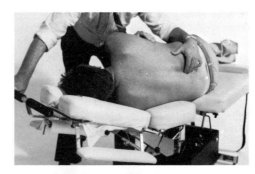

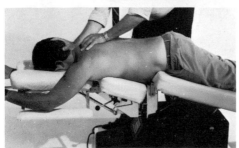

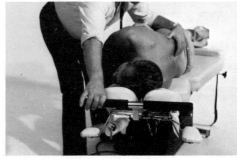

Figure 5.44. Checking upper thoracic interspinous mobility with the patient prone on a mobile adjusting table. *Top,* palpating the interspinous space; *bottom,* using the heel of the hand to determine if slight z-axis translation occurs.

Figure 5.45. Palpating flexion/extension mobility of the lumbar spine with the patient laterally recumbent. *Top,* step one; *bottom,* step two. Refer to text for explanation of each step.

Bibliography

Bachman DC, Noble HB: Helping the patient with low back pain. *Modern Medicine*, 46(4):34-37.

Beal MC: The sacro-iliac problem: review of anatomy, mechanics, and diagnosis. *Journal of the American Osteopathic Association*, vol 81, June 1982.

Bell GR, Rothman RH: The conservative treatment of sciatica. *Spine*, 9:54-56, 1984.

Bellamy N, Park W, Rooney P: What do we know about sacro-iliac joints? *Seminars in Arthritis and Rheumatism*, 12(3):282-305, February 1983.

Blower PW: Neurologic patterns in unilateral sciatica: a prospective study of 100 new cases. *Spine*, 6:175-179, 1981.

Bogduk N: The innervation of the lumbar spine. *Spine*, 8(3):286-291, 1983.

Bogduk N: Lumbar dorsal ramus syndrome. *Medical Journal of Australia*, 2:537-541, 1980.

Brewer BJ: Low-back pain. *American Family Physician*, 19:114-119, 1979.

Breig A: *Adverse Mechanical Tension in the C.N.S.* New York, John Wiley & Sons.

Brodin H: Inhibition-facilitation technique for lumbar pain treatment. *Manuell Medizin*, 20:95-98, 1982.

Brunarski DJ: Functional considerations of spinal manipulative therapy. *ACA Journal of Chiropractic*, May 1980.

Burton AK: Back pain in osteopathic practice. *Rheumatology and Rehabilitation*, 20:239-246, 1981.

Burton CV: Conservative management of low back pain. *Postgraduate Medicine*, 70:168-183, 1981.

Cailliet R: *Low Back Pain Syndrome*, ed 3. Philadelphia, F.A. Davis, 1981, pp 1-21, 44-51, 53-67, 69-78.

Cailliet R: *Soft Tissue Pain and Disability*. Philadelphia, F.A. Davis, 1980, pp 41-54.

Calin A: Back pain: mechanical or inflammatory? *American Family Physician*, 20:97-100, 1979.

Carmichael SW, Burkart SL: Clinical anatomy of the lumbosacral complex. *Physical Therapy*, 59:966-975, 1979.

Cassidy JD, Potter GE: Motion examination of the lumbar spine. *Journal of Manipulative and Physiological Therapeutics*, 2(3):151-158, September 1979.

Chusid JG: *Correlative Neuroanatomy & Functional Neurology*, ed 19. Los Altos, CA, Lange Medical, 1985, pp 150-161.

Cox HH: Sacro-iliac subluxation as a cause of backache. *Surgery, Gynecology, and Obstetrics*, 45:637-48, 1927.

Crock HV: Normal and pathological anatomy of the lumbar spinal nerve root canals. *Journal of Bone & Joint Surgery* (British), 63:487-490, 1981.

Cyriax E: Some common postural deformities and their treatment by exercise and manipulation. *British Journal of Physical Medicine*, June 1938.

D'Amico JC: The postural complex. *Journal of the American Podiatry Association*, August 1976.

Daniels L, Worthingham C: *Muscle Testing: Techniques of Manual Examination*, ed 4. Philadelphia, W.B. Saunders, 1980, pp 22-29, 34-35.

Dinnar U: Classification of diagnostic tests used with osteopathic manipulation. *Journal of the American Osteopathic Association*, 79(7):451-455, March 1980.

Drevet JG, Chirossel JP, Phelip X: Lumbago-lumbo-radiculalgia and posterior vertebral joints. *Lyon Medical*, 245:781-787, 1981.

Dvorak J: Neurological and biomechanical aspects of back pain. In Buerger AA, Greenman PE (eds): *Empirical Approaches to the Validation of Spinal Manipulation*. Springfield, MO, Charles C. Thomas, 1985, pp 241-262.

Ebel JN: Reflex relationships of paravertebral muscles. *American Journal of Physiology*, 200(5), May 1961.

Edgelow PI: Physical examination of the lumbosacral complex. *Physical Therapy*, 59:974-977, 1979.

Evans DC: Biomechanics of spinal injury. In Gonzna ER, Harrington IJ: *Biomechanics of Musculoskeletal Injury*. Baltimore, Williams & Wilkins, 1982, pp 204-212.

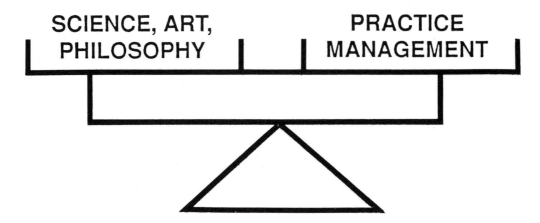

Figure 5.46. The ideal practice is well balanced.

Evans DP: *Backache: Its Evolution and Conservative Treatment*. Baltimore, University Park Press, 1982, pp 21-30, 40-43, 55-63, 161-165.

Evans FG: Some basic aspects of biomechanics of the spine. *Archives of Physical Medicine and Rehabilitation*, 51:214-226, 1970.

Farfan HF, et al: The effects of torsion on the lumbar intervertebral joints: The role of torsion in the production of disc degeneration. *Journal of Bone and Joint Surgery*, 52A:468, 1970.

Farfan HF: Symptomatology in terms of the pathomechanics of low-back pain and sciatica. In Haldeman S (ed): *Modern Developments in the Principles and Practice of Chiropractic*. New York, Appleton-Century-Crofts, 1980.

Farrell JP, Twomey LT: Acute low back pain: comparison of two conservative approaches. *Journal of the Australian Medical Association*, 1:160-164, 1982.

Faye LJ: Chiropractic Manipulation of the Lumbar Spine [Videotape]. Los Angeles, Dynaspine, 1987.

Faye LJ: Manipulation I [Cassette tape program]. Huntington Beach, CA, Motion Palpation Institute, 1983, 6 tapes.

Faye LJ: *Spine I: Motion Palpation and Clinical Considerations of the Lumbar Spine and Pelvis*. Huntington Beach, CA, Motion Palpation Institute, 1987, pp 15-20, 22-27.

Finneson BE: *Low Back Pain*. Philadelphia, J.B. Lippincott, 1973, pp 7-9, 93-132, 141-177, 256-287, 325-326.

Fisk JW: *The Painful Neck and Back*. Springfield, IL, Charles C. Thomas, 1977, pp 13-34, 91-114, 169-193.

Fosse M: A clinical study of lumbar spine movement using an external method of measurement. Brussels, Prestoprint, 1972. Anglo-European College of Chiropractic. Thesis.

Gehweiler JA Jr, Osborne RL Jr, Becker RF: *The Radiology of Vertebrae Trauma*. Philadelphia, W.B. Saunders, 1980, pp 267-273, 296-299, 401-429, 446-447.

Gillet H: Evolution of a chiropractor. *National Chiropractic Journal*, November 1945, January 1949, December 1949, January 1951.

Gillet H, Liekens M: *Belgian Chiropractic Research Notes*. Huntington Beach, CA, Motion Palpation Institute, 1984, pp 8-9, 15, 17-18, 36, 133-135.

Gillet H, Liekens, M: A further study of spinal fixations. *Annals of the Swiss Chiropractic Association*. Geneva, IV:41, 1967.

Gitelman R: A chiropractic approach to biomechanical disorders of the lumbar spine and pelvis. In Haldeman S (ed): *Modern Developments in the Principles and Practice of Chiropractic*. New York, Appleton-Century-Crofts, 1980, pp 297-299, 314-320.

Gottlieb HJ, Alperson BL, Koller R, Hockersmith V: An innovative program for the restoration of patients with chronic back pain. *Physical Therapy*, 59:996-999, 1979.

Gowitzke BA, Gowitzke MM: *Understanding the Scientific Bases of Human Movement*, ed 2. Baltimore, Williams & Wilkins, 1980.

Gracovetsky S, Farfan HF, Lamy C: The mechanism of the lumbar spine. *Spine*, 6:249-262, 1981.

Grice AS, Fligg DB: Class notes: Spinal dynamics. Department of Biomechanics/Kinesiology, BK202. Toronto, Canadian Memorial Chiropractic College, date not shown, pp 36-41.

Grieve GP: *Common Vertebral Joint Problems*. New York, Churchill Livingstone, 1981, pp 17-29, 34, 48-55, 60-62, 143-158, 198, 200.

Grynbaum BB, Belandres PV: Managing low back pain. *Female Patient*, 3:43-45, 1978.

Gunn CC, Milbrandt WE: Early and subtle signs in low-back sprain. *Spine*, 3(3):267-281, September 1978.

Hadley LA: *Anatomico-Roentgenographic Studies of the Spine*. Springfield, IL, Charles C. Thomas, 1981, pp 230-252, 399, 401, 404.

Hasue M, Kikuchi S, Sakuyama Y, Ito T: Anatomic study of the interrelation between lumbosacral nerve roots and their surrounding tissues. *Spine*, 8:50-58, 1983.

Helfet AJ, Gruebel Lee DM: *Disorders of the Lumbar Spine*. Philadelphia, J.B. Lippincott, 1978, pp 3-25, 27-31, 38, 42-48, 51-61, 69-82, 116, 145-161, 170-182, 219-220, 237-242.

Hoehler FK: Low back pain and its treatment by spinal manipulation: measures of flexibility and asymmetry. *Rheumatology and Rehabilitation*, 21:21-26, 1982.

Howe JW: Determination of lumbo-sacral facet subluxations. *Roentgenological Briefs*, Council on Roentgenology of the American Chiropractic Association, date not shown.

Hviid H: Erect working posture. *Annals of the Swiss Chiropractors' Association*, VI:71-90, 1976.

Janse J: Differentiation and interpretation of spinal pain syndromes. *Notes on Correlative Techniques*. Chicago, National College of Chiropractic, date not shown.

Janse J: *Principles and Practice of Chiropractic*. Lombard, IL, National College of Chiropractic, 1976, pp 45-46, 116, 187-196.

Jayson MIV, et al: Mobilization and manipulation for low back pain. *Spine*, 6:4, July-August 1981.

Jayson MIV, Sims-Williams H, Young S, Baddeley H, Collins E: Mobilization and manipulation for low-back pain. *Spine*, 6:409-416, 1981.

Johnston WL: The role of static and motion palpation in structural diagnosis. In Goldstein M (ed): *The Research Status of Spinal Manipulative Therapy*. NINCDS Monograph No. 15, DHEW Publication No. (NIH) 76-998, Stock No. 017-049-000607, Washington, DC, U.S. Government Printing Office, 1975.

Kanse J: The clinical biomechanism of the sacro-iliac mechanism. *ACA Journal of Chiropractic*, 12:S-1, January 1978.

Kapandji IA: *Physiology of the Joints: Lower Limb*, ed 2. New York, Churchill Livingstone, 1981, vol III, pp 54-57, 68, 74-78, 80-82, 86, 88-106, 114-118, 120.

Kirkaldy-Willis WH: Five common back disorders: How to diagnose and treat them. *Geriatrics*, December 1978.

Kirkaldy-Willis WH: A more precise diagnosis for low back pain. *Spine*, 4(2), March-April 1979.

Kirkaldy-Willis WH: The relationship of structural pathology to the nerve root. *Spine*, 9:49-52, 1984.

Kirkaldy-Willis WH, Wedge JH, Young-Hing K, Reilly J: Pathology and pathogenesis of lumbar spondylosis and stenosis. *Spine*, 3(4):319-328, December 1978.

Kuo PP, Tang HF: Manipulation as a treatment of low back pain. *The Journal of the Western Pacific*

Orthopaedic Association, 2:31-34, 1983.

Lamb DW: The neurology of spinal pain. *Physical Therapy*, 59:971-973, 1979.

Leavitt F, Garron DC, D'Angelo CM, McNeill TW: Low back pain in patients with and without demonstrable organic disease. *Pain*, 6:191-200, 1979.

LeVeau B: *Williams and Lissner: Biomechanics of Human Motion*. Philadelphia, W.B. Saunders, 1977.

Lewit K: Post-isometric relation in combination with other methods of muscular facilitation and inhibition. *Manuell Medizin*, (2:101-104, 1986.

Macnab I: *Backache*. Baltimore, Williams & Wilkins, 1977, pp 19-23, 44-63, 69-74, 98-104, 133-207.

Malik DD, et al: Recovery from radiculalgia by chiropractic adjustment and physical therapy. *ACA Journal of Chiropractic*, June 1984.

Manipulation in lumbar intervertebral disc protrusion. *Chinese Medical Journal*, 3(1):31-36, January 1977.

Markey LP: Markey distraction technique: new protocol for doctor and patient safety, part I. *The Digest of Chiropractic Economics*, September-October 1985.

Markolf KL: Deformation of the thoracolumbar intervertebral joints in response to external loads. *Journal of Bone and Joint Surgery*, 54A:511-533, 1972.

Martin L, et al: A comparative study between loss of joint play by evaluating (1) a patient in active sitting palpation as described by L. Faye, DC, as compared to (2) passive joint play using the Hill table. Canadian Memorial Chiropractic College, Toronto, 1982. Thesis.

McAndrews JF: Spinal motion examination. *ACA Journal of Chiropractic*, May 1969.

McCall IW, Park WM, O'Brien JP: Induced pain referral: posterior lumbar elements in normal subjects. *Spine*, 4(5):441-446, September/October 1979.

McGregor M, Cassidy JD: Post-surgical sacro-iliac joint syndrome. *Journal of Manipulative and Physiological Therapeutics*, 6(1), March 1983.

McKenzie RA: *The Lumbar Spine: Mechanical Diagnosis and Therapy*. Waikane, NZ, Spinal Publications, 1981, pp 1-2, 4-5, 87-90.

McRae R: *Clinical Orthopaedic Examination*, ed 2. New York, Churchill Livingstone, 1983, pp 71-96.

Mensor M, Duval G: Absence of motion at the fourth and fifth lumbar interspaces in patients with and without low-back pain. *Journal of Bone and Joint Surgery*, 41-A(6):1047-1054.

Mior SA, Cassidy JD: Lateral nerve root entrapment: pathological, clinical, and manipulative considerations. *The Journal of the Canadian Chiropractic Association*, 26(1):13-20, March 1982.

Molloy RD: A correlation between muscle testing and chiropractic treatment. Anglo-European College of Chiropractic, 1976. Thesis.

Moore KL: *Clinically Oriented Anatomy*. Baltimore, Williams & Wilkins, 1980, pp 127-137, 617-618.

Morris JM: Biomechanics of the spine. *Archives of Surgery*, 107:418-423, 1973.

Mumenthaler M: *Neurology*, ed 2. Translated by EH Burrows. New York, Thieme-Stratton, 1983, pp 361-363.

Murphy KA, Cornish D: Prediction of chronicity in acute low back pain. *Archives of Physical Medicine & Rehabilitation*, 65:334-337, 1984.

Nachemson AL: The lumbar spine, an orthopaedic challenge. *Spine*, 1(1):59-68, March 1976.

Nash CL, Moe JH: A study of vertebral rotation. *Journal of Bone and Joint Surgery*, 51:223, 1969.

Ng SY: Sacro-iliac lumbar mechanism. *ACA Journal of Chiropractic*, pp 51-59. April 1983.

Offierski CM, Macnab I: Hip-spine syndrome. *Spine*, 8(3):316-321.

Olsen GA, Hamilton A: The lateral stability of the spine. *Clinical Orthopaedics*, 65:143, 1969.

Olsen RE: Acute lumbosacral angle. *Roentgenological Briefs*, Council on Roentgenology of the American Chiropractic Association, date not shown.

Panjabi MM, Goel VK, Takata K: Physiologic strains in the lumbar spinal ligaments. *Spine*, 7:192-203, 1982.

Park WM, McCall IW, O'Brien JP, Webb JK: Fissuring of the posterior annulus fibrosis in the lumbar spine. *British Journal of Radiology*, 52:382-387, 1979.

Parke WW: Applied anatomy of the spine. In Rothman RH, Simeone FA (eds): *The Spine*. Philadelphia, W.B. Saunders, 1975, vol I, p 27.

Pennal GF, et al: Motion study of the lumbar spine: A preliminary report. *Journal of Bone and Joint Surgery*, 54B:3, August 1972.

Peters RE: The facet syndrome. *Journal of the Australian Chiropractors' Association*, 13:15-18, 1983.

Poole PB: Considerations of neurogenic pain. *Ortho Briefs*, Council on Chiropractic Orthopedics of the American Chiropractic Association, Fall 1982.

Porter RW, Hibbert C, Wellman P: Backache and the lumbar spinal canal. *Spine*, 5:99-105, 1980.

Roaf R: A study of the mechanics of spinal injuries. *Journal of Bone and Joint Surgery*, 42B:810-823, 1960.

Rothman RH, Simeone FA: Lumbar disc disease. In Rothman RH, Simeone FA (eds): *The Spine*. Philadelphia, W.B. Saunders, 1975, vol II, pp 443-506.

Ruge D, Wiltse LL (eds): *Spinal Disorders: Diagnosis and Treatment*. Philadelphia, Lea & Febiger, 1977.

Sandoz R: New trends in the pathogenesis of spinal disorders. *Annals of the Swiss Chiropractic Association*, V:93, 1971.

Sandoz R: Some reflex phenomena associated with spinal derangements and adjustments. *Annals of the Swiss Chiropractic Association*, VII:45, 1981.

Schafer RC: *Chiropractic Management of Sports and Recreational Injuries*. Baltimore, Williams & Wilkins, 1982, pp 283-286, 442-452

Schafer RC: *Chiropractic Physical and Spinal Diagnosis*. Oklahoma City, Associated Chiropractic Academic Press, 1980, pp IV: 7, 10, 29; XIII:1-8, 15-19.

Schafer RC: *Clinical Biomechanics: Musculoskeletal Actions and Reactions*. Baltimore, Williams & Wilkins, 1983, pp 375-388, 412-431.

Schafer RC: *Physical Diagnosis: Procedures and Methodology in Chiropractic Practice*. Arlington, VA, American Chiropractic Association; Chapter 20, Physical Examination of the Lumbar Spine and Pelvic Girdle. In development; scheduled to be released in 1989.

Schafer RC: *Symptomatology and Differential Diagnosis*. Arlington, VA, 1986, pp 788-840.

Sharpless SK: Susceptibility of spinal roots to compression block. In Gold stein M (ed): *The Research Status of Spinal Manipulative Therapy*. NINCDS

Monograph No. 15, DHEW Publication No. (NIH) 76-998, Stock No. 017-04900060-7, Washington, DC, U.S. Government Printing Office, 1975.

Simons DG, Travell JG: Myofascial origins of low back pain. *Postgraduate Medicine*, 73(2):66-108, February 1983.

Stonebrink RD: Palpation for vertebral motoricity. *ACA Journal of Chiropractic*, February 1969.

Sunderland S: Anatomical perivertebral influences on the intervertebral fora men. In Goldstein M (ed): *The Research Status of Spinal Manipulative Therapy*. NINCDS Monograph No. 15, DHEW Publication No. (NIH) 76-998, Stock No. 017 049-00060-7, Washington, DC, U.S. Government Printing Office, 1975.

Sweere JJ: A method of physiological testing in the differential diagnosis of acute mechanical low back pain. *Orthopedic Brief*, ACA Council on Chiropractic Orthopedics, September 1984.

Travell J: Myofascial trigger points: Clinical view. In Bonica JJ, Albe Fessard D (eds): *Advances in Pain Research and Therapy*. New York, Raven Press, 1976.

Triano J: Significant lumbar dyskinesia. *ACA Journal of Chiropractic*, February 1980.

Turek SL: *Orthopaedics: Principles and Their Application*, ed 3. Philadelphia, J.B. Lippincott, 1977, pp 1322-1333, 1339-1341, 1350-1353, 1356-1358, 1362-1366, 1383-1389.

Van Dusen LG: *Chiropractic Relationship to Gravitational Force*. Sodus, NY, published by author, 1968, pp 87, 91, 93, 97, 103,

Voloshin A, Wosk J: An in vivo study of low back pain and shock absorption in the human locomotor system. *Journal of Biomechanics*, 15:21-22, 1982.

Waddell G, McCulloch JA, Kummel E, Venner RM: Nonorganic physical signs in low back pain. *Spine*, 5:117-125, 1980.

Wax M: Procedures in elimination of trigger points in myofascial pain syndromes. *ACA Journal of Chiropractic*, October 1962.

Weitz EM: The lateral bending sign. *Spine*, 6:388-397, July-August 1981.

West HG Jr: Physical and spinal examination procedures utilized in the practice of chiropractic. In Haldeman S (ed): *Modern Developments in the Principles and Practice of Chiropractic*. New York, Appleton-Century-Crofts, 1980, p 283.

White AA, Panjabi MM: *Clinical Biomechanics of the Spine*. Philadelphia, J.B. Lippincott, 1978, pp 78-81, 166-178, 184, 212, 251-264, 272, 295, 292-293, 297-302.

Wigh RE: The transitional lumbosacral osseous complex. *Skeletal Radiology*, 8:127-131, 1982.

Wilson FC: *The Musculoskeletal System: Basic Processes and Disorders*, ed 2. Philadelphia, J.B. Lippincott, 1983, pp 67-69.

Wyke BD: Articular neurology and manipulative therapy. In *Aspects of Manipulative Therapy*. Proceedings of Multidisciplinary International Conference on Manipulative Therapy, Melbourne, Lincoln Institute of Health Sciences, Carlton, Victoria, Australia, August 1979, pp 67-72.

Yang KH, King AI: Mechanism of facet load transmission as a hypothesis for low back pain. *Spine*, 9:557-565, 1984.

Chapter 6

The Pelvis

This chapter draws attention to the effects of fixations occurring within the pelvis (viz, the sacroiliac and pubic joints). Basic biomechanical, diagnostic, and adjustive considerations are described, along with some important points that will be helpful during differential diagnosis.

BASIC CONSIDERATIONS

Illi reported that sacroiliac fixation of any degree inhibits the compensatory torsion capacity of the spinal segments. When the mobile spine is flexed forward, there is always a degree of related lumbar torsion. If the sacroiliac joint is locked, however, normal torsion is restricted and axial torsion of the cord and nerve roots is produced. If this occurs, far-reaching neurologic and biomechanical manifestations can manifest.

From a purely biomechanical viewpoint, the greater the degree of sacroiliac fixation, the greater degree of stress placed upon the primary load-transferral points; ie, the lumbosacral and hip joints. If this stress cannot be spread to other adaptable links in the kinematic chain, local symptoms will arise.

Any degree of sacroiliac fixation or hypermobility disturbing reciprocal motion bilaterally can be associated with:

• The direction of excessive rotary forces to the lumbar spine, leading to disc protrusion and potential rupture.

• An adaptive lumbar scoliosis away from the side of pain, leading to compensatory biomechanical changes in the thoracic and cervical regions.

• Compensatory overstress at the acetabulum, leading to hip pain and arthritis.

• Rotational overstress at the knee to widen the base of support, leading to chronic sprain. Such effects may extend as far distal as the ankle and foot.

Applied Anatomical Considerations

The mechanical link between the axial skeleton and the lower extremities is the pelvic basin. Each half of the pelvic girdle consists of the ilium, ischium, and pubic bones that are three separate bones during early life that, through custom, retain their separate identity in adulthood even though they become completely fused and function as one bone. Although the hip joint is classically considered part of the lower extremity from an anatomical viewpoint, it is so closely linked functionally to the innominates, sacrum, and lumbar spine that it must be considered in any discussion of the pelvis.

The anterior superior iliac spine (ASIS), anterior inferior iliac spine (AIIS), posterior superior iliac spine (PSIS), posterior inferior iliac spine (PIIS), and symphysis pubis are the common landmarks of the pelvis (Fig. 6.1).

The summit of the iliac crest is typically listed as being on a level with the L4 spinous process and the PSIS on a level with the S2 spinous (near the midline of the lower third of the sacroiliac articulation. This textbook ideal, however, varies greatly from observations seen in clinical practice.

In our previous descriptions of the articular surfaces in the spine, we were dealing primarily with fairly flat or ovoid surfaces that met congruently unless pathologic changes or congenital deformities existed.

Spinal mechanisms of motion, thus, were not especially difficult to comprehend. Unfortunately, this is not true for the complex sacroiliac joints.

From an architectual design viewpoint, the pelvis consists of several interlocking triangles, resembling an inverted pyramid from the front, back, and sides. The dorsal surface of the sacrum is convex, and its anterior surface is concave. To meet with the ilia, which are forced to flare laterally (P-A) because of the angle of the upper and lower sacral facets, the S1—S3 segments are wider anteriorly than posteriorly (Fig. 6.2). It is within this area, from S1 to approximately between S2 and S3 that the sacroiliac joint extends.

The concave sacral articulations with the ilia are congruently bootshaped, and numerous bumps and depressions of the articulating surfaces help to offer stability and limit motion. The ridges and furrows of the sacrum, however, are not always ideally reciprocal with those of the ilium nor are the bilateral planes of articulation commonly symmetrical. The ilia resemble an inverted triangle when viewed laterally.

The Sacroiliac Joint Complex

The Ilia. The ilia are the broad superior portions of the innominate. They are fused with the pubic bones that articulate anteriorly with the symphysis pubis and posteriorly with the sacrum. The flared wings (upper aspect) of the ilia forms the *major pelvis* (false pelvis), which supports the contents of the lower abdominal quadrants. The lower half of the pelvis forms the *minor pelvis* (true pelvis), which is surrounded by the pubes, lower ilia, ischia, sacrum, and coccyx (considered inconsequential). Cups within the inferior aspects of the ilia form the superior aspects of the acetabula.

The Iliac Facets. Anterolateral to the PSIS and PIIS of the ilia are the complex facets that articulate with the sacrum. These facets resemble rough, concave, bony ears that face backward or forward, depending upon the area being considered. Some authorities refer to these facets as being *boot shaped*, with the toes of the boots pointing backward. Regardless of the descriptive sim-

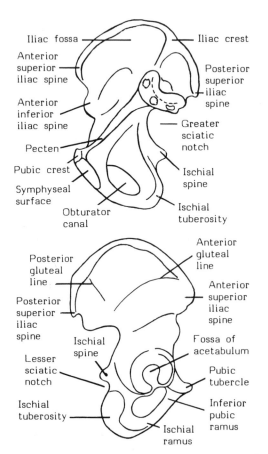

Figure 6.1. Major features of the medial aspect of the pelvis, *top,* and the lateral aspect of the pelvis, *bottom* (Courtesy ACAP).

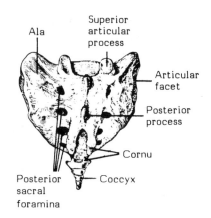

Figure 6.2. Posterior view of the sacrum, pointing out some major features (Courtesy ACAP).

iles used, the iliac facets are slightly wider than their mates on the sacrum.

The "foot" of the articulation allows a slight sliding motion anterior-inferiorly or posterior-superiorly and a distinct rotating action about the pit. The leg of the boot articulates at the level of the S1 tubercle. The foot of the boot articulates between the S2 and S3 segments. This design has a distinct influence on traumatic iliosacral motion. The upper pit also serves to offer osseous relief to the relatively weak superoanterior sacroiliac ligaments. Another important role of this design is to prevent sacral displacement during loaded movements. Superior and posterior to the articular surface is a larger area of rough bone that serves for the attachment of strong sacroiliac ligaments.

The articular surfaces of both the sacrum and ilium are fairly smooth during childhood and do not exhibit their rough ridges and furrows until after puberty. Like fingerprints, their exact design is unique to the individual. In the child, stability is essentially ligamentous.

According to Boorsma, the boot-shaped design of the sacral facets is typically deep, oblique, and mobile, and it is especially related to a hyperlordotic spine. When associated with a flattened lumbar spine, the sacroiliac articulation is generally more bean shaped, vertical, shallow, and less mobile.

The most important point to remember about the sacroiliac joints is this boot-shaped design (when viewed from the side), in which two distinct articulations are found: one above the ankle of the boot, which articulates with the S1 segment, and one at the foot of the boot that articulates between the S2 and S3 segments. An oversimplified comparison of these two areas of articulation (at the superior and inferior aspects of the joint) would be a link in a bicycle chain. The upper joint is more influenced by body weight descending via the lumbosacral articulation, and the lower joint is more influenced by forces ascending from the lower extremity via the head of the femoral-ilial articulation. When mobile, these two articulations act reciprocally; when one rotates in one direction, the other rotates in the reverse direction. However, if either the superior sacroiliac articulation or the inferior sacroiliac articulation becomes partially fixed,

the other can only pivot in an arc around the abnormal axis of the fixated articulation.

The Sacroiliac Joints. The sacroiliac joints are uniquely both diarthrotic and amphiarthotic. Gehweiler is one of several authorities who states that the sacral facet is covered by hyaline cartilage and that the iliac facet is covered by fibrocartilage. Others, however, report a variety of different findings. The inferior two-thirds of each joint is a true synovial articulation; the superior third is a fibrocartilaginous amphiarthrosis supported by the short but strong sacroiliac ligaments. Thus, a true polysynovitis can involve only the caudad aspect of the joint. Synovial membrane blankets the whole joint cavity except at its posterior aspect where it is replaced by large ligaments that attach to the articular cartilage. See Figure 6.3.

The slight but important rotating, sliding, gliding, and pivoting action of the sacroiliac facets serve as the singular link point where the axial skeleton is attached to the pelvis; thus the necessity of this joint being bilaterally strong and slightly mobile to adapt for biomechanical impairments deficiencies above and and below.

By puberty, in adaptation to walking and the imposed stress of daily living, the articulating bony surfaces develop a variety of acquired incongruities and small projections where dynamic stress would be concentrated if not for the smoothing effect of articular cartilage. Of all articulations, the sacroiliac joint contains a large array of reciprocal

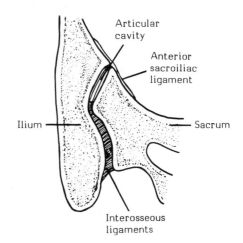

Figure 6.3. Schematic of the left sacroiliac joint as viewed from above.

bony hills and valleys. This joint surface roughness, more prominent in males, is generally considered the result of its segmental heritage; ie, the fused lateral tips of the transverse processes and the intertransverse spaces.

During aging degeneration, calcium infiltration of the joint appears within the fibrocartilage of the ilium long before changes occur in the hyaline coated sacral facet. This is attributed to the fact that the sacral cartilage is three times thicker than the iliac cartilage.

Grieve reports that more than 30% of the population possess accessory sacroiliac joints formed between the PSIS area and either S2 or S1. These accessory articulations, which are lined with fibrous cartilage or sometimes synovial membrane, are common sites of early osteoarthritic changes.

Sacroiliac Innervation and Referred Pain Patterns. The posterior aspect of the sacroiliac joint is innervated by posterior rami of the L5—S2 spinal nerves. Inflammation at the posterior aspect of the joint usually refers pain to the buttocks and back of the thigh, following dermatomal distribution. The anterior aspect of the joint is innervated by both posterior branches from the L3—S2 roots and the superior gluteal nerve (L5—S2). Irritation of the joint anteriorly commonly refers pain to the groin and anterior thigh. If the sciatic nerves pierces the piriformis rather than exiting the pelvis over or under the muscle (a common occurrence), sacroiliac distortion or inflammation may involve any of the numerous sciatic fibers.

The Sacrococcygeal Joints

The joint between the last sacral segment and the first segment of the coccyx is atypical. It is usually considered a symphysis, united by a rudimentary IVD and tough ligamentous bands around its circumference. Slight motion posteriorly is normal during defecation, gait, and more so during parturition.

Ligamentous Changes During Pregnancy

During pregnancy, all pelvic ligaments normally loosen. This is attributed to natural hormonal changes that occur at this time. Although this is beneficial for enhancing a less painful delivery, two adverse clinical effects of this hypermobility can occur. Many clinicians have found that: (1) the hypermobile joints may not fully return to their normal positioning following delivery; (2) as it takes several months for the relaxed ligaments to shorten to their prepartum state, sacroiliac and sacrococcygeal instability will predispose the mother to chronic sacroiliac irritation that frequently leads to a state of fixation if not properly monitored. The constant lifting of the child by the mother, often from awkward positions, plus other forms of loading, is certainly a contributing factor. This adds to the list of factors of why chiropractic postnatal care of both mother and child is important as a preventive procedure. [See Clinical Comment 6.1]

The Symphysis Pubis

Pubic innervation is achieved from branches of the L1—S4 fibers, thus referred pain can be diffuse or unpredictably specific. The forward portions of the hyaline coated pubes join at the fibrocartilaginous pad (anuclear disc) of the pubic symphysis. Slight but important movement takes place at this joint by the yielding of the interpubic fibrocartilage. For this reason, the plasticity, flex-

---

DR. FAYE'S CLINICAL COMMENT #6.1

The postpartum symphysis pubis often remains hypermobile as described by Sandoz in the **Annals of the Swiss Chiropractors' Association.** A special roentgenographic view taken with the patient standing on a 4-inch block under one foot and the other limb hanging will show a rise of the pubis superiorly on the side of groin pain or severe episodic sacroiliac pain. In chronic cases, a traction spur commonly forms at the sacroiliac joint inferiorly. During the past year, our practice has revealed three cases; thus, this condition is not rare.

ibility, and elasticity properties of the fibro-cartilaginous pad are important in the maintenance of normal pelvic biomechanics. Excessive pubic movement is normally restrained by the superior and inferior pubic ligaments. Clinically, what is more important is the fact that iliac motion imposes reciprocal compression, tensile, and torsional forces on the joint. Although fixation is often found, complete fusion is rare even in old age. [See Clinical Comment 6.2]

Biomechanical Considerations

The *three-joint complex* of a vertebral motion unit has been previously described. This complex consists of the disc anteriorly and the apophyseal facets posteriorly. A similar three-joint complex is seen in the pelvis. This complex consists of the symphysis pubis anteriorly and the sacroiliac facets posteriorly. Thus, the pelvis viewed as a unit has six degrees of freedom just as a vertebral motion unit. See Figure 6.4.

Kinematics of the Pelvis: General Considerations

The pelvic articulations are located fairly central to the kinematic chain that extends from the cranium to the feet. Thus, changes in normal pelvic dynamics such as a unilateral sacroiliac fixation can readily produce biomechanical inadequacies above and below the involved joint. As a general rule, motion impairment at a link or links of any kinematic chain forces hypermobility on the nearest possible adaptable segments.

When an individual is standing, body weight and any extrinsic loading of the upper body are transmitted from L5 to the sacral base, the sacroiliac joints, ilia, and ischia. Impact forces from below arise from the foot via the tibia and femur. These axial forces meet at the acetabulum and are dispersed transversely (primarily), to be absorbed by the cartilages and ligaments of the hip joints, sacroiliac joints, symphysis pubis, and the spongiosa of pelvic bone. The gross effect is locking of the involved joints by the opposing forces traveling around each side of the pelvis anteriorly and posteriorly from the acetabulum. If these counterdirected axial forces are not equalized, the pelvis cannot be in a state of equilibrium according to Newtonian principles. When the force from below is greater, the head of the femur tends to jam within the acetabulum. If the force from above is greater, the L5 and S1 end plates or sacroiliac joints tend to displace from their normal resting position (subluxate). Thus, the sacrum influences and is influenced by

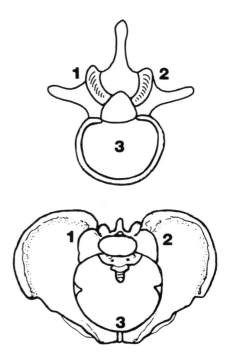

Figure 6.4. The three-point articular complex in a vertebral segment, *top*, as compared to that of the pelvis, *bottom* (Courtesy ACAP).

DR. FAYE'S CLINICAL COMMENT #6.2

Hypermobile or hypomobile symphysis pubis joints will not only produce pain locally, they can also cause severe stress at the sacroiliac joints. In athletes that complain of recurring groin strains, it is necessary to obtain roentgenographs of the symphysis pubis to see if it is stable during the special proedure described in Clinical Comment #6.1. Alternately pulling one knee toward the chest and holding this position for about 30 seconds while sitting will help to mobilize a fixated symphysis pubis.

the trunk and lumbar spine, and the ilia influence and are influenced by the heads of the femur. These are important facts to remember when analyzing postural distortions.

Lumbosacral Motion. The transitional junction between L5 and S1 is a unique "universal joint." If the sacrum rotates anteroinferiorly on one side within the ilia, for example, L5 tends to rotate in the opposite direction because of the restraint of the iliolumbar ligament. A mechanical accommodation of the lumbar spine is produced above; viz, a posterior rotation on the side of the unilateral sacral anteroinferiority. It also tends to assume an anteroflexed position, thus producing the three-dimensional movements of the lumbar spine. Owing to the biomechanical intricacy of the lumbosacral junction, anomalies such as asymmetrical facets have a strong influence on predictable movements in this area. Such asymmetry is far more common than generally suspected.

Classes of Intrapelvic Motion. Gillet classifies intrapelvic mobilities into three categories: (1) the P-A and A-P rotations of the ilia relative to the sacrum, and to each other at the pubis, (2) the various movements of the sacrum itself in relation to the ilia, and (3) the sitting-standing changes that affect the relationship of the ilia to the sacrum and to each other. Another mobility important to consider is the motion of the sacrum at the lumbosacral joint where it moves passively with the ilia; eg, as seen in lateral flexion of the pelvis during gait. Weisl, Gonstad, and others report of an inferior or superior gliding motion along the caudal aspect of the sacroiliac facet.

Sacroiliac Motion

It was the strong conviction of the medical community for many years that there was no normal sacroiliac or pubic motion in the absence of disease or pregnancy and that the sacrum and innominates moved as a whole. This opinion was disputed by empirical evidence submitted by chiropractic and osteopathic physicians since the turn of the century and in recent years the allopathic assumption has been proved a fallacy through cineroentgenographic studies and reports submitted by objective scientists. Only since the 1970s has sacral motion been recognized in allopathic literature (an embarrassment never mentioned).

According to Illi, a human being is the only vertebrate with a movable sacroiliac articulation. At birth, the joint is only slightly movable. Sacroiliac function is the effect of bipedism. However, because sacroiliac and pubic articulations are readily subject to fixation, normal movement is not always exhibited in the adult within modern society where physical activity is minimal. Nevertheless, several autopsy studies report freely movable joints in individuals over the age of 80.

Faye mentions that since the sacroiliac joints form their shape as a child matures as a biped, it is absolutely necessary that all children be examined periodically to assure normal sacroiliac function. He states that "Sacroiliac dysfunction in the young leads to abnormal gait and muscle development."

For the sake of study, specific sacroiliac motions will be described. In vivo, however, these motions are always coupled when the articulations are mobile. There is no *one* normal movement of the sacrum upon the ilia. Not recognizing this point can lead to many analytical errors.

Slight but smooth sacroiliac motion occurs upward, downward, forward, and backward, and axial rotation occurs about a transverse axis to allow pelvic tilting. Because the sacrum does not have distinct articular planes but moves (floats) within the pelvic ring, its motion is multidirectional for 1—3 mm rather than in restricted specifically defined paths. This multidirectional movement of the sacrum is likely the result of (1) the wider iliac facet, (2) the longer sacral facet, and (3) the thick articular cartilage of the sacrum. As described previously, this diverse motion is especially passive in the non-weight-bearing positions and influenced above by lumbar forces and/or laterally and below by iliac-ischial forces.

Sacroiliac motion is a consequence of trunk or hip motion and must be able to accommodate both of these movements at the same time. For this reason, it is clinically important to be able to restore restricted sacroiliac function in all directions.

Axis of Rotation. Where the exact axes of rotation for the sacroiliac joints are has not been definitively determined. Farabeuf and DeJarnette place them posterior to the center of the whole joint's surface, posterior to the ankle of the boot (Fig. 6.5). Bonnaire and Cassidy place them anteriorly within the joints, near the heel of the boot. Weisl locates an axis for sacral rotation below the foot of the boot and a plane of transition that moves horizontally through the foot of the boot (Fig. 6.6). Shrader's model indicates that they are likely to be in a common plane that extends from the torsional center of the symphysis pubis through the center of each femoral head. Illi's studies arrived at a combination of Farabeuf's, Bonnaire's, and Weisl's findings. Gillet's findings will be described with various topics within this chapter.

Sacral Changes from Recumbent to Standing Positions. The sacrum approaches its nearest state of static equilibrium in the slightly flexed prone position where inferior and superior forces are removed. This is probably why sacral (eg, Logan Basic) and para-anal (eg, Watkins') reflex techniques achieve their greatest effect in this position. Several studies have shown that there is distinct sacral position alterations when changing position from the recumbent, to the sitting, to the standing postures. Gillet describes these changes in detail.

During forward flexion of the trunk in either the standing or sitting position, the sacral base pivots farther anteriorly and inferiorly, and the apex of the sacrum moves posteriorly and superiorly. Simultaneously, the

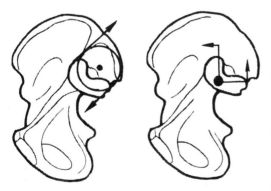

Figure 6.5. Farabeuf's axis (*left*) and Bonnaire's axis (*right*) of sacral rotation (Courtesy ACAP).

PSISs of the ilia move posteriorly, inferiorly, and obliquely medial so that the space between the spines is reduced. The ischia concurrently move obliquely anteriorly, superiorly, and fan laterally. During backward bending of the trunk, these pelvic actions are reversed. Note the reciprocal action between the A-P and P-A motions of the sacrum and the ilia and the reciprocity between the inward and outward flaring of the superior aspect of the ilia above and the ischia below.

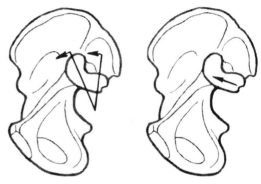

Figure 6.6. Weisl's axis of sacral rotation, *left,* and Weisl's plane of translation, *right* (Courtesy ACAP).

Standing P-A/A-P Sacroiliac Motion. During erect weight bearing, the base of the sacrum tends to rotate (pivot) anterior and inferior about the lateral S2 tubercles. When a standing subject lifts the right knee to a maximum, for example, as in taking a high step, the right ilium tends to follow the femur in its motion, rotating in the P-A/A-P plane with the approximate center of movement being at the head of the femur. Simultaneously, the right pubic bone moves upward in relation to its partner. This is palpable. The iliac portion of the sacroiliac articulation glides backward and downward relative to its contact with the sacrum. After this, the sacrum arcs posteriorly and inferiorly with the left ilium; ie, it is passively carried along by the active ilium. If both the pubic and sacroiliac articulations reach their limits of mobility and the knee is lifted still further, the pubic joint begins to serve as the center of rotation and, at the posterior aspect of the pelvis, the ilium start to pull the sacrum downward in its course, forcing it to compress against the opposite ilium. Because this latter movement does not follow the plane of the sacroiliac facets, a degree of joint separation must occur. If the knee lifting test is carried still further, the normal limit of the other articulation (the left in this example) will be reached, and then the whole pelvis becomes involved.

In the standing position described, motions of the sacrum relative to the ilia are sometimes difficult to detect because of coupled acetabular changes. Thus, it may be necessary to seat the patient to restrict these movements. Sitting fixes the pelvic base (the ischia), alters its shape, and allows a completely different type of motion than that seen in the standing position.

Sitting P-A/A-P Sacroiliac Rotational Motion. The sacrum readily flexes in the sitting position, turning between the two ilia. To produce this movement, the stabilizing arm of the examiner grasps the opposite shoulder of the patient across the chest and rotates the patient to a maximum while the examiner's palpating fingers follow the sacral spinous processes in their course. The lumbar region also rotates and flexes to follow the line of the thoracic vertebrae that move laterally in a wide arc. The placement of the sacrum can roughly be judged by the direction of the buttocks line.

Rotation and flexion of the sacrum in the sitting position carries the ilia along with it to a degree. Sacroiliac motion in the sitting position can be palpated by placing the thumb on the iliac crest or on the PSIS and following it forward and downward as the thorax is rotated in that direction. Note that most authorities agree that any degree of sacral rotation has a related translatory component.

Sacroiliac Motion During Lateral Flexion. During lateral bending, movement of the sacrum takes place with a maximum of tilting and a minimum of rotation. To palpate this movement, the shoulders of the patient must be put into a complete lateral bending posture, concentrating the movement in the area being palpated. Again, the ilia make an effort to follow this movement into lateral flexion.

Sacroiliac Motion During Walking. Axial or lateral rotation of the pelvis about a fixed femoral head is produced by actions of the muscles of the thigh, loin, and the abdominal obliques. This is exhibited in walking. Illi has shown that sacroiliac motion provides reciprocal action of the ilia and a gyroscopic motion of the sacrum during gait (Fig. 6.7). These motions tend to dampen the axially directed forces of heel strike. Illi reports that as the heel strikes, the ilium rotates posteriorly and inferiorly, the sacral base reciprocally rotates anteriorly and inferiorly, and the ipsilateral transverse of L5 is pulled backward. This vertebral action of the functional lumbar scoliosis diminishes cephally. During midstance, the pelvis moves over the femoral head in a neutral position. As the contralateral extremity is abducted forward, the sacrum is pulled backward and upward on that side. This reciprocal motion between the sacrum and ilium describes a horizontal figure 8 between the ilia when viewed during gait. One side of the sacral base arcs downward, forward, and rotates toward the ipsilateral side, while the other side swings upward, backward, and the sacral apex rotates toward the contralateral side. The path of this arc appears to be the product of (1) sacral translation and torque

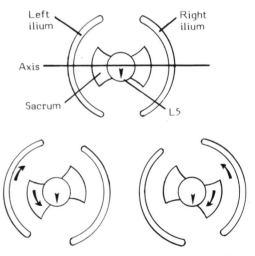

Figure 6.7. The normal gyroscopic motion of the sacrum during gait. *Top,* neutral position; *bottom left,* left swing phase; *bottom right,* right swing phase. Note that L5 normally maintains a relatively stable position over the sacrum (Courtesy ACAP).

having various components, depending on the planes of the bilateral facets, (2) the force vectors, and (3) the bilateral integrity of the involved restraining ligaments.

Sacral Motion During Breathing. The majority of references to this mechanism have been published by DeJarnette, Goodheart, and a number of osteopaths researching cranial manipulation and reflexes. They have found that there is slight sacral P-A and A-P motion during respiration and Valsalva maneuvers. The base of the sacrum tends to pivot posteriorly during inspiration (or increased intra-abdominal pressure) and anteriorly during expiration of 1—7 mm. The rate is about 14 excursions per minute. This mechanism, synchronized with a reciprocal cranial action, appears to produce a "pumplike action" on cerebrospinal fluid circulation, made possible by the continuous dural sheath that descends from the cranial vault through the spinal canal to insert near S2. This helps to explain why sacral and upper cervical dysfunctions are so frequently associated.

Pelvic Changes During Sitting

During sitting, where weight is borne essentially by the ischial prominences, the body attempts to broaden its base of support by slightly separating the ischia, which in turn slightly close the iliac crests superiorly. As the sacroiliac joint space opens inferiorly, the apex of the sacrum juts backward to remain in contact. That is, because of the oblique slant of the sacral facets, the sacral base nods anteriorly and the apex moves posteriorly. The axis of this motion is commonly a horizontal plane located at or near the S2 level. Articulation for this motion takes place at both the pubic and sacroiliac joints.

In arising, however, the ischia are passively brought together to permit body weight to lie directly over the heads of the femurs. The iliac crests then open laterally (flare). This closes the inferior sacral angle and opens the joint space that holds the base of the sacrum. In adaptation, the sacral base moves slightly backward and the apex nods forward. In considering A-P and P-A nodding of the sacrum, keep in mind that the position of the

ilia are not rigid and that the slant of the articulations force the ilia to adapt themselves to sacral flexion by lateral flexion of their own. Thus, we rotate each hip backward and forward each time we walk. Each time we sit and arise, we cause our ilia to flare outward and inward. Each time we bend or turn in a seated position, we cause the sacrum to turn within the interiliac space.

Anterior and Posterior Pelvic Tilt

In the neutral standing position, the ASISs normally lie in the same vertical plane as that of the symphysis pubis. The motions of the pelvis as a whole are (1) forward and backward tilt around the transverse interfemoral axis, (2) lateral tilt (associated with lumbar scoliosis), and (3) rotation in the horizontal plane. None of these motions are produced by intrinsic pelvic muscles; rather, they are produced by the muscles of the trunk and/or hip that attach to the pelvis or sacrum. These motions primarily occur at and affect the lumbosacral junction and the heads of the femurs. They involve the sacroiliacs to a much lesser degree.

Forward and backward pelvic tilts describe an arc that normally follows the arcuate (bow-shaped) ridge and groove of the sacroiliac facets.

• Forward tilt is related to lumbar hyperlordosis and hip flexion. The anterior thigh muscles are also a strong component in this motion, thus the frequent involvement of these muscles in pelvic distortions.

• Backward tilt is associated with lumbar flattening and hip extension. The major actions come from the posterior pull of the hamstrings and the anterior pull of the rectus abdominis, with help from the obliques.

If an individual shifts most body weight to one leg, passive lateral pelvic tilt occurs. The pelvis on the unsupported side is restricted actively by the gluteus medius and minimus and passively by the iliotibial band. When body weight is distributed bilaterally, lateral tilting of the pelvis is associated with lumboscoliosis, sacroiliac distortion, and a unilateral short leg, and likely a combination of these factors. [See Clinical Comment 6.3]

Lateral Pelvic Inclination

After studying 200 patients with a presenting complaint of low back pain, Greenman found that 64% exhibited lateral pelvic tilt (sacral base unilaterally inferior). A pelvic sag, as viewed from the anterior or posterior, can be the effect of several factors. The most common causes are unilateral lower extremity deficiency, muscle shortening or weakness, sacroiliac dysfunction, and hip or lower extremity alignment problems. Muscle fixation from lack of stretch is the second most common cause, second only to the common unilateral leg-length deficiency. See Figure 6.8.

From a biomechanical viewpoint, lateral pelvic inclination directs the lumbar curvature and that pelvic inclination is essentially determined by posture of the hips. Thus, the muscles of the hips are important factors in controlling pelvic inclination and the lumbar curve. During standing, the thighs are fixed points from which the hip muscles act. For example, shortening of the pelvic extensors (eg, glutei, hamstrings) reduces the dimension of the lumbar curve from front to back and rotates the pelvis posteriorly. Shortening of the pelvic flexors (eg, iliopsoas, rectus fe-

---

DR. FAYE'S CLINICAL COMMENT #6.3

In all low-back pain cases, it is essential to test for hamstring, quadriceps, and psoas length. Shortening of any of these muscles should be treated with PNF or spray-and-stretch techniques as a pre- or post-manipulative procedure. Stretching exercises at home should be prescribed as tolerated during active management as well as a preventive procedure.

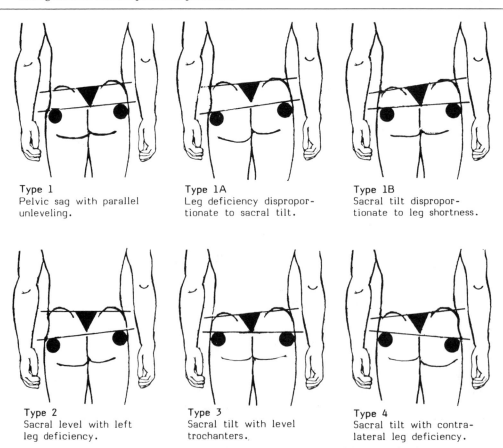

Type 1
Pelvic sag with parallel unleveling.

Type 1A
Leg deficiency disproportionate to sacral tilt.

Type 1B
Sacral tilt disproportionate to leg shortness.

Type 2
Sacral level with left leg deficiency.

Type 3
Sacral tilt with level trochanters.

Type 4
Sacral tilt with contralateral leg deficiency.

Figure 6.8. Greenman's classification of lateral pelvic tilt (Courtesy ACAP).

moris) increases the lumbar lordosis and tips the pelvic basin forward. Weakness of the antagonists would have the same effect. Thus, rehabilitation should be directed to relax and stretch muscles shortened by spasm or contracture and strengthen counterparts weakened by inactivity or constitutional factors. In mild—moderate cases, this need not be a dual activity as a muscle relaxes as its antagonist contracts against resistance.

In bilateral muscle checking during posture analysis, applied kinesiologists believe that most patients presenting with postural defects have muscle weakness rather than primary spasm. It is their contention that it is this weakness that causes the contralateral muscles to contract into an apparent spasm. Thus, the weakness is said to be primary and the spasm to be secondary. The spasm is thought to be the result of the prime-mover/antagonist reciprocal relationship. For example, an elevated iliac crest on the right may be due to weakness on the right of the psoas, gluteals, and tensor fascia lata or weakness on the left of the adductors, quadratus lumborum, rectus or transverse abdominis, or the sacrospinalis. Likewise, an elevated shoulder on the right may be due to weakness on the right of the latissimus dorsi, lower trapezius, anterior serratus, pectoralis major and minor, subscapularis, teres minor, infraspinatus, and levator scapulae or weakness on the left of the upper trapezius. These viewpoints, originated by Goodheart, have not been accepted by several authorities. Nevertheless, they do help to broaden our perspective.

Gillet's Comments on the Sacroiliac Articulations

There are four possible movements in the pelvic articulations (sacroiliac, sacrococcygeal, and pubic). The primary considerations are (1) movements of the sacrum in relation to the ilia in which the sacrum is active and the ilia try to follow the movement, (2) movements of the ilia relative to the sacrum, (3) and movements of the ilia relative to each other (at the pubic joint) in which the sacrum is passive and the ilia are active.

Pelvic Movements: General Considerations

In all movements of the trunk, upper body motion forces are transmitted from the structures to the lower ones in a decreasing degree since the motion must end upon a solid nonmoving structure, usually the floor or the seat of a chair. In all movements in which the trunk is almost passive, as in walking and running, the structures that move the most are the lower extremities, and this motion is transmitted to the upper structures in diminishing degrees. In these movements, therefore, the ilia move the most and the sacrum serves as a connecting link between the ilia and the spine. Farfan has shown a counter-rotation occurs by the swinging arms and pelvic swing that counterrotates to produce a kinetic energy of forward propulsion.

Another factor tends to complicate this study; ie, the functioning of each articulation is often different in weight bearing. Gillet has done little work on this subject but "a priori" feels that this would only show some articulations capable of physiologic locking according to the weight borne. In the study of fixations, therefore, it is necessary to keep this in mind and to analyze the spine without weight bearing, as far as this is possible.

The best known movement in the pelvis is the forward-backward rotation of an ilium. No definitive attempt has been made, as far as we know, to determine the exact pivot around which this motion takes place. In Belgium, the study group has tried to do so by palpation of a great number of cases. They are certain that this motion takes places around a point at or near the head of the femur. This means that the movement occurring at the pubis is a gliding motion of one articular surface upward and backwards. On the other hand, the contact of the ilia with the sacrum moves down and backward in its superior aspect and down and *forward* in its inferior aspect.

Standing Relationships

Normally, with the patient standing, and in spite of the amount of weight bearing that this movement applies to the opposite artic-ulation, the sacrum remains vertical. This means that, at least in its first part, the sacrum does not participate in this move-ment. Illi shows this in his motion x-ray films of the patient walking. If the articular sur-faces at the sacroiliac and pubic joints are completely free, not only will the sacrum re-main vertical during walking, it will remain so when the knee is pulled up flexed to an easy maximum height. In fact, it can be given as a rule that if on doing this movement the sacrum tilts to one side, there must be at least a partial fixation between the sacrum and the ilia.

The first part of iliac rotation posteriorly takes place with the moving ilium gliding down and backward on the surface of the sacrum. Soon, however, the end of the range of motion is reached. If the knee is lifted higher, the moving ilium carries the sacrum down with it. At this time, therefore, the mo-tion takes place between the sacrum and the opposite ilium: the sacrum moving down and the ilium remaining in its place relative to the limb bearing the weight of the body. It is important to understand this movement for we will see it again when all the possibilities of partial fixations have been described. [See Clinical Comment 6.4]

The second type of movement possible between the ilia and the sacrum and at the pubic joint is one that has practically never been described outside the literature of *dy-namic chiropractic*. During *standing*, the weight of the body is transmitted to the low-er extremity and then to the floor via the heads of the femurs. To do so, the pelvis changes its shape: the crests of the ilia sep-arate laterally and the ischia come closer together. This movement takes place around the pubis (which opens and closes at its su-perior and inferior aspects) and the sacrum.

Keep in mind that the shape of the sacrum resembles an inverted wedge when viewed from the anterior or posterior and also re-sembles a wedge when viewed from above because of the obliquity of the sacroiliac articulations. The movement of the ilia just described must necessarily produce a relat-ed movement of the sacrum for it to main-tain contact with the iliac facets. This move-ment is an anterior-posterior flexion, in which the sacral base moves posteriorly and its apex anteriorly during standing, and vice versa when during sitting. This, once more, necessitates free mobility at the sacroiliac and pubic facets. It also brings into function two sets of muscles: the quadratus lumbo-rum and coccygeus, for it is principally these muscles that produce the motion described.

Forward Flexion Considerations

Another movement, which has been de-scribed by Grice, is that which occurs when the patient bends forward. It is widely known that most of this motion takes place in the hip joints and that the lumbar region participates by forward flexion. There is, however, a movement between the sacrum and ilia in which the sacrum glides deeply forward between the ilia. This motion can readily be felt in the standing patient by placing your thumb on some portion of the sacral apex and the tip of your forefinger on one of the PSISs. When the subject flexes for-ward, this space opens up, usually about 1 cm at least if the articulation is free. One articulation may function normally and the other not because of fixation. We then see, on the side of fixation, that the PSIS holds back and the two PSISs are then misaligned.

Lateral Flexion and Rotation Considerations

We will now describe two movements that have given the Belgium group a great deal of difficulty in their studies: that of pelvic rota-tion and lateral flexion in the sitting posture.

DR. FAYE'S CLINICAL COMMENT #6.4

It has been my experience that the loss of this second motion of the sacrum against the motionless weight-bearing ilia can produce excruciating sacroiliac pain, the sciatica of the sacroiliac syndrome, and be significant in acute lumbosacral facet syndrome. The specific adjustment for this disorder will be described later in this chapter.

These two movements are important because we do much of our examining in this position. In these two movements, as stated previously, the sacral part of the pelvis is active and the ilia are passive; ie, they take up the space between the moving sacrum and the immobilized ischia.

Lateral Flexion. Here we must take the lumbar vertebrae into consideration to make the whole motion clearer. In lateral bending, we know that the lumbar region is forced into flexion-rotation. The intervertebral space is flattened on the concave side and opened on the convex side of the lumbar curve. This is pure lateral flexion, a movement that takes place in spite of what the physiologists say. It takes place normally if the sidebending is made in the sitting posture with the lumbar region in forward flexion; ie, in slight kyphosis. If the normal lordosis is retained, there is a certain amount of rotation that takes place also. The maximum of rotation occurs if the lateral flexion is done with the subject standing.

To reveal these movements in the sitting position, it is necessary to concentrate the motion in the region to be studied. This is done by pushing the shoulder of the patient down as far as possible on the concave side of the curve. This is especially important in the study of the motion of the sacrum. In this

movement, the relative motion of the sacrum and the two ilia is complex. The two ilia assume a slanting position toward the convexity of the lumbar curve, with the related side of the pubis gliding upward and laterally. This forces the ilium on that side to shift laterally, with the iliac crest and ischium moving sideward from 5 to 19 mm, respectively. The ilium on the concave side of the lumbar curve just flexes; ie, the ischium serves as a pivot, and the crest moves slightly laterally toward the convex side. This forces the sacrum (and the lumbars) to sway laterally to the same side. The sacrum remains nearly vertical, with only a slight amount of flexion. The base of the sacrum moves a little more laterally than the apex. The difference in movement between the flexing ilia and the swaying sacrum produces a composite motion between the two in which there are two lateral motions: the ilium moving downward on the sacrum on the concave side and upward on the sacrum on the opposite side. Some investigators believe that this movement is not a "natural" one. In fact, it is probably rarely done in everyday life. But as a test for mobility, it is extremely useful.

Rotation. During pelvic rotation, there is another complex movement. To make the description clear, let us suppose we are rotating the patient's torso anteriorly on the

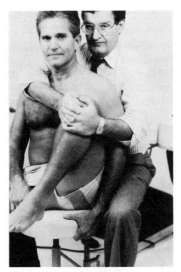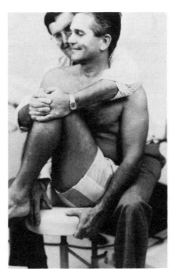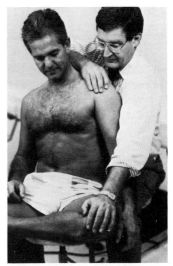

Figure 6.9. Dr. Faye demonstrating Gillet's three 30-second stretches for patients with sacroiliac fixations and/or hip joint dysfunction.

right. It will be readily apparent that the patient's right shoulder will move both anteriorly and to the left relative to the patient's midline. The patient's left shoulder will rotate posteriorly and toward the median line of the patient. This forces the T12 area of the spine to sway to the right from 5 to 10 cm, depending on the general suppleness of the patient's spine. The reason for this is that rotation in the thoracic region does not take place in the spine itself but around a pivot point that Gillet believes is located at the sternum.

This lateral sway of the lower thoracic vertebrae forces the lumbar region into a mixture of rotation and flexion toward the side of rotation. This movement gave Gillet's group another problem to solve because several authorities teach that the center of rotation in the lumbars is at the tip of the spinous processes. If this were true, we would find all the tips of the lumbar vertebrae in perfect alignment during rotation and the T12 spinous process in line with the sacrum. This is evidently not the case in the typical human spine. In our hypothetical subject, we find (if no fixations exist) that the lumbar spinous processes in rotation produce a straight slanting line that extends from T12 to the tip of the sacrum. In fact, variations of the line can be used to indicate the vertebrae in fixation. This has been described by Gillet in the *Annals of the Swiss Chiropractors' Association.*

In this movement, the sacrum assumes a flexion-rotation to the right around a pivot point that is located slightly inferior to the tip of the coccyx. The right ilium follows this movement, the crest moves to the right and anteriorly, the ischium moves very little, and there is probably a torsion at the pubic joint. The left ilium moves in the opposite direction but to a lesser degree.

At this point it may be necessary to excuse the length of this description but it must be considered a necessity to build, once and for all, our chiropractic theories and practices on facts—pure science, if you will—and not do like some of our predecessors: slap on any old theory that might support their findings.

Total (articular) fixation in the pelvis is rare. Total fixations due to the presence of several degenerated taut ligaments are, in contrast, prevalent. [See Clinical Comment 6.5]

Considerations with the Patient Supine

One last short description: the movement that takes place when the subject is in the supine position and lifts one extended leg without bending the knee. Here the pelvic motion takes place to a greater degree at the pubic joint and to a lesser degree around the head of the femur.

Sacral Motion

As mentioned elsewhere in this chapter, there is no *one* movement of the sacrum in relation to the ilia. The sacrum appears to "float" in the pelvic ring; it does not have a specific "groove" that directs its movements. Indeed, pressure on a supple sacrum can make it move upward, downward, forward, etc, in any direction for at least from 1 to 2 mm. The sacrum shifts easily from side to side, with the base usually moving farther laterally than the apex. The sacrum is usually passive in its movements, being influenced either by the lumbars if the force comes from above or by the ilia if it comes from below.

When the lumbars bend sideward, the sacrum follows their movement in flexion and

---

DR. FAYE'S CLINICAL COMMENT #6.5

It is for this reason Gillet taught three 30-second-hold stretches to his patients with sacroiliac fixations. I also use the same regimen for my patients with hip dysfunction. The procedure with a patient sitting on a hard chair is as follows: (1) Pull the knee toward the chest, being sure that the femur rather than the tibia is the lever arm. (2) Pull the knee toward the opposite shoulder. (3) Place the lateral malleolus of the ipsilateral ankle on the opposite knee in a "figure 4" fashion and push the knee laterally and toward the floor with the hand on the same side as the externally rotated hip. Repeat these three stretches on the opposite side all for 30 seconds each. See Figure 6.9.

rotation, and the ilia rotate in a reciprocal opposite direction. With the patient sitting, and especially if flexion forces are concentrated in the lumbar region by pushing the shoulder of the patient downward and inward toward the opposite side, flexion of the sacrum takes place toward the side of convexity. The ilia will then also flex laterally in the same direction, with a shearing motion taking place at the pubis. This produces a paradoxical change of position of the coccyx toward the convexity of the lumbar curve.

Sacral Rotation. The sacrum turns within the iliac cavity almost around a vertical axis, but the base moves more than the apex. This gives the impression of lateral flexion of the sacrum, made in order to follow the line of the lumbars. At the same time, the ilia rotate on a horizontal axis: moving forward on the far side and backward on the near side. This movement causes a torsion-like movement at the pubis; and, if fixation exists in this articulation, the sacrum will then turn on a more vertical axis and to a greater degree (hypermobility).

Pure sacral movement without subsequent movement of the lumbars or of the ilia normally does not occur. The sacrum can move in spite of certain fixations of the lumbars or of the ilia to each other at the pubis.

Sacroiliac Reciprocity

The ilia move relative to the sacrum and to each other. We have described that the ilia may flex laterally in relation to the sacrum upon lateral flexion of the latter. There is another iliac flexion that occurs when changing from the sitting to the standing position, and vice versa. In this movement, the ilia, instead of flexing to the same side, flex together but in opposite directions. Allow us to review some important points for emphasis.

Sitting. In the sitting position, the weight of the body is distributed to the ischia. The body therefore does its best to widen its base by separating these processes. As they separate, the iliac crests come closer together, thus producing a medial flexion of both ilia. This movement also takes place around the pubis, and due to the diagonal slant of the sacral articulations, the sacral base is pushed forward and the apex is drawn backward,

thus producing a forward flexion of the sacrum. The sacrum is passive, and movement in this bone usually takes place around an horizontal axis that is near the S2 tubercle.

Standing. On standing, the pelvis transmits its weight to the head of the femurs. In order to do so efficiently, the ischia move toward each other. A separation of the iliac crests therefore occurs. The sacrum then flexes, base posterior to maintain contact with the iliac articular surfaces. Normally, when the standing patient stoops forward, this same opening and closing takes place but now the sacrum is forced inferiorly as if to be drawn down and wedged deeper into the pelvis.

Iliac A-P and P-A Rotation

Iliac mobility has been the subject of numerous controversies. This is understandable because in Gillet's studies he found that it can also be influenced by a great many partial fixations of a muscular or ligamentous nature.

Total motion of the different bones of the pelvis takes place in two parts. With the patient standing and lifting the flexed knee, the ilium on the side of the knee will follow the movement until its sacral articulation has reached the end of its range of motion. It will then continue to rotate backward and downward at its sacral aspect, but now it will pull the sacrum down with it. As the opposite ilium is weight bearing, it will not move, and as a consequence, the sacrum will glide downward in relation to it, thus producing an anterior rotation of this ilium. Paradoxically, this movement does not seem to follow intimately the surfaces of the sacroiliac articulations. They probably gap open to a certain degree. In this movement, the two arms of the *pubic articulation* glide one over the other in the anterior-superior direction.

Apart from these multiple movements of the different part of the pelvis relative to each other, it is evident that there also exist the three fundamental movements of the whole pelvis. For all practical purposes, they can be considered as movements of the sacrum in relation to the L5. From the fixation point of view, L5 must be considered as part of the pelvis, and it must be seen in its relationships of lateral flexion and, principally, rotation between the crests of the ilia.

Why Investigators Differ in Their Conclusions

One of the reasons for the disagreement among investigators who have studied the function of the pelvic bones in various positions (eg, standing, sitting, bending forward, etc) is that, unfortunately, the pelvis functions differently in each of those positions. Another cause for data discrepancies is that some authors did not clearly define the different positions they described. They often mention a change of position of an ilium or a sacrum in relation to what they considered to be the ideal position in space. For many authors, an ilium was "superior" or "inferior" if it moved "up" or "down." Little or no mention was made of whether this movement was a sliding motion, a rotation, or if the sacrum followed the movement or not.

Some authors studied the movement of the sacral articulations relative to the iliac articulations and described them as moving in relation to the ilia, when, in fact, it is the opposite that usually happens, especially in walking. It can be argued that this does not matter much for practical purposes. Unfortunately, when one wants to do fundamental research, it *does* matter. How often have we seen would-be men of science argue for hours and not be able to agree for the simple reason that they had not defined correctly the words they used.

Another mistake often made in spinal research is to consider that the only "normal" position of a spine is upright, standing, and facing forward—the anatomical position used in textbooks. That is not true. *All* possible positions of the human body are "normal," at least if the joints are supple.

Humans sit today more than they stand, ride more than they walk, and recline for about a third of their lives. Why then the emphasis of the necessity to expose x-ray films of the spine in the standing position? There may be great changes between the standing and sitting postures, and these changes can have important clinical meaning. This is also true for the changes occurring in the recumbent posture.

Gillet's group was therefore forced to take into consideration all the studies published on the subject, invent many different ways of checking their accuracy, and push their studies still further to be sure that they had not missed something. This has taken us years of work; in fact, they were terribly confused most of the time because they could not put all our findings into a coherent whole. Today, they hope they have succeeded in solving this problem.

A certain type of chiropractor likes to draw conclusions from anatomical data. He likes to decide what motion is possible in a joint by looking at the plane lines of the articulations and at the characteristics of the muscles and ligaments of the joint. This may sometimes lead the investigator astray as we have previously shown for the occiput-atlas-axis articulations. Some still maintain that normal occipitoatlantal rotation is not possible, despite the fact that it can easily be proved by stress films and motion palpation.

DIAGNOSTIC CONSIDERATIONS

Pelvic Fixations

Total Sacroiliac Fixations

We know today that there are relatively few total fixations of the articular type at the sacroiliacs. By far, most of them seem to be ligamentous. This region is complicated further by the fact that the superior or inferior portions of the sacroiliac ligaments can become tightened quite separately one from the other. The pubic articulation can also appear to be in total fixation, which is also due, it would seem, to shortened ligaments.

Sacroiliac Muscular Fixations

The primary muscles that Gillet has found to influence the lumbopelvic region are the lower portions of the quadratus lumborum, the fibers extending from the L5 transverses to the crest of the ilia and the two coccygeous muscles coursing from the inferior part of the sacrum and the superior aspect of the coccyx to the corresponding part of the ilium. Two other important muscle groups to consider here are the hamstrings and the lumbar extensors.

The Hamstrings. Shortened hamstrings are common, and they may be found either bilaterally or unilaterally. Taut hamstrings prevent pelvic rotation at the hip anteriorly by fixing the ischium and destroying normal lumbosacropelvic rhythm; thus, any motion achieved is forced upon the lumbar segments, often with compensatory stretching of the posterior longitudinal ligaments. If movement is sharply forced, avulsion may occur that leads to further degenerative changes. [See Clinical Comment 6.6]

The Lumbar Extensors. Shortening of the lumbar extensors has the opposite effect as that of hamstring shortening. This is a common cause and/or effect of hyperlordosis. If the hamstrings are normal and the perivertebral muscles are tight, it will be found that pelvic motion is free but lumbar flexion is restricted. If movement is forced, overstress is placed on the hips, sacroiliac joints, and posterior soft tissues of the lumbar region. This leads to chronic strain, sprain, avulsion, spurring, and degenerative arthritis.

The effects of shortened iliopsoas or piriformis muscles upon the hip and lumbar spine will de described later in this chapter.

In a certain number of purely muscular fixations, the contracted or hypertonic muscle will have a tendency to degenerate and become fibrosed. For all practical purposes, it becomes a "ligament" and, as most muscles are accompanied by a ligament, it is often difficult to determine which structure is responsible for the fixation. Fortunately, the type and direction of a corrective thrust is practically the same, and even the amount of change to be expected from a fibrosed muscle or a shortened ligament is the same. Both of these types of fixations can therefore be considered "ligamentous." From the point of view of correction, this fixation is the most common, although it is not the most irritative.

Correction of Anterior or Posterior Pelvic Tilt

Forward Tilt. An anterior tilt of the ilium is primarily the product of (1) weak abdominals, hamstrings, or both, (2) hypertonicity of the lumboextensors or hip flexors, (3) contractures of the rectus femoris, or a combination of these factors. Some authorities believe that the resulting distortion is "the most common postural fault of muscular origin." Strengthening the inferior pull of the hamstrings posteriorly and the rectus abdominis superiorly offers an in-line force couple to correct anterior pelvic tilt. The erector spinae, quadratus lumborum, and iliopsoas usually need stretching.

Backward Tilt. Conversely, posterior tilt of the ilium is typically the result of (1) hypertonic abdominals, (2) shortened hamstrings, or (3) weakened lumboflexors or hip extensors, or a combination of these factors.

In either cases of forward or backward pelvic tilt, biomechanical correction should incorporate (1) mobilization of fixated facets, (2) strengthening of weak musculature, (3) stretching of contractures, and (4) relaxation of hypertonicity.

The Sacroiliac Ligaments

The Posterior Sacroiliac Ligaments. White/Panjabi state that the interosseous sacroiliac ligaments supporting the thin

---

DR. FAYE'S CLINICAL COMMENT #6.6

Failure of the hamstrings to elongate normally produces stress on the posterior elements of the lumbar spine because the extensors muscles are at the end of their eccentric contraction and the lumbar spine is hanging on its ligaments. Repeated stress from this scenario causes hypermobility of the zygapophyseal joints and increased intradiscal pressure. Anular tears and the pathogenesis of disc degeneration develop from the faulty biomechanics of the hamstrings. This is just one etiologic factor but an often overloooked point in treatment programs. PNF or spray-and-stretch of the hamstrings, quadriceps, and psoas muscles should be a priority consideration with all patients except those that are in the acute stage and cannot withstand the stretches. Chiropractors should declare war on shortened back and thigh muscles.

joint capsule posteriorly and inferiorly are the strongest of the body. These ligaments, considered the major bond between the sacrum and ilia, are so thick that they fill the roughened space between the sacral and iliac tuberosities behind the sacroiliac joint. There is an upper portion that spans between S1—S2 and the anterior medial iliac crest. Immediately below is the lower part of the ligament that arises from S3 and inserts into the iliac crest. The strength of these ligaments helps prevent displacement of the sacrum even during forceful jumping.

The Anterior Sacroiliac Ligaments. The primary ligament straps anteriorly are the thinner anterior sacroiliac ligaments at the superolateral aspect of the sacrum and the stronger sacrospinous ligaments that extends from the inferolateral aspect of the sacrum and coccyx to the spine of the ischium. The superolateral ligaments appear to be little more than extensions from the anterior capsule.

Sacroiliac Ligamentous Fixations

According to Gillet, no other area of the axial skeleton is prone to fixation from ligamentous shortening more than the sacroiliac articulations. In fact, he feels that it is almost impossible to find a state of clinical imbalance that does not reflect this state. This is probably because few occupations require pelvic motion throughout the maximum range of possible motion. However, generalized bilateral ligamentous shortening in itself is not necessarily a cause of clinical concern even if a state of mobility is considered ideal. Gillet believes that the clinical state of the sacroiliac ligaments is determined by the habitual positions the articulations are required to maintain in the patient's lifestyle. See Figure 6.10.

The iliolumbar, sacroiliac, and sacrotuberous ligaments are common sites of ligamentous shortening that affect pelvic dynamics, and they appear to become involved in that order according to Grieve. Gillet, however, reports many cases of iliolumbar and sacrotuberous fixation without involvement of the sacroiliac ligaments.

The Iliolumbar Ligaments. The iliolumbar ligaments connect the transverse processes of L5 to the crests of the ilia and sacral base. As an iliolumbar ligament becomes shortened, the iliac crest tends to be pulled medially while the ischium is forced outward. In response to the load above, the sacral base is pushed forward and the sacral apex is pulled backward. Thus, the patient's pelvis will exhibit the normal state of the sitting pelvis in the standing position. This same condition may be the result of a fibrotic or reflexly contracted quadratus lumborum.

Aside from the articular facets, the iliolumbar ligaments are often the most important structures limiting axial rotation of L5 on the sacrum and preventing forward gliding of L5 on the sacrum. Because of its deep position below the iliac crests and the strong strapping by the iliolumbar ligaments and spinal extensors, L5 is only as movable as the sacral base will allow. Thus when lipping or spurs at the inferior aspect of the centrum of

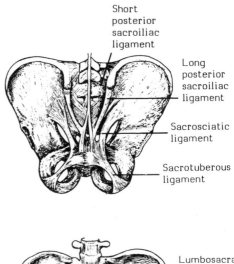

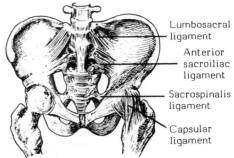

Figure 6.10. Major ligaments of the pelvis. *Top,* view from the posterior; *bottom,* view from the anterior (Courtesy ACAP).

L5 are seen (signs of overstress), a history of instability can be presumed.

In Gillet's studies of fixation, as mentioned in the previous chapter, he found that the 5th lumbar acts as part of the pelvis and there the most common ligament at fault is the iliolumbar.

The Sacroiliac Ligaments. When the posterior ligaments shorten, they tend to push the sacral base forward so that the PSISs appear more prominent and closer together. When the anterior ligaments shorten, the sacral base has a tendency to bulge posteriorly, with an unusual mass palpable medial to the PSISs that have flared further apart.

The Sacrotuberous Ligaments. The sacrotuberous ligaments have a strong tendency to shorten. When tight, the sacrum displaces deeper between the two ilia like a driven wedge. With the patient in the lateral recumbent position, deep gluteal palpation will reveal the taut cords. Grieve reports that ipsilateral calf and heel numbness is often associated, thus suggesting sciatic nerve involvement.

Shortening of the sacrotuberous ligaments can also be palpated through the relaxed gluteal muscles when the patient is prone. They will be felt as short, taut, tough cords. The pull of the ligament is usually not total, reports Gillet. In the knee lifting test, the sacrum is capable of moving downward towards the ischium somewhat but it does not move back into its normal location. Furthermore, this motion takes place in one articulation only, the one opposite the side of the lifted knee instead of moving harmoniously in each articulation. This is another example of the hypermobility that usually accompanies partial fixations (ligamentous or muscular).

Shortening of the Sacroiliac Capsular Ligaments. Shortening of the capsular ligaments should give us an "articular" fixation, but here again the amount of fixation is not total for there is still a certain amount of torsion possible in the fixed articulation.

This characteristic of capsule ligament shortening is especially found in extraspinal articulations; eg, in the feet where there are many fixations between the calcaneus, the metatarsals, and the tarsals. These same fixations can also be found in the superior articulation of the fibula with the tibia, in the metacarpals, and in the lateral and medial articulations of the clavicle. Remember that these fixations have noxious effects either in themselves or through the reflex fixations they produce in the spine.

Gillet and associates have found few spinal fixations that can be explained by shortening of capsular ligaments. On the other hand, practically all other spinal ligaments seem to be involved in fixations. In fact, ligament shortening should be a characteristic of all articular fixation, for it is a normal function of ligaments to take up the slack and adapt themselves to the amount of motion produced in an articulation.

Sacroiliac Motion Palpation

It has just been explained that covering the sacroiliac articulations are a host of ligaments which, if normal in tension and elasticity, control sacroiliac motion and assure that the articular surfaces remain within normal limits. Unfortunately, most people use a majority of specific and specialized

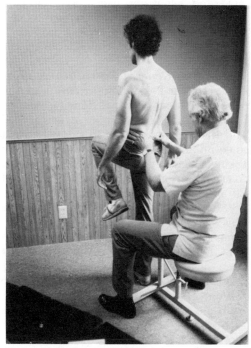

Figure 6.11. Conducting the knee-raising test.

movements rather than maintaining a healthy mobility in all possible ranges of motions. This causes one or several of these ligaments to shorten and tighten, which in turn causes the involved ligament to serve as a new, but abnormal, center of rotation that may restrict mobility in one or several directions. The pubic joint, for example, may tighten and effectively hinder A-P and P-A rotation of the ilia. In the sitting position, however, the sacrum will still be able to move between the ilia; in fact, hypermobility of both sacroiliac joints in the sitting position will occur, and at the same time, a total fixation of the ilia will be found in the standing knee lift test described earlier in this chapter.

Some of Gillet's postulates described previously in this chapter will be summarized in this section for emphasis.

The Standing Flexed-Knee-Raising Test

The sacroiliac and the lumbosacral joints should be palpated in the standing and/or sitting positions. Several sacroiliac tests are suggested below, and each should be conducted bilaterally. The thumbs are usually used for palpation because deep pressure is necessary to hold firm contact during the tests.

Standing General Sacroiliac Motion. To screen iliac flexion and extension on the sacrum in the standing position, the examiner's thumbs are placed on the patient's PSISs and the patient is asked to raise the right knee up and down, bending the knee as if taking a high step. The right PSIS will be felt to arc posteriorly and inferiorly. After about 20° of leg raise, the patient's left sacroiliac PSIS also drops backward and downward. This is normal sacroiliac motion. Any motion other than this indicates a problem in this joint. Repeat the test by having the patient raise the left flexed knee up and down (Fig. 6.11). If the joint is fixated, the pelvis tends to move as a whole and the ipsilateral thumb will tend to remain level or possibly raise rather than drop. These signs of thumb movement can be seen as well as felt.

Standing Superior Joint Motion. Place one thumb on the sacral base of the patient and your other thumb on the right PSIS. Ask the patient to raise the right flexed knee as if taking a high step, and note the separation of the thumbs. The sacral base will normally be seen and felt to arc ¼—½ inch anteriorly and inferiorly. Or, conversely, the PSIS will move backward and downward. Repeat the test with the patient raising the left flexed knee. During these tests, the tissues over the sacroiliac joint should relax. If the superior sacroiliac joint or the symphysis pubis is locked, the sacrum and ilium will move as a unit, the thumbs will not separate appreciably, and the sacral tissues (ligaments and spinal muscle attachments) will remain taut. This, states Gillet, is probably the most common pelvic fixation found. Invariably, there is a degree of forward tilting of the pelvis and associated lumbar hyperlordosis.

Standing Inferior Joint Motion. Place a thumb on the patient's sacral apex and your other thumb on the ischial protuberance. Ask the patient to raise the knee on the side first being tested. A ¼—½-inch excursion should be felt as the ischium moves anterosuperior and slightly lateral on the sacrum. If the inferior sacroiliac joint is locked, the ischium and sacral apex move as a unit (Fig. 6.12). Fixation of this motion is most often associated with a contralateral sacral base fixation. The direct cause is usually failure of the muscles acting on the sacral apex to stretch. Piriformis contracture is a common cause, but the iliopsoas or deep glutei may be the cause or a contributing factor.

Anterior Sacral Fixation. In some patients, the anterior sacroiliac ligaments will have shortened but not the posterior ligaments. These anterior ligaments can be divided into superior and inferior straps. If one is short, A-P rotation in the knee lifting test will still take place, but the center of sacroiliac rotation will have changed. Instead of taking place at the head of the femur, it will be found at the offending ligament. A related hypermobility will exist at the pubic articulation. This A-P mobility or immobility can be palpated by placing one thumb on a PSIS and the other thumb on the corresponding part of the sacrum. When the patient lifts the knee, the ipsilateral ilium will normally arc backward and downward. If the contacts are taken on the inferior part of the ilium and sacrum, the former will be felt to move forward and upward. During fixation, both of these movements will be sluggish, quickly reaching their limits and pulling the sacrum into a visible distortion.

Posterior Sacral Fixation. Fixation at the posterior ligaments is more difficult to palpate because the palpating thumbs are over the actual center of rotation, thus unable to register perceptible movement. However, if the patient is turned around and the ASISs are contacted, the knee lifting test will show abnormal mobility. It appears that these forms of sacroiliac fixations also insult the movement of the sacrum itself between the ilia, as tested in the sitting patient, making the motion sluggish or even nonexistent. Bilateral shortening of these ligaments also alters the in- and out-flaring of the ilia when the patient is either standing or sitting.

Gillet's Standing Straight-Leg-Raising Test

With the patient standing, it is also helpful to have the patient lift the leg with the knee extended. This will produce a decided change in the movement found in partial fixations, for, as previously explained, the normal movement of the ilium on the side of the *flexed knee* is a rotation around a point

that is about the head of the femur. When the knee is not flexed, the pull of the posterior muscles will change the center of rotation to a point at or near the pubic articulation (contrary to that seen in the supine position). This will make no practical difference if these articulations are completely free, but it may cause a partial sacroiliac fixation to appear as a total fixation. To make this clear, it will be necessary to describe all possible points of fixation in this area.

Differential Analysis

It seems that the different sacroiliac ligaments can shorten individually. Four of these points can be found on each side, two anterior (one superior and one inferior) and two posterior (one superior and one inferior). Any combination of fixation at these four points on each side can be seen; any two or three points being simultaneously in fixation would be considered a "total" fixation. See Figures 6.13 and 6.14. For this reason, a detailed differentiating form of analysis in this region should be used.

Let us take as an example a sacroiliac fixation at the anterior-inferior portion of the sacroiliac articulation. It is evident that when the patient's knee is raised (patient standing), the ilium rotates around this fixed point rather than around an axis at the head

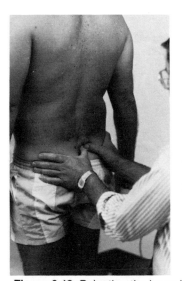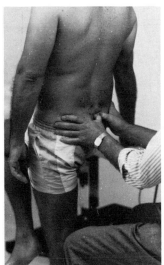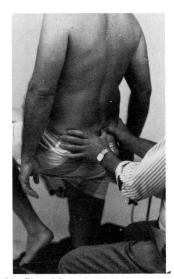

Figure 6.12. Palpating the lower left sacroiliac joint, using the standing flexed-knee tests.

of the femur. There will be motion, but the motion will be around an abnormal axis. Furthermore, the posterior part of the ilium opposite the fixed point will appear to move, although the amount of motion will be smaller than normal. In some cases, especially if the palpator is in a hurry, this half movement may be mistaken for total motion.

There are other ways of revealing such a fixation for confirmation. One will be described later when the patient is in the sitting position. In the standing position, which is our present topic, the following two tests can be made:

1. When lifting the leg straight, the pubis is blocked physiologically, forcing the facet of the ilium to glide downward on its sacral counterpart. Thus, any fixation in the joint will effectively stop this gliding and the fixation will be more evident.

2. It is also possible to have the patient lift the *opposite* knee, while you maintain your

palpation contacts on the ilium and the part of the sacrum on the side of the weight-bearing limb.

To fully grasp the purpose of this, it is necessary to review the normal movement of these articulations. When the unfixated subject lifts a knee, the first part of sacroiliac motion occurs in a gliding manner, in the articulation that does not bear body weight. If, however, the knee is forced a little higher, the first articulation to come to the end of its range of motion is the opposite joint, the weight bearing one that is forced to move. That is, the active ilium continues its motion by pulling the sacrum with it, forcing the sacrum to move on the opposite ilium.

This motion can be felt and seen when the palpating thumbs are put in contact with the sacrum and ilium on the weight-bearing side. It is thus necessary, in this test, to have the patient raise the knees one after the other, putting your thumbs alternatively over the

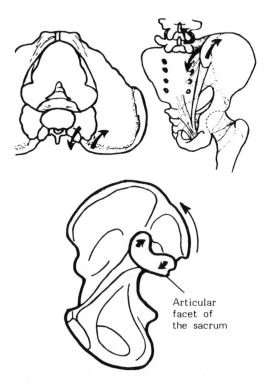

Figure 6.13. Direction of sacral and iliac motion when the sacral base is fixated in a posterior position, anterior motion restricted (Courtesy ACAP).

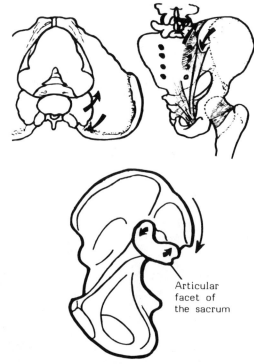

Figure 6.14. Direction of sacral and iliac motion when the sacral base is fixated in an anterior position, posterior motion restricted (Courtesy ACAP).

right, left, superior, and inferior portions of the articulations. There must be palpable-visible movement at all points when each knee is raised to be sure that these articulations are completely free of fixation.

When an articulation is completely free, it must be remembered that the sacrum will remain vertical. If it tips laterally, it is a sign that there is a partial fixation somewhere. If the point of partial fixation is at the posterior aspect of the joint, all rotation occurs around that point. No motion will be felt when either the patient's right or left knee is lifted, or even when the limb is lifted straight. This may give the impression of a total fixation, but it is not; for if contact points far removed from the area of fixation are used (ie, the ischia, the iliac crests, or the ASISs of the ilia), a definite motion will be felt.

Readers of Gillet's early notes may be surprised that he does not mention here the test in which the standing patient flexes laterally. The lateral flexion test can be used, but the amount of mobility in a normal pelvis is relatively small in this movement and it is difficult to evaluate correctly.

Gillet's Standing Straight-Leg-Extension Test. It is also sometimes helpful to have the patient lift the leg backward. Theoretically, this movement should produce the opposite movement to those described above. In practice, however, this test is not used frequently because, in the standing position, the sacrum comes to rest near one end of its range of motion—the ischia are close together, the crests are separated, and the sacral base has moved backward to fill the space between the crests. Posterior movement is therefore *normally* restricted. This is not true in the sitting position, where the sacrum "floats" at or near the center of its range of motion. This permits the palpator to evaluate motion in the different parts of the pelvis quite easily when the patient is in the *sitting* position.

Evaluating Horizontal Parallel Sway. Faye attributes the following test for horizontal parallel sway to Grice: The patient stands with legs parallel and is asked to bend sidewards and run the palm of his or her ipsilateral hand down the lateral aspect of the thigh. During the maneuver, the examiner should feel the patient's PSIS glide parallel

to the floor in the opposite direction of the patient's lateral flexion. Hip or sacroiliac fixation, however, will cause the PSIS to raise on one side of the pelvis and rotate around one hip joint. Possible quadratus lumborum or psoas imbalance is given as a primary cause.

Gillet's Comments on Palpation in the Sitting Position

Several alternative contacts taken from Gillet's writings will be described in this section. The important thing is to understand what you are palpating and why, then you may select the contacts of your preference.

According to the principle of palpating the major fixations first, it is helpful to use the back of your hand to generally perceive sacroiliac fixation. As during a *spinal screen*, your fingers are placed vertically to cover the whole surface of the sacrum. Your forearm may be reinforced by your thigh, which can be used to push your palpating hand forward against the patient's sacrum. This is especially helpful with the patient whose spine has not been corrected to any great degree because its resistance may fatigue your palpating arm.

The sensation of sacroiliac fixation is evident after it has been felt on several patients. It can be described as the difference in sensation that is felt when the hand is pushed against the knee cap (fixation) or the muscles of the thigh (no fixation, or at least, no total fixation). A total fixation will be perceived as a resistance to movement at all points of the articulation. Partial, though important, fixations can be felt if the contact is moved to the superior or inferior parts of the sacrum, or also to the right and left articulations. It has been noticed that some students neglect to palpate the inferior parts of this joint.

Sacral Lateral Flexion During Sitting. Many palpators prefer changing the contact from the back of the hand to the thumb to find the principal area of fixation. In fact, it is even possible to perceive lateral flexion and rotation of the sacrum between the ilia by placing the thumb in the sacroiliac groove at the four points of contact. To judge medial and lateral glide of the upper sacroiliac joint,

Gillet palpates just medial to the PSIS and asks the patient to open and close the legs. The ilium should glide medially and laterally over the lateral border of the sacrum.

Lateral flexion and rotation can be felt in still another way, by placing the lateral aspect of the forefinger vertically against the tips of the sacral spinouses. The patient is flexed to one side and then to the other with your free hand on the patient's shoulders. The sacral spinouses should be felt to glide towards the convexity of the lumbar curve. This movement is normally a wide and free one. In fact, an abnormal amount of motion may be felt in some cases. This occurs when there is a total fixation of the *pubis*.

For palpators who have difficulty in palpating the movement of the whole sacrum in this way, it is possible to feel the mobility of the superior part of the joint by contacting the first sacral tubercle with the thumb and then the mobility of the inferior part of the joint by palpating the end of the coccyx with the tip of your second finger. The back of the hand is anchored on the palpating stool, with the tips of the fingers pressed up against the tip of the coccyx (through the patient's underclothes). On lateral flexion of the patient, the coccyx will be felt to glide right and left over your finger. Care must be taken to concentrate the lateral flexion of the patient's lower back by pushing down and centrally against the patient's shoulder on the side of lateral flexion.

In lateral bending of the spine, there is also a tilting of the ilia toward the convexity. This distorts the pelvis into a sort of leaning capital M in which the two upright lines represent the ilia and the two others (forming the internal V) represent the sacrum. In this movement, the pubis is forced into lateral gliding. If there is any fixation in this articulation, the sacral motion will occur, but the ilia will not tip. This movement (or the lack of it) can easily be felt by placing the palpating thumb on the iliac crest on the side opposite to the lumbar flexion. Upon forced flexion, this crest flares laterally.

Contact may also be taken on the ischium of the same side. The palpating hand is placed as in palpation of the coccyx, with the back of the hand on the palpation stool and two fingers on either side of the ischium. Upon forced lateral flexion of the patient, the patient's ischium should normally be felt to glide laterally.

Sacral Rotation During Sitting. Normal rotation (or its absence) can be felt: (1) on the sacrum by evaluating the lateral movement of the upper sacral tubercles, (2) in the ilium, by contact on the iliac crest and feeling its forward rotation. The ASIS can also be palpated (from the back or the front) and felt to move downwards. Torsion-rotation of the different parts of the pelvis in the sitting position normally takes place around one ischium. The sacrum flexes to the anterior side of rotation, the anterior ilium rotates forward, and the posterior ilium rotates backward but to a lesser degree—almost as if all the movement takes place around it.

General Effects of Partial Fixations. Apart from fixations resulting from shortening of the various sacroiliac ligaments, there also exists a certain number of partial fixations in this area that are due to hypertonicity of the sacroiliac muscles mentioned elsewhere in this chapter (especially the coccygeous and the lower portion of the quadratus lumborum). The coccygeous muscles will pull the ischia together, and their hypertonicity will block these two bones in the position that they normally have when the subject is standing. The patient will then prefer to stand rather than sit and will not feel comfortable when sitting for any length of time.

Both coccygeous muscles are not necessarily hypertonic at the same time. When only one is "spastic," the related ilium is functionally as it is in the standing position. When the patient stands, the pelvis seems to be normal because the other ilium takes the same position naturally. When the patient sits, however, one ilium, the mobile one, changes to the sitting position (crest in, ischium out), while the other remains as in the standing position. In this case, the patient's lumbar region will be scoliotic in the sitting position but be straight when standing.

The opposite is true when the lower part of the quadratus lumborum is taut and fails to relax. This pulls the crests of the ilia together and, naturally, pushes the ischia outward. As with the case described above, but in the opposite direction, the patient will feel more comfortable in the sitting posture. In fact, while standing, the patient will rapidly tire and feel pain. Here the lumbar scoliosis will appear in the standing position, and the lumbars will straighten when the patient sits. This point should be quite important to those who radiograph the patient in the standing posture only.

L5 Motion During Sitting. Fixations due to any part of the quadratus muscle or iliolumbar ligament will have also a partial effect on the A-P and P-A rotation of the ilia on the sacrum as seen with the knee lifting test. The knee-raising test will show a characteristic sign of the ilium rotating posteriorly, pulling L5 into rotation with it. With the patient sitting, it is also possible to feel the *normal* movement between L5 and the ilium on either side by placing the palpating thumb in the space between these two structures and rotating the patient's thorax with your free hand. Normally, the thumb can be pushed relatively easily into this area. The tissues should feel fairly relaxed. If this ligament is shortened, the tissues in the area will feel hard and taut and this will not change when rotating the patient's thorax.

At the other end of the sacrum, we have previously described how the ischia will separate upon lateral flexion and how the coccyx-iliac space will open on one side and close on the other.

Sacral Apex Motion During Sitting. To test forward flexion freedom of the sacral apex with the patient sitting, place a thumb on one PSIS and the other thumb on the sacral apex. Keep in mind that the PSISs are normally about ¼ inch closer together in the sitting position than the standing position due to ischial spread. Note the separation of the thumbs as the patient flexes forward enough to flatten the lumbar curve. This separation will normally be about a half inch if the dynamics are normal. The tissues over the sacrum will be felt to tighten. If either the spinal extensors (multifidi, sacrospinalis) or pelvic extensors (hamstrings, gluteus maximus) fail to elongate during flexion, the sacroiliac joint will be inhibited from above or below, or both, and the lumbars will remain somewhat lordotic. Thus, this type of fixation can be secondary to failure of the lower thoracic and lumbar muscles to stretch. Gluteal lengthening can be further evaluated by flexing the thigh of the supine

patient diagonally towards the opposite shoulder. To test motion during spinal extension, take the same contacts described above and have the patient arch the back. The distance between your thumbs should reduce and the tissues overlying the sacrum should relax.

Sacroiliac End-Play Motion During Sitting. The degree of translatory motion (end play) at the end of voluntary motion reflects ligamentous elasticity. The test, originally suggested by Mennell, is made at the end of extension by firm thumb pressure on the sacral apex while the other thumb is on the PSIS. This palpation should elicit further tissue relaxation.

Summary Review of Highlights

Lateral Flexion of the Pelvis During Sitting. Place both thumbs on the patient's PSISs so that your fingers firmly grip the crests of the ilia bilaterally. As the patient curves his trunk laterally, the lumbar spine should arc smoothly. The sacrum will normally tilt towards the side of the concavity, but the PSISs should remain almost level even though there is some bilaterally reciprocal iliac rotation. The tissues overlying the sacrum on the side of lateral flexion should relax while those on the side of the convexity should tighten. At the end of voluntary motion, added thumb pressure on the sacrum in the direction of its movement should reveal further tissue relaxation. This will not occur if the ligaments have stiffened. If one PSIS raises during lateral flexion, it suggests elongation failure of the lumbar extensors (multifidi, erector spinae) or lateral stabilizers (iliopsoas, quadratus lumborum). If there is bilateral sacroiliac fixation, there will usually be associated lumbar fixations.

In the standing position, lateral sacral flexion is difficult to differentiate from pelvic lateral rotation about the weight-bearing head of the femur.

Position-Change Iliac Alterations. Place your thumbs on the PSISs of a sitting patient. Note the distance between the contacts, and then have the patient stand. Observe the distance between your thumbs. On standing, the PSISs normally open laterally (like a book) so that the inter-PSIS distance increases. If a firm contact can be held on the ischial spines, a reverse reaction will be revealed; ie, the ischia tend to close medially when arising to the standing position. If fixation is present, these iliac and ischial motions will not be felt.

Sitting Iliac Horizontal Rotation. With the patient sitting, place your thumbs on the patient's PSISs and ask the patient to fan his knees open and close several times. As the knees are abducted laterally, the PSISs normally move medially so that they are closer together. Frequently, one PSIS will be felt to move less than the other, indicating a fixation at the inhibited base of the sacrum.

Sitting and Standing Pelvic Changes. Keep in mind the various pelvic changes that occur between the sitting and standing postures that vary with different occupations. These changes are essentially controlled by the sacroiliac-ligament complex. If the superior ligaments are tightened, the crests will be pulled together and actually fix the pelvis in the shape characteristic for the sitting position. Such a patient will feel more comfortable when seated, and spinographs taken in the sitting posture appear quite normal. On standing, however, the crests of such a pelvis would be incapable of separating and the ischia will not approximate. The opposite may also occur; ie, the inferior sacroiliac ligaments may shorten and pull the ischia toward each other, locking the pelvis in the standing position and making sitting uncomfortable if not painful. There are many such states of fixation; eg, one ilium may be blocked or one fixed in a position of flexion on one side and one in a position of extension on the other. Careful analysis is necessary in differentiation.

It is interesting to see that in Gillet's explanation of his findings in sacroiliac fixation many concepts of sacroiliac dynamics taught by Hugh Logan and his son from the 1920s through the 1950s in *Basic Technique* (and generally ignored by the profession as a whole) are confirmed. Gillet received his initial training at Palmer.

Static Palpation

Theoretically, if your thumbs are placed on the patient's PSISs and one thumb is more posterior and inferior or anterior and superior than the other when the patient is either standing or sitting, it would indicate a fixed unilateral pelvic rotation. Likewise, if the thumbs are placed on the patient's PSISs and one thumb is more superior and anterior or inferior and posterior than the other when the patient is prone, it would indicate unilateral pelvic rotation. However, because osseous asymmetry is so common, these static signs are frequently misleading. Dynamic tests, such as those described in motion palpation, correlated with other signs and the patient's symptoms are much more reliable during analysis.

Palpating the Lumbosacral Junction

Gillet frequently adds words of caution about palpating the lumbosacral area. He states that the posterior articulations of L5 are probably those in which errors of palpation can most easily arise. This is because of the wide range of motion of the sacrum. For instance, if there is movement in the lumbosacral articulation during lateral flexion toward the left, the sacral apex tilts to the right and the spinous process of L5 glides a little less laterally to the right than the process of the first sacral segment. However, if L5 is fixed to S1 and the sacrum is freely movable, L5 and the sacrum must move as a whole.

The 5th lumbar vertebra has a great range of movement under the skin but no appreciable movement relative to the sacrum. Special care must be taken to feel the scissor-like movement between the *spinous process of L5* and the *1st sacral process* and not be misled by the general movement of the sacrum and L5 felt under the skin.

There are other combinations of fixations of the 5th lumbar and the sacrum. As soon as you are capable of palpating the dynamics in this area, you will be able to appreciate the different combinations of fixations of this highly important articular complex.

In the palpation technique described above, Gillet takes into consideration the local movement between two contiguous bones. Palpation of the general movements of the spine also shows resistance to movement, sometimes of several spinal segments.

In addition, as described in a previous chapter, palpation of the perivertebral region will usually indicate fixations in the lower thoracic costovertebral and costocostal complex.

At this point in his teaching, Gillet reviews two points of caution in the hope of preventing his students from committing serious errors in palpating the lumbosacral area. The first error is the gliding of the skin over the spinous process, which may give the impression of movement between the spinous process of L5 and the 1st sacral tubercle even if there is a complete fixation. Therefore, you must concentrate sufficiently to avoid this error. Secondly, in rotation and lateral flexion, lateral bending of the whole spine may give the impression of *local* movement. Constantly keep in mind that the local movement between two spinous processes is a scissor-like movement. This mistake, states Gillet, is commonly made in the following areas of the spine: from C7 to T2, T10 to T12, and L5 to S1.

Differentiating Sacroiliac from Lumbar Fixations

To differentiate sacroiliac from lumbar fixations, Faye offers the following comments for consideration.

With the patient sitting and their hands placed behind their head, rotate the patient's trunk first to the right and then to the left. Special care should be taken not to lift the patient's pelvis. Motion restriction of the patient's left lumbar facets or left sacroiliac joint will reduce rotation to the left (positive theta Y). Motion restriction of the patient's right lumbar facets or right sacroiliac joint will inhibit rotation of the patient's trunk to the right (negative theta Y).

To discern between a lumbosacral or sacroiliac lesion, the patient is allowed to relax against the doctor (patient's hands are still behind their head). In this position, the lumbosacral joint is relatively stress free. Next, twist the patient's trunk into posterior rotation on the right until the patient's left ischial tuberosity lifts slightly (buttocks remaining on palpation stool). In this position, there is a marked posterior torsion strain on the right sacroiliac joint. If pain arises in the

right sacroiliac that can be relieved by pushing the left ilium posteriorly, then the pain can be assumed to arise from the right sacroiliac joint. Reverse the doctor-patient positions to differentiate fixations on the left. This is Mennell's modified Kemp's test for the lumbosacral area.

Here are some helpful clues: The patient suffering from sacroiliac dysfunction gets up in the morning with stiffness that improves with activity. The patient suffering with facet inflammation and/or an IVD lesion arises improved, but the condition worsens as the day goes on. Fixation produces a sharp pain on certain movements that is relieved when the site is not stressed. Other points characteristic of a sacroiliac lesion are:

1. There is usually unilateral pain in the sacroiliac joint.

2. The patient may describe an onset involving a lifting or twisting maneuver upon which a "catch" in the back is felt.

3. The patient has difficulty rising from bed, and the disability is worse in the morning, improving with activity.

4. The patient has difficulty getting into or rising from a chair because the joints fail to accommodate the normal pelvic changes that occur from changing from a sitting to standing posture.

5. The associated pain may refer to the (a) ipsilateral buttock, (b) ipsilateral posterior thigh (usually no further than the knee), (c) ipsilateral groin, and/or (d) ipsilateral anterior thigh (rare). See Figure 6.15.

6. The pain is usually an "achy" type, but it may be sharp on certain movements.

7. There is usually no severe pain on coughing or sneezing.

8. There is usually no abnormal neurologic signs, but there may be some current or recent history of paresthesia in the ipsilateral buttock and thigh.

9. The most common sites of pelvic fixation are found within the sacroiliac joints themselves or the hip joints.

10. A corrective adjustment frequently results in dramatic relief immediately.

Pubic Fixations

Pubic fixation offers a clinical dilemma that awaits resolution. The pubic articula-

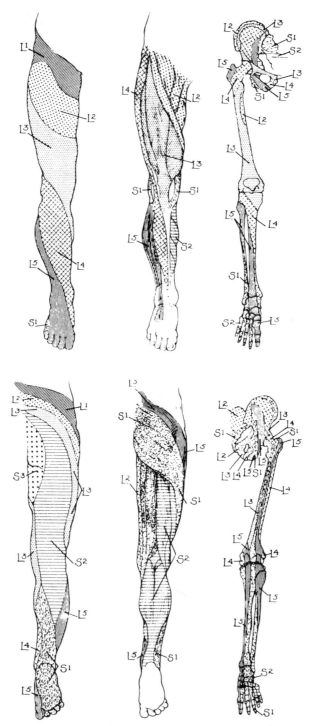

Figure 6.15. Innervation of the lower extremity. *Left,* dermatomes; *middle,* myotomes; *right,* sclerotomes (Courtesy ACAP).

tion is not a gliding type as seen in the spine, thus, states Gillet, one would think it would be prone to only a ligamentous type of fixation. If this were true, a degree of torsion would be possible in spite of fixation. However, motion palpation demonstrates that (1) normal A-P and P-A iliac rotation does not take place when the pubis is fixated, and (2) a fixation-mobilizing adjustment results in a rapid improvement in mobility. Neither of these characteristics are typical of ligamentous fixation. See Figure 6.16.

Myofascial Pain Syndromes

Muscles can undergo changes that of themselves are primary components of a subluxation complex. If this abnormal state is not treated specifically, it can severely hinder recovery.

Apart from obvious trauma, states Faye, the examiner must discern if there are any areas of myodysneuria that serve as a trigger point and/or if there is a shortening of the overall length of a group of muscles. The iliopsoas, hamstrings, quadriceps, and tensor fascia lata muscles often have areas of myofascitis.

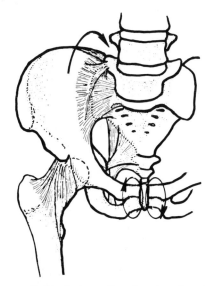

Figure 6.16. Schematic showing the torque forces that must occur at the symphysis pubis when the right ilium rotates; in this instance, posteriorly (Courtesy ACAP).

Proprioceptive neuromuscular facilitation (PNF) and postisometric relaxation (PR) are two effective stretching techniques. It has been Faye's experience that shortened muscles respond best to PNF, PR, or Travell's "spray-and-stretch" technique. A trigger point refers pain outside its neuromere and should respond to two or three treatments utilizing pressure, spray and stretch, ultrasound, electrotherapy, etc. PNF is contraindicated for active trigger points because it is too painful.

Significant Neurologic and Orthopedic Tests

Any patient subjected to pelvic pain should be given a thorough physical, orthopedic, and neurologic examination, plus any other tests directed by clinical judgment. Evaluating the possibility of hernia; pelvic, genital, and rectal lesions; and testing light touch and pain perception should be routine. Anal, adductor, cremasteric, obliquus, patellar, and Achilles reflexes should be checked, as well as gross and segmental motions of the lumbar spine, pelvis, and hips. Following are several additional clinical tests that are applicable for syndromes involving the pelvis. Only a few will be necessary to apply in any particular case, depending on early clinical suspicions.

Goldthwait's Test. The patient is placed supine. Place one hand under the patient's lumbar spine, with each fingerpad pressed firmly against the interspinous spaces. Your other hand is used to slowly conduct an SLR test. If pain occurs or is aggravated before the lumbar processes open (0°—30°), a sacroiliac lesion should be suspected. In general, Goldthwait believed that if pain occurred while the processes were opening at 30°—60°, a lumbosacral lesion was suggested; at 60°—90°, an L1—L4 disc lesion. If pain is brought on before the lumbar spine begins to move, a lesion, either arthritic or a sprain involving the sacroiliac joint, is probably present. If pain does not come on until after the lumbar spine begins to move, the disorder is more likely to have its site in the lumbosacral area or less commonly in the sacroiliac areas. The test should be repeated with the unaffected limb. A positive sign of a lumbosacral lesion is elicited if pain occurs at about the same height as it did with the first limb. If the unaffected limb can be raised higher than the affected limb, it is thought to be significant of sacroiliac involvement of the affected side. These specific points in differentiation, however, are difficult to explain biomechanically.

In reference to Goldthwait's test, Faye mentions that "The examiner, of course, would have already conducted the SLR test and once pain was experienced would have lowered the leg 5° and then dorsiflexed the foot to see if root stress caused the pain. The examiner must also remember that facet, radicular, and trigger-point syndromes can also be present."

Smith-Peterson Test. If it is possible during Goldthwait's test to raise the limb on the unaffected side to a greater level without pain than the involved side, a positive Smith-Peterson's sign is found, which helps to confirm a sacroiliac lesion; ie, pain usually occurs at the same level for either leg when a lumbosacral lesion is present.

Nachlas' Test. The patient is placed in the prone position. Flex the patient's knee to a right angle, then, with pressure against the anterior surface of the ankle, the patient's heel is slowly directed straight toward the patient's ipsilateral buttock. Stabilize the patient's contralateral ilium with your other hand. If a sharp pain is elicited in the patient's ipsilateral buttock or sacral area, a sacroiliac disorder should be suspected. If pain occurs in the patient's lower back or is sciatic-like in nature, a lower lumbar disorder (especially L3 or L4) is suggested. If pain occurs in the patient's upper lumbar area, groin, or anterior thigh, quadriceps shortening (spasticity or contracture) or a femoral nerve lesion should be suspected.

Erichsen's Test. With the patient supine, place your hands on the patient's iliac crests, and localize your thumbs on the lateral aspect of the patient's ASISs (Fig. 6.17). Forcibly compress the pelvis toward the midline. This tends to separate the sacroiliac joints posteriorly. If conducted very carefully, this test can be quite specific. Pain experienced in the sacroiliac joint suggests a joint lesion (postural, traumatic, or infectious).

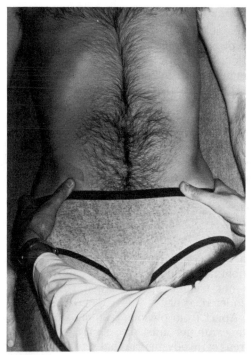

Figure 6.17. Conducting Erichsen's test (Courtesy ACAP).

Iliac Compression Test. The patient is placed on the side with the affected side up. Place yours forearm over the patient's iliac crest and apply pressure downward for about 30 seconds. This tends to compress the sacroiliac and pubic joints. A positive sign of joint inflammation or sprain is seen with an increase in pain; however, absence of pain does not necessarily rule out sacroiliac involvement. This test is usually contraindicated in geriatrics and pediatrics or with any sign of a hip lesion or osseous pelvic pathology.

Hibb's Test. The patient is placed in the prone position. Stand next to the patient on the side of involvement. Stabilize the patient's contralateral uninvolved hip, flex the patient's knee on the involved side toward the buttock, and then slowly adduct the leg, which internally rotates the femur. Pain initiated in the hip joint indicates a hip lesion; pain rising in the sacroiliac joint but not the hip points to a sacroiliac lesion.

Sacroiliac-Lumbosacral Differentiation Test. To differentiate these two common disorders, the patient is placed supine on a firm flat table. A folded towel is placed transversely under the small of the patient's back. The doctor stabilizes the patient's pelvis by cupping the hands over the ASISs and exerting moderate pressure. The patient is instructed to raise both extremities simultaneously with the legs held straight. If the patient senses discomfort or an increase of discomfort in the low back or over the sacrum and gluteal area at about 25°—50° leg raise and before the small of the back wedges against the towel, sacroiliac involvement is suspected. If, on the other hand, discomfort is experienced or augmented only after the legs have been raised beyond 50° and the small of the back wedges firmly against the towel, lumbosacral involvement should be the first suspicion.

Mennell's Tests. The patient is placed prone, and one hand of the examiner is used to stabilize the contralateral pelvis. With your palpating hand, place a thumb over the patient's PSIS and exert pressure, then slide your thumb outward and then inward. The sign is positive if tenderness is increased. When sliding outward, trigger deposits in structures on the gluteal aspect of the PSIS may be noted. If when sliding inward tenderness is increased, it suggests sprain of the superior sacroiliac ligaments. Confirmation is positive when tenderness is increased when you pull the patient's ASIS posterior when standing behind the patient or when you pull the patient's PSIS forward when standing in front of the supine patient. These tests are helpful in determining that sacroiliac tenderness is due to overstressed superior sacroiliac ligaments.

Sacroiliac Stretch Test. The patient is placed supine. Stand facing the patient, cross the patient's arms, place one of your hands on the patient's contralateral ASIS, and place your other hand on the patient's ipsilateral ASIS. Apply oblique (posterolateral) pressure to spread the anterior aspects of the patient's ilia laterally. A positive sign of sacroiliac sprain is a deep-seated pelvic pain that may radiate into the buttock or groin. While the iliac compression test is designed to stretch the posterior sacroiliac ligaments, this test stretches the ligaments on the anterior aspect of the joints.

Gillis' Test. With the patient prone, stand on the side of involvement. Reach over and stabilize the uninvolved sacroiliac joint while the patient's thigh on the involved side is extended at the hip. Pain initiated by this maneuver in the sacroiliac area of the involved side is a positive sign of an acute sacroiliac sprain/subluxation or sacroiliac disease.

Belt Test. The standing male patient, with feet about 12—15 inches apart, flexes forward while you hold the patient's belt at the back. If bending over without support is more painful than with support, it suggests a sacroiliac lesion. Conversely, if bending over with support is more painful than without support, it suggests a lumbosacral or lumbar involvement. A variation of this test is to stand behind the patient and place your hands so that they firmly support the patient's innominates. Some examiners brace a hip against the patient's sacrum while the patient flexes forward to stabilize the pelvis.

Yeoman's Test. The patient is placed prone. With one hand, apply firm pressure over the patient's suspected sacroiliac joint, fixing the patient's anterior pelvis to the table. With your other hand, flex the patient's leg on the affected side to the limit. The patient's thigh is hyperextended by your lifting the patient's knee off the examining table. If pain is increased in the sacroiliac area, it is significant of a ventral sacroiliac or hip lesion because of the stress on the anterior sacroiliac ligaments. Normally, no pain should be felt on this maneuver.

Piedallu's Sign. When a sacral base is locked unilaterally anteroinferior and lateral so that the adjacent ilium is found to be more posteroinferior and medial than normal, the ipsilateral PSIS on the side of inferiority will be low in the standing and sitting positions. If this PSIS becomes higher than the contralateral PSIS during forward flexion, the phenomenon is called a positive *Piedallu's sign.* Such a sign signifies either ipsilateral sacroiliac locking where the sacrum and ilium move as a whole or muscular contraction that prevents motion of the sacrum on the ilium. Regardless, it shows that sacral dysfunction is probably present.

Laguerre's Test. With the patient supine, the thigh and knee are flexed and the thigh is abducted and rotated outward. This forces the head of the femur against the anterior portion of the coxa capsule. Increased groin pain and spasm are usually positive signs of a lesion of the hip joint, iliopsoas muscle spasm, or a sacroiliac lesion. This test can help to differentiate a hip or sacroiliac disorder from a lumbar disorder.

Gaenslen's Test. In this test, the patient is placed supine with knees and hips acutely flexed by the patient who clasps his knees with both hands and pulls them toward the abdomen. This brings the lumbar spine firmly in contact with the table and fixes both the pelvis and lumbar spine. Standing at right angles to the patient, bring the patient well to the side of the table and slowly hyperextend the patient's opposite thigh by gradually increasing force by pressure of one hand on top of the patient's knee while your other hand is on the patient's flexed knee for support in fixing the lumbar spine and pelvis. Some examiners allow the hyperextended limb to fall from the table edge (Fig. 6.18). The hyperextension of the hip exerts a rotating force on the corresponding half of the

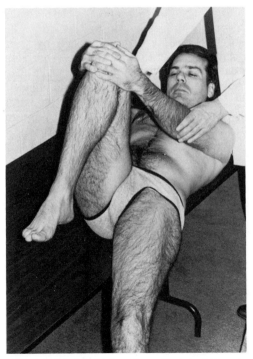

Figure 6.18. Conducting Gaenslen's test (Courtesy ACAP).

pelvis. The pull is made on the ilium through the Y ligament and the muscles attached to the AIISs. The test is positive if the thigh is hyperextended and pain is felt in the sacroiliac area or referred down the thigh, providing that the opposite sacroiliac joint is normal and the sacrum moves as a unit with the side of the pelvis opposite to that being tested. This test should be conducted bilaterally. A positive sign may be elicited in a sacroiliac, hip, or lower lumbar nerve root lesion. If the L4 nerve is involved, pain is usually referred anteriorly to the groin or upper thigh. If this sign is negative, a lumbosacral lesion should be the first suspicion. This test is usually contraindicated in the elderly.

Lewin-Gaenslen Test. The patient is placed in the sidelying position with the underneath lower limb flexed acutely at the hip and knee. Stabilize the uppermost aspect of the patient's hip with one hand. With your other hand, grasp the patient's leg near the knee and extend the patient's thigh on the hip. Initiated or aggravated pain suggests a sacroiliac lesion.

Lewin's Standing Test. With the patient standing with the back toward you, cautiously forces first the right and then the left knee of the patient into complete extension. Then both knees are straightened at the same time. In lumbosacral, lower lumbar, sacroiliac, and gluteal disturbances, these movements will be accompanied by increased pain and the knee will snap back into flexion.

Mazion's Step-Flex Test. A standing patient with low back pain is asked to take a large step forward, hold this position by keeping the toes in place, and then flex the trunk forward. According to Mazion, the initiation or aggravation of the patient's complaint on the contralateral limb (the one behind) exhibits a positive sign of a unilateral subluxated ilium in relation to the sacrum (ie, sacral base anteroinferior).

Neri's Bowing Sign. This sign is positive when a standing patient can flex the trunk further without low-back discomfort when the ipsilateral leg is flexed than when both knees are held in extension. A positive sign suggests hamstring spasm, contractures of the posterior thigh and/or leg muscles, sciatic neuritis, a lumbar IVD lesion, or a sacro-iliac subluxation syndrome.

Minor's Sign. Sciatic radiculitis is suggested by the manner in which the patient with this condition rises from a sitting position. Body weight is supported on the uninvolved side by holding on to the chair for firm support in arising or the patient places the hands on the knees or thighs while working into the upright position, balances on the healthy leg, places one hand on the back, and flexes the leg and extends the thigh of the affected limb. The sign is often positive in sacroiliac lesions, lumbosacral strains and sprains, lumbar fractures and disc syndromes, dystrophies, and myotonias.

Gillet's Comments on Common Fixations Found in Lumbago and Sciatica

The Relationship of Upper Cervical Fixation to Low-Back Pain

Gillet insists that a large percentage of low-back pain cases are not due primarily to lower back fixations. He states that this cannot be emphasized too strongly because there is a type of practitioner who has a tendency to read medical books and consider that everything written in them is true. Such a practitioner will invariably think that the only region to correct is the lower back. If he does not get rapid results in these cases, he feels that "chiropractic" has been applied in vain and that the case must be rapidly referred to an orthopedic surgeon.

Gillet maintains that the first region to correct before any other is the upper-cervical region, even if the trouble appears to be stemming from the lumbar spine. HIO practitioners have published statistics of these cases in which *only* the occiput-atlas-axis complex was adjusted with rapid and gratifying results. There is no reason to deny these statistics, as paradoxical as they may seem on the surface. The fact that they have sometimes been published by chiropractors who are a bit fanatically inclined does not eliminate all their value.

This type of case is often of an overly stressed, highly emotional patient who has had a mental conflict just prior to the onset of the low-back pain. The patient, usually, has had similar pains after other emotional conflicts, and this would tend to show there is an anatomical substratum in the lower back, one that is not great enough to cause the pain by itself but which would constitute some type of localizing cause. The occiput-atlas-axis complex is usually in articular fixation, and the correct adjustment should be given according to the rules laid down previously. Nothing more need be done at this time, for if a good correction is made at the top of the spine (the seat of primary righting reflexes), decided changes will take place in the remainder of the spine immediately. More changes will take place within the next 24 hours. In a certain number of cases, nothing more need be done at any time, for the next day the pain will have disappeared and the complete spine will be found to be moving normally. In other cases, either the atlas is, to start with, only in partial fixation or it has been corrected. Then an examination should be made of the pelvis, and thereafter the lumbar spine, searching for total or at least important fixations in this area.

The Feet

Another part of the body to be taken into consideration in low-back pain cases is the feet. Gillet recommends that foot fixations should be corrected last, when the spine shows no signs of recurrent fixations. However, foot fixations must be investigated and corrected earlier if the spinal fixations that have been corrected have a tendency to return.

Closing Remarks on Diagnostic Considerations

After motion palpation of the pelvis, often several fixations, complete and partial, will have been found. Experience shows that it is best to adjust the articulation that shows the greatest evidence of fixation and contracture, then the next one in order of importance. Empiric evidence also shows that it is *not* the most powerful thrust that is the most corrective. The least force necessary to move a vertebra is the best because excessive force may lead to trauma and a reaction contracture. The force of the thrust should be proportional to the resistance of the joint, and it is always best to act prudently.

This method described for spinal analysis is not complete (it is constantly evolving), but it gives today valuable information concerning the mechanical state of the spine. It eliminates the mistake of adjusting a bent spinous process, it permits an immediate signal that the correction has been made, it eliminates the danger of repeated x-ray studies, it may be used easily as a preventive method of examination and correction, and it gives answers to the questions of *when to adjust* and *when not to adjust* (ie, when a segment is freely movable, there is no need to force movement).

To master the art of motion palpation is not an easy job; but with time, concentration and steadiness, it gives valuable information on the functional state of the spine and the way to better and more stable correction. Based on this principle, chiropractic becomes more scientific and practitioners are led to a better understanding of the true phenomena that occur in the spine and how to achieve better results.

THERAPEUTIC APPROACH

Muscular Fixations

Muscle spasms in the pelvis generally reflect themselves in the trunk, thigh, or both. Shortening of most major muscles acting on the pelvis has a restrictive influence upon the mobility of the femur and an effect upon an individual's stance. When evaluating relative muscle function, note that mild unilateral hypertonicity is difficult to differentiate from contralateral hypotonicity. In differentiation, static palpation may reveal more than kinetic tests.

Piriformis Hypertonicity

If a patient has deep gluteal pain, sciatic neuralgia, and walks with the foot noticeably everted on the side of involvement, involvement of the piriformis should be suspected. Abnormal piriformis tone tends to pull the sacrum anteriorly and to externally rotate the thigh.

The sciatic nerve should pass under the piriformis and follow the "wisdom" of the textbooks. In many cases, however, the nerve takes a different course and is found on surgery to be stretched over or even pass through the muscle in 15%—20% of the population (ie, about one of every 5—7 patients). This common "anomaly" and its consequences are often overlooked.

Piriformis Myofascitis Test. The patient is seated on a table with the hips and knees flexed. Apply resistance as the patient attempts to separate the knees. In piriformis myofascitis, pain and weakness will be noted on resisted abduction and external rotation of the thigh. Inflammation will be confirmed by rectal examination exhibiting acute tenderness over the lateral pelvic wall proximal to the ischial spine.

Iliopsoas Hypertonicity

In the normal erect posture, only about 12% of the weight of the abdominal organs is borne by the suspensory ligaments. The majority of weight is supported by the inclined iliopsoas and held there by the abdominal wall.

Increased tone of the psoas major muscle tends to pull the lumbar spine into anterior and inferior flexion, and externally rotate and flex the thigh. The psoas minor, which spans between T12 and L1 to the arcuate line of the hip bone, assists the psoas major.

In psoas spasm, the thigh is flexed to some degree on the trunk, but this is usually concealed by forward bending of the trunk. Hypertonicity can be confirmed by tension and pain during deep palpation of the abdomen below the umbilicus, lateral to the linea alba, medial to and slightly inferior to the ASIS. The psoas will feel as a taut longitudinal bundle. It is also palpable in the upper sulcus of the pubic arch.

Bilateral psoas shortening results in lumbar rigidity, anterior pelvic tilt, and hip flexion. When associated with acute back pain, the patient tends to flex the knees and hips to help decrease the degree of pelvic tilt and lordosis. When the hip flexors are short, the lumbar region does not flatten in the supine position unless the knees and hips are flexed. In psoatic sciatica, states Faye, the patient walks on their toes on the ipsilateral side of involvement.

Electromyographic studies conducted by Nachemson showed that the iliopsoas is just as important a lumbar stabilizer against gravitational forces in standing as it is a hip flexor during gait. Some authorities feel that the psoas is the key to postural correction.

Michelle, who asserts that 30% of the population has an iliopsoas imbalance, boldly charges that any and all defects of the spine and hip structures should be evaluated in terms of iliopsoas dysfunction. His studies present some evidence that practically all conditions working against the "straight child" are attributable to the failure of the iliopsoas to elongate during bipedal maturation. He claims: "When the abnormal force of the nonelongated iliopsoatic musculature is presented bilaterally, the directional force is symmetrical, with the formation of an exaggerated dorsal kyphosis."

Ely's Test. To support iliopsoas spasm suspicions, the patient is placed prone with the toes hanging over the edge of the table, legs relaxed. Either heel is approximated to the opposite buttock. After flexion of the knee, pain in the hip will make it impossible to carry out the test if there is any irritation of the psoas muscle or its sheath. The buttock will tend to rise on the involved side. However, a positive Ely's test can also be an indication of rectus femoris contraction, a lumbar lesion, a contracture of the tensor fascia lata, or an osseous hip lesion. Few singular orthopedic maneuvers will isolate a specific lesion.

Thomas' Test. This is another test to determine excessive iliopsoas tension. The supine patient holds one flexed knee against the abdomen with the hands while the other limb is allowed to fully extend (Fig. 6.19). The patient's lumbar spine should normally flatten. If the extended limb does not extend fully (ie, the knee flexes from the table) or if the patient rocks the chest forward or arches the spine, a fixed flexion contracture of the hip is indicated, as from a shortened iliopsoas muscle. Michelle uses the degree of pain elicited on forceful extension of the flexed knee as his criteria of iliopsoas tension. This test should always be conducted bilaterally.

Psoas Abscess

If the urogenital complex, colon, appendix, pancreas, or lumbar lymph nodes or nerves are diseased, the sheath of the psoas is likely to be secondarily inflamed and painful. As the psoas muscle also crosses the sacroiliac joint, inflammation is likely to lead to a protective reflex to fix the joint from irritating motion.

Buttock Sign. To conduct this test, a lower extremity of a supine patient is passively flexed at the hip with the knee extended as in an SLR test. If the flexion of the limb on the trunk is restricted by local or radiating buttock pain (rather than pain in the hip or lower back), it is significant of an inflammatory pelvic lesion such as ischiorectal abscess, osteomyelitis of or near the hip joint, coxa bursitis, sacroiliac septic arthritis, or an advanced pelvic neoplasm.

Baron's Sign in Appendicitis. The patient is placed supine, relaxed, and instructed to breath deeply. The examiner's 2nd, 3rd, and 4th fingers are placed on the patient's Poupart's ligament and pressure is made in the direction of the psoas muscle. The patient is then told to elevate the leg of the same side with the knee extended, forming about a 45° angle at the hip. In this position, the palpating fingers can readily palpate the now tensed psoas muscle. Similar palpation should be made bilaterally for comparison.

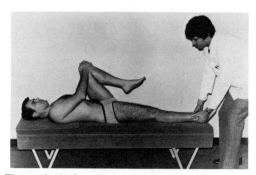

Figure 6.19. Conducting Thomas' test (Courtesy ACAP).

In suspected cases of chronic appendicitis, Baron found that the right psoas muscle was frequently hypersensitive to pressure. Even in the healthy individual, a tensed psoas may be tender, but when the appendix is involved, the tenderness is more marked on the right side. It is also important to realize that because the psoas is covered by peritoneum it can be painful in the presence of sacrospinal and gluteal myalgias; in lumbar, lumbosacral, and iliosacral arthrosis; and sometimes in sciatica.

General Hip Hypertonicity

Two forms of spasm are common in the hip joint: (1) that which is due to irritation of the psoas alone, and (2) that in which all the muscles moving the joint are more or less contracted. The normal range of hip flexion is 120°. In isolated psoas spasm, motions of the hip (rotation, adduction, abduction, and flexion) are not impeded.

General spasm of the hip muscles is tested with the patient supine and the limb flexed at a right angle, both at the knee and at the hip. A child may be tested on its parent's lap. Using the asymptomatic limb as a standard for comparison, draw the patient's knee away from the midline (abduction), toward and past the midline (adduction), and toward the patient's chest (flexion). Rotation is tested by holding the knee still and moving the patient's foot away from and toward the median line of the patient.

Physical Tests for Hip Pathology

Patrick's F-AB-ER-E Test. This test helps to confirm a suspicion of hip joint pathology. With the patient supine, grasp the patient's ankle and flex knee. The patient's thigh is flexed (F), abducted (AB), externally rotated (ER), and extended (E). Pain arising in the hip during the maneuvers, particularly on abduction and external rotation, was attributed by Patrick to be a sign of hip pathology. [See Clinical Comment 6.7]

Hip Abduction Stress Test. The patient is placed in the lateral recumbent position with the underneath lower limb flexed acutely at the hip and knee. With the upper limb held straight and extended at the knee, the patient is instructed to attempt to abduct the upper limb while you apply resistance. Pain initiated in the area of the uppermost sacroiliac joint or the hip joint suggests an inflammatory process of the respective joint.

Trendelenburg's Hip Test. If the hip and its muscles are normal, the iliac crest and sacral dimple will be slightly low on the weight-bearing side and high on the leg-elevated side when one leg is lifted. To test this, have the patient with a suspected hip involvement stand on one foot (on the side of involvement), and raise the other foot and leg in hip and knee flexion. If there is hip joint involvement and muscle weakness, the iliac crest and sacral dimple will be markedly high on the standing side and low on the side the leg is elevated. A positive sign suggests that the gluteus medius and minimus muscles on the supported side are weak. The gait will exhibit a characteristic lurch to counteract the imbalance caused by the descended hip. The sign is is not specific, however, It is also commonly positive in a developing Legg-Calve-Perthes disease, poliomyelitis, muscular dystrophy, coxa vara, Otto's pelvis, epiphyseal separation, pathology of the superior gluteal nerve, coxa ankylosis, hip dislocation, fracture, or chronic subluxation of L4, L5, or the sacrum.

Ligamentous Fixations

Gillet reports that there are three common ligamentous fixations that occur in the pelvis: (1) sacrotuberous ligament fixation,

---

DR. FAYE'S CLINICAL COMMENT #6.7

While doing this test, I find it clinically significant to differentiate capsular restriction from muscular fixation. At the end range of the F-AB-ER-E maneuver, I spring the joint by pressing on the knee. A springy end feel warrants a stretching technique. The loss of springiness demands a hip joint manipulation that produces an audible movement and muscle stretching.

(2) posterior sacroiliac ligament fixation, and (3) anterior sacroiliac ligament fixations. These fixations are extremely common and tend to recur unless proper exercises are conducted frequently.

It should be remembered that, contrary to what is found in muscular hypertonicity, ligaments can he "pulled" into shape; ie, a *slow* forcing of the articulation in fixation can often be sufficient to stretch the shortened ligament. A dynamic thrust is not always indicated.

Sacrotuberous Ligament Fixation

To elongate a shortened sacrotuberous ligament, Gillet recommends a strong thrust on the apex of the sacrum that is directed cephalad. He states that this type of maneuver is usually effective, rarely needs to be made more than once, and that the postadjustive change should exhibit at least a 50% improvement. In contrast, Faye has found that knee-chest stretching exercises are the most effective.

Posterior Sacroiliac Ligament Fixation

Shortening of the ligaments binding the posterior surface of the sacrum to the iliac crest is found far more often than sacrotuberous shortening. Tight posterior sacroiliac ligaments tend to pull the iliac crests posteromedially, closing the distance between the PSISs (which would indicate movement of the sacral base anteriorly). Thus, the adjustive thrust should be directed to separate the joint to allow the sacrum to move posteriorly. A short, stiff adjustment is recommended by Gillet on the fixated aspect of the sacrum (base or apex) or on the superior or inferior aspect of the ilium, depending on where the major fixation is found. The points of contact

will vary according to the particular planes of motion determined to be restricted. Preadjustive thrusts will help determine whether the major site of fixation is on either the superior or inferior aspect of the sacroiliac complex.

Anterior Sacroiliac Ligament Fixation

Shortening of the anterior sacroiliac ligaments tends to pull the iliac crests anterolaterally, increasing the distance between the PSISs, and push the sacral base posteriorly. The adjustment should be designed to move the sacral base forward, relative to the ilia, allowing the two ilia to glide backward. This type of fixation can often be felt by the resistance of the inferior or superior aspect of the sacrum during preadjustive thrusts.

Supportive and Rehabilitative Exercise

To assist in the elongation process of shortened soft tissues, instruct the patient to: (1) Lie supine on a firm surface, flex the right knee toward the chest, grasp it with both hands, pull the thigh firmly against the abdomen, hold this position for 30 seconds, and then slowly return the limb to the extended position. During this maneuver, the other limb should remain in contact with the surface on which the patient is recumbent. The same exercise is then conducted with the contralateral limb. (2) After this, both knees are flexed toward the chest in a similar manner. (3) Each knee is then pulled diagonally toward the opposite shoulder and held there for 30 seconds. (4) Last but not least, the sitting patient places the lateral side of the ipsilateral ankle on the opposite knee in a figure 4 manner and pushes down on the medial side of the knee to the point of firm re-

DR. FAYE'S CLINICAL COMMENT #6.8

In acute low-back pain cases, marked relief can often be achieved by the doctor, seated behind the sitting patient, reaching around the patient and pulling the patient's ipsilateral hip into flexion by using a knee as a fulcrum. This pull should be held for 30 seconds. The relief obtained is often enough to get a house-confined patient into the office for roentgenography and further care.

sistance and holds the knee there for 30 seconds. This exercise should be conducted once each morning and evening to assure that corrected fixations will not return. If the patient can effectively conduct this exercise initially, states Gillet, it is likely that a diagnosis of pelvic ligamentous fixation is in error.

This exercise will, unfortunately, not have any important effect on total sacroiliac fixations. It is also evident that the effect of this exercise will only be momentary in cases where the pelvic fixations are due to fixations elsewhere, principally those of the feet.

Faye teaches the same technique with the patient in the sitting position. Little modification is required, and the stretching exercise conducted in either position will be equally effective. [See Clinical Comment 6.8]

Total vs Partial Sacroiliac Fixations

Total Sacroiliac Fixations

It is well to repeat here that in total articular fixation of both sacroiliac articulations, all the tests devised by Gillet will be positive. Even if the pubis is free, it is evident that a total lack of movement in the sacroiliac articulations will not permit motion in the pubic joint. The contrary is also true. In pubic fixation, the normal sitting-standing changes in the pelvis will not be found, the knee-lift test will show no motion, but the sacrum will still be able to rotate between the ilia (in fact, to a degree of hypermobility.

Partial Sacroiliac Fixations

Partial fixations of a sacroiliac joint show up differently. The pubic test will show movement, and the knee raising test will show movement if the palpatory contact is taken on both ilia but will indicate fixation if the contacts are taken individually; ie, one thumb on the sacrum and the other on the ilium. Obviously, if the two contacts are made on the articulation in fixation, no movement of the ilium will be felt.

The technique of pelvic palpation is man-

dated by the great number of potential partial fixations. This makes it necessary to use multiple contacts to correctly analyze the type of fixations being palpated (Figs. 6.20 and 6.21). In the first knee-lifting palpation, it is often necessary to use some eight different points, two on the superior posterior iliac spines, two on the crests, two near the inferior end of the sacroiliac articulations, and two underneath on the ischia. These last contact points are somewhat difficult to maintain and especially to follow if movement is normal.

In bilateral articular fixation of the sacrum or total fixation of the pubis, all contact points will show no movement, whether the right or left knee is raised. In unilateral total articular fixation, all points will show a diminished amount of motion, because only one articulation is functioning. It will then be necessary to change contacts to the sacrum and each ilium separately to determine the articulation responsible.

Considerations in the Lateral-Recumbent "Roll" Adjustment

The most popular adjustment in this region is the side-position "lumbar roll." It is known that this adjustment, as it is usually given, does not restrict its force to one articulation, much less to one part of an articulation. It is also evident that the same adjustment position can often be used for many different types of pelvic fixations. Fortunately also, and contrary to the observations made in other regions of the spine, a poorly delivered adjustment in this area will have far less adverse effect, either locally or in the remainder of the spine, not forgetting the highly sensitive uppercervical region. This should, however, not be interpreted that no harm can be produced by a traumatizing "cracking" adjustment on the pelvis. We always desire to use the minimal amount of force necessary to correct the fixation, no more.

Gillet asks us to remember that an adjustment in any region may be used to do one of three things: (1) break up adhesions in the articulation by opening it, (2) force it to glide in the plane lines of its articular surfaces (in

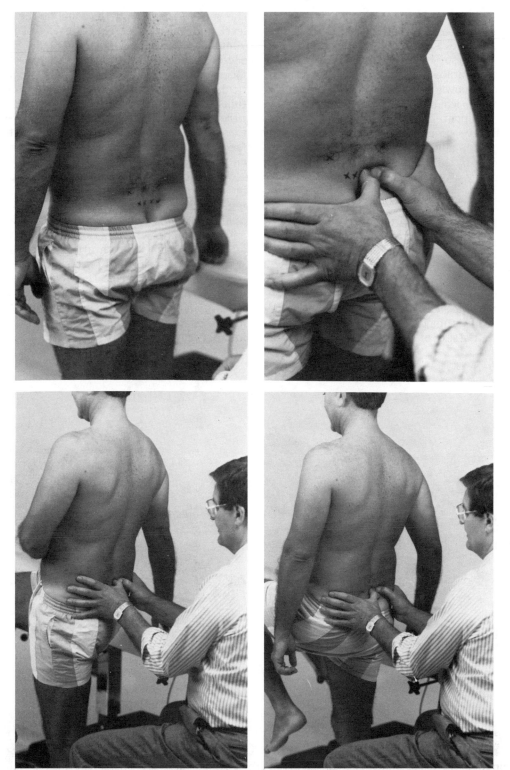

Figure 6.20. *Upper left,* contact points of the sacral triangle; *upper right,* securing palpation contacts for the upper right sacroiliac joint; *lower left,* patient lifting right knee; *lower right,* patient lifting left knee.

any direction that is restricted) but with a preference for the direction that will "replace" the "subluxated" bone, and/or (3) move the two bones in fixation in such a way that separates the two ends of the muscle to "break down" the hypertonicity or apply a force at right angles to the shortened muscle or ligament to elongate it. In fact, these adjustive effects may explain the different types of adjustments that have been invented by chiropractors since the turn of the century.

Summary of Sacroiliac Pathodynamics from an Adjuster's Viewpoint

Because of the boot or bean-shaped design of the sacroiliac joint and the architecture of its major ligaments, there are two potential sites of fixation on each side: one at the superior aspect of the joint at the S1 level, and one at the inferior aspect of the joint near the superior aspect of S3. The sacral facets of each of these articulations faces anterolaterally. Between these two articulation, at the S2 level, is a rounded protuberance on the sacrum that serves as a *pivot* for the joints above or below if either of these joints are fixated. The surface of the facets on the ilium are reciprocally congruent with those of the sacrum. See Figure 6.22.

With this understanding of the sacroiliac articulations, we see that there are four functional articulations to consider in sacroiliac analysis: the right superior and inferior joints, and the left superior and inferior joints. Inasmuch as each articulation participates in anterior and posterior rotation of the ilium on the sacrum, there can be eight motions that may be restricted, any one of which can greatly disturb pelvic dynamics and that of the spine above the pelvic foundation. See Table 6.1.

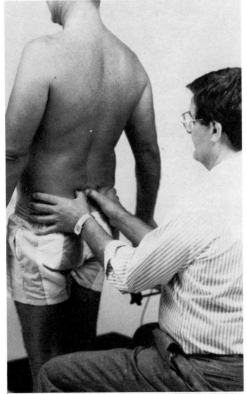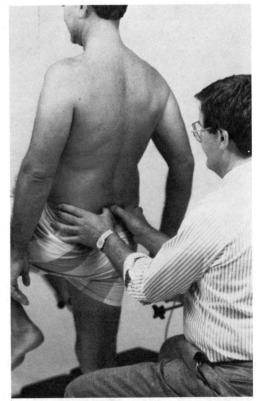

Figure 6.21. Palpating the upper left sacroiliac joint. *Left,* neutral position; *right,* during the left leg-raising test.

Some points in communication should be kept in mind when sacroiliac motion is described:

1. Normal iliac and sacral actions are reciprocally opposite. That is, one might say that the PSIS of the ilium normally rotates backward and downward relative to the sacrum during the knee-raising test. One might also say, and be just as correct, that the sacral base unilaterally rotates forward and downward relative to the ilium. Conversely, if a free ilium rotates upward and forward on the sacrum, the sacrum can be said to have rotated backward and downward on the ilium. Always keep in mind that these terms of rotatory motion are relative. You need no longer be confused when the points of reference (ilium or sacrum) are interchanged.

2. Inasmuch as iliac and sacral action are reciprocally opposite, it rarely matters whether the adjustive contact is taken on the ilium or the sacrum. For example, a thrust delivered anterosuperiorly on an ilium's PSIS will have the same biomechanical effect as a thrust delivered anteroinferiorly on the sacral apex of that side or anterosuperiorly against the contralateral ischium. Thus, you frequently have the option of taking an iliac, sacral, or ischial contact, depending on how the joint motion is restricted. One exception to this is the obvious fact that it is difficult to move the sacral base backward; much easier to move the ilium forward.

3. Iliac and ischial actions are reciprocally opposite because they are just different aspect of the same bone, the innominate. When

the ilium moves backward and downward on the sacrum, the ischium on the same side must move forward and upward, and vice versa. It has been explained previously that as the iliac crests rotate backward, as in

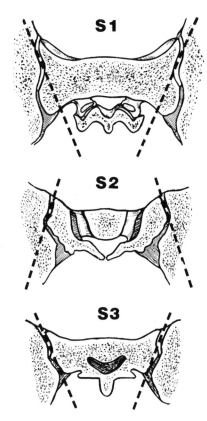

Figure 6.22. Coronal sections through S1, S2, and S3 segments, showing the typical planes of sacroiliac articulation (Courtesy ACAP).

Table 6.1. Sites of Potential Sacroiliac Motion Restriction

Articulation	Motion
Left superior	Iliac rotation posteroinferiorly
Left superior	Iliac rotation anterosuperiorly
Left inferior	Iliac rotation posteroinferiorly
Left inferior	Ischial rotation anteroinferiorly
Right superior	Iliac rotation posteroinferiorly
Right superior	Iliac rotation anterosuperiorly
Right inferior	Iliac rotation posteroinferiorly
Right inferior	Iliac rotation anteroinferiorly

sitting, the sacral base nods forward and the ischia flare laterally. Conversely, when the iliac crests rotate forward, as in standing, the sacral base slides backward and the interischial space decreases.

4. The options in chiropractic technic are usually not based on mechanical principles, but on their ease of administration. For example, rotating the iliac crest forward has the same mechanical effect as moving the sacral base backward. However, the former is much easier to apply than the latter. Conversely, moving a sacral base or ischium forward has the same mechanical effect as moving the iliac crest backward, but the former is much easier to apply that the latter.

5. The superior and inferior articulations of the sacroiliac joint on each side resemble a toggle switch. That is, as the sacral base nods forward the sacral apex juts backward. Conversely, as the sacral base slides backward, the sacral apex arcs forward. This toggle effect between the sacral base and sacral apex can be utilized in a large number of sacral technics. It is much easier to move the sacral base posteriorly by a thrust directed anteroinferiorly against the sacral apex than attempt to directly move the sacral base posteriorly. The pressure required anteriorly would undoubtedly injure the pelvic organs and be highly painful to the patient because of the intervening plexus. This toggle effect between the superior and inferior sacral articulations is afforded by the interarticular proturberance on the sacrum that serves as a fulcrum. It is not applicable, however, if the both the superior and inferior aspects of the joint are fixated.

Once these basic principles are understood, chiropractic sacroiliac technics will no longer be a confusing subject. You will immediately see that they are either logical for the situation at hand or in error.

Adjusting Pelvic Articular Fixations

It is Gillet's opinion that total sacroiliac fixations are second in importance only to total occipitoatlantal fixations. The lesion may be bilateral or unilateral. If unilateral, the con-

tralateral joint will usually be hypermobile in compensation and be the site of pain and tenderness.

Patient Laterally Recumbent

Gillet recommends the standard side-posture "roll" for releasing sacroiliac fixations, but special care must be made to deliver the thrust in the proper plane against the site of fixation. The adjustment may be made with the patient in the lateral recumbent position by placing the patient so that the fixated side is upward and taking contact on the the involved iliac crest or ischium, depending upon what intra-articular motion is to be achieved. This is the common application. An alternative method is applied by placing the patient so that the fixated side is downward and taking contact on the contralateral aspect of the sacrum; base or apex, depending upon what intra-articular motion is desired.

In either position, there is no need in most cases to produce heavy pressure on the patient's flexed knee—just enough to stabilize the patient during the adjustment. It will sometimes be found, however, that a firm pressure on the flexed knee will be beneficial in opening the superior aspect of the joint. Each adjustment must be adapted to the needs of the situation and patient at hand.

The following technics are described by Faye:

1. *Fixation at the Upper Aspect of the Sacroiliac Joint: Involved Side Upward.* Place the patient in the lateral recumbent position with the involved ilium facing upward. The patient's uppermost knee is flexed to the maximum. Assure that the patient's lumbars and shoulders are in the neutral position, and apply the contact of the active hand on the PSIS of the involved joint. Support the patient's uppermost shoulder with your stabilizing hand (Fig. 6.23). Open the posterior aspect of the sacroiliac joints by applying downward pressure against the patient's flexed knee with your knee, and with your active hand, deliver an impulse with a body drop directed to mobilize the area of fixation.

2. *Fixation at the Upper Aspect of the*

Sacroiliac Joint: Involved Side Downward. Place the patient in the lateral recumbent position with the involved ilium against the adjusting table. Assure that the patient's lumbars and shoulders remain in the neutral position. Flex and depress the patient's uppermost knee to stretch the posterior aspect of the sacroiliac joints. Support the patient's uppermost shoulder with your stabilizing hand (Fig. 6.24). Apply contact on the upper quadrant of the sacrum just medial to the PSIS that is closest to the table, and deliver an impulse with body drop directed against the fixation.

3. *Fixation at the Lower Aspect of the Sacroiliac Joint: Involved Side Upward.* Place the patient in the lateral recumbent position with the involved ilium facing upward. The patient's uppermost knee is flexed to the maximum (Fig. 6.25). Support the patient's uppermost shoulder with your stabilizing hand. Assuring that the patient's lumbars and shoulders are in the neutral position, apply an ischial contact, depress the

patient's knee to open the sacroiliacs posteriorly, and deliver an impulse with body drop to rotate the involved ilium.

4. *Fixation at the Lower Aspect of the Sacroiliac Joint: Involved Side Downward.* Place the patient in the lateral recumbent position with the involved ilium against the adjusting table. Assure that the patient's lumbars and shoulders remain in the neutral position. Flex and depress the patient's uppermost knee to stretch the posterior aspect of the sacroiliac joints. Support the patient's uppermost shoulder with your stabilizing hand. Apply contact on the lower quadrant of the sacrum (on the side closest to the table), and deliver an impulse with body drop directed against the fixation (Fig. 6.26).

Patient Prone

If posterior intra-articular adhesions are suspected, the joint may be opened by "springing" the joint open in either the side

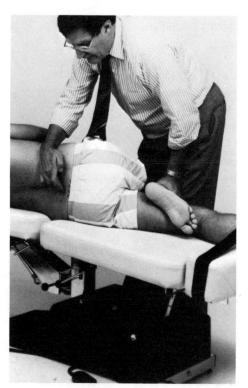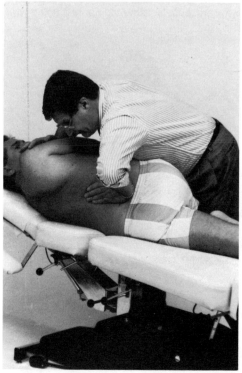

Figure 6.23. Adjusting a fixation at the upper aspect of the sacroiliac joint, involved side facing upward. *Left,* isolating the contact point; *right,* delivering the thrust.

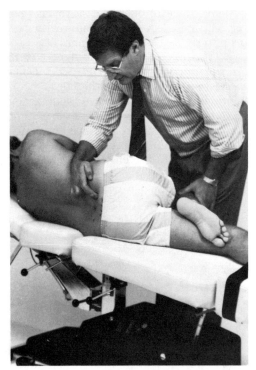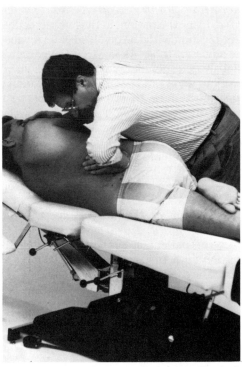

Figure 6.24. Adjusting a fixation at the upper aspect of the sacroiliac joint, involved side facing downward. *Left,* isolating the contact point; *right,* delivering the thrust.

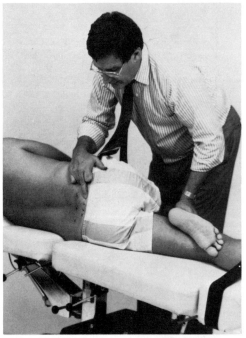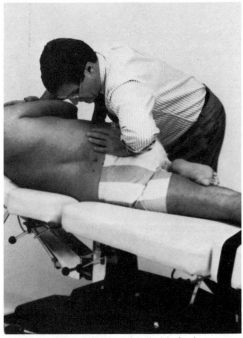

Figure 6.25. Adjusting a fixation at the lower aspect of the sacroiliac joint, involved side facing upward. *Left,* isolating the contact point; *right,* delivering the thrust.

position or with the patient prone. In adjusting a unilateral fixation, the contacts made on the ilium or ischium are bilateral; ie, one serving as the contact hand and the other as the stabilizing hand. The thrust should be firm, rapid, and short, with the abdominal piece of the adjusting table relieved of firm tension.

Lateral flexion mobility of a sacroiliac joint may still be restricted after A-P and P-A mobility has been restored.

Using Muscle Tension as an Aid During an Adjustment

Schafer advocates using muscle tension as an aid to sacroiliac adjustments whenever possible. For example, when rotating an iliac crest anteriorly on the sacral base with the patient in the side position, he does not flex the patient's uppermost knee. Rather, he flexes the patient's underneath knee and moves the extended upper limb backward to produce tension on the quadriceps and hamstring relaxation, which passively helps to rotate the iliac crest anteriorly. He only flexes the patient's uppermost limb when an ischial contact is taken so that tension on the hamstrings will assist in rotating the innominate posteriorly. This, states Schafer, is the approach frequently used in pioneer chiropractic. The more commonly applied flexed uppermost limb positioning taught today is of osteopathic heritage.

The same principles of using muscle tension as a passive aid can be used when the adjustment is applied with the patient prone. For example, when a contact is taken on an iliac crest, the patient's extended lower limb can be raised at the knee with the stabilizing hand to produce tension on the quadriceps and relax the hamstrings. Unfortunately, the advantage of a contralateral stabilizing hand will be lost. To prevent the contralateral side of pelvis from raising during the adjustment, a 2-inch-wide leather strap across the patient's pelvis just below

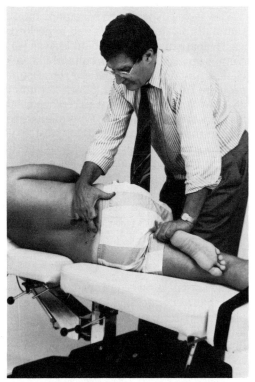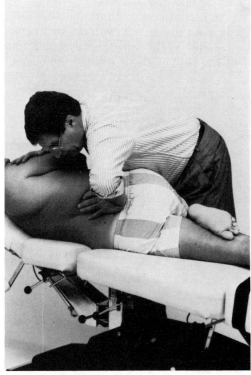

Figure 6.26. Adjusting a fixation at the lower aspect of the sacroiliac joint, involved side facing downward. *Left,* isolating the contact point; *right,* delivering the thrust.

your contact can be used. An alternative is to have a clinical assistant apply the stabilizing counterpressure.

Patient Supine

The following techniques are taught by Faye:

1. To perform general posterior rotation of an ilium on the sacrum with the patient supine, flex the patient's knee and hip on the side of involvement. The patient's foot should rest flat and comfortably against the tabletop. Stand on the side of involvement, apply a palm contact over the near ASIS, support the patient's contralateral hip with your stabilizing hand, lean against the patient's flexed knee to bring it toward the medial line and open the sacroiliac joint posteriorly, and then deliver a stiff-arm body drop upon the ASIS. This will rotate the ilium posteriorly (extend) on the sacrum. In stubborn fixations, it may be helpful to place your stabilizing hand under the patient's ischium and lift upward as your active hand applies the thrust against the iliac crest.

2. To perform general anterior rotation of an ilium on the sacrum with the patient supine, stand on the side of involvement, and shift the patient's body near to the edge of

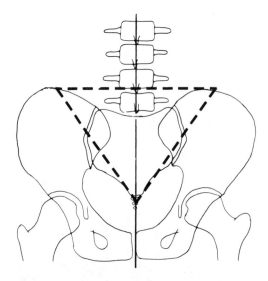

Figure 6.27. The lumbosacral triangle. It is this area that most low-back pain syndromes are expressed (Courtesy ACAP).

the table where you are standing. Flex the patient's knee and hip on the side of involvement, raise the patient's leg, extending the knee, bring the limb laterally past the side of the tabletop, and allow the limb to lower by its own weight below the level of the tabletop. This will place a stretching force on the anterior muscles of the thigh attached to the ilium that will tend to rotate the ilium anteriorly.

The above technique, not advised for the elderly patient or a patient afflicted with osteoporosis or coxa pathology, should be applied as a slow stretching maneuver. If the limb is allowed to drop suddenly in other than a supple youth, it is easy to produce a groin strain or an anterior dislocation of the head of the femur. It is also contraindicated in the supple child whose acetabulae are shallow.

Gillet's Method of Correcting Lumbosacral Kyphosis or Hyperlordosis

This leaves us with two remaining lumbosacral distortions: kyphosis and hyperlordosis. The patient who enters bent forward and cannot straighten up is frequently seen in clinical practice. Such a patient represents a problem to the chiropractor who wants to give the usual "adjustment to replace a subluxated vertebra." In this type of case, the lumbar muscles will usually react so strongly to a rapid thrust that not only will nothing "move," but the patient's pain will be greatly exacerbated immediately. Specific correction of lumbar kyphosis and hyperlordosis will be described in a following section of this chapter. See Figure 6.27.

Lumbosacral Kyphosis

The patient is placed prone on the adjusting table, as comfortable as possible (ie, the abdominal support is raised and/or cushions are inserted anteriorly to fit the forward flexion of the spine. Pressure is then applied to the apex of the curve to a degree that produces discomfort but not enough to set up a defensive reaction on the part of the patient's lumbar muscles. This pressure is applied in a series of short "kneading" thrusts, always to the degree that the patient can stand without producing a "splinting" reaction in the patient's lumbar and abdominal muscles. Little by little, the thrusts will become less painful, and the patient's lumbar muscles will be felt to relax under your hands. After 4 or 5 minutes of this, it will be possible to lower the abdominal piece or remove one cushion after another until the lumbars, instead of being kyphotic, will actually be in normal lordosis. At this time, a vigorous recoil thrust can be given at the point where the apex of the kyphosis was previously. Upon arising slowly, the patient will be able to walk out far straighter than when he came in.

In a few cases, the above technique will not be applicable; ie, no amount of easy thrusts on the lumbars will produce relaxation. On the contrary, the more "kneading" done, the more the lumbar muscles will contract. It will then be necessary to leave this region alone and to correct all the major and secondary fixations in the remainder of the spine. Remember that fixations as a whole summate the amounts of irritation that they produce. This causes a general tightening of all the spinal muscles. Therefore, every time a fixation anywhere in the spine is corrected, the amount of residual tone of all the spinal muscles is lessened. Little by little, day by day, the lumbar muscles will slowly relax without early local treatment, the kyphosis will reduce, and the associated pain will disappear.

Lumbosacral Hyperlordosis

In contrast to lumbosacral kyphosis is the *chronic* low-back fixation that exhibits as a local hyperlordosis. This usually occurs in the lower lumbars and is clearly seen by moving the sitting patient into full forward flexion. In this position, the whole spine should form a smooth curve posteriorly. The lordotic fixation, however, will exhibit as two or three vertebrae that do not follow the general curve. They will remain flat or lordotic. A dimple may be seen in the skin, indicating some degree of spondylolisthesis.

It is possible to "motion palpate" this fixation by placing the palpating finger or thumb in the interspinous space. This space will be unusually small, and it will not open when the spine is flexed forward or close during extension.

Gillet reports that this fixation is due in most cases to hypertonus of the interspinous muscles or shortened ligaments. In many cases, the muscular hypertonicity is such that the spinouses of the two consecutive vertebrae are pulled against one another. In many cases, the pre- and post-zygapophyses will be in an abnormal position relative to each other, leaving a triangular space with the inferior articulation jutting into the IVF. This condition often gives the typical picture of a facet syndrome or radiculitis.

In the beginning, states Gillet, it is always the muscle that pulls the spinouses together. It is only later that the ligament shortens and the muscle degenerates and atrophies. A recoil adjustment with a contact on the inferior spinous, or in between the spinouses (abdominal piece free) according to the principle of thrusting at right angles to the muscle, will usually release the muscle hypertonicity.

There is no way to determine whether it is the muscle or the ligament that is pulling the vertebrae together. If the recoil does not succeed, then the patient must be placed on the back, the knees pulled up toward the chest, and then forced a little farther. If the knees flex easily to the chest, you can place the palm of your free hand under the patient's buttocks and force that part of the spine inferior to the fixation backward. In chronic fixations of this type, it is necessary to ask the patient to continue this lumbar-curling exercise at home.

Schafer notes that this exercise may also be done in the sitting position, and that the typical patient is more apt to apply it several times a day while watching television than attaining the supine position. Forward flexion of the trunk on the pelvis while sitting has the same biomechanical effects on the lumbar spine as hip and knee flexion in the supine position. Instruct the patient to slowly curl forward, stretching the arms downward between abducted knees. When the maximum range of passive motion is reached, tightness and a soft motion block will be perceived in the lower back. When this point is reached, the patient is instructed to bob up and down in a small arc (about 6 inches) several times rhythmically to slowly stretch the posterior spinal tissues and increase the range of motion. The patient then slowly returns to the neutral position and repeats the stretching exercise two or three times. This exercise bout should be repeated at least three times daily during rehabilitation; every 2 hours during the acute stage. [See Clinical Comment 6.9]

Measuring the Amount of Correction Obtained. An effective way to measure the amount of correction obtained, states Gillet, is to place a ruler (about 10 inches long) under the back of the supine patient while he is in full forward flexion. The mid point of the ruler should be centered as nearly as possible over the mid point of the patient's lordosis. A mark is then made on the patient's skin over the two ends of the ruler. After the adjustment, the patient is again put into full forward flexion (sitting), and the distance between the two points described above is remeasured. If the involved spinouses now separate more than before the adjustment, the two points on the skin will be farther apart. In muscle fixations, the change may be as large as a centimeter. In ligament fixations, however, it will rarely exceed 8 millimeters because the involved ligament(s) cannot "relax" like a muscle. It is normal, therefore, to expect a slower change in a ligamentous fixation than in a muscle-induced hyperlordosis.

Correcting Pubic Fixations

Pubic fixations are of the ligamentous type. The supine exercise previously described for sacroiliac fixations is usually quite effective in correcting and maintaining pubic fixations. If the pubic fixation is strongly fixed, the following adjustment should be considered: Place the patient supine and select the ASIS that has rotated the most anteroinferiorly. Flex the patient's hip and bring the corresponding knee toward the patient's chest, adding some body weight of your own if necessary. Stabilizing the patient's contralateral ilium with your nonactive hand. This is a slow stretching maneuver. A heavy sharp thrust should never be applied.

Gillet's Comments on Cases of Low-Back Pain

In this concluding section, we will describe the routine of palpation and correction used by Gillet in all cases of low-back pain of neuromusculoskeletal origin.

In Gillet's practice, for all cases, he searches for total fixations of the first two cervical vertebrae and corrects them first. In a large number of cases, nothing else is required if the results are complete and rapid. This does not mean that the patient's "lumbago" or "sciatica" was simulated or that it was some type of psychologic "revenge." The upper-cervical fixation did exist, and it was probably brought on by an emotionally induced contraction of the muscles at the base of the skull. Any lower lumbar fixation found would therefore be a localizing factor and the cervical fixation would be the precipitating focus of the patient's pain.

True, these cases would probably get well eventually if these fixations were corrected in inverse order, or even if they were adjusted during the same visit. It has been Gillet's experience, however, proved time and again, that the best, the most rapid, and the most lasting results are attained when the fixations are corrected in the order suggested (upper cervical, pelvis, and lower lumbars), with at least several hours between the two

---

DR. FAYE'S CLINICAL COMMENT #6.9

In countries where people frequently squat on their heels flat footed, much less degenerated disc disease exists. This squatting posture produces interspinous separation of the lumbar spine. Patients with lumbosacral hyperlordosis should be asked to practice this posture until they can remain comfortable for at least 3 minutes. If they cannot achieve this posture easily, instruct them to hold on to the edge of a desk or a sink until balance is easily achieved. The worse they are at this exercise initially, the more they need it.

corrections to give time to the body to adapt itself to the corrections made.

Gillet employs the following two palpations: (1) palpation for total occipitoatlantal fixation (A-P and P-A movement with the palpation contact placed just below the rim of the occiput, on the two sides of the posterior arch; (2) palpation for total pelvic fixation (A-P and P-A movement, using the back of the hand). Once fixations within these two structure have been corrected, the lumbar vertebra are examined, first for total fixations and then especially for partial fixations.

A question has often been asked about the difficulty of producing the necessary movements of the spine in palpating for fixations in patients that are in considerable pain. This is not an insurmountable difficulty. It is easy to produce small movements that are revealing: motion that is not enough to exacerbate the patient's pain but enough to reveal any fixations present.

In the lumbar region, three different types of fixation are often found. In fact, as muscular hypertonicity can be severe in this region, it is not difficult to see the type of fixation likely present just by recognizing the characteristic shape of the spinal distortion.

Low-Back Pain on the Convex Side of Lumbar Scoliosis. The most common "distortion" is one of lateral flexion-rotation. This constitutes the basis for the typical "antalgic" posture, which is caused principally by a contraction of the quadratus lumborum that pulls the lumbar vertebrae towards the iliac crest and rotates them posteriorly on the same side. In this type of distortion, the patient's local pain or sciatica will be on the side of lumbar laterality and posteriority. The mechanism of subluxation, states Gillet, will be due to a rotation of L5 on the sacrum, or L4 on L5, in which the pre- and post-zygopophyses have separated, leaving a space between the articular surfaces and forcing the lower facet into the IVF to produce a classic "pressure on nerve." In this type of fixation, it is the lumbar rotation toward the concave side that should take priority consideration because the articulation on that side is still able to function partially. On rotation to the convex side, the movement will immediately be stopped by the hypertonic

muscle.

The most efficient adjustment, if the patient can relax enough to permit it, is a "roll" with the patient lying on the concave side. The contact is applied on the iliac crest to exert a rapid traction on the quadratus lumborum. If this is not possible, the muscle may be relaxed by applying a rapid thrust directly on it when the patient is prone and the abdominal piece is free.

Low-Back Pain on the Concave Side of Lumbar Scoliosis. Another type of "sciatica" described by Gillet is one in which the pain is on the concave side of the lumbar scoliosis. Here the mechanism is different. Instead of being separated by muscle hypertonicity, the articulations are pulled together. The offending muscle is invariably the intertransverse. It pulls the vertebrae into lateral flexion and flattens the disc on one side. The patient's pain is on the concave side of the curve, and there is little or no vertebral rotation. Inducing movement (lateral flexion) towards the concave side will be easier in spite of the fact that it is the side of pain. On the contralateral side, however, there will be restriction because of the taut intertransverse muscle (this is typical of all muscle fixations). In this type of fixation, as it is difficult to invent an adjustment that will pull the two ends of the muscle apart, the best thrust is one at right angles to the point of fixation when the patient is prone.

IVD Lesions. The reader may have noticed that little emphasis has been placed on IVD lesions. Gillet's believes that the role of this factor, or its very existence in many cases, has been vastly overplayed. There are probably two types of discal hernias seen clinically: (1) the true rupture, which can be described as an anular "tumor" invading into the spinal canal; (2) and the false one, which is a posterolateral "bulging" of the disc as the result of abnormal pressure exerted on it by severe muscle contraction. With the second type, anything that will lessen the chronic muscular contraction will relieve the "hernia." Thus, reflex techniques, modalities, or even the anesthesia administered before an operation will have the necessary relaxing effect of the muscles responsible for a "false" hernia.

A great amount of information has been

described in this chapter. It is suggested that you review it frequently. We are sure that with each reading you will discover a new idea, a new viewpoint, that will contribute to your clinical proficiency. [See Clinical Comment 6.10]

Bibliography

Banks SD: Sacro-iliac biomechanics and its effect on gait. *Journal of the ACA Council on Sports Injuries*, 1(3):9-14, April 1983.

Barge FH: *Tortipelvis*. Davenport, IA, Bawden Bros, 1980, pp 104-120.

Beal MC: The sacroiliac problem: review of anatomy, mechanics, and diagnosis. *Journal of the American Osteopathic Association*, 81:667-679, 1982.

Boorsma JD: Architecture of the sacro-iliac joint. In *Biomechanics of the Pelvis*. Council on Technic of the American Chiropractic Association, Denver Conference, June 17-20, 1980, pp 5-7.

Brunarski D: Sacroiliac concomittants of the iliolumbar syndrome: a case report. *Journal of the Canadian Chiropractic Association*, 24:19-20, 1980.

Campbell JR: Gonstead analysis of pelvic biomechanics. In *Biomechanics of the Pelvis*. Denver Conference on Biomechanics of the Pelvis, June 17-20, 1980, Spears Chiropractic Hospital, published by the Council on Technic of the American Chiropractic Association, Des Moines, IA, 1982, pp 9-18.

Cassidy JD, Bowen CV: Anatomy and biomechanics of the sacroiliac joint. In *Biomechanics of the Pelvis*. Denver Conference on Biomechanics of the Pelvis, June 17-20, 1980, Spears Chiropractic Hospital, published by the Council on Technic of the American Chiropractic Association, Des Moines, IA, 1982, pp 20-22.

Colachis SC Jr, Warden RE, Bechtol CO, Strohm BR: Movement of the sacroiliac joint in the adult: a preliminary report. *Archives of Physical Medicine & Rehabilitation*, pp 490-498, September 1963.

Davis P, Lentle BC: Evidence for sacroiliac disease as a common cause of low backache in women. *Lancet*, 2:496-497, 1978.

De Jarnette MB: *Chiropractic Manipulative Technique: Sacro Occipital Technic;* 1975 Seminar Notes. Publication data not shown, privately distributed.

De Jarnette MB: *Sacro Occipital Technic 1977*. Publication data not shown, privately distributed.

De Jarnette MB: *Subluxation Patterns: Sacro Occipital Technic;* 1975 Seminar Notes. Publication data not shown, privately distributed.

Denton DG: Sacro-occipital technique biomechanics of the pelvis. In *Biomechanics of the Pelvis*. Denver Conference on Biomechanics of the Pelvis, June 17-20, 1980, Spears Chiropractic Hospital, published by the Council on Technic of the American Chiropractic Association, Des Moines, IA, 1982, pp 24-42.

DonTigny RL: Function and pathomechanics of the sacroiliac joint: a review. *Physical Therapy*, 65:35-44, 1985.

Epstein MC: Causes of low back problems. *Digest of Chiropractic Economics*, January-February 1983.

Esch D, Lepley M: *Musculoskeletal Function: An Anatomy and Kinesiology Laboratory Manual*. Minneapolis, University of Minnesota Press, 1974, pp 11-12.

Fairbank J, O'Brien J: The iliac crest syndrome: a treatable cause of low-back pain. *Spine*, 8:220-224, 1983.

Faucret BH: Introduction to pelvic biomechanics. In *Biomechanics of the Pelvis*. Council on Technic of the American Chiropractic Association, Denver Conference, June 17-20, 1980, pp 51-75.

Faye LJ: Manipulation I [Cassette tape program]. Huntington Beach, CA, Motion Palpation Institute, 1983, 6 tapes.

Faye LJ: Motion Palpation and Manipulation of the Sacro-iliac [Videotape]. Los Angeles, Dynaspine, 1983.

Faye LJ: *Spine I: Motion Palpation and Clinical Considerations of the Lumbar Spine and Pelvis*. Huntington Beach, CA, Motion Palpation Institute, 1987, pp 10-14.

Finneson BE: *Low Back Pain*. Philadelphia, J.B. Lippincott, 1973, pp 9, 15-17, 325-326, 332.

Fisk JW: *The Painful Neck and Back*. Springfield, IL, Charles C. Thomas, 1977, pp 39-47, 54-76, 176-187.

Gatterman B: Motion palpation of the sacroiliac joints. In *Biomechanics of the Pelvis*. Council on Technic of the American Chiropractic Association, Denver Conference, June 17-20, 1980, pp 76-80.

Gatterman MI: Sacroiliac motion and pelvic tilt. In *Biomechanics of the Pelvis*. Council on Technic of the American Chiropractic Association, Denver Conference, June 17-20, 1980, pp 81-92.

Gehweiler JA Jr, Osborne RL Jr, Becker RF: *The Radiology of Vertebrae Trauma*. Philadelphia, W.B. Saunders, 1980, pp 85-88, 379-398.

DR. FAYE'S CLINICAL COMMENT #6.10

As stated in the chapter concerning the thoracic spine for all low-back pain cases determined amenable to manipulation, be sure to include restoring motion to the hip joints and the thoracolumbar junction if these areas are fixated. Both of these sites of fixation can produce hypermobile L4—L5 or L5—S1 function that can readily lead to lower lumbar disc bulging. Upper lumbar and lower thoracic fixations can also produce tension on the spinal cord that results in less angulation of the L5 and S1 nerve roots as they exit from the spine. This more obtuse angulation allows the roots to press against an otherwise tolerable disc protrusion. Such cases will be much more sensitive to Lindner's test, the Soto-Hall test, or a Valsalva maneuver. Thoracolumbar adjustments relieve the root tension, and antalgic postures improve quickly.

Gillet H: Clinical measurements of sacro-iliac mobility. *Annals of the Swiss Chiropractors Association.* 6:59-70, 1976.

Gillet H: The Gillet-Liekens mobility test. *Journal of Clinical Chiropractic,* 1(2):21-30, 1968.

Gillet H, Liekens M: *Belgian Chiropractic Research Notes.* Huntington Beach, CA, Motion Palpation Institute, 1984, pp 9-10, 14-15, 17, 22-23, 47-61, 101-106, 128-129.

Gillet H: Movement palpation—measurements. *Bulletin of the European Chiropractors Union,* 23(2), 1974.

Gillet H: A multiple purpose technique for pelvic correction. *Journal of Clinical Chiropractic,* 2(4):57-62, 1969.

Gillet H: Normal and abnormal pelvis mechanics. *Kentucky Kyrogram,* date unknown.

Gitelman R: A chiropractic approach to biomechanical disorders of the lumbar spine and pelvis. In Haldeman S (ed): *Modern Developments in the Principles and Practice of Chiropractic.* New York, Appleton-Century-Crofts, 1980, pp 297-299, 304-307.

Goodheart GJ: *Applied Kinesiology.* Place of publication not shown, published by author, privately distributed, 1964, pp 11-12, 23-24, 38-43.

Goodheart GL: The psoas muscle and the foot pronation problem. In *Collected Published Articles and Reprints.* Montpellier, OH, Williams County Publishing, 1969, pp 72-73.

Granger CV: The clinical discernment of muscle weakness. *Archives of Physical Medicine,* 44:430-438, 1963.

Greenman PE: Lift therapy: use and abuse. *Journal of the American Osteopathic Association,* December 1979.

Grice AS, Fligg DB: Class notes: Introductory Concepts to Clinical Analysis of Joint Movement and Muscle Testing. Department of Biomechanics/Kinesiology, BK101. Toronto, Canadian Memorial Chiropractic College, date not shown, pp 100-102, 105-109.

Grice AS, Fligg DB: Class notes: Spinal dynamics. Department of Biomechanics/Kinesiology, BK202. Toronto, Canadian Memorial Chiropractic College, date not shown, pp 12-23, 91-101.

Grice AS: Clinical analysis of the sacroiliac joint. In *Biomechanics of the Pelvis.* Council on Technic of the American Chiropractic Association, Denver Conference, June 17-20, 1980, pp 96-109.

Grieve DW: The sacroiliac joint. *Physiotherapy,* 62(12):384-400, 1976.

Grieve GP: *Common Vertebral Joint Problems.* New York, Churchill Livingstone, 1981, pp 29-31, 34-35, 151-158, 279-295, 309, 328-334.

Helfet AJ, Gruebel Lee DM: *Disorders of the Lumbar Spine.* Philadelphia, J.B. Lippincott, 1978, pp 24-25, 191-196, 211, 219.

Hemauer JD: Sacroiliac anatomy, movement, and subluxation. In *Biomechanics of the Pelvis.* Council on Technic of the American Chiropractic Association, Denver Conference, June 17-20, 1980, pp 112-119.

Hoehler FK, Tobis JS: Low back pain and its treatment by spinal manipulation: measures of flexibility and asymmetry. *Rheumatology and Rehabilitation,* 21:21-26, 1982.

Howe JW: Determination of lumbo-sacral facet sublux-ations. *Roentgenological Briefs,* Council on Roentgenology of the American Chiropractic Association, Des Moines, IA, date not shown.

Illi FW: The phylogenesis and clinical import of the sacroiliac mechanism. *Journal of the National Chiropractic Association,* September-October 1963.

Illi FW: *The Vertebral Column: Life-Line of the Body.* Chicago, National College of Chiropractic, 1951, pp 11, 13-14, 19, 61-73.

Janse J, Houser RH, Wells BF: *Chiropractic Principles and Technic.* Chicago, IL, National College of Chiropractic, 1947, pp 456-492.

Janse J: Clinical biomechanics of the sacroiliac mechanism. *ACA Journal of Chiropractic,* February 1978.

La Ban M, et al: Symphyseal and sacroiliac joint pain associated with public symphysis instability. *Archives of Physical Medicine and Rehabilitation,* 59:470-472, 1978.

Michelle AA: *Iliopsoas: Development of Anomalies in Man.* Springfield, IL, Charles C. Thomas, 1962.

Milne RA, Mierau DR: Hamstring distensibility in the general population: relationship to pelvic and low back stresses. *Journal of Manipulative and Physiological Therapeutics,* 2(3):146-150, September 1979.

Mitchell T: Structural pelvic function. *Yearbook of Applied Osteopathy,* 1965.

Nachemson AL: Electromyographical studies of the vertebral portion of the psoas muscle (with special reference to its stabilizing function of the lumbar spine). *Acta Orthopaedica Scandinavica,* 37:177-190, 1966.

Ng SY: The significance of psoas myospasm in the lordotic compared to the kyphotic sacrolumbar spine. *ACA Journal of Chiropractic,* October 1978.

Ng SY: Sacroiliac lumbar mechanism. *ACA Journal of Chiropractic,* April 1983.

Otter R: A review study of the differing opinions expressed in the literature about the anatomy of the sacroiliac joint. *European Journal of Chiropractic,* 33(4):221-241, December 1985.

Pace JB, Nagle D: Piriform syndrome. *Western Journal of Medicine,* 124:435-439, 1976.

Parke WW: Applied anatomy of the spine. In Rothman RH, Simeone FA (eds): *The Spine.* Philadelphia, W.B. Saunders, 1975, vol I, pp 27-28.

Pinkenburg CA: A study of the sacroiliac articulations. *ACA Journal of Chiropractic,* November 1978.

Pitkin HC, Pheasant HC: Sacroarthrogenetic tekalgia: a study of referred pain. *Journal of Bone and Joint Surgery,* vol 18, 1936.

Reinert OC: *Chiropractic Procedure and Practice,* ed 3. Florissant, MO, Marian Press, 1972, pp 82-85, 116-118, 144-151.

Reinert OC: *Fundamentals of Chiropractic Techniques and Practice Procedures.* Chesterfield, MO, Marian Press, 1983, pp 9-12.

Retzlaff EW, et al: The piriformis muscle syndrome. *Journal of the American Osteopathic Association,* 73:799-807, 1984.

Reynolds HM: Three dimensional kinematics in the pelvic girdle. *Journal of the American Osteopathic Association,* 80:4, December 1980.

Rosse C: The hip region and the lumbosacral plexus. In Rosse C, Clawson DK (eds): *The Musculoskeletal System in Health & Disease*. Hagerstown, PA, Harper & Row, 1980, pp 253-254, 256-257, 268-272.

Salter RB: *Textbook of Disorders and Injuries of the Musculoskeletal System*. Baltimore, Williams & Wilkins, 1981, pp 257-258.

SantoMauro A: Bio-statics of the pelvis. In *Biomechanics of the Pelvis*. Council on Technic of the American Chiropractic Association, Denver Conference, June 17-20, 1980, pp 139-141.

Sashin D: A critical analysis of the anatomy and the pathologic changes of the sacroiliac joints. *Journal of Bone and Joint Surgery*, vol 12, 1930.

Schafer RC: *Chiropractic Management of Sports and Recreational Injuries*. Baltimore, Williams & Wilkins, 1982, pp 263-264, 286-287, 454-456, 458-460.

Schafer RC: *Chiropractic Physical and Spinal Diagnosis*. Oklahoma City, American Chiropractic Academic Press, 1980, Chapter XIII: Physical examination of the lumbar spine and pelvic girdle.

Schafer RC: *Clinical Biomechanics: Musculoskeletal Actions and Reactions*. Baltimore, Williams & Wilkins, 1983, pp 451-484.

Schafer RC: *Physical Diagnosis: Procedures and Methodology in Chiropractic Practice*. Arlington, VA, American Chiropractic Association, 1989.

Schafer RC: *Symptomatology and Differential Diagnosis*. Arlington, VA, American Chiropractic Association, 1986, pp 827-839.

Schmidt WH Jr: The psoas sitting test: key to hidden lumbosacral problems. *The Digest of Chiropractic Economics*, September-October 1983.

Shrader TL: A model for simulation of pelvic biomechanics. In *Biomechanics of the Pelvis*. Council on Technic of the American Chiropractic Association, Denver Conference, June 17-20, 1980, pp 143-151.

Shunke GB: Anatomy and development of the sacroiliac joint in man. *Anatomical Record*, 72:3, 1938.

Simons DG, Travell JG: Myofascial origins of low back pain. *Postgraduate Medicine*, 73(2):66-108, February 1983.

States AZ: *Spinal and Pelvic Technics*, ed 2. Lombard, IL, National Chiropractic College, 1968, pp 2, 12-15.

Stierwalt DD: *Fundamentals of Motion Palpation*. Davenport, IA, published by author, 1977, p 31.

Taylor RG, Fowler WM Jr: Electrodiagnosis of musculoskeletal disorders. In D'Ambrosia RD (ed): *Musculoskeletal Disorders: Regional Examination and Differential Diagnosis*. Philadelphia, J.B. Lippincott, 1977, p 84.

Travell J: Myofascial trigger points: Clinical view. In Bonica JJ, AlbeFessard D (eds): *Advances in Pain Research and Therapy*. New York, Raven Press, 1976.

Turner JA, Robinson J, McCreary CP: Chronic low-back pain: predicting response to nonsurgical treatment. *Archives of Physical Medicine and Rehabilitation*, 64:560-563, 1983.

Weisl H: Ligaments of the sacro-iliac joint examined with particular reference to their function. *Acta Anatomica*, 20:201-213, 1954.

Weisl H: Movements of the sacro-iliac joints. *Acta Anatomica*, 23:80-91, 1955.

Weisl H: The articular surfaces of the sacro-iliac joint and their relation to movements of the sacrum. *Acta Anatomica*, 22(1)1-14, 1954.

West HG Jr: Physical and spinal examination procedures utilized in the practice of chiropractic. In Haldeman S (ed): *Modern Developments in the Principles and Practice of Chiropractic*. New York, Appleton-Century-Crofts, 1980, pp 281-282, 283-284.

White AA, Panjabi MM: *Clinical Biomechanics of the Spine*. Philadelphia, J.B. Lippincott, 1978, pp 264-270, 272.

Wilder DG, et al: The functional topography of the sacroiliac joint. *Spine*, 5:60, 1980.

Wiles MR: Reproducibility and interexaminer correlation of motion palpation findings of the sacroiliac joints. *Journal of the Canadian Chiropractic Association*, 24(2), 1980.

Wood J: Motion of the sacroiliac joint. *PCC Research Forum*, 1(3):95-101, Spring 1985.

Chapter 7

Spinal Fixation Complexes

This chapter describes various spinal complexes that the Belgium group of researchers have found to be clinically consistent. A spinal complex, as used in this sense, can be defined as a focal point of fixation that is commonly associated with one or more remote fixations.

INTRODUCTION

Many reflexes are modulated within the spinal cord. Their potential interrelationship with a subluxation complex, and vice versa, cannot be ignored when it is considered that a vertebral lesion can be a focus for either neuronal hyperexcitability or hypoexcitability. All afferent fibers entering the IVF and all structures receiving efferent fibers via the IVF are therefore potentially exposed to excessive stimulation or inhibition by some factor producing irritation, pressure, or tension at this vulnerable gateway. We have described in previous chapters how articulation fixation can be one such factor—possibly one of the most common factors.

A somatosomatic reflex develops when a sensory receptor in joint articular surfaces, striated muscle, tendons, ligaments, fascia, subcutaneous tissue, or the skin is stimulated to trigger a volley of impulses to another anatomical location of this type via efferent sensory, motor, or autonomic fibers. In this context, Korr has shown that muscle spindles in which the "gain" has been turned up by intensified activity in their gamma motor innervation may, together with other sensory inputs, account for many of the motion characteristics and palpatory features of a spinal subluxation complex. "Turning down" the gain seems to be a common denominator in a variety of manipulative procedures.

This chapter will not be a review of the theoretical neurologic implications involved in such reflex reactions. It will, from a musculoskeletal viewpoint, describe certain primary and remote secondary manifestations that empirically appear to be neurologically linked.

FIXATION COMPLEXES

Readers of Gillet's earlier "Notes" will recall his use of the term "reflex fixations." Since then, the term *reflex fixations* has developed into what he now calls fixation complexes. The reason behind this is that, instead of one fixation being linked reflexively to another, he and his associates have found whole series of fixations that consistently appear to be specifically complimentary to each other, hence the term *complex*.

Following is a brief summary of Gillet's thoughts on this subject, as taken from his published notes.

Background

It is of interest to the chiropractor to know of all the series of fixations that have a tendency to exist together. There seems to be at least twelve of these linked to pelvic phenomena; ie, twelve types of local pelvic fixations that have related lumbar, thoracic, costal, and cervical fixations associated.

We are slowly beginning to understand that the concept of a single spinal subluxation, or of a local fixation between any two spinal structures, is only partially true. A localized state can be easily shown in acute conditions; but once the spinal disorder becomes chronic, there will practically always be found a series of fixations, or more often several series, with each series containing somewhere within it a focal (causative) fixation-subluxation to which several secondary ones that have added themselves to it.

A new concept of the subluxation could be logically proposed from our findings, one in which we would have a fixation complex that would be considered as being a "subluxation" from the viewpoint of the total individual. This concept will have far reaching implications, as we shall see later in this chapter.

We have as yet no plausible explanation for these observations, as they do not always follow known neurologic pathways. Yet in clinical practice in which hundreds of patients have been examined and a large variety of tests have been used, all tend to prove the one-for-all and all-for-one law. We have found this to be eminently true in all living matter, thus completely true in the reciprocal effects of fixations on each other.

The Belgian Chiropractic Research Team discovered quite rapidly the great corrective effect of the adjustment of total fixations on partial fixations. It has recently been a surprise to find that the opposite, a reciprocal effect, is also true. Yes, the correction of partial fixations on more total ones is possibly much greater than previously thought. It remains true, however, that the advantage of correcting the "major" is still considerable. But the opposite effect appears to be considerable enough to explain why certain systems of adjusting in which only one spinal area was used could, aided by an enthusiastic personality, be propagated and be quite successful in many cases.

In a practice where clinical attention is restricted to one area of the spine, the corrected fixation will actually be the primary one in a certain percentage of cases. These cases will be the foundation for the "excellent results" reported, those put forward to prove the theory of the practitioner or school of thought. Other cases, however, will prove to be more difficult, and it is of these that the "specialized" practitioner will argue that his analysis or his line of drive must have been not exactly correct, etc. In the first instance, the case will thus need to be adjusted only once, while the other cases, those in which the focal fixation exists remote from the restricted area of specialization, necessitate repeated adjustments to make the correction "hold"—this being the real criterion between primary and secondary fixations.

This concept of fixation complexes has not only simplified somewhat our motion-palpation analysis, it has also permitted us to discover new technics of adjustment. These technics have proved to be not only far more effective than the usual thrust in many cases but also methods that are also far less traumatizing, both to the patient and to the chiropractor.

In the following sections, these complexes will be described. As all basic elements necessary for understanding have been described in previous chapters, each description will be brief.

SACROILIAC LIGAMENTOUS ANTERIOR COMPLEX (SILA)

When the anterior ligaments joining the sacrum to the ilia are shortened, they tend to push the sacrum backwards. The sacral base will bulge posteriorly between the ilia, either at its apex inferiorly and or at its base superiorly. This can sometimes be seen, or it can be palpated by the back of the hand or with the palpator's thumb trying to push the sacrum forward between the ilia. This fixation reflexively produces a hypertonus of the *anterior intercostal muscles*, which "bunch up" the ribs anteriorly and cause the thoracic spine, in part or in toto, to distort into some degree of associated hyperkyphosis.

In the superior SILA, the anterior rectus capitis becomes tightened next, pulling the reflexively connected part of the occiput down onto the atlas and opening the posterior occiput-atlas space. Another cervical component of the superior SILA will be found at the anterior aspect of the C2—C3 intertransverse space (Fig. 7.1).

The lumbars have not been mentioned in this complex because Gillet's group has not been able to find specific muscles responding to the fixated state of the sacroiliac ligaments. We are sure, however, that there are some muscles that are influenced but possibly not affected in the same manner as other spinal muscles. This influence can readily he seen and measured by rotating the sitting patient's trunk on the pelvis and noting the vertebral level at which the rotation starts to take place.

Readers may have noticed that all shortening effects in this complex are found on the *anterior* side of the body and that all the normal kyphoses are increased and all the lordoses are diminished.

SACROILIAC LIGAMENTOUS POSTERIOR COMPLEX (SILP)

The contrary of the above is true in the posterior sacroiliac ligamentous fixation complex.

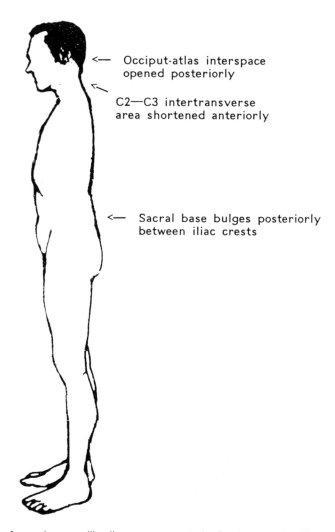

Occiput-atlas interspace opened posteriorly

C2—C3 intertransverse area shortened anteriorly

Sacral base bulges posteriorly between iliac crests

Figure 7.1. Major effects of superior sacroiliac ligamentous anterior fixation complex (Courtesy ACAP).

In *superior SILP*, the sacral base will be pushed *forward* and the PSISs of the ilia will be pulled medially. An associated hypertonicity of the superior costo-costal muscles posteriorly push the thorax forwards to flatten the normal thoracic kyphosis, and the atlas can be easily palpated as being posterior; ie, its transverse processes will jut backwards and be found under the mastoids (Fig. 7.2).

In *inferior SILP*, it is the apex of the sacrum that is pushed anteriorly. The lower half of the thorax will be flattened at the ribs, and the posterior C2—C3 intertransverse area will be tightly contracted anteriorly (Fig. 7.3).

In both of these types of complexes (SILA and SILP), as in many others, the fixations tend to be bilateral but one side is often in greater fixation than the other. This will show itself in the whole complex, but possibly more easily in the positioning of the atlas or axis, giving us interesting indications for a corrective thrust. In addition, these two fixation complexes are quite visible in all spinographs taken in profile. In fact, it is surprising that they have not already been observed and reported by chiropractic roentgenolo-

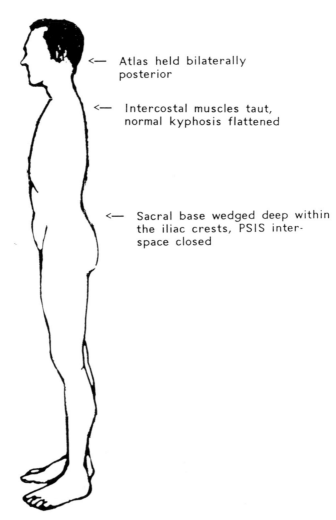

<— Atlas held bilaterally posterior

<— Intercostal muscles taut, normal kyphosis flattened

<— Sacral base wedged deep within the iliac crests, PSIS interspace closed

Figure 7.2. Major effects of superior sacroiliac ligamentous posterior fixation complex (Courtesy ACAP).

gists.

The thoracic component of the complex can be palpated in lateral flexion movement of the thoracic spine. It will then be noticed that these thoracic fixations take place in series and that each series will tend to include the upper *or* lower thoracics, corresponding to the location of the sacral fixation; ie, whether it is at its base or at its apex.

Fixation at both sacral *base* and *apex* will produce a related general tightness of the whole thorax, and this will readily be felt and observed as soon as the doctor tries to rotate or laterally flex the patient's spine. Hypertonic findings in the cervicals, at the occipitoatlantal or C2—C3 area, and lumbars will manifest accordingly.

PUBIC FIXATION COMPLEXES

Fixation at the pubic joint will also have a comparable effect on the whole spine, along with hypertonicity of the abdominal muscles. No specific cervical part of the pubic complex has yet been found.

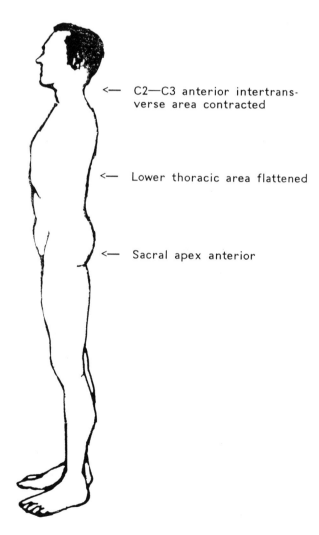

← C2—C3 anterior intertransverse area contracted

← Lower thoracic area flattened

← Sacral apex anterior

Figure 7.3. Major effects of inferior sacroiliac ligamentous posterior fixation complex (Courtesy ACAP).

THE SACROILIAC LIGAMENTOUS OBLIQUE COMPLEX (SILO)

There also seems to exist distinct groups of sacroiliac ligament fibers, both anteriorly and posteriorly, that ascend and descend obliquely from the sacrum to the ilium.

The Anterior Obliques (SILOA)

Anteriorly, they can produce what seems to be an associated fixation between the ribs and the sternum. This fixation can be felt by passing the palpating hand over the sternum. A characteristic forward bulge will be felt, which gives the perception of it being a part of the sternum itself. This impression cannot be true for in its greater part of the sternum is just a single plate. There are, however, the costosternal and the costocostal articulations to consider.

The Posterior Obliques (SILOP)

If the posterior oblique ligaments are tightened, the related thoracic fixation will

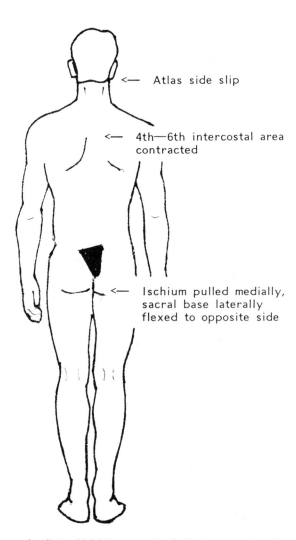

Figure 7.4. Major effects of unilateral (right) sacrospinalis fixation complex (Courtesy ACAP).

exhibit as a hypertonicity of the short lateral muscles in the midthoracic region. These can easily be palpated within the costospinal grooves. This complex also seems to affect the midcervical anterior intertransverse muscles. They are sometimes difficult to palpate; the patient's neck must be put into posterior rotation to feel them. The midcervical part of the posterior oblique fixation (SILOP) is felt more easily by following the line of the transverses as the neck is rotated forwards. The effect on the lumbars is evident, but it has not been codified as yet.

THE SACROTUBEROUS COMPLEX

The sacrotuberous complex is a small one it seems, involving only the sacrotuberous ligament and the rotatores muscle specifically at the 7th cervical. This complex is frequently unilateral, in which case the ligament in question will pull the corresponding ilium into rotation so that the iliac crest moves anteriorly and the ischium posteriorly. If the fixation is bilateral, the sacrum will be pulled downward and spread the ilia apart.

The sacrotuberous ligament is a tough

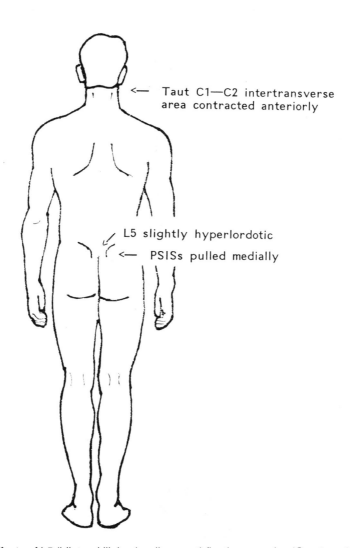

←— Taut C1—C2 intertransverse area contracted anteriorly

L5 slightly hyperlordotic
←— PSISs pulled medially

Figure 7.5. Major effects of L5 (bilateral iliolumbar ligament) fixation complex (Courtesy ACAP).

mass of fibers. It can be palpated through the outer tissues of the buttocks when the patient is prone. It can also be "adjusted" in this position.

The related C7 fixation can be felt when the base of the patient's neck is in lateral flexion and the tips of two palpation fingers are placed firmly against the spinous process of C7. This palpation is delicate, for normal movement is not large but it is extremely specific. It should feel springy.

THE SACROSPINOUS COMPLEX

Moving from the sacrotuberous ligaments, we isolate the *sacrospinous ligaments*. When these are shortened bilaterally, they pull the ischia medially, thus blocking the pelvis in the standing posture. If it is blocked *unilaterally*, which is often the case, it will pull the apex of the sacrum into lateral flexion and along with it the lumbars (Fig. 7.4).

The thoracic component of this complex is a specific rib-rib fixation at the lateral aspect of the 4th—6th intercostal spaces, almost under the shoulder and scapula. This site of fixation feels hard and refuses to open during lateral flexion.

The cervical component of the sacrospinous complex is a small but important one. It is perceived as a hypertonicity of the later-

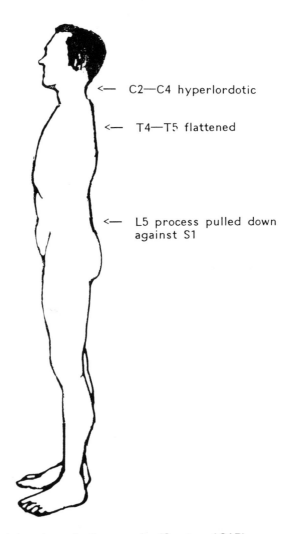

<— C2—C4 hyperlordotic

<— T4—T5 flattened

<— L5 process pulled down against S1

Figure 7.6. Major effects of the interspinous fixation complex (Courtesy ACAP).

alis muscle (obliquus capitis superior) that courses from the mastoid process to the transverse process of the atlas. This is the muscle responsible for the famed "atlas side slip" of HIO days. This atlas fixation can indeed be adjusted with, sometimes, an important effect on the whole complex, including the pelvis.

THE L5 COMPLEX

We have previously described that L5 forms a functional part of the pelvis when fixations are considered, so we will now take into consideration the fixations between this foundation vertebra and the ilia (iliolumbar ligament), and between it and the sacrum (the sacrolumbar and interspinous ligaments).

Shortening of the iliolumbar ligaments will pull the posterior aspect of the iliac crests medially and block the pelvis in the sitting posture. It will also force L5 into a slight local hyperlordosis, which is characteristic in that this segmental lordosis seems to extend laterally to the crests (Fig. 7.5). This distortion naturally has an effect on the lumbars, but Gillet and associates have not as yet found it in the thoracic region.

From these local manifestations, we can move to the Atlas-Axis area where the anterior intertransverse muscles will be tightened, rendering C1—C2 rotation restricted. Tightening of the posterior muscles in question is, on the other hand, part of the *lumbosacral* fixation complex. Differentiation between the two is often difficult, but fortunately the adjustment used will be effective in either type of fixation.

THE INTERSPINOUS FIXATION COMPLEX

The *interspinous fixation complex* (Fig. 7.6) is another easy one to determine for it always manifests in the same manner:

1. *Local effect.* The spinous of L5 will be pulled down against the process of S1, causing the typical subluxation described by Fox.

2. *Thoracic effect.* There will be a short local flattening in the T4—T5 region, which can be both palpated and observed with the patient in total forward flexion.

3. *Cervical effect.* There will be a shorter local hyperlordosis in the C2—C4 area in which the tightened muscles can also be felt.

ANTERIOR BODY FIXATION COMPLEX

Upper-thoracic anterior body fixations in the spine, especially in the upper-thoracic region (Fig. 7.7), will have a hypertonic effect on the rectus capitis major muscles. The occiput will be pulled down against the posterior rim of the atlas.

CORRECTION OF PELVIC FIXATION COMPLEXES

The different pelvic fixation complexes are by far the more frequent and far reaching. Fortunately, we have devised a system of pelvic correction that might dethrone the famous "million dollar roll." The principle is simple: we use the leg and primarily the knee of the patient as a lever to stretch the offending ligaments in the following manner.

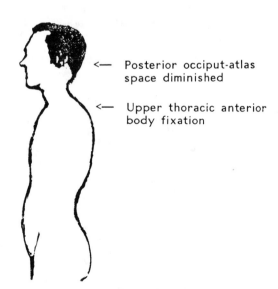

← Posterior occiput-atlas space diminished

← Upper thoracic anterior body fixation

Figure 7.7. Major effects of upper-thoracic anterior body fixation complex (Courtesy ACAP).

Anterior Sacroiliac Ligament Complexes

To correct a bilateral anterior sacoiliac ligament fixation (SILA), we request that the patient to sit and open the knees as far as possible. Sitting behind the patient, we reach over and strongly abduct the knees a little farther. There will be no feeling of release, but on repalpating the previously fixated area in this complex, a great change will be felt. If necessary, the patient may be asked to do this exercise at home once or twice a day (Fig. 7.8).

Posterior Sacroiliac Ligament Complexes

The opposite fixation complex (SILP) will be treated in a similar fashion, but it will be the posterior ligaments that will be stretched. We ask the patient to cross one knee over the other. We then reach over from behind and force the patient's knee into greater adduction (Fig. 7.9). Hold for 30 seconds while the patient exhales.

If, as described previously, one ligament is in greater tension, only the ipsilateral limb will be stretched. If the fixation is bilateral, both limbs will be stretched, one after the other. This exercise can also be prescribed as a regimen to be conducted at home by the patient. Assure that the patient holds the

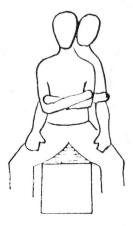

Figure 7.8. Stretching anterior sacroiliac ligament fixation.

stretch for 30 seconds and exhales during at least the final 10 seconds.

Both of the exercises described in this section can be conducted with the patient supine, but they are awkward to do in that position.

Sacrotuberous Ligament Fixation Complexes

Sacrotuberous fixations are, in the Belgium studies at least, nearly always unilateral, tending to be more strongly involved on the right side. Typically in sacrotuberous fixation, the right PSIS will palpate higher on the right. If this is true, we will reach under or over the right shoulder of the patient, and take hold of the patient's right knee and pull it up strongly against the patient's chest for 30 seconds (Fig. 7.10).

Sacrospinous Fixation Complexes

The sacrospinous ligament fixation usually pulls the tip of the sacral apex unilaterally, usually to the right, so we will use the same knee-chest "adjustment" previously described (refer to Fig. 7.10). This is usually highly effective.

Iliolumbar Ligament Fixation Complex

The same maneuver shown in Fig. 7.10 can be used for a tightened iliolumbar ligament, which usually forces the lower lumbars to deviate to the *left*. A marked change in this deviation will frequently be observed immediately after the corrective stretch.

In these fixations if they are bilateral and of even strength on both sides, *both* knees should be brought up against the patient's chest, one after the other.

We have also used the old gymnastic stand-by: full forward flexion when standing (Fig. 7.11). This exercise has lost its previous reputation since it has become widely known that it produces considerable strain on L5, but here we explain that we use it only once

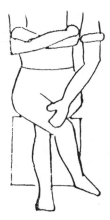

Figure 7.9. Stretching posterior sacroiliac ligament fixation.

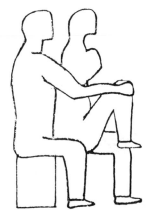

Figure 7.10. Stretching sacrotuberous ligament fixation.

or twice at the most. Should we have to prescribe it to the patient, we ask him to do it while supine.

No attention should be paid to the ease or difficulty with which the patient can touch the floor. There are several other articulations, especially the hips, involved in this motion, but we are not trying to measure their suppleness at this time. What we want to use is that last inch of movement that the patient is asked to apply against the shortened ligaments. Faye mentions that exhalation helps all such stretching exercises.

CONCLUDING REMARKS ON SPINAL FIXATION COMPLEXES

This is the point of advancement of the Belgium group's spinal research to date. They openly admit that they still have much to do. We will conclude this section of investigation with the following thought that has also appeared previously in Gillet's writings:

"We can even extend this concept of a fixation complex to areas and structures, and even functions, *far from* the spine. We have written in various papers of the "adjustment" of the cranial bones and their effect on the spine. In other cases, we have found that the primary cause may be in the long muscles (as described by Goodheart, Nimmo, and others), while in still other instances, the mental state of the patient could be

just another "handle" through which the doctor may influence the whole fixation complex.

"Thus, our horizon widens continually, and those of you who have enough vision will one day be able to encompass the whole landscape, and will learn to choose the best technic applicable—not only for each patient but at each stage of treatment of that patient. Who knows, some day we may be able to encompass *all* therapy, *all* medicine, into our synthesis."

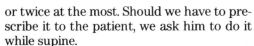

They drew a circle that shut me out. I drew a circle that brought them in!

RELATED EXTRASPINAL FIXATIONS

The unsatiable curiosity of the Belgium researchers spurred them into the study of not only the spine but of *all* body articulations. This was necessary because not only were they interested in subluxations but also in their causes, and we have explained how these causes can sometimes be located far from the spine.

Gillet's studies led him to the general conclusion that one of the primary reasons why vertebrae have a tendency to not regain normally and easily their "place," after they have been mobilized to the limit of the range of

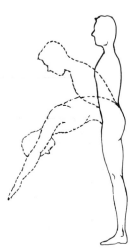

Figure 7.11. Full forward flexion stretch (Courtesy ACAP).

motion, is a general overall tenseness of all spinal and, possibly, extraspinal muscles of the body.

We have also seen that this tension can be changed momentarily by different methods—reflexes, drugs, heat, etc—with the spontaneous correction of certain fixations. We believe that we have found the reason for this abnormal tension, at least one reason. This is the general tendency of human beings, especially manual workers, to overuse their articulations, especially their extraspinal joints, far more in *flexion* than extension. The effect is to produce, after a while, a dysequilibrium between the structures that force and those that maintain these articula-

tions in their position of work.

Our studies have found that there is a reflex effect of fixations at the tibiofibular articulations on L5, and of those of the clavicals on the lateral muscles over the first and second ribs. There also seems to be a fixation that takes place at the junction of the manubrium with the remainder of the sternum. This appears to have an effect on the axis, but we have not been able to bring this out on a consistent basis.

This study has unearthed some important facts concerning the upper and lower extremities and the fixations to be found in them. Furthermore, we have found that these extremity fixations are extremely important to the correction and the maintenance of the functional state of the spine. This area of study, extraspinal fixations, will be our subject within the concluding two chapters of this manual. [See Clinical Comment 7.1]

Bibliography

Gillet H, Liekens M: *Belgian Chiropractic Research Notes.* Huntington Beach, CA, Motion Palpation Institute, 1984, pp 81-85.

Jirout J: Persistence of the synkinetic patterns of the cervical spine. *Neuroradiology,* 18:167-171, 1979.

Jirout J: Studies in the dynamics of the spine. *Acta Radiology,* 46:55-60, 1956.

Korr IM: Proprioceptors and Somatic Dysfunction. *Journal of the American Osteopathic Association,* 74(3):638-650, 1975.

DR. FAYE'S CLINICAL COMMENT #7.1

Fixation complexes should not be used as "diagnostic crutches." Most patients do not have simple complexes, and it has been my experience that each patient must be treated as an individual and examined without bias. However, once an area continues to re-fixate visit after visit, it is essential to find the causative factor. Most often, the cause will be a remote spinal, pelvic, or extremity major fixation. Correction of the remote fixation will prevent the secondary, constantly returning, spinal fixation (erroneously chosen as the major) from recurring. Lasting beneficial clinical results often depend on the manipulation of a cuboid, navicular, superior tibiofibular, or some other less known culprit.

As a rule, do not repeat the same adjustment of the spine week after week if the fixation keeps returning. Seek the significant major. On adjusting the true major, the secondary fixation will spontaneously release within 24 hours, and you will find that the relationship has been confirmed.

Chapter 8

The Extraspinal Axial and Upper Extremity Joints

Extraspinal joint fixations have been shown by practitioners of *dynamic chiropractic* to produce local symptoms, remote symptoms in the spine, or both. The reason for the remote effects, as described in the previous chapter, are unclear. They cannot be fully explained by either reflex or biomechanical hypotheses. This interesting topic will be the subject of this and the following chapter.

This chapter has two major subjects: (1) extraspinal axial joint considerations and (2) fixations of the upper extremities. Within each topic, practical biomechanical and motion restriction considerations of specific joints will be described, including dynamic palpation, significant neurologic and orthopedic testing, and adjusting procedures. Numerous aids in differential diagnosis are listed.

BASIC CONSIDERATIONS

The phrase *joint stiffness* is a subjective term that refers to an individual's or an examiner's perception of motion restriction. Extremity stiffness or motion restrictions are common complaints that can often signal progressing muscle or joint dysfunction or disease. As in the spine and pelvis, extremity joint pain arises when a joint is forced to move in a restricted plane.

If a patient reports that joint stiffness is a frequent experience, its distribution and duration should be discussed. Questions should also be directed to related activities and circumstances that relieve or aggravate the stiffness and associated discomfort. Refer to Table 2.1, which lists typical questions that should be asked during the investigation of joint pain.

Review of Reactions Within and About an Injured Joint

Trauma produces an inflammatory reaction that is one of the earliest steps of nature to set up the healing process. This initial inflammatory reaction is almost identical whether the irritation is traumatic in origin or the result of an invasion by pathogenic organisms. If traumatic in origin and the skin has not been broken to allow entry of bacteria, the site of injury is referred to as a *sterile inflammation*, unless, of course, septicemia exists which would produce a superimposed secondary infection. The cardinal signs of inflammation, pathogenic or sterile, are revealed in the following signs:

• Local heat (calor) from increased metabolic activity
• Local redness (rubor) from increased circulation and arteriole dilatation
• Local swelling (tumor) from impaired venous and lymph drainage and arteriole dilatation
• Local pain (dolor) from chemically, mechanically, or thermally stimulated nociceptors (usually irritated free nerve endings).

The initial reaction of joint inflammation usually occurs within 30 minutes of onset and it reaches its maximum in 6—8 hours. During this time, if it is possible for body defenses to react, the injured cells are walled off to prevent the spread of infection and serve as a target for leukocytes, platelets, and fibrinogen whether the need exists or not. For some unknown reason, this defensive reaction is usually greater than its need (ie, an overreaction).

If the skin is not broken to allow the invasion of bacteria and if septicemia is not present during the injury to predispose a secondary infection, the primary consequences of trauma are, in varying degrees, the following potential subtypes of inflammation:

• *Exudative inflammation*, distinguished by a large accumulation of serum and blood cells with vascular congestion and circulatory stasis.

• *Reactive inflammation*, which surrounds dead tissue or a foreign body.

• *Hemorrhagic inflammation*, distinguished by a conspicuous quantity of blood cells in the exudate. Note that blood debris is highly irritating to free nerve endings.

• *Interstitial inflammation*, principally involving the noncellular or supporting elements of a joint or organ.

• *Fibrinous inflammation*, in which the exudate is rich in fibrin.

• *Adhesive inflammation*, characterized by opposing tissues or sides of a cavity adhering to each other.

• *Chronic inflammation*, which progresses slowly and is of long duration, featuring the formation of scar tissue.

From a chiropractic viewpoint, one of the greatest concerns in the management of sterile injuries is that the normal resolution of inflammation (any subtype) is fibrosis which progresses to the development of scar tissue. Scar tissue restricts normal joint motion and produces its biomechanical, neurologic, and circulatory consequences. This adverse process can only be minimized by treating each type of injured tissue specifically and *thoroughly* until *all* signs of inflammation have been removed.

Faye underscores the fact that, in the treatment of joint trauma, partial correction is not good enough. Treatment must be thorough to assure that all joint play is restored. The abatement of pain, tenderness, spasm, and swelling is not adequate. Full end play mobility must be restored.

Differentiating Various Types of Motion Restrictions

Joint stiffness can be produced by either periarticular or intra-articular structural changes or swelling.

Structural Changes: General Considerations

Joint stiffness due to structural changes can usually be traced to taut soft-tissues (eg, hypertonic muscles, shortened ligaments), cartilage degeneration, insufficient lubrication, or capsule tears. In many cases of fixation, inflammation may have resulted in intra-articular adhesion formation or tight periarticular soft tissues.

Mennell explains that a tough "springy" block with some rebound at the end of motion suggests soft-tissue shortening or a deranged cartilage. Mobility may be normal in one direction and completely absent in another. A firm "leathery" arrest occurring before the end of normal motion in some directions but not others suggests fibrotic ligamentous restraint, adhesions, or capsule thickening as is often seen in subacute arthritis.

If a sudden protective spasm occurs at some point during the arc of motion (felt as a firm resistance), an active localized lesion should be suspected. To distinguish muscular spasm from bony outgrowth as a cause of limited joint motion, keep in mind that bony outgrowths allow free motion up to a certain point and then motion is suddenly halted without pain. Muscle spasm, on the other hand, checks motion somewhat from the onset. The resistance and pain gradually increase until the examiner's efforts are arrested at some point that feels like a "thick rubber" block.

If the extent of joint limitation depends on the position of another joint, it can generally be assured that the cause is extra-articular; ie, the cause is within a structure spanning between the two joints. Hip flexion, for example, may be limited with the knee extended but not with the knee flexed, indicating shortened hamstrings. Another example is Volkmann's ischemic contractures in which the fingers cannot be extended unless the wrist is first flexed. Contractures usually feature limited motion in one direction and painless motion in other possible directions.

Motions limited by capsular thickening and adhesions are generally not as painful after a conditioning process. There is no sudden arrest after a space of free mobility, but motion is limited from the first and usually in all directions even if the muscles around the joint are not taut. The possibility of "limbering-up" after exercise (or passive stretching) distinguishes this type of limitation. Restricted mobility from capsule restriction usually follows inadequately treated degenerative joint disease, acute trauma, arthritis, or prolonged immobilization. Stiffness from degenerative diseases becomes pronounced when muscle compensation in the area fails to protect thinning cartilage. The stiffness associated is greater after rest but is quickly relieved by mild exercise.

A "snapping" sound results when a tendon abruptly slips over a bony prominence or fibrotic soft tissue. This is often seen in tendon displacements, lax joints, osteoma, and trigger fingers.

Swelling

A swollen joint is frequently the result of inflammatory edema, thickening of the synovial membrane, or an excess fluid in the joint cavity. Such swelling, when deep, is often obscured by bones, muscles, and tendons that overlie the joint cavity or its pouches; however, it is noticeable over thinly covered areas of the joint. For instance, swelling in the hip joint is almost impossible to detect. Swelling in the elbow is observed only at the posterior aspect on the sides of the olecranon process because the anterior surface of the elbow joint is thickly covered with muscles and the lateral aspects by strong collateral ligaments that prevent protrusion. For the same reasons, a wrist swelling is least noticeable when viewed from the front and radial side and a knee swelling is least noticeable when viewed from the medial or posterior aspect.

Associated Pain and Tenderness

Joint nerve irritation is characterized by pain on active motion but a full passive range of movement exists unless the joint is splinted by spasm. Pain induced by passive motion in one direction and active motion in the opposite direction suggests a muscle or tendon lesion; ie, the muscle becomes painful when passively stretched by manipulation or by contraction of its antagonists or by its own contraction against resistance.

Pain brought forth by external pressure commonly results from one or more trigger points, traumatic lesions of sensitive subdermal tissue, or the development of a toxic accumulation or deep-seated inflammatory irritation. The myogenic features of cervical root and peripheral nerve lesions reflected in the upper extremity are shown in Table 8.1.

Motion resistance produced by a periarticular lesion will frequently be felt before passive motion induces pain. If passive motion produces sharp pain far before the end of normal motion occurs and little internal resistance is felt to further motion, an acute inflammatory process, a mass (eg, a neoplasm), or possibly a psychosomatic disorder should be suspected. Tenosynovitis expresses pain during both stretch and relaxation as the roughened tendon slides within its inflamed sheath.

Mild cases of joint involvement invariably have points of maximum tenderness that correspond to those endothelial regions that are most superficial. For example, they are elicited in the extremities (1) in the ankle at the anterior surface of the joint, (2) in the knee on both sides of the patella, (3) in the wrist over the anatomical snuffbox, and (4) in the elbow over the radiohumeral joint.

Joint trauma is sometimes profiled by a cool periarticular swelling that is extremely tender. Trauma or inflammation may result in hemorrhage or effusion. Painless bony lumps and asymptomatic joint swelling can often be traced back to forgotten trauma, especially when associated with sports injuries (eg, karate lumps, surfer's nodes). In degenerative joint diseases, the trauma may be only normal activity on sensitive tissues that is sufficient to elicit effusion.

Differential Pointers

From 50% to 60% of the pains and discomforts that the average ambulatory patient has are the direct or indirect result of involuntary muscle contraction. Thus, the relationship of spasm to pain must be considered in both diagnosis and therapy. Several other important points are described below.

Joint Degeneration. Peripheral joint degeneration within the extremities follows a pattern that is similar to that found in the axial skeleton. See Table 8.2.

Table 8.1. Myologic Features of Cervical Root and Peripheral Nerve Lesions

Site	Muscle Sign
C6 root	Shoulders are held abducted Elbow flexors weak Elbow extensors weak Forearm pronators weak Forearm supinators weak Wrist extensors weak
C7 root	Elbow extensors weak Forearm pronators weak Wrist flexors weak Wrist extensors weak Grip weak
C8 root	Elbow extensors weak Wrist extensors weak Grip weak Thumb flexion weak Thumb pressure weak Thumb—little finger apposition poor Finger extensors weak Finger spread poor
Radial nerve	Elbow extensors weak Forearm supinators weak Wrist extensors weak Finger extensors weak
Median nerve	Forearm pronators weak Wrist flexors weak Grip weak Thumb pressure weak
Ulnar nerve	Grip weak Thumb pressure weak Finger spread poor

Muscle Tone. The typical feeling of a normal muscle on palpation is one of resilience. An increased perception of tone by the examiner denotes a hypertonic muscle; decreased tone, a hypotonic muscle.

Spasticity. The major function of muscle is contraction. When shortening occurs involuntarily, the cause can usually be traced to neuropathy or a protective reflex (splinting). This splinting reaction to inhibit movement is not always beneficial, especially when the disorder becomes chronic. When muscles become acutely spastic or chronically indurated from overstress, normal movement is impaired and foci for referred pain are frequently established. Spastic and indurated muscles feature circulatory stasis that is essentially the effect of compressed vessels. This circulatory deficit leads to poor tissue nutrition and the accumulation of metabolic debris. Palpation will often reveal tender areas that feel taut, gristly, ropy, or nodular.

A spastic resistance is primarily a stretch reflex induced at the muscle-spindle level. In common spasticity disorders, the contracted muscles relax when the part is comfortably rested with support and contract again with volitional movements, tendon tapping, vibration, or even startling noises.

Muscle Mass. Palpation and mensuration are used to determine extremity muscle volume. When palpating a resting muscle, there should be a pliable mass that is symmetrical bilaterally. If not, a measurement should be made with a flexible tape from a bony prominence to the belly of a suspected muscle and the point marked with a skin pencil. The circumference of the part should then be measured at that point and then compared with a contralateral measurement. The two sides should be approximately the same circumference unless there is a history of unilateral occupational or sports activity. A decrease in size indicates atrophy and is usually associated with some degree of hypotonicity. However, differentiating ipsilateral enlargement from contralateral atrophy is no easy task, especially when no overt muscle weakness exists on the atrophic side.

Myoedema. The term *myoedema* refers to an edematous muscle or group of muscles in which a contractual "lumping" or "mounding" occurs within a wasted muscle after it is sharply struck. This fatigable "knot" is usually located at the margin of percussion. The cause is unknown, and the phenomenon is always symmetric. It is a common occurrence in atrophied pectoral muscles overlying a tubercular cavity in a lung. Other wasting disorders featuring myoedema are acute infections, peripheral neuropathy, chronic alcoholism, malnutrition, malignant cachexia, and myxedema.

Pitting. Pitting from palpation is a sign of liquid infiltration into the underlying tissues. The pressure should be maintained for at least 10 seconds. The depression is often palpable with the fingertips even if it is not visible. Tenderness associated with pitting is indicative of inflammatory edema. While edema gives rise to a soft pitting, a degree of induration can be felt if pus is present.

Fluctuation. If a mass fluctuates in one plane but not in another, it is negative for swelling because a swelling fluctuates in opposite planes. Although fat and muscle also transmit a percussion impulse, they do so in a less perfect manner than fluid.

Hyperthermia. The presence of local heat is a sign of inflammation. It may be noted by passing the outstretched hand rapidly over the affected part to an unaffected part and back again. Any difference in warmth from the affected area to the unaffected area signifies an increase in local temperature.

Neuralgia. *Neuralgia* is a general term that refers to any sharp, stabbing, extremely severe pain, with temporary periods of abatement in severity, that travels along the course of one or more nerves. The term *neurodynia* is sometimes used to describe a similar pain that is less severe, ie, a deep ache. The pain of neuralgia is usually associated with tenderness along the course of the

Table 8.2. Phases of Chronic Peripheral Joint Degeneration

Features	Dysfunction ⟶	Instability ⟶	Stabilization
History	Strain/sprain.	Strain/sprain with likely history of previous injury.	Chronic episodes of pain.
Signs and symptoms	Periarticular muscle spasm, pain that is aggravated by certain movements (eg, "catches"), tenderness, motion restriction, slight swelling at times.	Like features of dysfunction, except feelings of weakness and periodic tendency toward collapse are usually reported; a segmental shift may be seen during active motions.	Pain, area stiffness, incapacitating attacks after minor trauma, muscle weakness.
Biomechanics	Tension or compressive overstress leading to subluxation.	Hypermobile joint motion with frequent subluxation, cartilages likely malpositioned.	Hypomobile joint motion.
Pathology	Small cartilage fissures, possible disc displacement, synovitis leading to fixation due to intra-articular adhesion and/or articular cartilage degeneration, probable subluxation.	Lax capsule, coalesced disc tears, possible nipping of a synovia.	Fibrosis, cartilage degeneration, loose bodies, severe joint-space thinning, marginal osteophytes leading to ankylosis.

nerve and violent episodic spasms in the muscles innervated. Although the term neuralgia is nondiagnostic, it is often acceptable in situations where the exact etiology and pathology involved are unknown. Neuralgia rarely subsides spontaneously.

Analyzing a Swollen Joint

A mushy "boggy" sensation perceived at the end point of motion is the typical feature of chronic joint effusion in which synovitis is minimal. Periarticular edematous swelling around the joint capsule is characteristic of inflammatory disorders. Intra-articular edema within the capsule secondary to inflammation features being worse after rest such as in the morning or upon arising after sitting. Swelling and stiffness lasting more than a half hour, often for several hours, suggests one of the inflammatory arthritides.

The key features of any joint swelling will be noted in its character, its effect on motion restriction and positioning, and its shape.

Character. Swelling around a joint can be caused by painless edema (fluid overload) or venous insufficiency. Infiltration, effusion, or inflammation can cause direct joint swelling. Localized infiltration is seen in leukemia and amyloid disorders. Swelling around a joint that is warm and tender is characteristic of sprain, gout, and rheumatic arthritis. Synovial inflammation is characteristic of the nonspecific arthritides, rheumatic fever, septic arthritis, gout, and various collagen-vascular diseases. A gonococcal wrist or ankle joint will usually be associated with nearby tenosynovitis.

Motion Restriction. In general, joint motion becomes restricted from either pain or mechanical disability. Intra-articular swelling impairs both active and passive movements, while extra-articular swellings impair only one type of movement or none. Foreign bodies or fragments within a joint resulting in effusion are associated with intermittent motion restriction.

Positioning. Because of the relative position of various bones and associated relaxation of the muscles around joints, each joint has one position in which the synovial cavity attains the greatest dimensions. When tension increases in the synovial cavity because

of effusion, the patient will unconsciously adopt an antalgic position that gives the greatest relief.

Shape. The shape of a swollen joint corresponds to that of the synovial membrane distended in toto. For example, distention of the tabular process of endothelium about the long head of the biceps in the shoulder may exhibit enlargement over the surgical neck of the humerus. In the lower extremity when a subcrural pouch becomes dilated, swelling of the knee joint may extend as much as 7 inches above the joint line.

Closed-Packed Joint Positions

Most long-bone joints are in the ovoid class in which the cross-sectional surface curves so that it has a smoothly changing radius. As an opposing articular surface moves along an ovoid surface, the apposing surfaces will not fit closely except at one particular point, which every joint has, where congruency is close (the closed-packed position). It is at this point that movement stops.

Some joint movements are accompanied by compression, others by distraction, and others by compression and distraction—depending upon the range and angle of motion. The term *closed-packed position* refers to a specific joint position in which the articular surfaces are at their maximum point of congruency.

Opposing articular surfaces may be either in a state of (1) approximation (compression) such as when moving toward the closed-packed position or (2) separation (distraction) such as when moving away from the closed-packed position. Alternating compression and distraction within a joint has a beneficial influence on articular surface nutrition and lubrication. Such alternating motions also form the basis of *proprioceptive neuromuscular facilitation* techniques.

Knowledge of the closed-packed position of each joint in which movements involve compression and/or distraction can be determined (Table 8.3). Most subluxations, dislocations, and fractures occur when a joint is in the closed-packed position. In contrast, most sprains occur when the joint is in a loose-packed position because the force is imposed more on the supporting periarticular structures of the joint than on the intra-articular structures.

Conjugate rotation is required when an impure swing occurs during joint motion. This unusual rotation produces a twisting action upon the joint's capsule and major ligaments that, in turn, causes the joint surfaces to approximate until the closed-packed position is reached. For example, a fall upon an outstretched hand throws most joints of the upper limb, shoulder girdle, and thoracic cage into a closed-packed position (two exceptions are the metacarpophalangeal and acromioclavicular joints). If the force is greater than the structural strength of the bony links involved, either a dislocation or fracture occurs.

Resisted Joint Motion

If resisted motion in opposite or incompatible directions induces pain, a muscle lesion is highly unlikely; rather, an acute nonmuscle lesion should be suspected near the site of attachments of the involved muscle. For example, resisted motion exhibits pain in periosteal tears, fractures, bursitis, or when a tender mass (eg, an abscess, neuroma) is compressed by a muscle.

The purpose of evaluating passive resistance to active motion is to reveal and isolate hypomobility, hypermobility, weakness, pain, and associated patient reactions. During such tests, the joint must be held near midrange, the resistance must be strong enough to avoid joint motion, and, when possible, specific muscles should be isolated. The general interpretation of responses to resisted motion are shown in Table 8.4. Such responses can be extremely helpful during differential diagnosis if confirmed by other tests.

Myalgia and Its Evaluation

Myalgia, whether it is associated with fixation or not, has peculiar characteristics.

Table 8.3. Closed-Packed Joint Positions*

Joint	Closed-Packed Position
Temporomandibular	When the heads of the condyles are at their most retruded position.
Glenohumeral	When horizontal adduction, abduction, and external rotation are fully achieved.
Acromioclavicular	During elevation and horizontal adduction of the arm; combining upward scapular rotation and narrowing of the scapula-clavicle angle (as seen from above).
Elbow	Full extension.
Wrist (as a whole)	Full dorsiflexion and radial deviation.
Trapezio metacarpal	Opposition.
Metacarpophalangeal	Full flexion.
Interphalangeal	Full Extension.

*Modified from Kessler/Hartling.

Pain arising from an injury to muscle may be elicited by forcing the muscle to contract against resistance without allowing it to shorten; ie, preventing movement of adjacent joints. This test, even if it is helpful in differentiating muscle pain from pain due to other causes, is not absolute because it is not always possible, even with great care, to avoid some indirect pressure or tension on adjacent structures. Another feature of myalgia is that pain arising from a chronic contraction of an involved muscle is not increased by contracting the muscle further.

Excessive motor fiber stimulation produces involuntary painful muscle contraction, and severe spasm will place considerable tension on highly sensitive periosteum via tendon attachments. Keep in mind that it is one thing to determine existing hypertonicity or spasm and another to determine if it is protective, primary, compensatory, or hysterical in origin. Spasm may be caused by:
• Irritation, stretching, or pressure on a nerve trunk, a nerve plexus, or peripheral nerve branches
• Traumatic irritation directly or that of

Table 8.4. General Interpretation of Resisted Motion Signs

Response	Probable Cause
Strong with excessive range of motion	Capsule laxity, ligamentous instability.
Strong and painful in a specific direction	Minor musculotendinous lesion.
Strong and painful in all directions	Neurosis.
Strong with pain on repetitive resisted movements	Arterial flow deficit.
Strong and unchanged pain in all directions	Referred pain syndrome.
Strong, painful, and hypomobile	Guarded joint for some reason.
Strong, painless, and hypomobile	Contracture, adhesion.
Weak and sharply painful	Fracture, dislocation, rupture, gross pathology.
Weak without aggravation of pain (painless or unchanged constant pain)	Neurogenic disorder, muscle or tendon rupture.
Weak and painless in all directions	Nonmusculotendinous deficit, probable neurogenic lesion.
Pain only at specific point of arc	Functional entrapment, lax joint, dislocated tendon, loose body.
Pain at one range extreme	Subluxation-fixation, tissue entrapment, eroded cartilage.
Painful with gross hypermobility	Severe sprain.
Painless with gross hypermobility	Ruptured tissues with interrupted sensory path.

an adjacent structure
- Toxic irritation of the anterior horn cells
- Psychogenic origins.

As described above, peripheral spasm can be the result of encroachment irritation of a nerve root. It is for this reason that chiropractic spinal adjustments have corrected many cases of chronic upper- and lower-extremity pain that have been previously treated medically or surgically only at the site of pain. Common examples of this in the upper extremity are cases of subdeltoid bursitis, tennis elbow, or carpal tunnel syndrome that are produced or contributed to by lower cervical fixations.

Painful Splinting

The myotatic stretch reflex uses a single sensory neuron and is initiated by stretching the muscle spindle's annulospiral receptors. A reflex contraction is produced that is designed to protect sensitive tissues against further stretch so that the muscle may maintain a constant length. This reflex action is several times more severe if initiated by a sudden stretch (eg, jerk, dynamic thrust) than by a slow stretch. Inhibitory impulses are transmitted to the motor neurons of the antagonists (reciprocal inhibition) and facilitating impulses are sent to synergists, and both of these involuntary reactions enhance the response. A stretch reflex is not normally initiated by voluntary contraction.

Striated muscles, especially the erectors, become painfully splinted (intrinsically immobilized) by spasm (active, involuntary, or both) when they are fatigued. In time, trophic changes occur and normal tone is lost. Splinting differs from ordinary spasm in that relaxation of the affected muscles occurs at rest. Prolonged pain from bone, muscle, tendon, and joint lesions with resultant long-term splinting or pseudoparalysis may lead to eventual osteoporosis in involved and possibly adjacent bones. Joint contractures may also develop and thus produce a typical myogenic fixation. This is an example, similar to a psychic conversion symptom, where a sensory symptom may lead to definite structural changes.

If spasm exists after trauma, the irritating

focus can usually be attributed to irritating ischemia initially and blood debris later. For some unknown reason, prolonged states often establish a self-sustaining reflex spasm that continues long after the initial cause has been erased. The noxious cycle appears to resemble some form of habitual conditioning process within the spinal cord. For this reason, local therapy must always be combined with spinal therapy when indicated.

Cramps

Neuromusculoskeletal disorders are often associated with muscle cramps. These powerful involuntary muscular contractions severely shorten the flexor muscles and produce extreme pain, often incapacitating, that is directly initiated by ischemia and hypoxia of muscle tissue.

Lymph Stasis

Skeletal muscle tissue lacks an intrinsic lymph supply, but a muscle's connective-tissue sheath and tendon sheaths are richly endowed with lymphatic vessels. During the normal physiologic exchange of fluids through capillary walls, the quantity of fluid leaving the capillary is usually greater than that entering the venule. The related lymphatic network takes up the excess and eventually delivers it to the venous system. It is this process that allows a continuous exchange of tissue fluids and maintains a constant pressure of interstitial fluid. A deficit in this process is thought to be the basis of Bennett's neurovascular and Chapman's neurolymphatic points.

Lymph flow is increased during activity as is capillary circulation, but the flow can be impeded by excessive pressure exerted by a constantly hypertonic or phasic contracted muscle. Inhibited lymph drainage contributes to muscular pain during prolonged activity by (1) causing a buildup of interstitial fluids that increase hydrostatic pressure and (2) encouraging the accumulation of metabolic waste products that would normally be drained by the lymphatics and venules.

Fibrositis

A large number of localized, tender, widely dispersed, and symmetrical sites suggests fibrositis. These sites resemble trigger points, but they are more superficial; ie, around muscle in its fascia rather than within the body of muscle. In contrast to fibrositis, a small number of tender points that are clustered in a single region and not associated with a diffuse aching stiffness and fatigue suggests a referred pain syndrome (eg, similar to a trigger point syndrome).

Basic Adjustive Considerations

The first phase of treatment of posttraumatic injury to a joint is to relieve the associated pain and swelling yet not interfere in the natural healing processes. Emphasis here should be on cold, compression, rest, and possibly elevation. The second phase is to enhance the natural healing processes and avoid adverse consequences by restoring normal movement (viz, by adjustment, passive stretching, active exercise, and interrupting any noxious reflex cycle). As mentioned previously, the latter is often thought to be a somaticosomatic spinal reflex that tends to perpetuate itself spontaneously long after its initial cause has been removed. Thus, spinal foci should not be neglected even if the site of injury is far removed from the spine. And, as we shall see in this and the following chapter, the opposite is also true: the extraspinal joints should not be neglected even if the pain is localized in the patient's spine. The nervous system is not a one-way street.

Restoring End Play

Two general categories of abnormal motion in any joint must be considered:

1. The hypermobile (unstable) joint in which the supporting ligaments have been severely stretched or torn. Such a joint requires temporary immobilization to promote tissue shortening. Manipulation of such a joint would be contraindicated unless the joint later acquires hypomobility, which is a common occurrence.

2. The hypomobile (fixated) joint in which the supporting ligaments and/or associated muscles and other soft tissues have shortened or in which intraarticular changes have occurred that restrict motion. Manipulation of such a joint to restore normal end play is indicated. If this is not accomplished, a state of chronic inflammation from dyskinesia will be established. Keep in mind the following characteristics of joint play:

• Joint play cannot be produced by voluntary action, yet voluntary motion depends on the integrity of joint play specific for each plane of motion.

• Loss of joint play produces pain on stressing the joint to the degree that joint play should be perceived.

• Muscles that move a joint exhibiting dysfunction become hypertonic due to intrinsic irritation (usually mechanical or chemical). This, in turn, contributes to restricting the normal range of motion.

Almost all extremity joints have more passive end points of motion than are indicated by their function during voluntary activity. For example, an interphalangeal joint's gross function is essentially flexion and extension. However, besides A-P/P-A glide, long-axis extension, lateral tilt, and rotational end play must exist for normal flexion-extension to occur. Each end play must be tested. It is doubtful that a true hinge joint exists in the human body, and this statement includes the elbow and knee. This fact is often overlooked in traditional orthopedic care where treatment is typically confined to restoring voluntary motion only.

Motion palpation is an art, a sensorimotor skill, and as any art or such skill, it must be learned by application. "One does not learn to ride a bicycle by reading about it," states Faye. Only the basic mechanics can be grasped by listening to lectures, watching videotapes, and reading textbooks. Understanding comes from practice: hands on application. Only by practice and concentration will an examiner be able to perceive minute ranges of end play, which sometimes may normally not exceed 1 mm. Only by practice will an examiner be able to distinguish the normal from the abnormal and all the variables associated with age, gender, history of trauma, genetic modifications, and so forth.

Appropriate Technic

The general principles described in previous chapters for correcting a spinal fixation are also true when applied to a fixation found in an extraspinal joint. Once a specific motion restriction has been isolated, it is necessary to adjust *into* the restriction plane of normal movement. If more than one plane of normal motion is restricted, each restricted plane should be released if possible. The ideal objective is to restore each joint's normal direction and degree of mobility into the range of passive end play.

Specific technics to correct extraspinal axial fixations and upper-extremity mobility restrictions will be described later in this chapter. Essentially, correction is made by testing the plane of normal movement, and if found to be restricted, applying a short dynamic thrust against the fixation to restore normal end play. The cardinal symptom of fixation is the arousal of pain or unusual discomfort when passive motion is attempted against the restriction.

The amount of force applied during correction should be just sufficient to achieve the mobility desired at a certain stage of rehabilitation, with amendments for the patient's age, physical status, discomfort, and the other factors commonly considered in adapting an adjustive thrust to the needs of a patient and the condition at hand. Faye states that a mild thrust followed by a moderate thrust is usually enough. If a moderate force is insufficient, then the force should be increased gradually to patient tolerance until an adequate amount produces mobilization (with or without an audible release).

The depth of an adjustment must be carefully controlled. The objective is to release restricted mobility, not produce hypermobility. If motion is forced beyond the end of the physiologic barrier, an inflammatory reaction will be produced. In many instances, the range of normal end play may be not more than 1—3 mm. Overcoming resistance within such a small range of motion is the advantage of the dynamic impulse.

EXTRASPINAL AXIAL JOINT CONSIDERATIONS

We usually think of the spine when the axial skeleton is mentioned. However, there are a few other extraspinal axial joints that need to be considered. The major joints in this category are the temporomandibular, sternoclavicular, sternocostal, and intercostal joints, and the articulation between the manubrium and the body of the sternum. From a clinical viewpoint, the interface between the scapula and the thoracic cage can also be placed in this classification. The one remaining extraspinal axial joint is the pubis, which has been described in a previous chapter.

Initial Considerations During Physical Diagnosis

It is assumed that prior to the investigation of mechanical dysfunction in the thorax that a complete physical examination has been conducted to rule out advanced pathologic processes as the cause of the patient's complaint. Routinely, all cardiac, pulmonary, diaphragmatic, and upper-abdominal signs brought out by inspection, auscultation, palpation, and percussion should be evaluated. The integrity of the pectoral, scapular, and

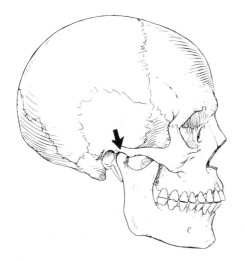

Figure 8.1. The temporomandibular joint (Courtesy ACAP).

abdominal reflexes (including Barkman's reflex) should be tested, along with tests for light touch, pain perception, and muscle strength (including Beevor's sign). Many clinicians knowledgeable in meridian therapy incorporate a check of all thoracic alarm points in their standard examination.

Following the physical examination, all suspicions or initial rejections of underlying pathology should be confirmed or rejected with appropriate roentgenographic, ECG, and laboratory findings when such procedures are indicated by clinical judgment.

The Temporomandibular Joint

As with many articular-dysfunction complexes, TMJ dyskinesia may be a cause or an effect. If primary, its effects may express itself through the whole functional-structural complex of the body. If secondary, its cause may be found as remote as in the feet.

According to Lay, the actions of muscles, ligaments, and fasciae from head to foot coordinate it as a functioning unit. Thus, a functional or anatomical short leg, sacroiliac fixation, lumbar fixation, fixed rib-cage distortion (especially with scalene shortening), fixated thoracic or cervical distortions, or occipitoatlantal dysfunction may be a cause of, contributor to, or an effect of TMJ dysfunction.

Applied Biomechanics

The TMJ hinges within the glenoid fossa of the mandible and glides anteriorly to the eminentia during normal motion (Fig. 8.1). The articular space contains a small amount of viscous fluid for lubrication. The head of the condyle and the glenoid fossa are covered with fibroid cartilage, which serves as a shock absorber. This cartilage tends to wear thin when subjected to prolonged overstress because it contains no direct blood supply that would enhance tissue regeneration. The blood supply to the TMJ is from the superficial temporal branch of the external carotid artery; the disc itself, however, is avascular. The meniscus of the joint divides the joint cavity into two divisions. The lower part of the joint cavity is used during gliding motion,

and the upper part is used for hinge-like movements.

TMJ motion is accomplished primarily by one head of the external pterygoid muscle pulling the meniscus forward while the second head opens the joint. Secondary assistance is provided by the mylohyoid, geniohyoid, and digastric muscles, and gravity is helpful in lowering the mandible when in the upright position. Thus, the two heads of the pterygoid muscle, primarily, act asynchronously to open the TMJ. In closing the jaw (approximating the teeth of the mandible and maxillae), the temporal, masseter, and internal pterygoid muscles are activated. All the muscles active during TMJ function assist in maintaining the mandible in its resting position.

Articular Disrelationships

Berkman reports that the jaw influences the stability of the atlas and axis, and, in turn, fixation-subluxations of the atlas and axis influence the stability of the TMJ. The fascia colli bind the jaw and cervical spine into a unit where a fault of any one part will influence the entire mechanism. Several papers by osteopaths have proposed that TMJ dysfunction is essentially caused by stress factors that distort the normal position of the temporal bone.

Two major forms of TMJ malposition and dyskinesia occur. They arise from either partial displacement or complete dislocation of the articular disc and occur in 10%—12% of the population. In partial anterior displacements, condyle translation is not blocked. That is, when the patient moves the closed jaw forward and/or toward the contralateral side, the condyle will snap forward (opening click) into its normal position so that the mouth can be fully opened. Farrar/McCarty state that when a jaw in such a state is retruded, the disc will displace with a snap (reciprocal click). This can often be heard without auscultation.

A dislocated disc is usually dislodged anteriorly toward the front of the condyle so that the condyle's translation is restricted when the mouth is opened, increasing the joint space. See Figure 8.2. Persistent condylar motion on a dislocated disc encourages irregular adaptive remodeling and osteoarthritis to develop within the joint because the dislocated disc can no longer cushion the articular surfaces. Crepitus will exhibit if bone-on-bone articulation occurs. In time, the collateral ligaments may perforate or tear and be drawn into the articular space and osteoarthritis will likely result.

The major signs and symptoms of TMJ dysfunction are shown in Table 8.5.

Inspection

Inspect active joint motion by having the patient open and close the mouth, and observe the movement of the mandible from the front and sides. Motion rhythm should be smooth, and the arc should be continuous and unbroken. The mandible should open and close in a straight line symmetrically, with the molars easily separating and joining. An awkward arc, a restricted range of motion, and/or lateral deviation toward one side during opening of the mouth suggest dyskinesia.

Ask the patient to slowly tap their teeth together and note the fit of the bite. The mandible normally moves backward during cervical extension and forward in cervical flexion, producing poor occlusion during flexion-extension. You can easily test this on yourself. Thus, a patient with a cervical spine in a chronic state of fixed hyperlordosis or kyphosis in the resting position will exhibit a constant state of malocclusion, which will lead to TMJ dysfunction and resulting symptoms.

Palpation

Bony Palpation. During the initial palpation of the TMJs, place your little fingers in the patient's external auditory canals and apply mild pressure anteriorly and downward while the patient opens and closes the mouth (Fig. 8.3). Motion of the mandibular condyles will be felt on the fingertips: normally felt to be smooth and equal on both sides. Normally, no crepitation will be perceived. Next, palpate the lateral aspects of the joints by placing the first and second fingers just anterior to the tragi. Have the patient open and close the mouth, and note any abnormalities. A palpable crepitus suggests traumatic synovial swelling or meniscal damage, and a slight dislocation (painful) may be felt when the patient widely opens the mouth. If there is any doubt as to the presence of crepitus, auscultate the joint for clicks or grating sounds.

Soft-Tissue Palpation. The middle fibers of the temporalis muscles should be palpated between the eye and the upper ear. Check the bellies of the masseter muscles. Palpate the external pterygoid muscle after the patient has opened the mouth. Point a gloved index finger posteriorly above the last molar, between the gum and the buccal mucosa, on the mandibular neck. The external

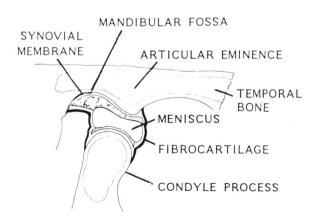

Figure 8.2. Close-up schematic of the temporomandibular joint (Courtesy ACAP).

pterygoid will normally be felt to tighten and relax as the patient opens and closes the mouth, and the patient will report tenderness and pain on palpation if the muscle has been strained or is in spasm. Palpate the internal pterygoid muscle intra- and extraorally simultaneously. Palpate the mylohyoid muscle beneath the tongue. You may wish to test the jaw and Chvostek's reflexes at this time if they haven't been checked previously. Then evaluate the posterior cervical, sternocleidomastoideus, and trapezius muscles for associated hypertonicity and tenderness.

Restricted Range of Motion

Impaired TMJ motion can be the result of muscle spasm, chronic hypertonicity, rheumatoid arthritis, osteoarthritis, scar tissue, trismus from spasm of the elevating muscles of mastication from hysteria, tetanus, congenital defect, or most any type of local inflammation. If a patient with a subnormal range of mandibular motion can suddenly open the mouth wider after the TMJ area has been sprayed with a vapocoolant, mus-

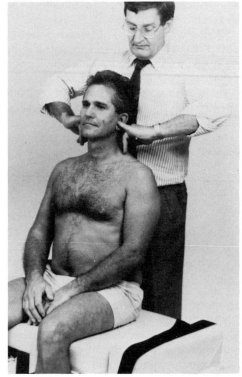

Figure 8.3. Initial bony palpation of the TMJs.

Table 8.5. Major Signs and Symptoms of TMJ Dysfunction

Local Effects	Remote Effects
Mandible deviates to one side when opened	Tenderness of posterior cervical muscles, usually unilateral
Joint click (palpable and/or audible) in displacement but not in dislocation	Pain radiates from TMJ area superiorly to temporoparietal region and/or inferiorly into the neck
Severe, unilateral, dull facial pain, aggravated by chewing and opening and closing the mouth.	Muscle spasm:
Crepitus of involved joint (sometimes)	Posterior cervicals
Tenderness at proximal mandible, usually unilateral	Sternocleidomastoid
Muscle spasm:	Trapezius
External pterygoids	Mylohyoid
Internal pterygoids	Scalenes
Masseter	Earache
Temporalis	Postural distortion (anywhere from the occiput to the feet)
Bruxism	Rib cage, spinal, and lower extremity sites of fixation and trigger points.
Malocclusion	Peripheral circulation disorders
Atypical facial neuralgia	Migraine

cle hypertonicity should be suspected as an important ingredient in the syndrome.

The adult range of mandibular motion is usually normal if (1) you are able to insert three finger widths between the incisor teeth when the patient's mouth is opened; (2) the patient is able to jut the jaw forward, without lateral deviation, and place the lower teeth in front of the upper teeth. If deemed necessary, an accurate measurement of the interincisal opening can be made with a Boley gauge.

Test TMJ muscle strength by placing one hand on the patient's occiput to steady the patient and the other hand, palm up, under the patient's jaw. Ask the patient to open the mouth while you apply resistance with your palm. The patient should normally be able to open the mouth against the increasing resistance of your palm.

Adjustive and Manipulative Approaches: General Considerations

If hypertonicity is found around one or both TMJs, apply gentle but firm passive pressure against the resistance until the tension releases. This is sometimes all that is necessary. Temporary correction will be indicated when free mobility is restored. The same technique can be applied if abnormal tension is found in the sphenomandibular and stylomandibular soft tissues, as determined by exerting pressure on the angle of the mandible downward and then upward, and comparing the resistance found bilaterally.

If intra-articular TMJ compression is a factor, and it often is, physical correction can be aided by the doctor inserting gloved thumbs against the patient's lower molars, with the doctor's fingers wrapped around the patient's jaw, and applying pressure and a short impulse to bring the mandible down and forward and then down and backward several times to open the joint space.

Motion palpation of the pubic and/or sacroiliac joints will frequently reveal a fixation when TMJ dysfunction is present. When this is found, the fixation should always be mobilized unless contraindications for adjustive therapy are found.

Mild Mobility Restriction (Fixation) Release

The basic working condylar motions of the TMJ essentially include (1) rotation with and without a lateral shift; (2) rotation with backward, upward, and lateral motion; and (3) rotation with forward, downward, and lateral motion. Assure that these motions are free and that end play can be perceived. Functional restriction may be the common result of local hypertonicity or shortened ligaments.

Active Stretching Exercise. Have the supine patient slowly and progressively open the mouth to a larger and larger degree but not to the degree of pain. During this exercise, instruct the patient to place the tongue against the hard palate as this will keep the motions essentially rotary and minimize protrusion. After the initial warmup, have the patient hold the full-open position for several seconds and follow this with complete jaw relaxation for several seconds in a hold-relax fashion. Kessler/Hertling state that ultrasound may be beneficial during this exercise.

Passive Stretching Exercise. When jaw opening is restricted, sustained passive stretching can be administered by almost any type of padded appliance (eg, a surgical mouth prop with a spring or rachet). Slowly inserting layers of tongue blades or a tapered cork (15—30 mm) between the molars are sometimes substituted during home treatments. Regardless of what appliance is used, this technique is best conducted with the patient in the relaxed supine position at first and then in the sitting position as improvement is achieved. Special care must be used to avoid too vigorous an application. Pretherapy moist heat applications to the involved TMJ(s) and cervical spine for 15—20 minutes is often helpful.

Reflex Relaxation. As described previously, a commonly used indirect technique can be conducted by applying slowly reducing resistance as the patient attempts to open the closed mouth. After several seconds of relaxation, active jaw motion (stretching) without resistance should be conducted several times. A reverse technique is then used by applying slowly reducing resistance as the patient attempts to close the opened mouth. These action-rest procedures should be repeated several times until function improves.

Moderate Fixation Mobilization Technics

Lateral mandibular movements are the most restricted jaw motions in bilateral TMJ capsule restrictions (eg, contractures, spasm, adhesions). Contralateral anterior-posterior gliding movements are the most restricted jaw motions in unilateral capsule restrictions, and the mandible will deviate toward the restricted side when the mouth is opened widely.

Caudad Traction. Place the patient in a relaxed full-supine or semi-supine position and stand to the side of the involved joint facing the patient. Place your cephalad stabilizing hand against the patient's forehead. Then place your active padded thumb (caudad hand) against the patient's rear molars with your fingers cupping the patient's chin. Slowly apply traction downward and ask the patient to swallow. Hold pressure for several seconds, add a mild impulse, and then allow a similar period for relaxation.

Mobilizing Restricted Protrusion (Anterior Glide). After caudal traction is administered several times, include anterior glide (protraction) and posterior glide (retraction) mobilization. This is best accomplished by standing on the contralateral side and grasping the angle of the mandible externally with your active hand's 1st and 2nd fingers with the thumb hooked around the patient's chin. Apply sustained traction anteriorly, ask the patient to swallow, and apply a mild impulse. After a period of relaxation and holding the same contact, apply sustained pressure posteriorly, ask the patient to swallow, and add a mild impulse. Repeat these action-rest procedures several times until function of anterior glide improves.

Mobilizing Restricted Medial-Lateral Glide. Stand behind the relaxed supine patient. Cup your active hand around the patient's chin, and support the patient's head with your stabilizing hand. With your active hand, slowly apply traction laterally,

hold it for several seconds, ask the patient to swallow, impulse, and then allow several seconds for relaxation. Reverse the procedure by applying pressure medially, hold it for several seconds, ask the patient to swallow, impulse, and then allow several seconds for relaxation. Repeat these procedures several times until medial-lateral glide improves.

Unilateral TMJ Inferior Malalignment Technic

One side of the mandibular articulation may become separated and fixed in a straight inferior position with the contralateral side normal. Prior to correction, place the patient in the sitting position facing forward. Stand behind the patient, slightly to the side of the lesion. If the lesion is of the patient's left TMJ, apply contact on the medial aspect of the mandible under the angle with the fingertips of your left hand. Your right stabilizing hand should be cupped under the patient's right mandibular ramus. Ask the patient to firm his or her occiput against your chest. The correction is made by asking the patient to force the mouth open while you apply pressure from the inferior to the superior. Apply sustained pressure, not a thrust, in this procedure.

Unilateral TMJ Anterior-Inferior Malalignment Technic

A fixated anterior-inferior malalignment of the mandible-temporal relationship may be found on one side while the other side tests normal. To correct this, place the patient in the sitting position facing forward. Stand behind the patient, and cup the patient's chin within your clasped fingers. Ask the patient to stabilize the occiput against your chest. The adjustment is made from the anterior-inferior to the posterior-superior. After all tissue slack is removed, the corrective impulse made should be short, rapid, wellcontrolled, and in accord with normalizing the fixated disrelationship.

Associated Medial Malposition. In some cases, there will also be a degree of fixed medial malalignment associated. If this is found, the line of correction should be diagonal toward the patient's eye on the side of fixed distortion rather than directly posterior-superior (ie, posterior-superior-lateral). This will require that you slightly rotate your shoulder anteriorly on the side contralateral to the lesion.

Unilateral TMJ Lateral Malalignment Technic

A TMJ joint may be found to be subluxated-fixated in an abnormal lateral position. This misalignment is usually accompanied by some degree of intra-articular jamming. Prior to correction, place the patient in the sitting position facing forward. Stand behind the patient, slightly to the side of the lesion. If the fixation is of the patient's right TMJ, place your right palm on the right side of the TMJ so that your thenar eminence is directly over the head of the affected condyle and the ramus of the mandible above the angle. Your left stabilizing hand is then placed in a sim-

ilar position on the patient's left mandible. Lean slightly forward so that your head is over the patient's head. In this position, your elbows will be flexed with your wrists extended. After tissue slack is removed, the extremely short dynamic adjustment is made from the superior-lateral to the inferior-medial against your stabilizing hand.

Faye prefers a similar technic with the patient in the supine position and the doctor at the head of the table facing the patient. The patient's ear and neck are cupped within the doctor's stabilizing hand on the contralateral side, and the patient's neck is then rotated so that the involved joint faces upward. A pisiform contact is taken on the mandible just below the TMJ, with the first metacarpal and little finger of the contact hand extending along the ramus of the patient's mandible (pointing toward the patient's chin). The patient is asked to open the mouth slightly, and a short sharp impulse is directed obliquely caudad, following an imaginary line drawn between the patient's chin and TMJ (Fig. 8.4). This is a highly ef-

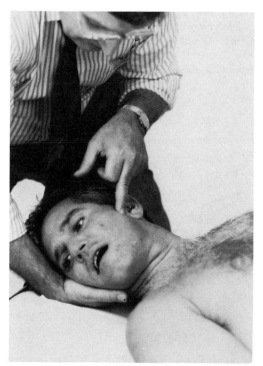 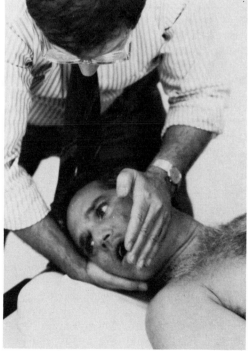

Figure 8.4. Adjusting a left TMJ lateral malalignment fixation with the patient supine. *Left,* isolating the contact point; *right,* applying the corrective thrust.

fective technic, but special care must be taken to assure that the thrust is extremely short and rapid.

The Manubrium-Sternal Body Joint

The hinge-like joint between the manubrium and the body of the sternum is normally active in forced breathing and extreme A-P and P-A movements of the trunk. Fixation at this joint will tend to restrict these motions to a minor degree. Gillet points out that such fixations are frequently mobilized spontaneously during an upper-thoracic double-transverse adjustment directed anteriorly on a prone patient. He checks motion in this joint by placing his palpating fingers over the joint and forcing the patient's trunk into full extension, noting the slight motion during extension and the return to neutral. The heel of the hand can also be used as the palpatory contact.

The Sternoclavicular Joints

Kessler/Hertling describe how free mobility of the sternoclavicular joint (Fig. 8.5) is necessary for normal shoulder mobility. For example, the clavicle must afford a degree of shaft rotation during elevation of the arm and somewhat during shoulder retraction and protraction. Anterior and posterior clavicular glide is necessary for normal shoulder retraction and protraction.

Mennell tests this motion in the supine patient by grasping the clavicle between his thumbs and index fingers at the junction of the clavicle's inner and middle thirds and carrying the clavicle upward and downward through its anterior-posterior range of motion. Superior and inferior clavicular motion is necessary for normal elevation of the arm and shoulder depression, but this is difficult to determine except by gross shoulder motion observation.

Many upper-thoracic symptoms may be directly or indirectly produced by sternoclavicular and acromioclavicular fixations, states Gillet. They may even be found in children, in which case they are probably caused by forward falls in which the child tries to reduce injury by extending the hands forward.

Dynamic Palpation

Gillet reports that clavicular fixations, especially at the sternoclavicular joints, are frequently related to readily palpable fixated ligamentous and muscular tissues in the C7—T1 area that extend laterally from the spine. To demonstrate to yourself the biomechanical relation of the cervical spine to the sternoclavicular joints, place your index and middle finger on one of the joints and move your neck into flexion, extension, rotation, and lateral bending. With each of these cervical motions, you should be able to perceive a distinct reciprocal motion in the sternoclavicular joint. The forces on the tendon of the clavicular head of the sternocleidomastoideus muscle are likely involved in this effect.

Immobility at either the medial or lateral joint of the clavicle can be easily screened by placing two fingers firmly on the joint and (1) moving the patient's shoulder back and forth in A-P/P-A directions (Fig. 8.6), and (2) then cupping the patient's flexed ipsilateral elbow with your stabilizing hand and moving the head of the humerus in superior-inferior directions (Fig. 8.7).

The normal tenseness of the muscles, states Gillet, should permit the palpating thumb to probe into the shoulder tissues easily, while hypertonicity will resist this motion to varying degrees; ie, the whole shoulder area may feel "hard" or possibly only certain areas will feel taut. This abnormal tension may be due

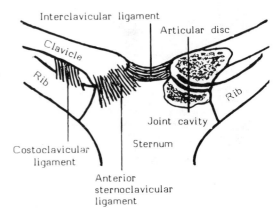

Figure 8.5. Diagrams of the sternoclavicular joints; right drawing is a coronal section (Courtesy ACAP).

to (1) fixation(s) at the spine, in which case it will be felt between the spinous and transverse processes; or (2) at one or more of the clavicular joints.

To start specific dynamic palpation of the sternoclavicular joint, your palpating hand can be brought around the sitting patient from behind and placed on the clavicle to be palpated. Your other hand will grasp the patient's arm or cup the patient's flexed elbow. After the patient is asked to relax the limb, slowly bring it upward and downward to a maximum degree without inducing undue patient discomfort. Any resistance to these two movements (in either degree or direction) that is not due to a reaction from the patient's pain or fear should be noted, for it will be indicative of a fixation in the superior-inferior plane. Next, bring the patient's arm to the forward horizontal position, cup the patient's flexed elbow, and check posterior-anterior mobility by pulling the patient's elbow toward you.

If a mobility block has been found, more specific palpation will then be necessary. For this, the palpating contact should be placed alternatively on the anterior, posterior, superior, and inferior aspects of the sternoclavicular joint while your free hand, in turn, forces, the patient's arm and elbow in each of these directions (ie, flexion, extension, elevation, and depression). These maneuvers are necessary because there are four major ligaments that hold the clavicle in its position with the sternum, and any one or a combination of these ligaments may be tightened (shortened) and restrict sternoclavicular mobility.

Sternoclavicular Dislocations. The sternoclavicular joint is said to be the least stable major joint of the body, yet, paradoxically, dislocation is rare. When dislocation does occur, it usually displaces anteriorly or posteriorly. The more common anterior luxations are actually displacement in an anterior, superior, and medial direction. Posterior dislocations, often hidden by local swelling, are sometimes associated with dyspnea and cervical edema from vascular compression. Such signs signal a medical emergency.

Adjusting Fixations

Faye recommends the following procedure. The patient's arm is placed in the relaxed position, the patient's elbow is flexed and cupped in the examiner's palm. The patient's elbow is then lifted upward and then pulled downward while the fingers of the doctor's other hand palpates the sternoclavicular joint. This maneuver uses the patient's humerus as a lever arm to spring the sternoclavicular joint downward and up-

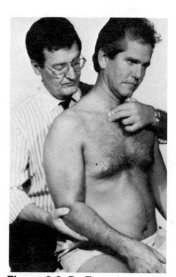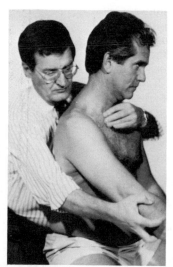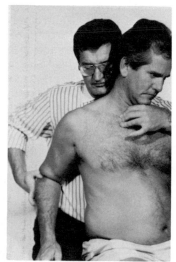

Figure 8.6. Dr. Faye demonstrating motion palpation of A-P/P-A mobility of the right sternoclavicular joint.

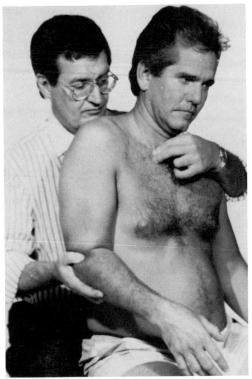

Figure 8.7. Palpating superior mobility of the right sternoclavicular joint.

imal aspect of the medial surface of your forearms should have firm contact with the anterior-superior surface of the patient's shoulders. In this position, spring (retract) the patient's shoulders backward (Fig. 8.9). This will pry the medial aspect of the patient's clavicles forward and release any restriction to anterior glide.

Releasing Restricted Anterior Glide with Patient Supine. Essentially the same maneuver can be conducted with the patient in the supine position. Stand at the side of the table and cup the patient's shoulders in your hands. Thenar contacts should be applied on the lateral aspects of the patient's clavicles. Apply pressure posteriorly and slightly lateral, and then add an impulse to spring (retract) the patient's shoulders backward to pry the medial aspect of the clavicles anteriorly. In stubborn fixations where greater leverage is necessary, it is helpful to place a small soft pad or pillow between the patient's upper thoracic spine and the adjusting table.

ward (superior-inferior). Next, the patient's elbow is passively flexed, raised forward to the horizontal level, and toggled forward and backward (posterior-anterior). This maneuver uses the patient's humerus as a lever arm to open and close the anterior and posterior aspects of the sternoclavicular joint. Movement should be felt under the palpating finger during these maneuvers. If not, an indication of fixation exists. If motion restriction is perceived in any of these directions, an impulse can be directed against the restriction during the testing procedure.

Two other technics to correct sternoclavicular fixations exhibiting restricted anterior glide are described below.

Double Wrist Adjustment of Restricted Anterior Glide with Patient Sitting. The patient is placed sitting, facing forward. From behind, locate the joints and reach around the patient so that your wrists are over the patient's sternoclavicular joints (Fig. 8.8). Your forearms should be in line with the shafts of the patient's clavicles, and the prox-

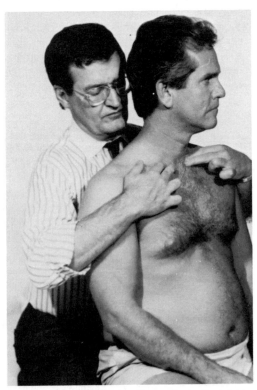

Figure 8.8. Locating the sternoclavicular joints.

Technics to correct sternoclavicular fixations exhibiting restricted posterior glide are described below.

Releasing Restricted Posterior Glide with Patient Supine. Faye releases posterior glide by applying a thenar contact over the joint, stabilizing the contralateral clavicle, and delivering a short impulse directed posteriorly (Fig. 8.10).

An alternative technic to release restricted posterior glide of the clavicle on the sternum, the same technic can be used as that classically applied for an anterior dislocation. Place the patient supine on a low table, and stand obliquely facing the patient on the contralateral side of the fixation. With your supporting hand, extend the patient's elbow and bring the limb to approximately a vertical position. Your palm and extended fingers should grip the lateral aspect of the patient's arm just above the elbow, your thumb should be hooked into the patient's antecubital space, and the patient's hand should be allowed to rest on your arm or shoulder. Place the pisiform of your active hand securely on the medial aspect of the patient's involved clavicle. In this position, apply traction to the patient's arm toward yourself (upward and slightly medial) while simultaneously applying pressure followed by a short dynamic thrust directed posteriorly and slightly laterally with your active hand.

Releasing Restricted Posterior Glide with Patient Sitting. Stand behind the patient who is sitting on a low stool. If the patient's right sternoclavicular joint exhibits restricted posterior glide of the clavicle, medially rotate your left arm so that you can cup the patient's trapezius between your thumb and index finger. The lateral aspect of the knuckle of your first metacarpal and proximal phalanx should be secured against the anterior aspect of the patient's clavicle just lateral to the patient's sternum. Your thumb will be hooked posteriorly over the soft tissues above the patient's scapula. Place

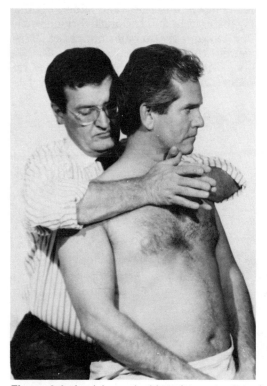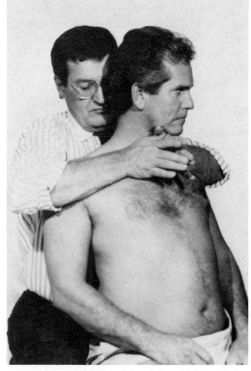

Figure 8.9. Applying a double wrist contact to release restricted anterior glide of the clavicle on the sternum.

the patient's ipsilateral flexed arm so that the palm is placed against the occiput. The patient's elbow will be supported between your stabilizing hand and your chest. With your active hand, apply pressure directed posteriorly followed by a short dynamic impulse while simultaneously leaning forward with your trunk to slightly adduct the patient's elbow.

Technics to correct sternoclavicular fixations exhibiting restricted inferior or superior glide are described below.

Adjustment of Restricted Inferior Glide with Patient Sitting. The technic described for releasing restricted posterior glide (patient sitting) can be readily adapted when inferior glide of the clavicle on the sternum is restricted. The only modification is that your contact will now be on the superior aspect of the medial clavicle near the sternum and your supporting hand will bring the patient's elbow upward rather than forward.

Adjustment of Restricted Superior Glide with Patient Supine. Restricted superior glide is a rare occurrence except in the elderly. When found, place the patient supine. Stand on the side of involvement, and apply a pisiform contact deeply under the medial aspect of the involved clavicle near the sternum with your medial hand. Your lateral hand should grasp the patient's ipsilat-

eral shoulder. Apply pressure cephalad with your active contact, and follow this with a short dynamic impulse while simultaneously applying traction caudad with your supporting hand.

The Sternocostal Joints

Lower cervical and thoracic rotation can be impaired by rib fixation(s) because the ribs must move with the rotating transverse processes. Similarly, unilateral or bilateral hypertonicity of the rotatores, multifidi, and/or levator costorum will restrict vertebral rotation. Such conditions are frequently found in the upper thoracic area. The intertransverse muscles may be a cause of fixation in the mid-to-lower thoracic area, states Gillet, and can be best determined by intertransverse palpation during lateral bending.

Inspection

When viewed laterally, the sternum normally moves anteriorly and superiorly during inspiration and the angle formed by the first rib and the manubrium closes. When viewed from above, the costosternal angles open. The costal cartilages of the true ribs rotate upward and forward, and the false

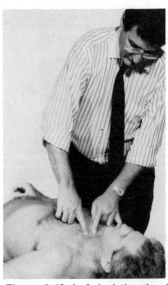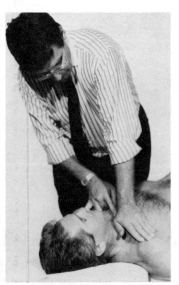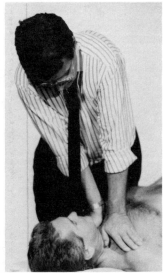

Figure 8.10. *Left,* isolating the right sternoclavicular joint; *center,* applying a thenar contact over the joint; *right,* position for delivering the corrective impulse to release restricted A-P glide.

ribs slide upon each other at their interchondral joints. These mechanisms are reversed during expiration.

Pectoralis Flexibility Test. With the patient placed supine and the hands clasped behind the head, the elbows are allowed to slowly lower laterally toward the table. If the elbows do not approximate the tabletop (ie, approach a horizontal position), shortening (eg, spasm, inflexibility, contracture) of the pectoralis group should be an early suspicion.

Applied Anatomy

The Costochondral and Sternocostal Joints. The anteriorly cupped T1—T7 rib ends join their costal cartilages at synovial synchondrotic costochondral joints. There is slight but important motion at these joints. The costal cartilages, in turn, articulate with the sternum at synovial synchondrotic joints. The sternocostal joints are similar to the costovertebral joints; ie, they are synovial joints divided by an intra-articular ligament. The capsules are thin but are strengthened by anterior and posterior radiate ligaments.

The T8—T11 ribs of the adult are held to the sternum by stiffened costal cartilage and anteriorly articulate (slide) superiorly and inferiorly within synovial-like joints that later become fibrous and then tend to fuse in old age. The fibrous capsules are thin but are strengthened by the interchondral ligaments. The interchondral articulations between T9 and T10 are united by an extremely tough fibrous joint.

Dynamic Palpation

Posterior Effects. Articular fixations at the costosternal articulations can produce hypermobility in the related thoracic vertebrae. This is usually manifested as an increased degree of spread of the spinous processes on full flexion. However, if a costosternal area is in a state of fixation and the corresponding anterior longitudinal ligament is shortened, the local area will be forced into an exaggerated state of kyphosis even in the erect neutral position.

Rib Pit Fixations. Rib fixations at their anterior aspect result in decreased chest excursion. They can be determined by motion palpation of the thoracic cage during deep inspiration with the patient in either the standing or supine position. First, traction the skin of the lateral thorax towards the midline with a broad bilateral palmar contact; then place your thumbs near the sternum on the rib being examined. As the patient inhales deeply, note if both of your thumbs move equally. Thumb motion restricted unilaterally suggests the side of fixation. Once identified, and the patient placed prone, a general rib mobilization technique with and without traction on the ipsilateral iliac crest or shoulder can then be applied on the angles of the ribs involved to generally loosen restrictions.

Releasing Specific Fixations

Sternocostal fixations can be released with the patient supine, utilizing a thumb,

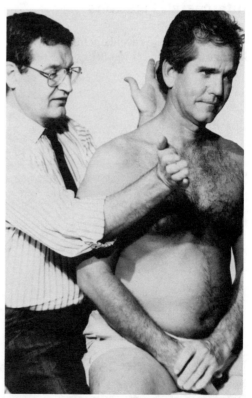

Figure 8.11. "Springing" the ribs with the patient in the sitting position.

thenar, or palm heel contact. Gillet suggests that they can also be corrected with the patient prone by applying a bilateral contact on the posterior aspect of the involved rib. Such a technique with the patient prone, however, would appear to increase the potential for rib fracture in patients past early adulthood. Nevertheless, it is likely that many sternocostal fixations are released inadvertently during the application of thoracic adjustments.

Faye and associates test sternocostal mobility by "springing" the ribs with the patient supine or in the sitting position (Fig. 8.11). Bilateral thenar contacts are usually applied. A corrective adjustment is made in the same manner if restrictions are found. With the patient supine, the patient's body weight and the applied A-P pressure will tend to immobilize the costotransverse and costovertebral joints.

Anterior Costocostal (Intercostal) Fixations

Palpation should reveal opening anteriorly during extension (Fig. 8.12), posteriorly

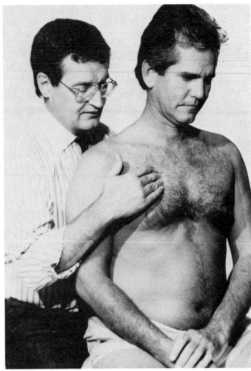

Figure 8.12. Position for evaluating costocostal mobility anteriorly during thoracic flexion and extension.

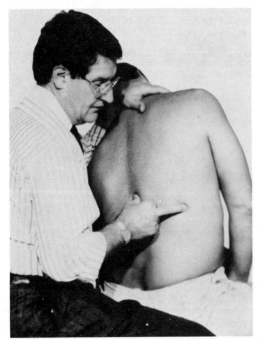 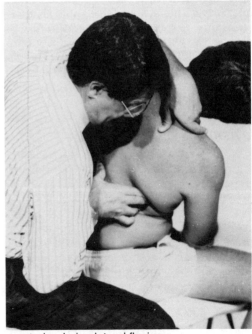

Figure 8.13. Evaluating intercostal mobility from the posterior during lateral flexion.

during flexion, on the convex side during lateral bending and on the side opposite to the direction of vertebral body rotation. If the intercostal muscles are hypertonic, the ribs will abnormally appose and the thoracic cage will exhibit an area of lateral flattening that restricts mobility on contralateral bending (Fig. 8.13). When bilateral, the patient will assume a somewhat "hunched" posture in the neutral position, states Gillet, depending on the extent of fixations. The fixations are best determined laterally near the rib angles.

Sternal Compression Test. If there is any suspicion of rib fracture, the sternal compression test should be conducted (Fig. 8.14): downward pressure is slowly applied against the sternum of a supine patient. A sudden, sharp, localized pain arising laterally suggests a fractured rib.

Dynamic Palpation

With the patient in the sitting position, Gillet recommends that the palpating fingers be inserted between the ribs at a lateral point in their arc. During passive lateral flexion, the palpating fingers should feel the intercostal spaces opening and closing.

Releasing Specific Fixations

With the patient supine, a pisiform contact may be taken so that an impulse can be delivered against the fixation. This will usually be on the inferior edge of the cephalad rib in which the intercostal fixation is found (Fig. 8.15). The direction of impulse is distinctively superior and the depth of the thrust is extremely shallow to avoid rib injury.

Lateral costocostal fixations can be released with the patient in the sitting position. A reinforced middle-finger contact is placed within the interspace of the fixated ribs, the patient's trunk is laterally flexed over your contact fingers, and an upward impulse is delivered as the patient is laterally flexed (Fig. 8.16). The direction of thrust is toward the patient's contralateral shoulder.

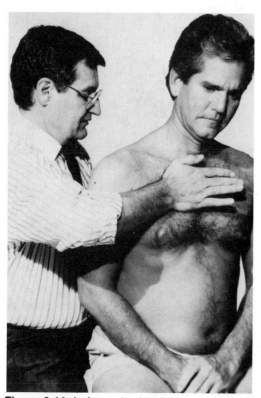 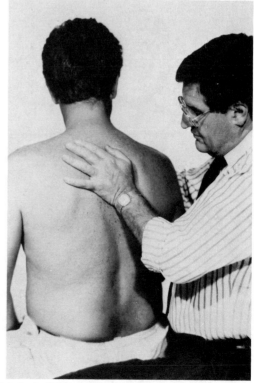

Figure 8.14. *Left,* conducting the sternal compression test; *right,* view from the back.

Gillet suggests that an anterior costocostal fixation can be corrected with the patient in the prone position. The thrust is directed obliquely toward the floor, in a slant that will follow the slope of the involved rib—so that the force will be transmitted around the rib to its anterior aspect. Such a technic is rarely recommended in this country, however, unless applied to children or patients in early adulthood, because of the danger of rib fracture. On this subject, Faye states, "There must be no pounding at the end of all slack. A very high velocity, short amplitude thrust of the impulse variety is used."

Alternative Technics When Fixed Malalignment Is Involved

Stand almost perpendicular to the supine patient on the opposite side of the fixation-subluxation. With your cephalad hand, take a pisiform contact over the anteriorly fixated rib slightly lateral to the sternum. Place

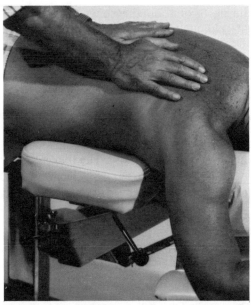

Figure 8.15. Applying a pisiform contact under the inferior edge of a cephalad rib involved in a costocostal fixation found at the posterior aspect of the thoracic cage.

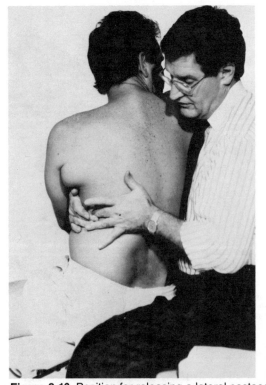
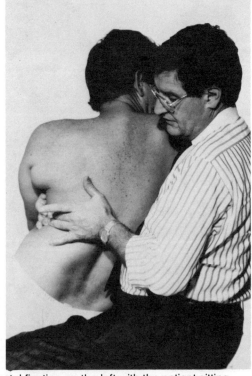

Figure 8.16. Position for releasing a lateral costocostal fixation on the left with the patient sitting.

your caudal stabilizing hand under the patient's scapula so that upward traction can be made during correction. Apply medial and slightly inferior traction with your stabilizing hand while your contact hand makes a light pushing-type thrust, at the end of patient exhalation, laterally and slightly superior to follow the curve of the rib. It frequently helps to have the patient internally rotate the ipsilateral humerus during the adjustment.

Another technic is a slight adaptation of the adjustment for an anterior medial clavicular deformity where contact is made on the medial rib angle rather than on the medial clavicle.

The Thoracoscapular "Articulation"

In the true sense of the word, there is no articular "joint" between a scapula and the thoracic cage. However, as the scapulae do move across the posterior surface of the upper thoracic cage in an arc, there is a potential for motion restriction that can affect the biomechanics of the shoulder girdle. For this reason, several authors refer to the scapulothoracic interface as an "articulation." This custom will be used in this section.

The site of restriction may be either shortening of the various muscles that attach to the scapula or adhesions between the scapula and the underlying ribs.

Gross Range of Motion Evaluation

For every 3° of lateral arm abduction, 1° occurs at the scapulothoracic articulation for every 2° at the glenohumeral joint. If you wish to check solely glenohumeral joint passive abduction, your stabilizing hand should anchor the scapula while your active hand passively abducts the patient's arm horizontally. The shoulder blade will normally not be felt to move until about 20° of abduction has occurred. Abduction should continue in this position to about 120°, at which point the surgical neck of the humerus meets the tip of the acromion. In the "frozen shoulder" syndrome, scapulothoracic motion will be normal but glenohumeral motion will be absent.

Then turn the patient's forearm to externally rotate the humerus and turn the surgical neck away from the acromion, and continue abduction to its maximum. Attempts of abduction against resistance will be painful in shoulder tendinitis.

Significant Clinical Tests

Teres Spasm Sign. When the relaxed standing patient is viewed from behind, the arms normally rest so that the palms face the thighs. If a palm faces distinctly backward (toward the examiner) on the involved side, a spastic contraction of the teres major muscle is suggested.

Comolli's Sign. Shortly after trauma to the upper posterior thorax, a triangular swelling may develop in the region of the involved scapula due to an accumulation of blood anteriorly and posteriorly to the scapula. For anatomical reasons, the blood cannot escape; hence, a cushion-like swelling develops more or less corresponding to the outline of the scapula that may persist for several days. This sign, which can be confused with an intramuscular hematoma (eg, of the rhomboideus major, infraspinatus, trapezius) is especially helpful in the initial physical diagnosis of fracture of the surgical neck and body of the scapula.

Dynamic Palpation

Restricted movements are often found in the scapular area. These can readily affect the dynamics of the shoulder girdle and thorax in both physical performance and posture. Their usual causes are (1) the consequence of injury, (2) spasm, or (3) viscerosomatic or somatosomatic reflexes. The somatic source of the difficulty may be local, at the spine, or at the shoulder. The common causes to search first are a costovertebral or upper-thoracic fixation, or contractions of any muscle that has a scapular attachment such as the rhomboids, trapezius, levator scapulae, supraspinatus, infraspinatus, or teres major and minor.

As described previously, complete motion of the scapula cannot be conducted without a reciprocal action at the glenohumeral joint.

To test involuntary scapular mobility, Mennell suggests that the patient be placed in a relaxed lateral recumbent position with the side of suspected mobility restriction upward. Stand behind the patient, and cup your caudad hand over the patient's shoulder. Grasp the apex of the scapula with your other hand. This requires that the scapular be "winged" somewhat so that you can get your fingertips slightly under the blade. With both hands in the positions described, rotate the apex of the scapular downward and laterally while bringing the shoulder tip upward and medially to test scapular rotation upon the chest wall.

Freeing Motion Restrictions

Scapular mobility should be found in all directions: superiorly, laterally, inferiorly, medially, and slightly clockwise and counterclockwise. If not, corrective manipulation is usually indicated. The procedure is conducted with the patient prone. Pressure is made with the base of the contact hand, the stabilizing hand is positioned on the wrist of the contact hand as in a dynamic recoil, and the direction of trust is into the fixation (restriction) on almost a horizontal plane so that the underlying thoracic cage is not greatly disturbed.

Rhomboid shortening will severely influence scapular mobility. Refer to Chapter 4. When the rhomboids are taut, it will be difficult to raise the medial border of the involved scapula. When this is found, flatten your hand and try to work it under the scapula while your supporting hand attempts to flare the scapula medially and posteriorly by retracting the ipsilateralshoulder.

With the patient in the prone position, stand on the involved side upward. Faye recommends the following technic: Stand fairly perpendicular to the patient, and grasp the medial border of the scapula with your caudad hand and the tip of the patient's shoulder with your cephalad hand (Fig. 8.17). Pull the scapula into rotation with your active hand while simultaneously applying pressure against the shoulder with your stabilizing hand. A similar procedure can be conducted with the patient in the lateral recumbent position, involved side upward.

In acute disorders, the manipulative procedure described above is often followed by chronic sprain therapy. Posttreatment in nonacute cases commonly includes deep heat and interferential therapy followed by muscle therapy and passive manipulation to a degree just below pain expression to stretch and relax the shortened connective tissues involved. To inhibit recurrence, therapeutic

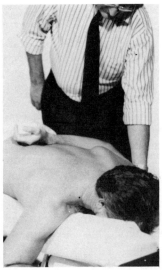 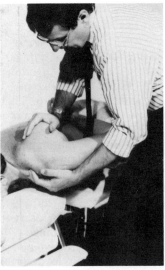 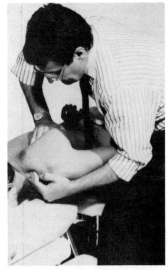

Figure 8.17. *Left,* positioning the patient to check for left scapula mobility; *center,* grasping the medial edge of the scapula and the shoulder firmly; *right,* pulling the scapula into rotation.

exercises can be prescribed that will stretch the shoulder in flexion, extension, adduction, and horizontal abduction.

THE UPPER EXTREMITIES

General Points of Significance During Joint Examination

Following is a review of major signs and symptoms that should be evaluated during joint examination. Most of these factors would be pertinent to any joint, not just those of the upper extremity.

Inspection

Check for:
• *Irregularities of contour.* Seek signs of abnormal contour due to osteophytes or lipping (attached to the bone); gouty tophi (not attached to the bone); constriction line opposite the articulation; or protrusion of joint pockets in large effusions that fill natural depressions. Irregularities of contour are easily recognized, provided that normal contour is familiar. Always compare bilaterally.
• *Telescoping of the joint with shortening.* Shortening of a limb as evidence of an advanced joint lesion is screened by careful measurements. The vast majority of such measurements are made with reference to a large joint (eg, the shoulder, hip), and then measuring the circumference of the limb at the same point bilaterally.
• *Trophic lesions.* Seek signs of trophic lesions over or near a joint (cold, sweaty, mottled, cyanosed, white, or glossy skin; muscle atrophy).
• *Sinus formation.* A sinus usually leads to necrosed bone, gouty tophi, or an abscess in or near the joint.

Static Palpation

Check for:
• *Tenderness and heat.* Tenderness and heat indicates inflammation; check in, near, and at a distance from the joint.
• *Abnormal shape.* Distortion or malposition due to muscle and/or ligament shortening near or around the joint, necrosis, exudation, or subluxation.
• *Enlargement.* Check for hard (probably bony), boggy (probably infiltration), thickening of capsule and periarticular structures, or fluctuating (probably fluid) in the joint. A joint capsule is not normally palpable. Enlargement is generally unmistakable; but when there is severe muscle atrophy between the joints, the joints may appear enlarged when they are not. Fluid or semifluid exudates in joints may fill up and smooth out the natural depressions around the joint, or, if the exudate is large, may bulge from the joint pockets.

Dynamic Palpation

Check for:
• *Limitation of motion.* This is usually due to pain and effusion, muscular spasm, thickening or adhesions in the capsule and periarticular structures, intra-articular blocks, obstruction by bony overgrowths or gouty tophi, or ankylosis.
• *Excessive motion as in a lax joint resulting from a dislocation that has been partially reduced spontaneously.* This is recognized simply by contrast with the limits furnished us by our knowledge of anatomy and physiology of joint motion at different ages. When the bone and cartilage appear normal or are not grossly injured, hypermobility may be due (eg, as in Charcot's joints) to destruction of bone and other essentials of the joint.
• *Crepitus and creaking.* These signs are detected simply by resting one hand on the suspected joint, with the other hand putting the joint through its normal range of motions while the patient remains passive. Free bodies in the joint are not palpable externally and are recognized only by their symptoms, by roentgenography, or during surgery.

Indirect Information

Check the course of the patient's dysfunction and the results of your treatment. Constantly monitor for general constitutional symptoms, their presence or absence.

334

Extremity Pain

Extremity pain may originate from nerves, muscle, skin, bone, ligaments, joints, arteries, and veins. Visualize these tissues during examination. See Figure 8.18. Muscle etiologies commonly include trauma, systemic infection, altered circulation, inflammation, and neoplasms. Pain from lesions of the nervous system commonly arise from CNS lesions, spinal roots and plexus lesions, or peripheral nerve disease from trauma, entrapment, reflex sympathetic dystrophy, or neuritis. Thus, limb pain may be the result of almost any structural disorder of the extremities or a disturbance elsewhere where the sensory phenomena are referred to the limbs. See Table 8.6.

History

As a general rule, normally mobile and ankylosed joints are functionally painless and partially fixated joints become increasingly painful with activity.

A thorough history will frequently reveal

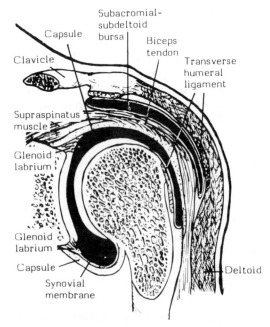

Figure 8.18. Coronal section of the shoulder joint showing some clinically significant structures (Courtesy ACAP).

the point of origin of extremity pain by its peculiar location and quality. The cause may be of mechanical, chemical, thermal, toxic, nutritional, metabolic, or circulatory origin, or a combination of several of these factors—depending on the nature of the dysfunctional or pathologic process involved. The most important clues toward determining cause —type of pain, its distribution, and its associated symptoms—are the result of a detailed case history.

Referred Pain

Pain and paresthesiae may be referred to the wrist or hand from the cervical spine, shoulder, or elbow such as from cervical disc disorders, osteoarthritis, brachial plexus syndromes, and shoulder and elbow entrapments. Cervical and upper-thoracic fixation syndromes, cervical pathology, rheumatoid arthritis of the wrist, a cervical rib, and neurovascular compression syndromes frequently refer pain to the shoulder. Sternocostal, upper rib, and many thoracic diseases may also refer pain to the upper extremity. Referred pain may also be projected along a somatic dermatome because of visceral inflammation, ischemia, or a tumor (eg, the shoulder-arm pain associated with myocardial infarction or angina). Although this subject will be explored further in this chapter in a subsequent section, it is well to mention here that such pains have two major features in common: (1) their distribution is limited to an anatomical dermatomal pattern and (2) the interruption of the nerve's function by any means will alleviate the symptoms (at least temporarily).

The Acromioclavicular Joints

If an acromioclavicular joint is hypermobile, conduct *Schultz's test:* Stand behind the sitting patient with a suspected acromioclavicular separation, facing the affected side. Place one hand under the patient's flexed elbow and push up while your other hand placed over the patient's acromioclavicular joint applies firm pressure. The more abnormal "give" that is felt in the joint, the greater the separation.

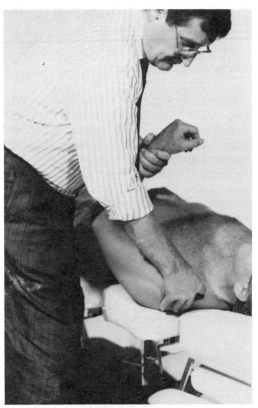

Figure 8.19. Faye applying Gillet's procedure for evaluating left acromioclavicular mobility.

Dynamic Palpation

Gillet recommends that motion palpation of the acromioclavicular joint for fixations not be attempted until after any fixation found at the sternoclavicular joint has been released. Once this has been accomplished, he recommends the following procedure: The palpating thumb is brought to the midpoint of the clavicle being examined and inserted as far posteriorly as possible without causing pain. With your free hand, take hold of the patient's arm and arc it forward and upward so that the head of the humerus rotates (Fig. 8.19). If fixation exists to any important degree, the clavicle will be perceived to move with arm motion almost immediately. Normally, specific clavicular motion should not be perceived until the arm is raised to about a 45° angle. Faye performs this maneuver with the patient in the supine position (Fig. 8.20). Positioning is a matter of personal choice once the underlying principles are understood.

Gillet also describes how fixations at the acromioclavicular joint can be evaluated from behind the sitting patient. Your palpating hand is placed lightly on top of the patient's shoulder, with the palpating fingers

Table 8.6. Major Upper-Extremity Joint Movements and Their Innervation

Segments	Joints	Movement/Roots
C2—T1	Scapulae	Elevation and retraction (C2—5) Depression and protraction (C5—T1)
C5—T1	Shoulder	Abduction (C5—6) Abduction and flexion (C5—T1) Extension (C5—8)
C5—T1	Elbows	Extension (C6—T1) Flexion (C5—6)
C6—T1	Wrists	Flexion (C7—T1) Supination, pronation, extension (C6—7)
C6—T1	Fingers	Extension (C6—8) Flexion (C7—T1)

on the clavicle and your thumb on the spine of the scapula. With your free hand (lateral), grasp the patient's ipsilateral elbow and bring it upward and backward to force the scapula to rotate. If the patient's acromioclavicular joint is free of fixation, the spine of the scapula should be felt to move upward and forward under your palpating thumb. Gillet also reports that it is easy to measure the amount of scapular movement by marking the placement of the superior spine of the scapula with a skin pencil in its resting position and at the end of the movement described. The difference between the points should normally be about a half an inch.

Faye also screens the mobility of this joint with the patient in the sitting position. The patient sits in a relaxed neutral position with the arms hanging loosely at the sides. The joint is then palpated with the index and middle finger of one hand while the other hand grips the patient's proximal forearm

and applies a mild pump-like action on the patient's limb. See Figure 8.21.

Releasing Fixations

Releasing Anterior Glide: Patient Sitting. Gillet relates that several different methods can be used to correct an acromioclavicular fixation, but he feels that the following method is the easiest to apply. The doctor hooks the forearms over the shoulders of the patient to bring the patient's shoulders firmly backward against the doctor's chest. The maneuver is then made by applying a brisk backward pull (Fig. 8.22). A series of dry cracks will be heard and post-adjustive palpation will indicate a distinct increase in mobility.

Opening the Joint Anteriorly: Patient Supine. This procedure is identical to that described for opening the sternoclavicular

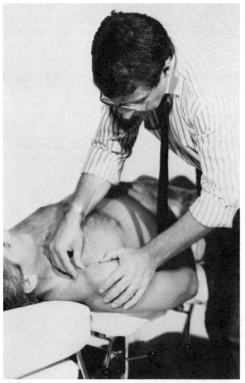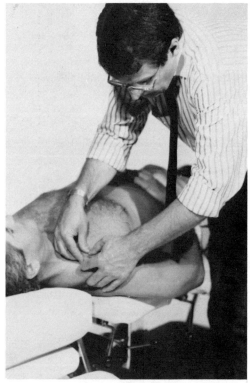

Figure 8.20. Evaluating acromioclavicular mobility with the patient supine. Thumb and index finger contacts are applied at the distal aspect of the clavicle. A pushing force is used to evaluate A-P motion, and a pulling force is used to test P-A mobility.

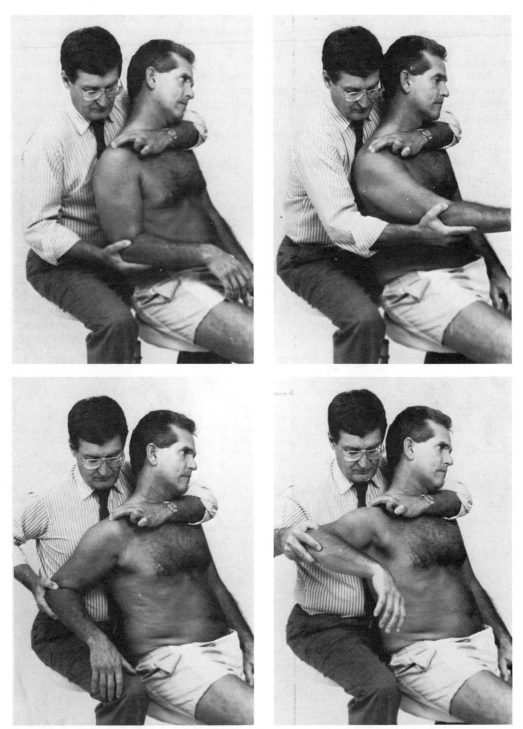

Figure 8.21. Dr. Faye demonstrating his method to test acromioclavicular function. Photos show the position of the examiner's palpating fingers and the patient's limb being maneuvered in a pump-like manner.

joint anteriorly except that the thenar contacts are taken against the heads of the humerus rather than on the lateral aspect of the clavicles. Stand at the side of the table and grasp the patient's shoulders (Fig. 8.23). Apply pressure posteriorly and slightly lateral, and then add an impulse to spring (retract) the patient's shoulders backward to pry the lateral aspect of the clavicles anteriorly.

Releasing Inferior-Superior Glide: Patient Supine. With the patient supine, Faye recommends grasping the involved clavicle between your index finger and thumb and applying an alternating arm pull superiorly and push inferiorly to test joint glide vertically (Fig. 8.24). If either motion is found to be restricted, a pisiform or double thenar contact is applied and the correction is made with an impulse and body drop against the fixation.

General Conditioning Maneuvers. The acromioclavicular ligament, glenohumeral capsule, coronoid ligament, and other soft tissues of the shoulder will generally be found to be shortened when shoulder dyskinesia exists. These soft tissues can be lengthened by almost any maneuver that will apply traction to the glenohumeral joint or pressure that will translate the humerus posteriorly in the glenoid fossa. Two simple conditioning maneuvers to accomplish this are:

1. Stabilize the patient's thorax with one hand (usually placed in the patient's axilla) and apply traction when the humerus has been (a) flexed forward, (b) abducted, (c) adducted, (d) raised upward, and (d) extended backward.

2. Stand behind the sitting patient on the side of involvement. Fully flex the patient's elbow on the involved side. Reach around and cup the patient's elbow with both hands. With the patient's arm in the neutral position, lift upward and impulse. Keep repeating this pressure and impulse as you raise the

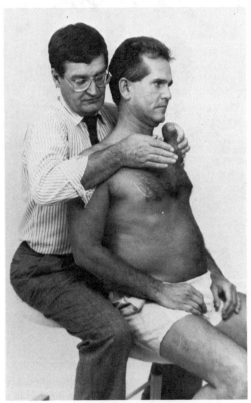

Figure 8.22. Releasing acromioclavicular anterior glide with the patient sitting.

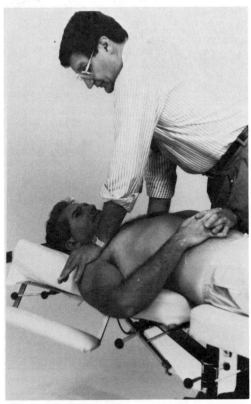

Figure 8.23. Releasing acromioclavicular anterior glide with the patient supine.

patient's elbow from the neutral to the forward horizontal position. This maneuver will translate the head of the humerus posteriorly in the glenoid cavity and stretch all tissues attached anteriorly. See Figure 8.25.

The Shoulders (Glenohumeral Joints)

Glenohumeral fixations may be a primary condition following intrinsic overstress or extrinsic trauma, or they may occur weeks or months after reduction of a primary dislocation. Thus, in cases of chronic shoulder pain, the history should be probed for possible shoulder dislocation and spontaneous reduction. As peripheral vascular injury may be involved, it is always a good policy to palpate the tone of the brachial and radial pulses, measure upper-limb blood pressure, and compare findings bilaterally. The major ligaments of the shoulder area are shown in Figure 8.26.

The effects of shoulder fixations are frequently nonacute and exhibit little or no swelling, but they present with chronic (often episodic) pain, stiffness or motion blocks, and other signs of local tissue fibrosis and intra-articular "gluing." From mild to moderate local muscle weakness and possible atrophy are characteristically associated. Postural distortions of the lower cervical and upper thoracic spine and musculoskeletal abnormalities of some aspect of the shoulder girdle are invariably related.

Tendinitis is not as common in the shoulder as it is in the elbow and wrist. However, because all tendons are relatively avascular, all are subject to chronic trauma and resulting microtears, slow repair, shortening, toughening, and aging degeneration.

Applied Anatomical Considerations of the Shoulder

The regional anatomy of the shoulder offers little to resist violent shoulder depression, and the shoulder tip itself has little protection from trauma. The length of the arm offers a long lever with a large head within a relatively small joint. This allows a

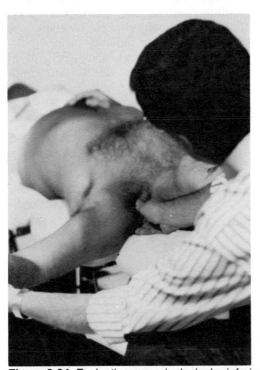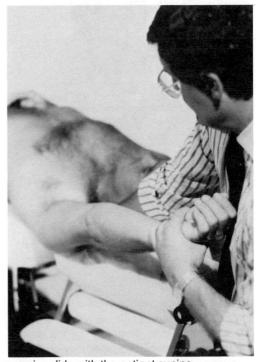

Figure 8.24. Evaluating acromioclavicular inferior-superior glide with the patient supine.

great range of motion with little stability. The stability of the shoulder is uniquely derived entirely from its surrounding soft tissues—an important point to remember.

The ball-and-socket glenohumeral joint is normally freely movable and lacks a close connection between its articular surfaces. Mennell points out that while only two bones comprise the glenohumeral joint, its function depends on the synchronous normal movement of the (1) acromioclavicular, (2) sternoclavicular, and (3) scapulothoracic articulations. Although the latter is not a synovial joint, it acts as one in many respects.

During correction of shoulder fixations, dynamic thrusts should be reserved for nonacute situations in which inflammation and swelling is minimal. When fixed displacement within the socket accompanies an acute sprain, attempts at articular correction should be more in line with gentle traction forces after the musculature has been relaxed and cooled. Obviously, the proba-bility of an underlying bone tumor, fracture fragments, osteoporosis, abscess, etc, must be eliminated prior to any form of manipulation.

Because the shoulder readily "freezes" after injury, treatment must strive to maintain motion *as soon as possible* without encouraging recurring problems. The key to avoiding prolonged disability is early recognition; early mobilization in all planes; normalization of neural, arterial, venous, and lymphatic circulation; and the elimination of contributing extrinsic contributions.

Shoulder Pain

Shoulder pain has a high incidence. Cailliet states that it is third only to low-back and neck pain. General intrinsic and extrinsic causes of common shoulder pain are shown in Table 8.7. Differentiation of dysfunctional causes from pathologic etiologies is the first clinical consideration, and either classification may have its origin in local or systemic causes. The differentiation of various pathologic causes of shoulder girdle pain can sometimes be made solely by its associated symptoms such as cough and expectoration, a neck or shoulder mass, swelling and tenderness, fever, or radiating ache.

Jaquet reports that about 95% of all shoulder disorders are due to four condi-

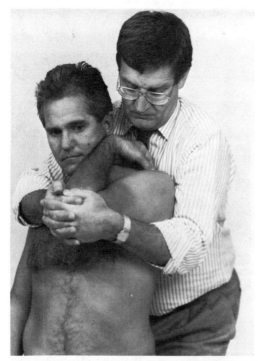

Figure 8.25. Position for classic adjustment of the left acromioclavicular joint in which the head of the humerus is mobilized posteriorly at varying degrees of flexion.

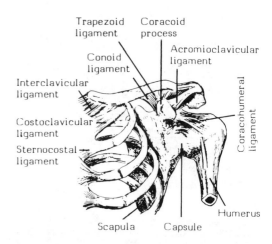

Figure 8.26. The major ligaments of the lateral clavicle and shoulder (Courtesy ACAP).

tions: (1) adhesive capsulitis (2) simple tendinitis, (3) tendinous perforation and rupture, and (4) hyperalgesic calcareous tendinitis. Note that three of these four conditions are tendinous in origin. All can readily lead to severe states of fixation. [See Clinical Comment 8.1]

Effects of Activity. Most shoulder syndromes involve a degree of either overuse or underuse:

• Overuse of poorly conditioned tissues is one of the most common cause of shoulder pain. Shoulder tendons are wide bands of collagen fibers, and if stress roughens a tendon, its tensile strength decreases. This leads to fibrinoid degeneration in and between the collagen fibers and later overt fibrosis. With necrosis and the initial inflammatory reparative process, the local tissues become alkaline and this induces precipitation of calcium salts. The deposits may invade an overlying bursa.

• Excessive postinjury immobilization leads to muscle atrophy and loss of capsular

elasticity, a predisposing factor to capsulitis and periarthritis. Lack of joint movement fosters retention of metabolites, edema, venous stasis, and ischemia—all leading to fibrous adhesions and nearby trigger-point development. It is for this reason that rehabilitation procedures should be instigated immediately after immobilization.

Cervical Disc Lesions. In cases of a herniated cervical disc (most common at C5–C6), pain may radiate from the neck into the arm, forearm, hand. The head and neck will be deviated to the affected side with marked restriction of movement. The shoulder will usually be elevated on the same side, with the arm slightly flexed at the elbow (protective position). Biceps and triceps reflexes will be lost or diminished. Paresthesias and sensory loss in the dermatome will be found corresponding to the disc involved.

Referred Pain and Tenderness. As the shoulder lies between the neck and the hand, pain from the neck or distal upper extremity may be referred to the shoulder,

---

DR. FAYE'S CLINICAL COMMENT #8.1

It has been my clinical experience that a major factor to rotator cuff tendinitis is the failure of the humerus to drop inferiorly and posteriorly in the glenoid fossa as the arm is raised above shoulder level and internally rotated. The loss of these joint-play movements causes compression of the rotator tendons that leads to the tendinitis. All nine joint-play movements can be involved. The correction with manipulation, described later in this chapter, is often delayed until physiologic therapeutics and rest have reduced the inflammation and pain to a tolerable level. Transverse massage is very effective in speeding the recovery time. It should also be emphasized that treatment must continue until all pain to pressure is eliminated. Recurrence is usually due to patients and doctors who discontinue treatment in haste after only a few weeks of care.

Table 8.7. General Intrinsic and Extrinsic Causes of Common Shoulder Pain

Intrinsic Origins	Extrinsic Origins
Arthritis	Contusions/lacerations
Bursitis	Neuropathy
Fracture/dislocation	Referred pain
Frozen shoulder	Diaphragm
Lax shoulder instability	Gallbladder
Nerve stretch/contusion	Heart
Osteochrondritis dessicans	Liver
Reflex sympathetic dystrophy	Lung
Rotator cuff lesion	Pleura
Strain/sprain	Trigger points
Subluxation/fixation	Tumor (eg, pulmonary)
Tendinitis	Vascular disorders

and a shoulder disorder may refer pain to the neck or hand. In shoulder disorders, as briefly mentioned previously, differentiation should include cervical problems, superior pulmonary sulcus tumor, and referred pain from viscera. Pain is also referred to the shoulder by brachial plexus involvement, pectoralis minor syndrome, anterior scalene syndrome, claviculocostal syndrome, suprascapular nerve entrapment, dorsal scapular nerve entrapment, cervical rib, spinal cord tumor, arteriosclerotic occlusion and other vascular disorders.

Many years ago, MacKenzie showed that both referred shoulder pain and tenderness may be of a visceral nature, especially when arising from (1) the liver, gallbladder, and right diaphragm to the right shoulder and (2) the stomach, left diaphragm, and heart to the left shoulder. Referred pain and tenderness, however, are not always predictable. If you are able to easily reproduce pain during joint motion, the condition is most likely structural or neuromuscular in origin. Pain that cannot be readily reproduced by passive motion suggests a visceral origin. Note, however, that it is untrue that visceral reflexes do not affect voluntary joint function. They may or may not produce musculoskeletal symptoms and signs.

Mercier reports that referred shoulder pain (unilateral or bilateral) often courses via the phrenic nerve (ie, the cutaneous branches of C4). For example, pain perceived on top of the shoulder, above the scapula, in the subclavicular fossa, or over the acromion or clavicle may be the only outward signal of a liver abscess that is threatening to perforate the diaphragm. Likewise, a perforated gastric ulcer might allow escaping stomach contents to cause irritation or pressure on the lower surface of the diaphragm. The same type of phrenic reflex can be set up by diaphragmatic pleurisy, subphrenic abscess, gallstones, acute pancreatitis, ruptured spleen, and the Fitz-Hugh-Curtis syndrome.

In many instances of localized referred

Table 8.8. Differentiation of Common Shoulder Disorders by Motion

Disorder	Active Motion	Passive Motion
Acromioclavicular arthritis	Acutely painful abduction above 110°.	Crepitus may be noted.
Adhesive capsulitis	Mild—moderate pain	Mild—moderate pain. Passive motion is limited in all directions.
Bicipital tendinitis and bursitis	More painful than passive motion at all levels of horizontal abduction.	Painful when the tendon or bursa becomes compressed beneath the acromion during abduction (approx. 60°). Arm pain increased by forearm pronation and supination against active resistance.
Rotator cuff tear (Grade 3 strain)	Able to hold horizontal abduction above 90° but not below 90°.	Unlimited motion without pain after the acute stage has subsided.
Synovitis	Acutely painful, increased by humeral rotation in the resting position.	Acutely painful at all levels of abduction.

pain, the location of the perceived pain correspondingly reflects the portion of the diaphragm being affected. For instance, it is generally thought that pain on top of both shoulders indicates a broad or median irritation of the diaphragm; pain on top of the left shoulder only, a left diaphragmatic irritation; and pain on top of the right shoulder only, a right diaphragmatic irritation. In upper-abdominal irritations, for example, a pyloric or duodenal ulcer or gallstone(s) usually refers pain to the right shoulder (commonly the right supraspinous fossa). A ruptured spleen, which may be spontaneous, can refer pain to the left shoulder. An anterior gastric perforation or midline diaphragmatic hernia can refer pain to both shoulders. Thus, shoulder pain should always substantiate the need for a complete thoracoabdominal examination.

Effects of Active vs Passive Motion. Several shoulder disorders can be differentiated by the characteristics of the pain associated with active and passive motion. See Table 8.8.

Initial Clinical Considerations

Prior to motion palpation of the shoulder area, inspect the upper limbs and conduct the standard tests for light touch perception, pain perception, muscle strength, and pectoralis flexibility. The following reflexes should be evaluated and graded: scapulohumeral, infraspinatus, pectoral, deltoid, triceps, biceps, and brachioradialis. Neri's arm sign will be positive in upper limb paralysis.

Note that the normal radial reflex produces forearm flexion. If a reverse reaction is found, it indicates a pathogenic reflex. The *inverted radial reflex*, exhibits hand and finger flexion rather than forearm flexion, indicating a C5 lesion.

To determine a lax capsule, the patient clasps the fingers behind the head and laterally abducts the elbows. The axilla is palpated high over the glenohumeral capsule while posterior force is applied on the patient's flexed elbow. While laxity of the anterior capsule can always be demonstrated by this maneuver, extra care must be taken not to dislocate the humerus within a loose capsule. It can be unexpectingly highly unstable.

Significant Neurologic and Orthopedic Tests

Glenohumeral dislocation is a common occurrence following a fall on an outstretched upper limb. If dislocation has occurred, Bryant's sign, Calloway's sign, Dugas' test, Hamilton's sign, and the shoulder apprehension test are likely to be positive.

Shoulder Apprehension Test. If chronic shoulder dislocation is suspected, slowly and gently abduct and externally rotate the patient's arm with the elbow flexed toward a point where the shoulder might easily dislocate. If shoulder dislocation exists, the patient will become quite apprehensive, symptoms may be reproduced, and the maneuver is resisted as further motion is attempted.

Dugas' Test. The patient places the hand of the involved side on the opposite shoulder and attempts to touch the chest wall with the elbow and then raise the elbow horizontally to chin level. If it is impossible to touch the chest with the elbow or to raise the elbow to chin level, it is a positive sign of a dislocated shoulder.

Bryant's Sign. A posttraumatic ipsilateral lowering of the axillary folds (anterior and posterior pillars of the armpit), with level shoulders, is indicative of dislocation of the glenohumeral articulation.

Calloway's Sign. The circumference of the proximal arm of a seated patient is measured at the shoulder tip when the patient's arm is laterally abducted. This measurement is compared to that of the uninvolved side. An increase in the circumference on the affected side suggests a dislocated shoulder, but consideration must be given to the individual who occupationally uses the involved arm almost exclusively (eg, tennis player).

Hamilton's Sign. Normally, a straight edge (eg, a yardstick) held against the lateral aspect of the arm cannot be placed simultaneously on the tip of the acromion process and the lateral epicondyle of the elbow. If these two points do touch the straight edge, it signifies a dislocated shoulder.

Evidence of biceps tendon instability and/or biceps tendinitis can be brought out by the Abbott-Saunders test, the Booth-Marvel test, Gilcrest's sign, Lippman's test, and Yergason's stability test.

Yergason's Stability Test. The patient flexes the elbow, pronates the forearm, and attempts elbow flexion, forearm supination, and humeral external rotation against the resistance of the examiner. The doctor stabilizes the patient's elbow with one hand while offering resistance to the patient's distal forearm with his other hand during the maneuver. Severe pain in the shoulder during this test is usually a positive indication of a bicipital tendon lesion, a tear of the transverse humeral ligament, or bicipital tendinitis.

Abbott-Saunders Test. This is a modification of Yergason's test that forces the biceps tendon against the lesser tuberosity which will stress an instable tendon. The arm of the sitting patient is brought into full abduction, rotated externally, and then lowered to the patient's side. A "click" felt or heard, frequently accompanied by pain and a reproduction of symptoms, indicates subluxation or dislocation of the biceps tendon.

Booth-Marvel Test. The examiner abducts the patient's arm laterally to the horizontal position, flexes the elbow to a right angle, and deeply palpates the bicipital groove as the humerus is passively rotated internally and externally. If the transverse humeral ligament has been stretched, a painful and palpable snap will be felt and sometimes heard as the tendon of the long head displaces from the bicipital groove.

Lippman's Test. In the relaxed seated position, the sitting patient is asked to flex the elbow on the involved side and rest the forearm in the lap. The examiner palpates for the tendon of the long head of the biceps about 3 inches distal from the glenohumeral joint. An attempt is made to displace the tendon laterally or medially from its groove. Pain, reduplication of other symptoms, and a palpable displacement of the tendon from its groove signifies tenosynovitis with instability.

Gilcrest's Sign. The patient is instructed to lift a 5-lb weight (eg, dumbbell) overhead and then to externally rotate the arm and slowly lower it to the lateral horizontal position. Pain and/or reduplication of symptoms during this maneuver (with or without tendon displacement from the groove) is said to indicate instability of the long head of the biceps and probable tenosynovitis.

Suspicions of a supraspinatus or rotator cuff lesion can usually be confirmed if three or more of the following tests and signs are positive.

Apley's Scratch Test. This is a two-phase test: (1) The patient (sitting or standing) is asked to raise the arm on the involved side overhead, flex the elbow, and then place the fingers as far down on the opposite shoulder blade as possible. (2) The patient is then asked to relax his arm at the side, then place the hand behind the back and attempt to touch as far up on the opposite scapula as possible. If either of these maneuvers increases shoulder pain, inflammation of one of the rotator cuff's tendons should be suspected. The supraspinatus tendon is most commonly involved. Restricted motion without sharp pain points to osteoarthritis or shortened soft tissues.

Shoulder Abduction Stress Test. The sitting patient is asked to abduct the arm laterally to the horizontal position with the elbow extended while the examiner applies resistance. If this causes pain in the area of the insertion of the supraspinatus tendon, acute or degenerative shoulder tendinitis is suggested.

Arm Drop Test. Hold the patient's arm horizontally at 90° abduction and then ask the patient to hold that position without assistance. If this cannot be done actively for a few moments without pain, it is a positive indication of a torn rotator cuff. In lesser tears, the patient may be able to hold the abduction (a slight tap on the forearm will make it drop) and slowly lower it against the side, but the motion will not be smooth.

Codman's Sign. This is a variation of the shoulder abduction stress test and the arm drop test. If the patient's arm can be passively abducted laterally to about 100° without pain, the examiner then removes support so that the position is held actively by the patient. This produces sudden deltoid contraction. If a rupture of the supraspinatus tendon or strain of the rotator cuff is present, the pain elicited will cause the patient to hunch the shoulder and lower the arm.

Impingement Syndrome Test. The patient is placed supine with the arms resting loosely at the sides. The elbow on the involved side is then flexed to a right angle and the arm is rotated internally so that it rests comfortably on the patient's upper abdomen. The examiner places one hand on the patient's shoulder and the other hand on the patient's elbow. A compressive force is then applied, which pushes the humerus against the inferior aspect of the acromion process and the glenohumeral fossa. Pain and/or a reduplication of symptoms indicates an impingement syndrome of the supraspinatus and/or bicipital tendon.

Supraspinatus Press Test. With the patient in the relaxed seated position, the examiner applies strong thumb pressure directed toward the midline in the soft tissues located superior to the midpoint of the scapular spine. The production of pain signifies an inflammatory process in the supraspinatus muscle (eg, strain, rupture, tendinitis).

A positive Dawbarn's test and subacromial button sign will isolate subacromial bursitis.

Dawbarn's Test. With the patient sitting, the examiner stands behind the patient and deeply palpates the area just below the acromion process to determine symptoms of focal tenderness or referred pain. Then, while still maintaining this palpatory pressure to patient tolerance, the examiner grasps the wrist of the patient with the other hand and brings the arm to the lateral extended position so that it is abducted to about 100°. If subacromial bursitis exists, the pain elicited on initial palpation should decrease substantially when the arm is raised because the deltoid will cover the spot below the acromion during abduction. If the pain remains unaltered or is increased by this abduction maneuver, subacromial bursitis can usually be ruled out.

Subacrominal Button Sign. The examiner stands behind the sitting patient, cups a palm over the involved shoulder, and applies finger pressure over the subacromial bursa. If this produces pain or unusual tenderness, subacromial bursitis is indicated.

Hypomobility of the Head of the Humerus

The head of the humerus is frequently flexed and abducted in most lifestyles and occupations, but it is less often used in maximum adduction and rarely used in maximum backward extension outside of athletics or unusual occupations. Likewise, internal rotation of the humerus is performed much more frequently than is external rotation. Lack of stretching exercise in any range of normal motion can readily lead to uncomfortable or painful motion restriction when unaccustomed movements are made with or without external loading. As in other fixations of the body, releasing such points of restriction will invariably relieve functional shoulder complaints as well as symptoms referred from the site of restriction.

Dynamic Palpation of the Glenohumeral Joint: General Considerations

The shoulder joint has a wide range of motion in flexion, extension, abduction, adduction, internal rotation, external rotation, and circumflexion. To assure normal dynamics, five translational joint plays must be evaluated to determine the point of possible fixation. These are:

• Posterior glide of the humerus relative to the glenoid cavity.
• Anterior glide of the humerus relative to the glenoid cavity.
• Medial glide of the humerus relative to the glenoid cavity.
• Lateral glide of the humerus relative to the glenoid cavity.
• Downward separation from the glenoid cavity.

Note that there is no appreciable end play directly superior because the acromion of the scapula, serving as an eave to the head of the humerus, blocks such motion.

Because pure rotation (internal and external) occur as a spinning action without perceptible shear or glide (ie, translation), rotational joint play is difficult if not impossible to perceive. The standard procedures for judging passive ranges of internal and external rotatory motion will accurately reflect the integrity of joint play. From a practical standpoint, if all the above listed joint play movements are normal, internal and external rotation joint play can be assumed to be normal.

Table 8.9. Differentiation of Various Shoulder Disorders by Motion Analysis

Characteristic Motion Pattern	Common Causes	
Painful arc	Acromion neoplasm Capsule laxity Cervical disc lesion Cervical subluxation syndrome Infraspinatus tendinitis	Intracapsular bicipital tendinitis Subdeltoid bursitis Subscapular tendinitis Supraspinatis tendinitis

Limited passive motion with capsule pattern	Arthritis
	  Bacterial
	  Immobilization
	  Monarticular rheumatoid
	  Osteoarthritis
	  Psoriatic
	  Traumatic
	Bone block
		Hemarthrosis
		Hemiplegia
		Neoplasm (primary or secondary)
		Neuropathic arthropathy
		Shoulder-hand syndrome
		Systemic lupus erythematosus

Limited passive motion without capsule pattern	Acromioclavicular sprain Capsule adhesions Costocoracoid contracture Clay-shoveler's fracture	First rib fracture Pulmonary neoplasm Subacromial bursitis Subdeltoid bursitis
Full passive motion with painful resisted abduction	Deltoid strain	Supraspinatus strain
Full passive motion with painful resisted adduction	Bicipital strain (long head) Latissimus dorsi strain	Pectoralis major strain Teres (major, minor) strain
Full passive motion with painful resisted internal rotation	Latissimus dorsi strain Pectoralis major strain	Subscapularis strain Teres major strain
Full passive motion with painful resisted external rotation	Infraspinatus strain	
Full passive motion with painful resisted forward movement	Bicipital strain	Coracobrachialis strain
Full passive motion with painful resisted elbow flexion and supination	Bicipital strain (long head)	

Table 8.9, continued

Characteristic Motion Pattern	Common Causes	
Full passive motion with painful resisted elbow extension	Triceps strain	
Full passive motion, painless weak deltoid	Axillary nerve lesion	
Full passive motion, painless weak deltoid, biceps, and spinatus group	C5 lesion Myeloma	Traction palsy
Full passive motion, painless weak spinatus group alone	Suprascapular neuropathy	
Full passive motion, solely painless weak supraspinatus alone	Supraspinatus tendon rupture	
Full passive motion, solely painless weak infraspinatus alone	Infraspinatus tendon rupture	
Full passive motion, painless weak serratus anterior	Long thoracic neuropathy	
Full passive motion, painless weak trapezius	Spinal accessory neuropathy	
Full passive motion, painless weak biceps and forearm muscles	C5 lesion	
Full passive motion, painless weak triceps and forearm muscles	C6 lesion	

A long bone is a cylinder, thus the motions of the distal and proximal aspects of the humerus are reciprocally opposite in rotation. This is also true for the relationship between the proximal humerus and the glenoid cavity. For instance, when the arm is raised forward and upward, the head of the humerus rotates in an opposite direction on the posterior aspect of the glenoid cavity. When the arm is extended laterally and raised, the head of the humerus rotates in an opposite direction on the medial aspect of the glenoid cavity. In a like manner, the site of articular fixation will determine the motion restricted. For example:

• Posterior glenohumeral fixation restricts flexion but not extension.

• Anterior glenohumeral fixation restricts extension but not flexion.

• Medial glenohumeral fixation restricts abduction but not adduction.

• Lateral glenohumeral fixation restricts adduction but not abduction.

• Downward (normal distraction) glenohumeral fixation of this important motion restricts all ranges of motion to some degree.

Visualize the site of restriction and the reason for these occurrences. Motion analysis is one of the most important procedures of physical diagnosis in differentiating lesions of the shoulder area. Table 8.9 lists a number of other helpful clues.

Mennell describes seven procedures that should be conducted during motion palpation of the head of the humerus. All can be conducted with the patient supine.

1. *Lateral translation.* Stand parallel to the patient on the side of involvement, flex the patient's elbow with the arm relaxed in the neutral position, and allow the patient's hand to rest upon his or her chest. With your medial hand, firmly grasp the medial surface of the patient's arm, high in the axilla. Your supporting hand should grip the lateral surface of the patient's elbow. To test lateral translation of the head of the humerus from the glenoid cavity, push the patient's humeral head laterally with your active hand while simultaneously applying pressure medially toward the patient's chest with your stabilizing hand (Fig. 8.27). Remove the soft-tissue slack and test end play.

2. *Anterior translation.* Maintain the same doctor-patient positions described above except slide your active hand under the posterior surface of the superior aspect of the patient's arm. The thumb of your supporting hand can be hooked into the angle (antecubital space) between the patient's arm and forearm. To test anterior translation of the head of the humerus on the glenoid cavity, firm the patient's elbow against the table by applying downward pressure with your stabilizing hand while simultane-

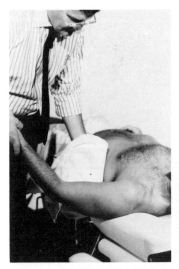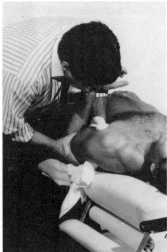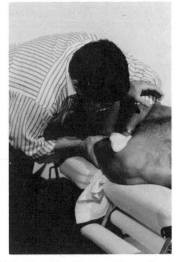

Figure 8.27. Evaluating lateral translation within the glenohumeral joint. *Left,* positioning the patient; *center,* securing the contact; *right;* testing lateral translation mobility.

ously bringing your active hand upward (Fig. 8.28). Remove the soft-tissue slack and test end play.

3. *Posterior translation at mild flexion.* To test posterior translation of the head of the humerus in the glenoid cavity with the humerus slightly flexed, you will need to reverse the positions of your hands as described above. Your active hand will cup the patient's shoulder tip so that the thenar eminence is directly over the greater tuberosity of the patient's humerus. Your supporting hand will cup the patient's elbow so that the thumb is hooked into the antecubital space of the patient's flexed elbow. Lift the patient's elbow slightly with your supporting hand so that the patient's arm is flexed. This will place the patient's ipsilateral scapula firmly flat against the table. With your active hand, push obliquely downward to test the degree of freedom of posterior shear (Fig. 8.29). Take care not to jam the head of the humerus against the acromial process.

4. *Inferior-Posterior Arcing.* With the patient in the same position, bend your knees so that the patient's raised elbow (about 45°) can be firmed against your medial shoulder. It can then be used as a fulcrum. Clasp both of your hands around the anterior surface of the patient's upper arm (Fig. 8.30). Your fingers can be intertwined to secure your grip. To test this motion, your active hands should pull the head of the patient's humerus downward and backward (toward you) in somewhat of a J-shaped motion, while simultaneously locking the patient's elbow against your shoulder by slightly flexing your trunk.

5. *Lateral-Posterior Arcing.* With the patient in the same position, remain in the crouched position but swing your body so that it is perpendicular to the patient and the patient's elbow is firmed against your other shoulder. Move your hands so that they are around the medial aspect of the patient's upper arm (Fig. 8.31). To test this motion, your hands should pull the head of the patient's humerus lateral and downward (to-

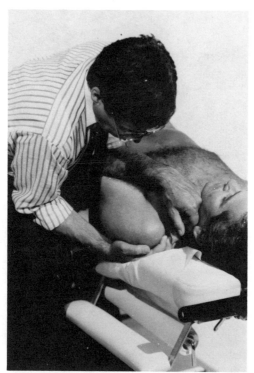

Figure 8.28. Testing anterior translation mobility of the glenohumeral joint.

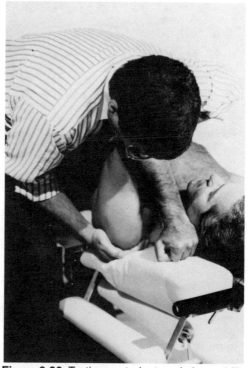

Figure 8.29. Testing posterior translation mobility of the flexed glenohumeral joint.

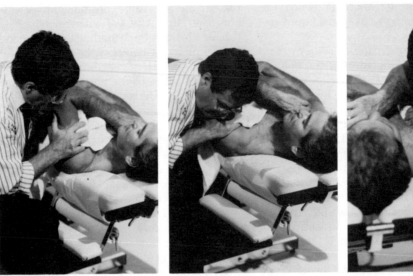

Figure 8.30. Position for checking glenohumeral inferior-posterior arching and releasing mobility restrictions. *Left,* positioning the patient; *center,* testing mobility; *right,* view of position from the front.

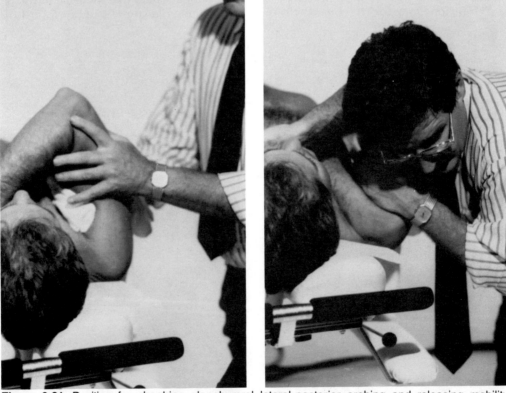

Figure 8.31. Position for checking glenohumral lateral-posterior arching and releasing mobility restrictions. *Left,* positioning the patient; *right,* testing mobility.

ward you), again in somewhat of a J-shaped motion, while simultaneously locking the patient's elbow against your shoulder by slightly flexing your trunk.

6. *Posterior Translation at 90° Flexion.* With the doctor-patient positions remaining approximately the same as described above, flex the patient's arm and elbow so that the elbow is pointing toward the ceiling and the patient's hand is resting near the opposite shoulder. The patient's humerus should be perpendicular to a line drawn through the patient's shoulders. Stand fairly perpendicular to the patient, and cup the patient's elbow with one hand and support this with your other hand. Apply pressure directly downward through the shaft of the patient's humerus to remove all tissue slack, and then check end play of posterior translation of the head of the humerus in the glenoid cavity.

7. *External Rotation.* With the doctor-patient position remaining the same, abduct the patient's forearm, keeping the elbow flexed. The patient's arm will be in the neutral resting position, but the head of the humerus will be rotated externally (Fig. 8.32). Support the patient's elbow with your caudad hand. With your active hand, reach over the patient's forearm and grasp the latero-anterior surface of the proximal aspect of the patient's arm. With your fingers grasping the patient's arm, externally rotate the humerus while simultaneously adding mild leverage pressure with your forearm against the patient's forearm. This is an excellent maneuver to test the end play of humeral external rotation after normal motion has reached its maximum.

Faye adds two more procedures to this list.

1. *Circumduction: Patient Prone.* Stand on the side of involvement, perpendicular to the patient positioned in the prone position. Bring the patient's flexed elbow (90°) to the

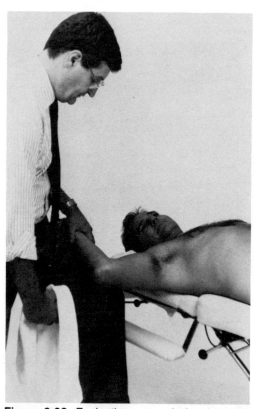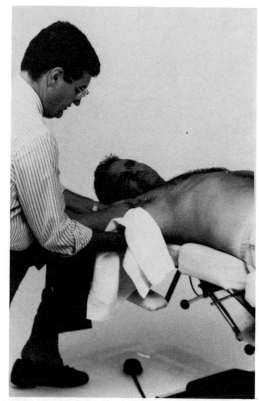

Figure 8.32. Evaluating external glenohumeral rotation of the right shoulder. *Left,* positioning the patient's arm; *right,* applying external rotation of the humerus in the glenoid cavity.

horizontal position. Insert the patient's elbow and forearm between your knees to prevent their motion while you grasp the patient's upper arm in both hands (Fig. 8.33). In this position, you will be able to circumduct the head of the patient's humerus within the glenoid cavity in all directions. Perform this motion in a wide circle counterclockwise and then clockwise. Keep in mind that the glenohumeral joint is of a ball-and-socket design, thus no specific planes of articulation exist. Thousands of planes exist. This maneuver will allow you to screen all possible areas of fixation.

2. *Internal Rotation: Patient Sitting.* Stand on the side of involvement of the sitting patient. The patient's arm and forearm should be hanging in a relaxed neutral position. Grasp the patient's distal forearm with both hands, and internally rotate the limb. Bend over obliquely so that you can firm your cephalad shoulder against the patient's shoulder for stabilization (Fig. 8.34). Apply traction to the patient's limb and add a short dynamic impulse after all soft-tissue slack has been removed.

When a mild or moderate motion block is found during any of the above nine tests, the release is simply made by adding a short dynamic impulse against the restriction.

The Elbows

The elbow is a complex joint. From a clinical viewpoint, the proximal ulna forms the most vulnerable articulation in the elbow and while the distal radius forms the most vulnerable articulation in the wrist. The major ligaments of the elbow area are shown in Figure 8.35.

Forearm injuries are generally the result of direct blows or falls. The most common injuries are avulsion-type trauma of the elbow as a result of acute or chronic strain at a site of tendon or ligament attachment. Any joint injury, if not properly monitored from the start, can readily lead to motion restrictions and advancing joint dysfunction.

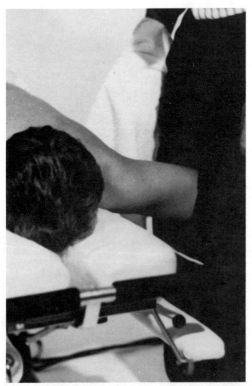
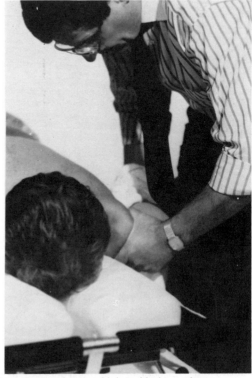

Figure 8.33. Position for testing circumduction of the left glenohumeral joint with the patient prone.

Many fixations in the elbow area will offer dramatic relief upon release. Generally, correction is made with a quick, short thrust or pull on the segment distal to the stabilized proximal segment. It is essential that the patient's muscles be relaxed or an attempt at correction will be inhibited and extremely painful. Naturally, quick thrusts are contraindicated in inflammatory arthritis or if adhesions are advanced. An attempt to stretch a large tough adhesion quickly, may produce acute periostitis if the attachment is to bone. Patience and pretherapy conditioning will prevent this from occurring.

Elbow Pain

The most common afflictions of the elbow are elbow bruises leading to bursitis and strain/sprain leading to fixation, malpositioning, and arthritis. Branch lists the most common causes of extrinsic elbow pain as medial or lateral epicondylitis and olecranon bursitis and of intrinsic elbow pain as synovitis, loose bodies, subluxations, dislocations, and fractures.

Initial Clinical Considerations

Inspection and static palpation of the entire limb should be conducted before motion palpation of the elbow is initiated. If not previously tested, check the integrity of the biceps, radial, and triceps reflexes; evaluate light touch and pain perception; and grade muscle strength if indicated.

General Clinical Tests

Elbow Abduction-Adduction Stress Tests. To roughly judge the stability of the medial and lateral collateral ligaments of the elbow, hold the patient's wrist with one hand

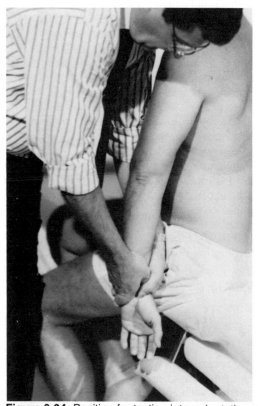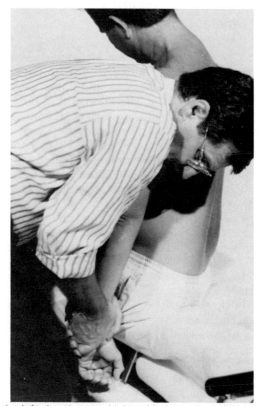

Figure 8.34. Position for testing internal rotation of the left glenohumeral joint with the patient sitting.

and cup your stabilizing hand under the patient's distal humerus. As the patient is directed to slightly flex his elbow, (1) push medially with your active hand and laterally with your stabilizing hand, then (2) push laterally with your active hand and medially with your stabilizing hand. With the fingers of your stabilizing hand, note any joint gapping felt during either the valgus or varus stress maneuver. Painful instability indicates torn ligaments.

Elbow Extension-Flexion Stress Tests. The patient's elbow is passively extended and flexed. Painful instability indicates sprain or destructive joint pathology, while discomfort with limited motion suggests contractures or degenerative arthritis.

Forearm Pronation-Supination Stress Tests. The patient's forearm is passively pronated and supinated. Painful instability indicates sprain or destructive joint pathology, while discomfort with limited motion suggests contractures or degenerative arthritis.

Dynamic Palpation: General Considerations

The elbow has long been considered a simple hinge joint. Soderberg, however, points out that biomechanical and kinesiologic studies have shown this viewpoint to be an oversimplification of the actual conditions required for normal elbow motion. Keep in mind that the relatively strong elbow complex consists of three joints: (1) the radiohumeral joint, (2) the ulnohumeral joint, and (3) the superior radioulnar joint. Because the elbow has such a wide range of motion in flexion, extension, supination, and pronation, freedom of joint play must be evaluated in detail to determine the sites of possible fixation.

Mennell describes three major motions in the elbow:
• Upward glide of the head of the radius on the head of the ulna
• Downward glide of the head of the radius on the head of the ulna
• Rotation of the head of the radius on the ulnar, a motion that is independent of forearm supination and pronation.

Other authorities add the following move-

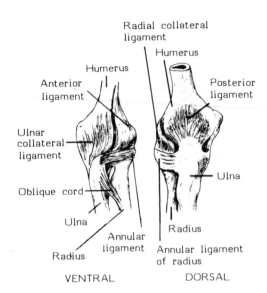

Figure 8.35. Schematic of the major ligaments of the elbow area (Courtesy ACAP).

ments:
• Medial glide of the olecranon on the distal humerus when the elbow is flexed.
• Lateral glide of the olecranon on the distal humerus when the elbow is flexed.
• Glide of the olecranon process of the ulna into the olecranon fossa of the humerus during elbow extension.
• Glide of the coronoid process of the ulna into the coronoid fossa of the humerus during elbow flexion.

Rotation of the head of the radius (internally and externally) on the head of the ulna and capitulum of the humerus and internal and external rotation of the olecranon of the ulna on the trochlea of the humerus are spinning actions. These actions are readily reflected in motion palpation procedures for evaluating passive ranges.

Humeroulnar Hypomobility

Distraction. The humeroulnar joint can be jammed by a fall on the outstretched hand or simply by severe periarticular muscle spasm. It is sometimes seen in patients whose occupations require repeated violent pushes with the heel of the extended hand (eg, football linemen, carpenters). Almost any type of axial traction will help to relieve this condition. A common procedure is to first place the patient supine, and sit at the side of the table on the involved side (obliquely facing the patient). Abduct the patient's shoulder to 90°, flex the elbow to 90°, and pronate the forearm. Place your medial knee in the patient's antecubital fossa to stabilize the humerus, grasp the under surface of the proximal forearm with both hands, slightly abduct the forearm so that more pressure will be applied to the ulnar than the radius, and apply axial traction toward your body. Slowly stretch to patient tolerance, hold, impulse if need be, and gradually release.

Medial-Lateral Tilt. With the patient placed supine, sit or stand at the side of the table on the involved side (obliquely facing the patient). The patient's involved limb should be resting loosely at the side, near the body, with the elbow extended and the wrist supinated. This is a two-phase procedure:

• *Phase One.* The first maneuver is to stabilize the patient's distal forearm with your medial hand and grasp the lateral surface of the patient's proximal ulnar with your active (lateral) hand. This position will allow you to apply a horizontal shearing force across the humeroulnar joint, from the lateral to the medial (Fig. 8.36). Slowly apply force to patient tolerance, hold, impulse if restricted, and gradually release.

• *Phase Two.* The second maneuver is just the reverse. Stabilize the patient's distal forearm with your lateral hand and grasp the medial surface of the patient's proximal ulnar with your active (medial) hand. This position will allow you to apply a horizontal shearing force across the humeroulnar joint, from the medial to the lateral (Fig. 8.37). Slowly apply force to patient tolerance, hold, impulse if restricted, and gradually release.

The same procedure can be conducted with the patient standing or sitting. See Figure 8.38.

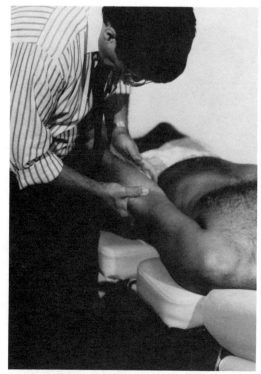

Figure 8.36. Evaluating lateral to medial humeroulnar mobility.

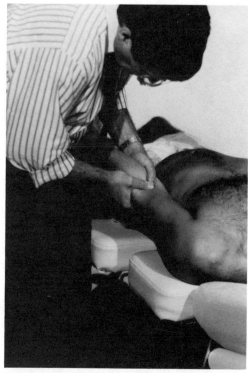

Figure 8.37. Evaluating medial to lateral humeroulnar mobility.

Radioulnar Hypomobility

Posterior Glide of the Proximal Radioulnar Joint. Place the patient supine, flex the elbow so that the patient's forearm is vertical, fully extend the patient's wrist, and grip the patient's hand. Lean over the patient's limb so that your body weight will be approximately centered over the shaft of the patient's forearm and apply pressure downward. Distinct motion should be perceived. If not, add some body weight and deliver a mild impulse. Assure that your pressure is over the heel of the patient's hand and not toward the fingers, else a wrist sprain may be induced. See Figure 8.39.

Inferior Glide of the Proximal Radioulnar Joint. Stand perpendicular to sitting patient, flex the patient's elbow to a right angle, and supinate the forearm. Grasp the patient's forearm with your active hand just above the wrist, anchor your stabilizing hand against the patient's distal humerus, and apply longitudinal traction with your active hand (Fig. 8.40). If end play is not perceived, hold the tension, impulse, and slowly relax the tension.

Rotation of the Radial Head on the Ulna. Pronate the standing patient's forearm. Place the thenar eminence of your medial hand over the anterior surface of the head of the radius. With your other hand, grasp the radial side of the patient's wrist. You should feel the proximal aspect of the radius against your thenar eminence. At this point, quickly rotate the patient's arm into full pronation (Fig. 8.41). You should feel the head of the radius spin backward on the ulna.

Pronation (Internal Rotation): Alternative Maneuver. With the patient placed supine, sit at the side of the table on the involved side (obliquely facing the patient). Abduct the patient's shoulder to 90°, flex the elbow to 90°, and supinate the forearm. Place your medial knee in the patient's antecubital fossa to stabilize the humerus, grasp under the patient's distal forearm with both hands,

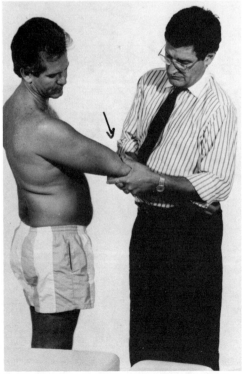 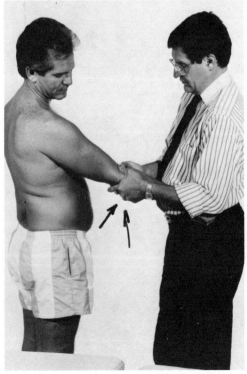

Figure 8.38. Evaluating humeroulnar tilt with the patient standing. *Left,* apply medial to lateral pressure; *right,* apply lateral to medial pressure.

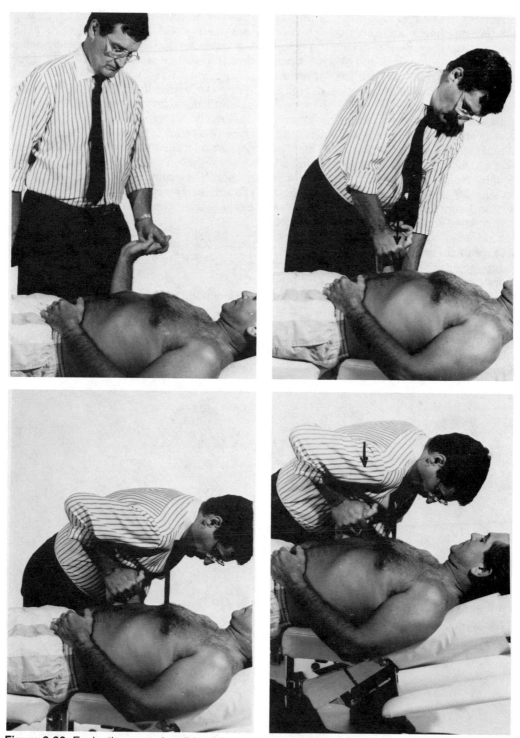

Figure 8.39. Evaluating posterior glide of the proximal radioulnar joint.

pronate the patient's forearm to tolerance by rotating your hands, and apply axial traction toward your body. Slowly stretch to patient tolerance, hold, impulse if end play is not perceived, and gradually release. Repeat several times, progressively increasing the degree of pronation possible.

Distraction. This technic is a variation of that described for a jammed humeroulnar joint. Place the patient supine, and sit at the side of the table on the involved side (obliquely facing the patient). Abduct the patient's shoulder to 90°, flex the elbow to 90°, and supinate the forearm. Place your medial knee in the patient's antecubital fossa to stabilize the humerus, grasp the upper surface of the proximal forearm with both hands, slightly adduct the forearm so that more pressure will be applied to the radius than the ulna, and apply axial traction toward your body. Slowly stretch to patient tolerance, hold, impulse if necessary, and gradually release.

Proximal P-A Glide of the Ulna on the Humerus. Stand perpendicular to the standing or sitting patient. Lift the patient's arm to about 45° degrees. Cup your stabilizing fingers around the patient's olecranon so that they will serve as a fulcrum, and grasp the patient's wrist with your active hand. With your active hand (lateral), move the patient's distal forearm downward to produce hyperextension at the elbow (Fig. 8.42). Once resistance is felt, slowly apply force to patient tolerance, impulse if restricted, and slowly release. This should be a rocking-type motion. The patient must completely relax the arm as any contraction of the patient's biceps against your thumb will produce pain.

Tests for Lateral Epicondylitis (Tennis Elbow)

Faye points out that tennis elbow is often a clinical triad involving the cervical spine, the proximal radius, and the distal radius. Fixation at the distal radius will produce hypermobility of its proximal aspect and predispose lateral epicondylitis.

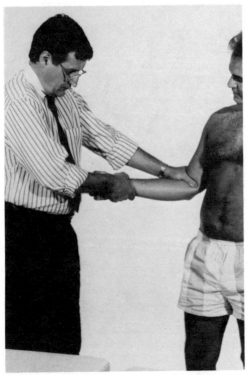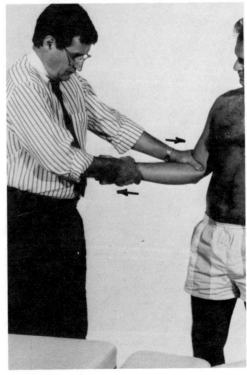

Figure 8.40. Evaluating inferior glide of the proximal radioulnar joint.

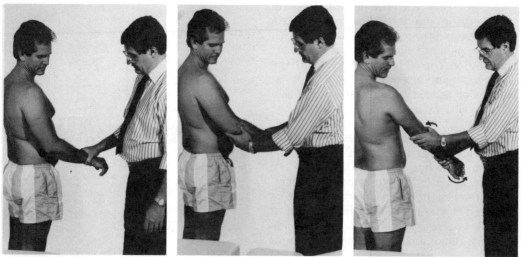

Figure 8.41. Evaluating rotation of the radial head on the ulnar. *Left,* positioning the patient; *center,* contacting the head of the radius; *right,* rotating the forearm.

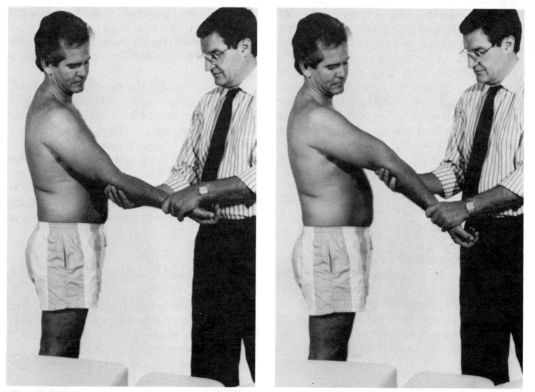

Figure 8.42. Evaluating proximal P-A glide of the ulnar on the humerus.

Cozen's Test. With the patient's forearm stabilized, the patient is instructed to make a fist and extend the wrist. The examiner then grips the patient's elbow with the stabilizing hand and the top of the patient's fist with the active hand and attempts to force the wrist into flexion against patient resistance. A sign of tennis elbow is a severe sudden pain at the lateral epicondyle area.

Mill's Test. The patient makes a fist; flexes the forearm, wrist, and fingers; pronates the forearm; and then attempts to extend the forearm against the examiner's resistance. This stretches the extensors and supinators attached to the lateral epicondyle. Pain at the elbow during this maneuver is an indication of radiohumeral epicondylitis (tennis elbow).

Kaplan's Test. This is a two-phase test: (1) The sitting patient is given a hand dynamometer and instructed to extend the involved upper limb straight forward and squeeze the instrument as hard as possible. Induced pain and grip strength are noted. (2) The test is then repeated except that this time the examiner firmly encircles the patient's forearm with both hands (placed about 1—2 inches below the antecubital crease). Induced pain and grip strength are noted. If the second phase of the test shows reduced pain and increased grip strength when the muscles of the proximal forearm are compressed, lateral epicondylitis is indicated.

Test for Medial Epicondylitis (Golfer's Elbow)

Medial Epicondyle Test. On the side of involvement, the patient is instructed to flex the elbow about 90° and supinate the hand. If severe pain arises over the medial epicondyle when the patient in this position attempts to extend the elbow against resistance, medial epicondylitis (golfer's elbow) is suggested.

The Wrists

Each wrist is composed of 16 synovial joints. The distal radius enlarges to form the

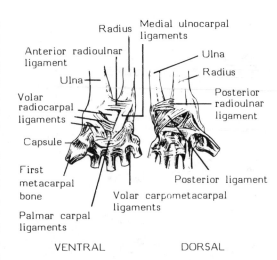

Figure 8.43. Schematic of the major ligaments of the wrist (Courtesy ACAP).

seat of the articulation of the proximal row of carpals. The proximal row of carpals articulate with the ulna only during extreme wrist adduction (ulnar deviation). The major ligaments of the wrist are shown in Figure 8.43.

As with any adjustive procedure, fracture, dislocations, and other contraindications to manipulation must be previously ruled out. If signs of swelling or inflammation are not evident, mild heat is frequently helpful before correction is made to allow maximum patient relaxation and rapid physiologic response to correction. Comparative bilateral P-A or A-P, oblique, and lateral x-ray films are helpful to diagnosis if fracture or pathology is involved.

Initial Clinical Considerations

If not conducted previously, perform standard tests for light touch and pain perception, muscle strength, and the integrity of the radial reflex. The ulnar reflex is highly unreliable. Some other general screening tests are described below.

Radial Stress Test. Pain over the medial aspect of the wrist is produced when the examiner forces the wrist into radial deviation. The sign is positive in posttraumatic disorders or pathology of the medial wrist.

Ulnar Stress Test. Pain arises over the lateral aspect of the wrist when the examiner forces the patient's wrist into ulnar deviation, indicating posttraumatic or pathology of the lateral wrist.

Wrist Flexion/Extension Stress Tests. The examiner moves the wrist firmly into flexion and extension. If pain is induced, wrist fracture, subluxation, sprain, acute tendinitis, or pathology are suggested. If negative, the movements are repeated against patient resistance. Induced pain then indicates wrist strain, rupture, acute or chronic tendinitis, or pathology.

The integrity of the median, ulnar, and radial nerves can be evaluated with the three following tests.

Ochsner's Sign. This refers to when clasping the hands so that the fingers intertwine, the index finger fails to flex. It is significant of a median nerve lesion affecting the flexor digitorum superficialis muscle.

Ulnar Tunnel Triad. Hypothenar wasting, tenderness of the ulnar tunnel, and flexion contracture of the ring finger are the three classic signs of entrapment compression of the ulnar nerve in the tunnel of Guyon. Froment's cone sign will also be positive.

Wrist Drop Sign. The two opposing palms are placed together with the hands in dorsiflexion. On separation, failure to maintain dorsiflexion indicates a positive test and is significant of radial nerve impairment.

When applicable, Allen's test for vascular occlusion, the bracelet test for rheumatoid arthritis, Finkelstein's test for DeQuervain's disease, and Finsterer's test for Kienbock's disease should be conducted.

Allen's Test. The sitting patient elevates the arm and is instructed to make a tight fist to express blood from palm. The examiner occludes the radial and ulnar arteries by finger pressure. The patient lowers the hand and relaxes fist, and the examiner releases the arteries one at a time. Some examiners prefer to test the radial and ulnar arteries individually in two tests. The sign is negative if the pale skin of the palm flushes immediately when the artery is released. The patient should be instructed not to hyperextend the palm as this will constrict skin capillaries and render a false positive sign. The sign is positive if the skin of the palm remains blanched for more than 3 seconds. This test, which should be performed before Wright's test, is significant in vascular occlusion of the artery tested.

Bracelet Test. In rheumatoid arthritis, compression of the distal ends of the radius and ulnar initiates acute pain in the forearm, wrist, and/or hand.

Finkelstein's Test. The patient is asked to make a fist with the thumb tucked inside the palm. The examiner stabilizes the patient's distal forearm with one hand and ulnar deviates the wrist with his other hand. Sharp pain in the area of the first wrist tunnel (radial side) strongly points toward stenosing tenosynovitis (De Quervain's disease) wherein inflammation of the synovial lining of the tunnel narrows the tunnel opening and causes pain on tendon movement.

Finsterer's Test. This is a two-phase test for Kienbock's disease. (1) If when clenching the fist firmly the normal prominence of the middle knuckle is not produced, the test is initially positive. (2) If percussion of the 3rd metacarpal just distal to the dorsal aspect of the midpoint of the wrist elicits abnormal tenderness, the test is confirmed.

Dynamic Palpation

Extension of the wrist occurs primarily between the carpal rows, and flexion of the wrist occurs essentially at the radiocarpal joints.

Joint play in the wrist should be evaluated to determine the point of possible fixation. These are:

• A-P and P-A glide of the ulnocarpal joints.
• A-P and P-A glide of the radiocarpal joints.
• A-P and P-A glide between the carpal rows.
• Lateral tilt of the triquetrum on the ulna.
• Lateral tilt of the navicular (scaphoid) on the radius.
• Long-axis traction separation of the ulnotriquetrum joint.
• Long-axis traction separation of the radiocarpal joint.
• Long-axis traction separation between the carpal rows.

• Long-axis rotational glide of the distal radioulnar joint.

• Approximation shear (induced by compression) of the distal radioulnar joint.

In testing any of the above motions, the proximal bone is stabilized and the distal segment is moved. The typical contact is to place the bone between the thumb and a crooked index finger. If end play is not perceived, apply a short quick dynamic impulse against the fixation.

Releasing Distal Radioulnar, Radiocarpal, and Ulnocarpal Fixations

Distal Radioulnar A-P/P-A Glide. Stand facing the standing or sitting patient. Straighten the involved limb, and pronate the patient's forearm. Place one thumb on the most distal dorsal aspect of the radius and the other thumb on the most distal aspect of the ulna. Flex your fingers so that the lateral surfaces of your respective index fingers are opposite your thumbs on the ventral side of the distal forearm. With the distal aspect of the radius and ulnar pinched between your thumbs and index fingers, slowly push forward with one hand while pulling backward with the other and then

reverse the maneuver in an alternating fashion. See Figure 8.44.

Faye states that the following technic is effective in general wrist mobilization. It is often used after a cast has been removed or as the first test of joint play motion in the wrist: The radius and ulna are clasped in one hand on the dorsum of the wrist and the metacarpals are clasped by the other hand. Short, sharp impulses are then made in A-P and P-A directions (Fig. 8.45).

Releasing Restricted Radiocarpal, Ulnocarpal, Intercarpal, and Carpometacarpal Distraction, Flexion, Extension, Abduction, and Adduction Mobility. While some authorities describe specific maneuvers for correcting each of these various fixations, it has been the experience of many clinicians that they all can be corrected by using one simple procedure. The doctor-patient positions are the same as described above with the exception that the contacts are taken approximately 1-½ inches more distal so that they are just beyond the last row of the carpals (over the metacarpal heads). Axial traction to patient tolerance is applied to the extended limb and the limb is slowly maneuvered through a small "figure 8" while holding the patient's hand firm with your fingers to prevent motion of the patient's metacarpals. This maneuver will pro-

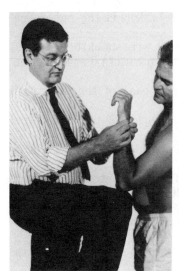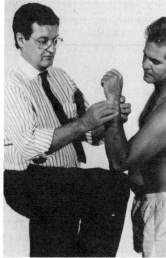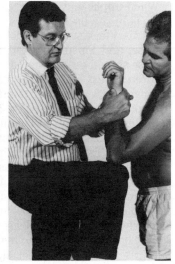

Figure 8.44. Evaluating distal radioulnar A-P/P-A glide. *Left,* neutral position; *center,* moving the distal radius forward on the ulnar; *right,* moving the distal ulna forward on the radius.

duce extension, flexion, abduction, and adduction within the radiocarpal, ulnocarpal, intercarpal, and carpometacarpal articulations. Repeat 20—30 times, progressively increasing the size of the "figure 8" to patient tolerance. This is a slow stretching maneuver, not a snapping or jerking procedure. See Figure 8.46.

Closing Separated Distal Radius and Ulna. This type of disorder is commonly seen in association with carpal tunnel syndrome, chronic wrist pain, and the posttraumatic effects of wrist sprain. Stand on the side of involvement, obliquely facing the standing or sitting patient. Grasp the patient's semipronated wrist with both hands so that your overlapping thumbs are crossed against the lateral aspect of the distal radius and your interlaced fingers cup the medial aspect of the patient's ulna. Apply a strong squeeze with your hands to approximate the distal radius and ulnar while simultaneously making a quick downward thrust with your thumbs by extending and adducting your elbows.

Opening Approximated Distal Radius and Ulna. Approximated distal radius and ulna are often found in cases of chronic wrist pain or following wrist and hand trauma. Obliquely stand on the side of involvement, facing the standing or sitting patient. Grasp the patient's pronated wrist with both hands

so that your overlapping thumbs cross between the dorsal aspects of the distal radius and ulna and your interlaced fingers cup under the lower forearm. Apply a strong thumb thrust inward and outward by extending your elbows while simultaneously using your fingers to separate the distal radius and ulna.

Carpal Tunnel Syndrome

Carpal tunnel syndrome can be simply defined as pain, tenderness, and weakness of the muscles of the thumb because of pressure on the median nerve at the point at which it passes through the carpal tunnel of the wrist. [See Clinical Comment 8.2]

Phalen's Test. The patient places both flexed wrists into apposition and applies moderate pressure for 30—45 seconds (Fig. 8.47). A positive sign of carpal tunnel syndrome is the production of symptoms (eg, pain, tingling).

Tinel's Wrist Test. The hand of a sitting patient is supinated, and the volar surface of the wrist is percussed. If this induces pain in all fingers except the first digit, carpal tunnel syndrome is indicated.

Wrist Tourniquet Test. A sphygmomanometer cuff is wrapped around the suspected wrist, inflated to a point slightly

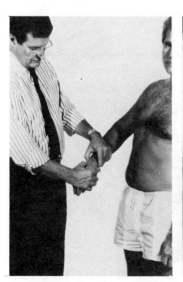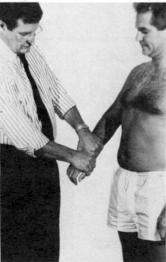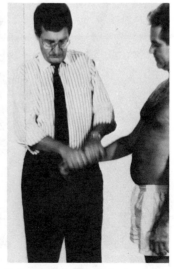

Figure 8.45. Faye's general A-P/P-A wrist mobilization technic. *Left,* localizing the contact points; *center,* firming the contacts; *right,* applying alternating A-P and P-A impulses.

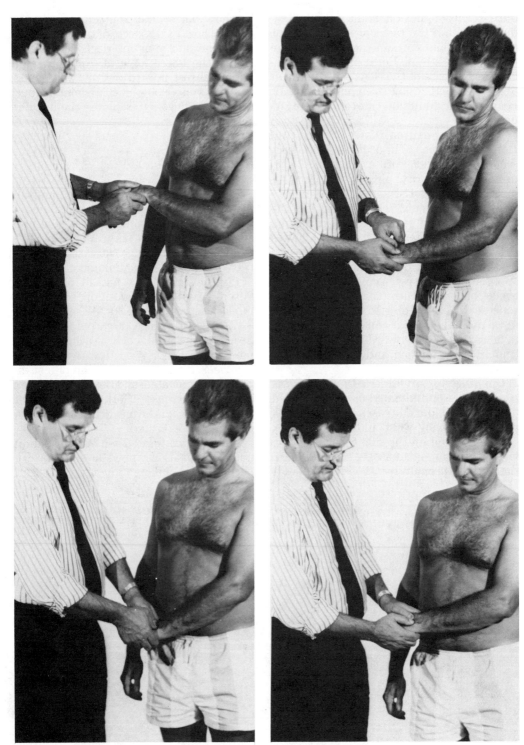

Figure 8.46. Conducting a "figure 8" maneuver of the left wrist. *Upper left,* wrist flexion; *upper right,* adduction; *lower left,* extension; *lower right,* abduction.

above the patient's systolic blood pressure, and maintained for 1—2 minutes. An increase in forearm, wrist, or hand pain indicates carpal tunnel syndrome.

The Hands

In terms of extraspinal fixations, Gillet believes that fixations of the hands are second in importance only to those of the feet, both of which can be linked to fixations in

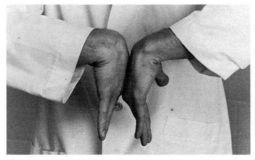

Figure 8.47. Phalen's test (Courtesy ACAP).

the spine. He also reports that (1) flexion fixations found in the hands are associated with a tightening of soft tissues on the anterior aspect of the spine and (2) flexion restrictions in the hands tend to produce spinal complexes that are characterized by tightening of soft tissues on the posterior aspect of the spine. He continues that, besides these nonspecific effects, extension blocks in the metacarpals appear to have a local influence in the T4—T6 region. The spinal fixation will be perceived during lateral flexion when the palpating fingers straddle the spinous processes in this area, and the fixation will be released by forcing metacarpal extension.

Hand and Finger Pain

Certain pain syndromes concerning the hands offer cardinal symptoms, especially those involving the ulnar, median, or radial nerves (Fig. 8.48).

• Pain radiating to the ulnar aspect of the

DR. FAYE'S CLINICAL COMMENT #8.2

It is worth mentioning again that most carpal tunnel syndromes are part of a "double crush" and fixation at the level of a C5—C6 (with severe tenderness palpable anteriorly). Motion palpation will reveal restricted intersegmental flexion and anterior to posterior rotation on the same side as the carpal tunnel syndrome. A positive doorbell sign is usual on this side as well. Stripping massage of the scalenius anticus muscles is very effective as a premanipulative procedure.

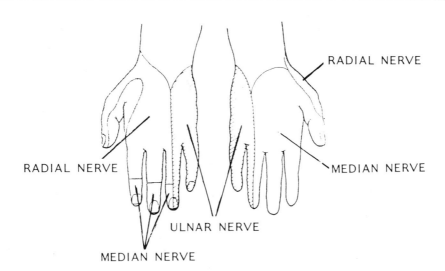

Figure 8.48. Schematic depicting the sensory innervation of the hand; *left,* dorsal view; *right,* palmar view (Courtesy ACAP).

hand extending to the ring and little fingers is characteristic of an ulnar nerve disorder.

• The median nerve supplies the radial side of the palm and the thenar muscles, and the origin of pain in this area may be at any point from the thumb to the cervical spine. In carpal tunnel syndrome where the median nerve becomes entrapped in its canal at the wrist, pain may be at the wrist or radiated up the forearm to the shoulder, and it is aggravated by wrist hyperextension.

• The radial nerve is excluded when pain is combined with weakness because this nerve has no sensory functions in the palm.

Associated Stiffness. The hands also express the effects of several of the arthritides. Early rheumatoid arthritis is often explained by the patient as morning stiffness of the hands and fingers that cannot be related to activity overuse. Rheumatoid stiffness, especially in the younger person, is often relieved with activity, while an older person with osteoarthritis will complain that activity aggravates the pain.

Associated Weakness. Progressive weakness in the hands suggests myasthenia gravis. The picture may progress to paralysis associated with repetitive muscle contractions because of the effect upon the intrinsic muscles of the hand. Neuropathic weakness is sometimes associated with diabetes mellitus. Increasing difficulty in releasing the grip is characteristic of amyotonia congenita (rare).

An absence of hand weakness when there is weakness elsewhere may also be an important clue. For instance, selective proximal weakness excluding the hands, forearms, and lower legs may suggest a neoplasm or one of the endocrine myopathies such as hyperthyroidism, hypothyroidism, adrenal hypofunction, or Cushing's syndrome.

Initial Clinical Considerations

Test hand and finger light touch and pain perception, grade muscle strength, and check the radial reflex if these procedures have not been conducted previously.

Significant Tendon Tests

Bunnel-Littler Test. Hold the metacarpophalangeal joint in slight extension and try to flex the proximal interphalangeal joint of any finger being tested (Fig. 8.49). If the joint cannot be flexed in this position, it is a positive sign that the intrinsic muscles are tight or capsule contractures exist. To distinguish between intrinsic muscle tightness and capsule contractures, let the involved metacarpophalangeal joint flex slightly, relaxing intrinsics, and move the proximal interphalangeal joint into flexion. Full flexion of the joint shows tight intrinsics; limited flexion indicates probable contracture of the interphalangeal joint capsule. This is sometimes called the *retinacu-lar test* or the *finger contracture test.*

Finkelstein's Test. The patient is asked to make a fist with the thumb tucked inside the palm. The examiner stabilizes the patient's distal forearm with one hand and ulnar deviates the wrist with his other hand. Sharp pain in the area of the first wrist tunnel (radial side) strongly points toward stenosing tenosynovitis (De Quervain's disease) wherein inflammation of the synovial lining of the tunnel narrows the tunnel opening and causes pain on tendon movement.

Extensor Digitorum Communis Test. The patient is instructed to flex and then extend a finger. The inability to extend any finger indicates a lesion of that extensor digitorum communis tendon.

Pollicis Longus Tests. The examiner stabilizes the proximal phalanx of the patient's thumb, and the patient is instructed to flex and extend the distal phalanx. Inability to flex the phalanx indicates an injury

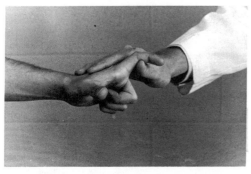

Figure 8.49. Conducting the Bunnell-Littler test (Courtesy ACAP).

to the tendon of the flexor pollicis longus. Inability to extend the phalanx indicates an injury to the tendon of the extensor pollicis longus.

Wartenburg's Sign. The patient is instructed to spread the hands out so that the palms face downward, the fingers are extended, and the thumbs are adducted; then raise the hands toward the face so that the palms appose. If the index fingers touch but the thumbs do not meet, paralysis of the abductor pollicis brevis is indicated.

Dynamic Palpation

Independent flexion, extension, abduction, and adduction motions of the metacarpal bases on the distal row of carpals are usually difficult to determine unless there is gross instability. Joint play occurs at the metacarpals, the interphalangeal joints, and the distal phalangeal joints as A-P/P-A glide, lateral tilt, rotation, and distraction. These joints function during finger and thumb flexion, extension, abduction, and adduction. See Figure 8.50.

Gillet points out that the hands exhibit fixations because the articulations are so frequently strongly flexed during daily activities yet many occupations rarely get strongly extended. It is for this reason that he attributes the resting "claw hand" of the manual laborer that resists extension. He reports that finger and wrist extension stretches lasting 30 seconds actually decrease cervical fixations of the muscular type.

When possible, joint play in the hand and fingers should be evaluated to determine the point of probable fixation. These are:

• Anterior and posterior glide of each proxmal phalanx on the middle phalanx, each metacarpal head on the proximal phalanx, and each middle phalanx on the distal phalanx.

• Abduction and adduction glide (lateral tilt) of each proximal phalanx on its apposed metacarpal head.

• Long-axis traction separation of the metacarpophalangeal and interphalangeal joints.

Note that a degree of interphalangeal side tilt and internal-external rotation normally

exists, but this motion is sometimes difficult to perceive.

Releasing Fixations

Flexion, extension, abduction, and adduction mobility restrictions may be found at the metacarpophalangeal joints and flexion-extension restrictions at the interphalangeal joints. Correction can be achieved simply by stabilizing the proximal bone and slowly moving the distal segment against the resistance, and then adding a brisk impulse. Repeat several times if necessary, gradually attempting to increase the range of motion up to patient tolerance.

Faye uses a manipulation for long-axis distraction of the thumb's carpometacarpal joint that is reported to be highly effective. See Figure 8.51.

Integrated Treatment Approach

One of the objectives of the teachings of *Dynamic Chiropractic* is to raise the competence of chiropractors in the art of extraspinal joint examination and the correction of fixations. Those doctors who have already become highly competent with motion palpation and adjustive treatment of the spine and pelvis realize the need for similar competency when extraspinal joints are involved in the patient's clinical picture.

There are many cases in which major biomechanical faults originate in the appendicular skeleton and produce spinopelvic symptoms and signs. When a clinician is able to diagnose and treat extremity dysfunction competently, it is common to find that difficult spinal conditions will clear and progressing chronic conditions will stabilize. For example, patients with chronic upper-thoracic disorders may have primary lesions in the shoulder, elbow, wrist, or hand. Likewise, a significant number of low-back and pelvic pain complaints are caused by or contributed to by articular hip, knee, ankle, or foot dysfunction.

Clinical evidence indicates that extraspinal motion restriction should be freed even if joint pain is not associated. The indication

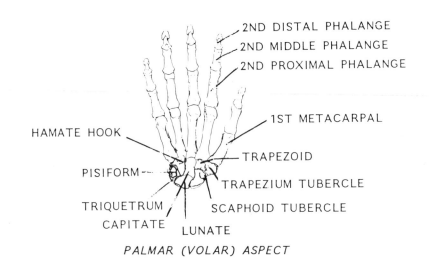

2ND DISTAL PHALANGE

2ND MIDDLE PHALANGE

2ND PROXIMAL PHALANGE

1ST METACARPAL

HAMATE HOOK

TRAPEZOID

PISIFORM

TRAPEZIUM TUBERCLE

TRIQUETRUM

SCAPHOID TUBERCLE

CAPITATE

LUNATE

PALMAR (VOLAR) ASPECT

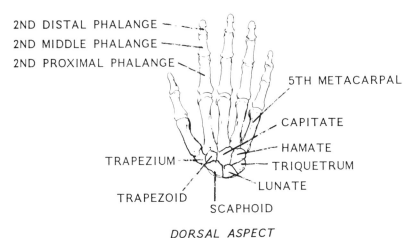

2ND DISTAL PHALANGE

2ND MIDDLE PHALANGE

2ND PROXIMAL PHALANGE

5TH METACARPAL

CAPITATE

HAMATE

TRAPEZIUM

TRIQUETRUM

LUNATE

TRAPEZOID

SCAPHOID

DORSAL ASPECT

Figure 8.50. The bones of the hand (Courtesy ACAP).

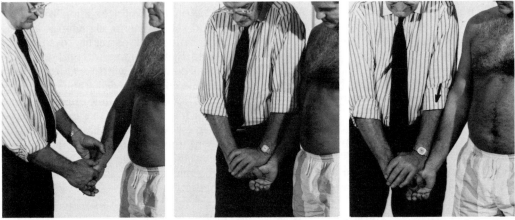

Figure 8.51. Position for long-axis extension of the thumb's carpometacarpal joint. *Left,* localizing the contact; *center,* firming the contact; *right,* applying the impulse.

for the adjustment is the mobility block. The ideal biologic model of health is the integrated harmony of normal joint, muscle, and neurologic mechanisms.

To learn and master the art of extraspinal joint examination and treatment should not be thought of as a subspecialty within chiropractic; it is an integral part of the basic chiropractic clinical approach.

Bibliography

Agostoni E, et al: Forces deforming the rib cage. *Respiratory Physiology*, 2:105, 1966.

An KN, Hui FC, Morrey BF, Linscheid RL, Chao EY: Muscles across the elbow joint: a biomechanical analysis. *Journal of Biomechanics*, 14:659-669, 1981.

Anon: Common sense management for TMJ troubles. *Patient Care*, pp 129-157, January 15, 1984.

Anon: "Doctor, my jaw hurts." *Patient Care*, pp 108-136, December 15, 1983.

Anon: When neuropathy underlies facial pain. *Patient Care*, pp 104-117, 121-135, February 15, 1984.

Barham JN, Wooten EP: *Structural Kinesiology*. New York, Macmillan, 1973, pp 202, 246, 247.

Basmajian JV (ed): *Grant's Method of Anatomy*, ed 9. Baltimore, Williams & Wilkins, 1975, pp 394-398.

Beatty HG: *Anatomical Adjustive Technic*, ed 2. Denver, CO, published by author, 1939, pp 200-204.

Belinghausen H, Gilula LA, Young LV, Weeks PM: Posttraumatic palmar carpal subluxation. *Journal of Bone & Joint Surgery*, 65:998-1006, 1983.

Bell WE: *Orofacial Pains: Differential Diagnosis*, ed 2. Chicago, Year Book Medical, 1979.

Berkman EH: The troublesome TMJ. *ACA Journal of Chiropractic*, June 1971.

Betge G: *Physical Therapy in Chiropractic Practice*. Via Tesserete, Switzerland, published by author, 1975.

Birnbaum JS: *The Musculoskeletal Manual*, ed 2. Orlando, FL, Grune & Stratton, 1986, pp 109-112, 338-340.

Bowerman JW: *Radiology and Injury in Sport*. New York, Appleton-Century-Crofts, 1977, pp 61-64, 87-94.

Branch WT Jr: *Office Practice of Medicine*. Philadelphia, W.B. Saunders, 1987, pp 898-922, 926-931.

Burns JR: *Extremities: Adjusting and Evaluation*. Published by author, 1984.

Cailliet R: *Shoulder Pain*, ed 2. Philadelphia, F.A. Davis, 1981, pp 125-136.

Cailliet R: *Soft Tissue Pain and Disability*. Philadelphia, F.A. Davis, 1977.

Chin WS, Oon CL: Ossification of the posterior longitudinal ligament of the spine. *British Journal of Radiology*, 52:865-869, 1979.

Chuinard RG: The upper extremity: elbow, forearm, wrist and hand. In D'Ambrosia RD: *Musculoskeletal Disorders: Regional Examination and Differential Diagnosis*. Philadelphia, J.B. Lippincott, 1977, pp 389, 391.

Craig AS: Elements of kinesiology for the clinician. *Physical Therapy*, 44:470-473, 1964.

Curwen IHM: Golf. In Armstrong JR, Tucker WE (eds): *Injury in Sport*. London, Staples, 1964, pp 200-204.

Dalinka MK: Fractures and dislocations about the shoulder. In Feldman F (ed): *Radiology, Pathology, and Immunology of Bones and Joints*. New York, Appleton-Century-Crofts, 1978.

Daniels L, Worthingham C: *Therapeutic Exercise for Body Alignment and Function*, ed 2. Philadelphia, W.B. Saunders, 1977, pp 66-71, 73-74.

Farrar WB: Dysfunctional centric relation of the jaw associated with dislocation and displacement of the disc. *Compendium of the American Equilibrium Society*, 13:63-67, 1973-1974.

Farrar WB, McCarty WL Jr: *A Clinical Outline of Temporomandibular Joint Diagnosis and Treatment*. Montgomery, AL, Normandie Publications, 1982.

Faye LJ, Weary B, Hooper P: *Motion Palpation and Clinical Considerations of the Upper Extremities*. Huntington Beach, CA, Motion Palpation Institute, 1986, pp 1, 13-30.

Faye LJ: Motion Palpation and Manipulation of Extremities [Cassette tape program]. Huntington Beach, CA, Motion Palpation Institute, 1981, 6 tapes.

Faye LJ: Motion Palpation and Manipulation of Hand, Wrist, Elbow [Videotape]. Los Angeles, Dynaspine, 1983.

Faye LJ: Motion Palpation and Manipulation of Shoulders, Scapula, and Clavicle [Videotape]. Los Angeles, Dynaspine, 1983.

Faye LJ: Motion Palpation and Manipulation of TMJ, Ribs, Babies and Children [Videotape]. Los Angeles, Dynaspine, 1983.

Gelb H (ed): *Clinical Management of Head, Neck and TMJ Pain and Dysfunction*. Philadelphia, W.B. Saunders, 1977.

Gertler L: *Illustrated Manual of Extravertebral Technic*, ed 2. Bayside, NY, published by author, 1978, pp 51-99.

Gillet H, Liekens M: *Belgian Chiropractic Research Notes*. Huntington Beach, CA, Motion Palpation Institute, 1984, pp 7-8, 16, 88-92, 107, 118-120, 147, 150-158.

Gillet H: Feet, hands, cranium, etc. *Bulletin of the European Chiropractors Union*, 26(3):28-30, 1978.

Grecco MA: *Chiropractic Technic Illustrated*. New York, Jarl, 1953, pp 171-185, 212-223.

Greene CS, Laskin DM: Long-term evaluation of conservative treatment for myofascial pain-dysfunction syndromes. *Journal of the American Dental Association*, 89:1365-1368, 1974.

Grice AS, Fligg DB: Class notes. Department of Biomechanics/Kinesiology, BK202. Toronto, Canadian Memorial Chiropractic College, date not shown, pp 81-82.

Grieve GP: *Common Vertebral Joint Problems*. New York, Churchill-Livingstone, 1981, pp 33, 235.

Grilliot JR, Staines MJ: Isolated rotary subluxation of the carpal navicular. *ACA Journal of Chiropractic*, February 1985.

Guralnick W, Kaban LB, Merrill RG: Temporomandibular-joint afflictions. *New England Journal of Medicine*, 299:123-129, 1978.

Hammer W: *Soft Tissue Diagnosis & Treatment*. Huntington Beach, CA, Motion Palpation Institute, 1987, pp 10, 12-15, 22-23.

Hearon KG: *What You Should Know About Extremity Adjusting*, ed 5. Place of publication not shown, published by author, 1981, pp 8-29.

Hertling D: The temporomandibular joint. In Kessler RM, Hertling D (eds): *Management of Common Musculoskeletal Disorders*. Philadelphia, Harper & Row, 1983, pp 233-271.

Hirata I Jr: *The Doctor and the Athlete*, ed 2. Philadelphia, J.B. Lippincott, 1974, pp 152-156, 177-180.

Hitchcock ME: Myofascial considerations in the thoracic area. *Osteopathic Medicine*, 85, December 1978.

Hoppenfeld S: *Physical Examination of the Spine and Extremities*. New York, Appleton-Century-Crofts, 1976, pp 128-132.

Hruby RJ: The total body approach to the osteopathic management of temporomandibular joint dysfunction. *Journal of the American Osteopathic Association*, 85(8):502-509.

Inman V, Saunders M, Abbott LC: Observations on the function of the shoulder joint. *Journal of Bone and Joint Surgery*, 26:1-30, 1944.

Iverson LD, Clawson DK: *Manual of Acute Orthopaedic Therapeutics*. Boston, Little, Brown, 1977, pp 129-133.

Janse J, Houser RH, Wells BF: *Chiropractic Principles and Technic*. Chicago, National College of Chiropractic, 1947, pp 523-558, 560.

Janse J: *Principles and Practice of Chiropractic*. Lombard, IL, National College of Chiropractic, 1976, pp 210, 222.

Jaquet P: *An Introduction to Clinical Chiropractic*, ed 2. Grounauer, Geneva, Switzerland, published by author, 1976.

Kent BE: Functional anatomy of the shoulder complex: A Review. Journal of the *American Physical Therapy Association*, 51:867-888, 1971.

Kent JM: Nailing the elusive Dx in shoulder pain. *Patient Care*, March 15, 1986, pp 136-154.

Kessler RM, Hertling D (eds): *Management of Common Musculoskeletal Disorders*. Philadelphia, Harper & Row, 1983, pp 135-155, 181-184, 187-191, 233-271, 533-537.

Larsen NJ: Osteopathic manipulative contribution to treatment of TMJ syndrome. *Osteopathic Medicine*, 3:15-27, August 1976.

Laskin DM: Etiology of the pain-dysfunction syndrome. *Journal of the American Dental Association*, 79:147-153, 1969.

Lay EM: The osteopathic management of temporomandibular joint dysfunction. In Gelb H (ed): *Clinical Management of Head, Neck and TMJ Pain and Dysfunction*. Philadelphia, W.B. Saunders, 1977.

London JT: Kinematics of the elbow. *Journal of Bone and Joint Surgery*, 63:529-535, 1981.

Magoun HI Sr: Dental equilibrium and osteopathy. *Journal of the American Osteopathic Association*, 75:981-991, June 1975.

Maitland GD: *Peripheral Manipulation*. Boston, Butterworths, 1976, pp 25-54, 59-91.

Mahan PE: Temporomandibular joint dysfunction: physiological and clinical aspects. In Rowe NH (ed): *Occlusion: Research in Form and Function. Proceedings of Symposium*. East Lansing, MI, University of Michigan, 1975, p 112.

Marbach JJ, Lipton JA: Treatment of patients with temporomandibular joint and other facial pain by otolaryngologists. *Archives of Otolaryngology*, 108:104, 1982.

Maurer EL: The thoraco-costal facet syndrome with introduction of the marginal line and the rib sign. *ACA Journal of Chiropractic*, X:S-158-159, December 1976.

Mennell JMcM: *Joint Pain*. Boston, Little, Brown, 1964, pp 32-90.

Mercier LR: *Practical Orthopedics*. Chicago, Year Book Medical, 1980, pp 44-65, 67-103, 136, 237-238, 274-278, 280-287.

Miyasaka K, Kaneda K, Ito T: Ossification of spinal ligaments causing thoracic radiculomyelopathy. *Radiology*, 143:463-468, 1982.

Nahum AM, et al: Deflections of human thorax under sternal impact. Paper delivered at the International Automobile Safety Conference, Detroit, 1970.

Ono M, Russell WJ, Kudo S, Yoshigoro K: Ossification of the thoracic posterior longitudinal ligament in a fixed population. *Radiology*, 143:469-474, 1982.

Orringer MB: Chest injuries in the athlete. In Schneider RC, Kennedy JC, Plant ML (eds): *Sports Injuries: Mechanisms, Prevention, and Treatment*. Baltimore, Williams & Wilkins, 1985, pp 826-827.

Poppen NK, Walker PS: Normal and abnormal motion of the shoulder. *Journal of Bone and Joint Surgery*, 58:195-201, 1976.

Quiring DP, Boroush EL: Functional anatomy of the shoulder girdle. *Archives of Physical Medicine*, 27:90-96, 1946.

Riggins RS: The shoulder. In D'Ambrosia RD: *Musculoskeletal Disorders: Regional Examination and Differential Diagnosis*. Philadelphia, J.B. Lippincott, 1977, p 336.

Robertson WE, Robertson HF: *Diagnostic Signs, Reflexes, and Syndromes*, ed 3. Philadelphia, F.A. Davis, 1947, p 261.

Rollis C: Motion palpation procedural manual. In Gillet H, Liekens M: *Belgian Chiropractic Research Notes*. Huntington Beach, CA, Motion Palpation Institute, 1984.

Rosse C, Clawson DK: *The Musculoskeletal System in Health and Disease*. New York, Harper & Row, 1980, p 129.

Rothman RH, Marvel JP, Heppenstall RB: Anatomic considerations in the glenohumeral joint. *Orthopaedic Clinics of North America*, 6:341-352, 1975.

Royder JO: Structural influences in temporomandibular joint pain and dysfunction. *Journal of the American Osteopathic Association*, 80:460-467, March 1981.

Schafer RC: *Chiropractic Physical and Spinal Diagnosis*. Oklahoma City, Associated Chiropractic Academic Press, 1980, Chapters IX and X.

Schafer RC: *Physical Diagnosis: Procedures and Methodology on Chiropractic Practice*. Arlington, VA, American Chiropractic Association. In preparation; to be released in 1989. Chapter 16.

Schafer RC: *Symptomatology and Differential Diagnosis*. Arlington, VA, American Chiropractic Association, 1986, pp 585-586, 603, 607.

Schoenholtz F: Conservative management of costovertebral subluxation. *ACA Journal of Chiropractic*, 14:S-77-78, July 1980.

Schultz AL: *The Shoulder, Arm, and Hand Syndrome.* Stickney, SD, Argus, 1969, pp 127-136, 146-161, 165, 183-192, 200-203, 206-219, 222-233, 254-256.

Shapiro BL: Changing views about temporomandibular pain-dysfunction. *Northwest Dentistry*, 60:6, 1981.

Smith SD: Head pain and stress from jaw-joint problems: diagnosis and treatment in tempororomandibular orthopedics. *Osteopathic Medicine*, 5:35, February 1980.

Smith SD: Vascular analysis in temporomandibular orthopedics: quantifying blood flow related to occlusal dynamics. *Osteopathic Medicine*, pp 29-32, 35-41, 71, October 1980.

Soderberg GL: *Kinesiology: Application to Pathological Motion.* Baltimore, Williams & Wilkins, 1986, pp 109-128, 131-147, 149-173.

Stierwalt DD: *Extremity Adjusting.* Davenport, IA, published by author, 1975, pp 8, 11, 13-24.

Stierwalt DD: *Fundamentals of Motion Palpation.* Place of publication not shown, published by author, 1977, pp 18-24.

Stoddard A: *Manual of Osteopathic Practice.* New York, Harper & Row, 1969, pp 203-219.

Stonebrink, RD: Palpation for vertebral motoricity. *ACA Journal of Chiropractic*, III:S-11-14, February 1969.

Sundstrom WR: Painful shoulders: Diagnosis and management. *Geriatrics*, 36(3):77-96, March 1983.

Turek SL: *Orthopaedics: Principles and Their Application*, ed 3. Philadelphia, J.B. Lippincott, 1977, pp 854-855, 857-858.

White AA, Panjabi MM: *Clinical Biomechanics of the Spine.* Philadelphia, J.B. Lippincott, 1978, pp 237-240, 250-251.

Williams JGP, Sperryn PN (eds): *Sports Medicine*, ed 2. Baltimore, Williams & Wilkins, 1976, pp 369, 387-390.

Zuidema GD, et al: *The Management of Trauma*, ed 3. Philadelphia, W.B. Saunders, 1979, 379-383.

Chapter 9

The Lower Extremity Joints

This chapter concerns the joints of the lower extremity; viz, those of the hip, knee, ankle, and feet. Within each topic, practical biomechanical and motion restriction considerations of specific joints are described, as well as concerns in dynamic palpation, neurologic and orthopedic testing, and adjusting procedures. Numerous aids in differential diagnosis are described.

BASIC CONSIDERATIONS

The chiropractic physician will find that there are many major biomechanical faults affecting the spine which have their origin in the lower extremities. When the clinician is able to accurately diagnose and efficiently treat joint dysfunction in the extremities as well as the spine, many difficult spinal conditions will be relieved and progressing degenerative disorders will be stabilized. In this

context, a significant number of low-back pain disorders will be found to have underlying hip, knee, ankle, or foot dysfunction.

This chapter underscores a point made in the previous chapter concerning the joints of the upper extremities: *To learn and master the art of peripheral joint examination and treatment should not be thought of as a subspecialty within chiropractic; rather, it should be considered an integral part of the chiropractic approach.* This point will be firmly established in this chapter as the lower extremities, unlike the upper extremities, are, with the exception of the fibula, weight-bearing structures that serve as the foundation for the spine.

Both primary and secondary joint disorders of the lower extremities are common, and they may have far-reaching biomechanical and neurologic effects. The major lower extremity joint movements and their innervation are shown in Table 9.1.

Table 9.1. Major Lower-Extremity Joint Movements and Their Innervation

L1—S2	*Hips*	Abduction (L4—S1) Adduction (L3—S1) Extension and rotation (L4—S2) Flexion (L1—S1)
L2—S2	*Knees*	Extension (L2—4) Flexion (L4—S2)
L4—S2	*Ankles*	Dorsiflexion (L4—S1) Plantar flexion (S1—2)

As in the application of any therapeutic procedure, diagnosis must precede therapy. The first concern is whether the patient's complaint is the result of pathological or dysfunctional origin and then to determine its cause—a cause that may be either local, remote, or systemic. For example, it is professionally embarrassing for the young practitioner (chiropractic, osteopathic, or allopathic) to unsuccessfully treat an apparently simple hip or knee strain only to find, on referral, that a half cup of pus was withdrawn from an infected joint—a condition that rarely exhibits itself on film. Never lose sight of the fact that a recent strain or sprain may be superimposed on a subclinical pathology.

In screening lower-extremity articular disorders for impairment, a priority concern is to seek muscle signs of atrophy or hypertrophy through inspection, palpation, and mensuration. Muscle strength should be tested against resistance and compared bilaterally. Abnormal tone (flaccidity, spasticity) can be determined by palpation and passive movements. Next, neurologic signs of fibrillations and abnormal movements such as tremors, myoclonus, chorea, athetosis, tics, etc, should be sought. Normal reflexes should be tested, and pathologic reflexes should be sought. Gross posture, structural attitude, and deformities should also be noted. Goniometry is often helpful. If there is even a remote suspicion that a underlying pathology may be involved, standard blood and urine workups and roentgenographic studies are almost mandatory. Referral for joint fluid analysis may also be necessary.

ARTICULAR CORRECTION: TECHNIC GUIDELINES

During lower-extremity articular analyses, the procedures are almost identical to those described for the upper extremity: test each range of motion for the integrity of end play, and adjust into the fixation when a restriction is found. Obviously, certain accommodations will have to be made for the larger size and weight of the lower-extremity segments. Most of the differences in examination, diagnosis, and treatment of articular disorders in the lower extremity in contrast to those of the upper extremity are effects from the fact that almost all the joints of the lower extremity are weight-bearing joints.

Almost any technic designed to release a fixation (total or partial) involving a synovial joint should apply a procedure (eg, manual axial traction) to assure slight physiologic distraction and biomechanical tissue adaptation prior to a corrective maneuver. If this precaution is not applied, there is a risk of injuring the cartilage of the articular surfaces and the periarticular soft tissues, thus adding to the development of further fixation. This principle is true throughout the appendicular and axial skeleton.

The act of injuring a joint during articular correction is almost always the result of inexperience. Obviously, from a purely mechanical viewpoint, distracted articular surfaces are much easier to move because friction is reduced to a minimum. In contrast, forcing motion on jammed articular surfaces will likely injure the apposed structures and the supporting elements and produce an imposed (iatrogenic) inflammation. This can lead to such complications as fibrosis, cartilage sclerosis, adhesion development, and pain and noxious reflexes from excited mechanoreceptors and effected splinting, etc—thus producing more harm than benefit to the patient.

A note of caution is worthy here: Any procedure to assure articular distraction can be overdone. If distraction is excessive, the articular surfaces might become so separated (eg, in an unstable joint) as to dislocate during a poorly controlled adjustment. In addition, stretched arthrosclerotic vessels are more likely to rupture when a strong longitudinal or rotational force is applied because structural plasticity is already at its limit. Even if the bleeding may be minute, a contribution to the adverse situation has been initiated.

Knowledge of just how much joint distraction to provide and how much force, velocity, and depth to apply during the adjustment in an individual situation is part of the *art* of chiropractic and is just one factor that differentiates the chiropractic physician from the therapist or technician.

Another common error among the inexperienced is to think of joint dysfunction in strict terms of either hypomobilty or hypermobility; ie, a joint may be either *hypermobile* as the result of the loss of ligamentous restraint or *hypomobile* as the result of something restricting motion. The experienced practitioner will always keep in mind that both conditions may exist in the same joint at the same time or in an adjacent joint at the same time. For example, a joint may exhibit hypermobility in extension and hypomobility in flexion, hypermobility in abduction and hypomobilty in adduction, or hypermobility in rotation in one direction and hypomobility in counterrotation—in fact, one state may be the cause of or in compensation to the other. In a like manner, the joints adjacent to a fixated joint in the kinematic chain frequently become hypermobile in compensation. These principles have previously been emphasized in the chapters of this book that concerned the spine. They are repeated here only to acknowledge that the same principles apply in the extremities, especially in the weightbearing segments.

The coexistence of hypermobility and hypomobility presents a therapeutic dilemma if we follow the formula of immobilizing a hypermobile joint temporarily and mobilizing a hypomobile articulation. Formulas cannot be applied globally with all patients. Patients and situations are often unique. Each patient and each condition must be judged individually. If the fixation can be mobilized within patient tolerance, then this should be done prior to immobilization and then re-evaluated when the immobilization is removed. However, if joint inflammation is so severe that mobilizing the fixation first would not be in the best interests of the patient (eg, acute sprain), then attention to the fixation should be delayed and management of the hypermobility should be given priority concern. Each case and each therapeutic regimen must be the result of clinical judgment in the situation at hand. Formula therapeutics should be left to the technicians.

These principles are just as applicable to adjustive technics involving spinal and other extraspinal joints. For example in treating cervical vertebrae, it is not difficult to dislocate an overly distracted joint that is unstable or normally exceptionally "loose." Such a situation is rarely found, however, with thoracic, lumbar, sacroiliac, or extraspinal axial articulations that have strong short ligamentous straps. Typical exceptions would be with acrobats, contortionists, and gymnists who are accustomed to performing somersaults, backflips, etc, and others whose occupations require extremely unusual postural distortions. The ligamentous restraints in these individuals may be lengthened, through prolonged conditioning and genetic predisposition to such a degree that dislocation (and spontaneous reduction) is commonplace.

THE COXA

The hip is the most proximal joint of the lower extremity and is a near-perfect ball-and-socket joint. It provides stability and agility for the body above and gross control for the extremity segments below (Fig. 9.1). It works as a functional unit with the pelvis and indirectly the lumbar spine, as well as with the knee, ankle, and foot—all of which have a direct influence on both adjacent segments and body structure as a whole.

It should be recognized that the hip joint is one of the most complex joints of the body in its role of providing both large ranges of mo-

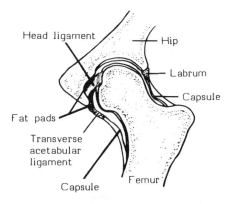

Figure 9.1. Frontal section of the hip showing the major structures associated with the head of the femur (Courtesy ACAP).

tion and large muscle torques in attempting to meet the requirements of imposed body weight during static and dynamic postures in the biped posture (Fig. 9.2). The major muscles of the hip and thigh and their functions and spinal level of innervation are shown in Table 9.2.

Biomechanical Considerations

The hip is highly stable because the head of the femur articulates deeply within the acetabulum. This attribute, unfortunately, excludes the advantages of direct palpation during examination. Thus, most of the physical clues of dysfunction must be analyzed indirectly from the effects expressed in the thigh or pelvis as a whole during passive motion studies in the nonweight-bearing position. See Figure 9.3. Other helpful clues can be found during gait and upright postural analyses, muscle strength testing, reflex testing, through questioning subjective symptoms (eg, pain, tenderness), and by superficial signs (eg, skin characteristics and temperature changes), and other standard physical and laboratory examination procedures.

Degenerative changes in bone and fractures predisposed by structural changes (eg, osteoporosis, biomechanical failures) within the hip are common. This is likely because the hip is frequently subjected to heavy repetitive loading that must be tolerated during function.

Muscle and ligament shortening affecting the hip is common in both the athletic and nonathletic individual, frequently producing complicating secondary effects in the musculoskeletal architecture above and below the hip (Fig. 9.4). Overstress imposed on such fixations (added to the large muscle torques required for hip function) appears

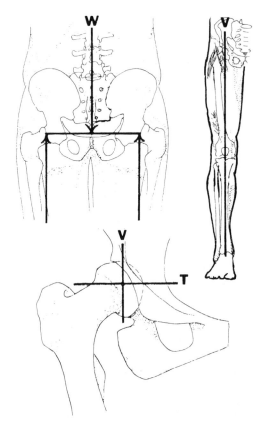

Figure 9.3. *Top left,* schematic of the static weight forces (W) that act on the femoral heads during bilateral stance. *Top right,* the vertical axis (V) for movement, extending from the hip through the lower tibia. *Bottom,* transverse axis (T) at the hip for hip flexion and extension, and vertical axis (V) at the hip for hip abduction and adduction (Courtesy ACAP).

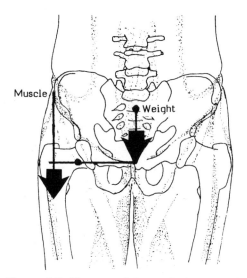

Figure 9.2. Diagram of the static forces acting about the axis of the femoral head during unilateral stance or the weight-bearing phase of gait (Courtesy ACAP).

to encourage the development of acute and chronic dysfunction. Although chronic hip fixations may exhibit themselves locally, they can also express themselves remotely in the kinematic chain (eg, lumbosacral area, sacroiliac joints, knee, ankles, feet, or even in the upper cervical spine). These areas can become either hypo- or hyper-mobile.

Hip Pain

Studies reported by Soderberg show that pain is a symptom common to most hip pathologies, regardless of etiology. "In such a circumstance, patients assume postures that diminish the force through the hip joint. During normal standing, the magnitude of the forces are low and are usually tolerable. However, single limb stance during gait significantly increases the joint force due to the abductor muscle force required to keep the pelvis from dropping on the opposite side." Thus, overstressed fatigued muscles from an adductor lurch are the common cause of hip pain, and it should be recognized that this soft-tissue injury, and the pain associated, is almost always a *secondary* condition.

Dermatomes, myotomes, and sclerotomes of the lower extremity are shown in Figure 9.5.

Table 9.2. Major Muscles of the Hip and Thigh

Muscle	Major Functions	Spinal Segment
Adductor brevis	Adduction, flexion, external rotation	L2-L4
Adductor longus	Adduction, flexion, external rotation	L2-L3
Adductor magnus	Adduction	L3-L4
Oblique fibers	Flexion	L3-L4
Vertical fibers	Extension, weak medial rotation	L3-L4
Gemelli	External rotation	L4-S2
Gluteus maximus	Extension, external rotation	L5-S2
Gluteus medius	Abduction, rotation	L4-S1
Anterior fibers	Flexion, internal rotation	L4-S1
Dorsal fibers	Extension, external rotation, abduction	L4-S1
Gluteus minimus	Abduction, medial rotation, flexion	L4-S1
Gracilis	Adduction	L2-L4
Hamstrings	Extension	L5-S2
Semitendinosus	Extension	L5-S2
Semimembranosus	Extension	L5-S1
Biceps femoris	Extension	L5-S2
Iliacus	Flexion	L2-L3
Obturators	External rotation	L3-L4
Pectineus	Adduction, flexion	L2-L3
Piriformis	External rotation	L5-S2
Psoas major	Flexion	L1-L5
Quadratus femoris	External rotation	L4-S1
Rectus femoris	Flexion	L2-L4
Sartorius	Flexion, abduction, external rotation	L2-L3
Tensor fasciae latae	Abduction, medial rotation, flexion	L4-S1

Note: Spinal innervation varies somewhat in different people. The spinal nerves listed here are averages and may differ in a particular patient; thus, an allowance of a segment above and below those listed in most text tables should be considered.

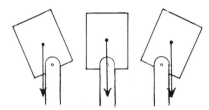

Figure 9.4. Mechanical model showing hip-pelvis relationships, as viewed laterally. Ideal balance is shown in the center diagram where the center of gravity is directly over its base of support. When the pelvis is abnormally inclined forward or backward, muscular action must be constantly active to maintain balance. In time, the involved muscles will become fibrotic because of the overstress (Courtesy ACAP).

Differentiation Clues

When hip pain is the primary complaint, the priority consideration in motion palpation during physical examination is to determine if joint mobility is restricted and if certain passive motions conducted in a non-weight-bearing position (eg, supine, prone) aggravate or initiate the patient's pain. Common causes of hip pain are shown in Table 9.3.

Gross evaluation should include internal and external rotation, abduction and adduction, flexion and extension, and circumduction. Branch feels that the loss of normal internal rotation is the most sensitive sign of hip disease. When hip flexion is tested with the knee locked (straight-leg-raising test), existing sciatic neuritis is aggravated. In contrast, when testing *full* hip flexion with the knee relaxed, a sacroiliac lesion may be aggravated. However, testing internal and external rotation of the hip with the hip and knee flexed to 90° should not normally initiate low-back or sacroiliac pain unless there is complicating psoas or piriformis spasm.

Referred Pain

Hip joint dysfunction often refers pain to the ipsilateral lower extremity. Although a lumbosacral lesion commonly refers pain to the area of the hip, rarely does a diseased hip joint refer pain to the lower back; ie, the tendency of a hip lesion is to refer pain caudad, especially to the knee.

Dynamic Palpation

Being a ball-and-socket joint, the hip normally moves freely in a multitude of directions; ie, multiple degrees in extension, flexion, abduction, adduction, circumduction, and distraction (Fig. 9.6).

Motion palpation of the hip is usually conducted immediately following the standard orthopedic/neurologic examination, including an evaluation of cerebellar function, leg-length analysis, gross range of motion tests, muscle strength grading, reflexes, and light touch and pain perception.

Hip Fixations

Many types of hip dysfunction will be associated with a limitation in joint distraction. Mennell considers long-axis (downward) joint play to be the most important motion of the hip joint. The gross degree of distraction available can easily be determined by placing the patient supine, in a position of rest, stabilizing one foot against your thigh and then applying traction on the thigh to be examined. The examiner's contact is usually applied just above the knee.

Forced flexion of the thigh on the involved side toward the abdomen will cause the contralateral thigh to raise from the table in osteoarthritic hip disease and certain adhesions. This is because motion restriction in the acetabulum will force the pelvis to rotate upward as a whole. Such movement suggests restricted hip flexion and points to shortened tissues posteriorly (eg, hamstrings) or a strong adhesion posteriorly. This same maneuver can also be used when testing forced extension with the patient in the prone position. If the contralateral thigh raises before normal full extension is reached, an anterior articular fixation or shortened quadriceps should be suspected.

Hip abduction, external rotation, and extension mobility can be tested by applying Patrick's test.

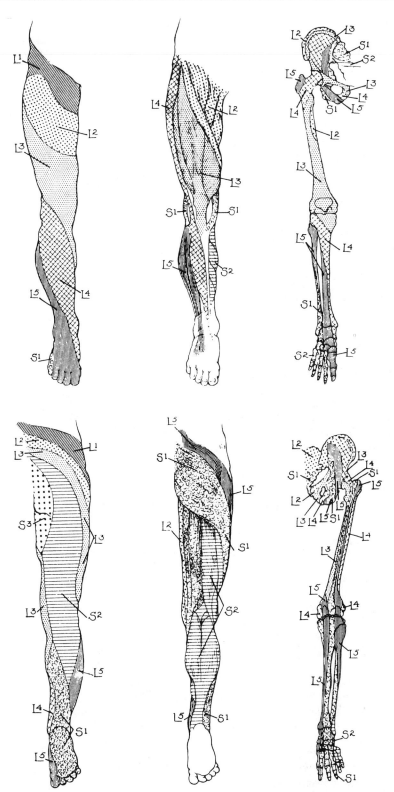

Figure 9.5. From left to right, dermatomes, myotomes, and sclerotomes of the lower extremity. *Top,* anterior view; *bottom,* posterior view (Courtesy ACAP).

Patrick's F-AB-ER-E Test. This test is often applied to help confirm a suspicion of hip joint pathology, but it is also an excellent set of maneuvers that can be used to appraise general hip mobility. The patient lies supine, and the examiner grasps the patient's ankle and the flexed knee. The patient's thigh is then flexed (F), abducted (AB), externally rotated (ER), and extended (E). Acute pain in the hip during the maneuvers, particularly on abduction and external rotation, is said to be a positive sign of coxa pathology. Passive end-play motion restriction without pain would indicate a fixation. [See Clinical Comment 9.1]

Significant Neurologic and Orthopedic Tests

Trendelenburg's Hip Test. If the hip and its muscles are normal, the iliac crest and sacral dimple will be slightly low on the weight-bearing side and high on the leg-elevated side when one leg is lifted. To test, have the patient with a suspected hip involvement stand on one foot, on the side of involvement, and raise the other foot and leg in hip and knee flexion. If there is hip joint involvement and muscle weakness, the iliac crest and sacral dimple will be markedly high on the standing side and low on the side the leg is elevated. A positive sign suggests that the gluteus medius and minimus muscles on the supported side are weak. The gait will exhibit a characteristic lurch to counteract the imbalance caused by the descended hip. The sign is also commonly positive in a developing Legg-Calve-Perthes disease, poliomyelitis, muscular dystrophy, coxa vara, Otto's pelvis, epiphyseal separation, pathology of the superior gluteal nerve, coxa ankylosis, hip dislocation, fracture, or chronic subluxation of L4, L5, or the sacral base. It is occasionally positive soon after a cervical "whiplash" if the sympathetic ganglion chain has been stretched.

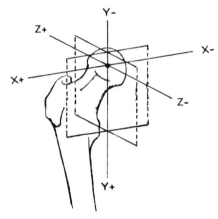

Figure 9.6. The coordinates pertinent to the hip joint's mechanical axis (Courtesy ACAP).

Table 9.3. Common Causes of Hip Pain

Chronic Hip Pain	Acute Hip Pain
Avascular necrosis	Arthritis
Congenital fault (eg, coxa vera)	Bursitis
Contractures/other fixations	Contusion and bone bruises
Degenerative joint disease	Dislocation
Fixation	Epiphyseal slip
Fugal infection	Fixation
Gout (rare)	Fracture
Meralgia paresthetica	Psoas abscess
Otto pelvis (protrusio acetabuli)	Referred pain
Referred pain	Sprain/strain
Rheumatoid arthritis	Synovitis
Transient synovitis	Tendinitis
Tuberculosis	

Hip Abduction Stress Test. The patient is placed in the side position with the underneath lower limb flexed acutely at the hip and knee. With the upper limb held straight and extended at the knee, the patient is instructed to attempt to abduct the upper limb while the examiner applies resistance. Pain initiated in the area of the uppermost sacroiliac joint or the hip joint suggests an inflammatory process of the respective joint.

Internal Femoral Torsion Signs. Internal femoral torsion can be observed if the patellae are marked with a skin pencil and these points are observed during gait. There will be toe-in, the patellae will face medially, an internal contracture of the hips will usually be found, and there will be excessive anteversion of the femur. If there is toe-in and the patellae face forward (as is normal), the cause of the toe-in will be distal to the knee. An internal rotation deformity can be considered to exist at the hip when internal rotation exceeds external rotation by more than 30°.

Lasegue's Differential Sign. This test is used to rule out hip disease. A patient with sciatic symptoms is placed supine. If pain is elicited on flexing the thigh on the trunk with the knee extended but not produced when the thigh is flexed on the trunk with the knee relaxed (flexed), coxa pathology can be ruled out, according to Laseque.

Gauvain's Sign. With the patient in the lateral recumbent position, the examiner stabilizes the patient's uppermost iliac crest with the heel of the hand and the fingerpads are firmed against the patient's lower abdomen. With the patient's uppermost knee extended, the examiner grasps the patient's upper ankle with the other hand, moderately abducts the limb, and firmly rotates it internally and externally. With the patient's knee locked in extension, these rotary maneuvers will affect the entire limb, as far superiorly as the head of the femur. A positive sign is seen when a strong abdominal contraction occurs, indicating a somatosomatic reflex spasm that is usually attributed to hip pathology (eg, coxa tuberculosis).

Note: Hibb's, Laguerre's, Nachlas', and Neri's bowing tests may also have significance in differentiating various hip complaints. Please refer to Chapter 6, which concerned the pelvis.

Muscle Tests

Thomas' Test. This test is used to determine excessive iliopsoas tension. The supine patient holds one flexed knee against his abdomen with his hands while the other limb is allowed to fully extend. The patient's lumbar spine should normally flatten. If the extended limb does not extend fully (ie, the knee flexes from the table) or if the patient rocks his chest forward or arches his back, a fixed flexion contracture of the hip is indicated, as from a shortened iliopsoas muscle. This should always be tested bilaterally. Some examiners use the degree of pain elicited on forceful extension of the flexed knee as their criterion of iliopsoas tension. If the heel is raised from the table along with the knee, check for shortened quadriceps.

Ober's Test. This is a common test for iliotibial band contractures. The patient is placed directly on his side with the unaffected side next to the table. The examiner places one hand on the pelvis or under the thigh to steady it and grasps the patient's ankle with the other hand, holding the knee flexed at a right angle. The thigh is abducted and extended in the coronal plane of the body. In the presence of iliotibial band contracture, the leg will remain abducted—the degree of abduction depending upon the amount of contracture present.

DR. FAYE'S CLINICAL COMMENT #9.1

Patrick's test should be modified. First, the examiner should note any loss of normal passive range of motion. When a range of motion is diminished, gently spring the joint against the restriction. If the resistance is springy, PNF or spray-and-stretch therapy is indicated for the involved muscles. If the restriction is completely blocked, capsule involvement is suggested and a mobilizing manipulation technic is usually called for—assuming that the diagnosis has ruled out any contraindications for such therapy.

Beery's Sign. This sign is positive if a patient with a history of lower trunk discomfort and fatigue is fairly comfortable when sitting with the knees flexed but experiences discomfort in the standing position. It is typically seen in spasticity or contractures of the posterior thigh and/or leg muscles.

Ely's Test. To support iliopsoas spasm suspicions, the patient is placed prone with the toes hanging over the edge of the table, legs relaxed. Either heel is approximated to the opposite buttock. After flexion of the knee, pain in the hip will make it impossible to carry out the test if there is any irritation of the psoas muscle or its sheath. The buttock will tend to rise on the involved side. However, a positive Ely's test can also be an indication of rectus femoris contraction, a lumbar lesion, a contracture of the tensor fascia lata, an osseous hip lesion, or femoral radiculitis (L2—L3).

Hip Spasm Differentiation Tests. In the hip joint, two forms of spasm are common: (1) that which is due to irritation of the psoas alone, and (2) that in which all the muscles moving the joint are more or less contracted. The normal range of hip flexion is 120°. In isolated psoas spasm, motions of the hip (rotation, adduction, abduction, and flexion) are not impeded. General spasm of the hip muscles is tested with the patient supine upon a table or bed and the leg flexed at a right angle, both at the knee and at the hip. A child may be tested on its parent's lap. Using the sound leg as a standard of comparison, the examiner then draws the knee away from the midline (abduction), toward and past the midline (adduction), and toward the patient's chest (flexion). Rotation is tested by holding the knee still and moving the foot away from the median line of the body or toward and across it.

Lewin's Knee Sign. If quick extension of a knee in the standing position produces pain and a sharp flexion response, hamstring spasm should be suspected.

Phelp's Test. The patient is placed in the prone position with both lower limbs extended in the relaxed position. In this position, the patient's thighs are abducted just short of the patient's threshold of pain, and then the examiner flexes the patient's knees to 90° angles with the thighs. If this flexion allows greater abduction of a thigh on the hip without undue discomfort, a contracture of the gracilis muscle is suggested.

Quadriceps Flexion Test. Scar tissue within muscle invariably limit the working length of all muscles in the group. Quadriceps contracture is exhibited by placing the patient prone, flexing the leg toward the buttocks, and measuring the distance from heel to buttock. Once the point of tolerance is measured, the lumbosacral spine will arch and the buttocks will rise to prevent further stretch. This test may prove a lesion too deep to palpate as well as evaluate progress during therapy.

Tripod Sign. The patient is placed prone with the knees flexed over the edge of the table, and active and passive muscle strength and range of motion of knee extension are evaluated. If the patient must lean back (extend the trunk on the pelvis) and grasp the table to support body weight on the arms when the knees are bilaterally extended, hamstring spasm is indicated. This may be the result of any lower motor irritation located between the midthoracic area and the lower sacrum.

Releasing Hip Fixations

Corrective adjustments should be applied gently and not beyond patient tolerance, with special caution used with the elderly and very young. The well-conditioned young athlete who can withstand, and possibly

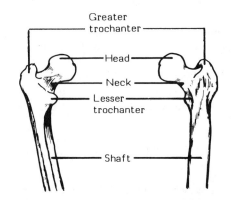

Figure 9.7. Major landmarks of the proximal aspect of the femur. *Left,* anterior view; *right,* posterior view (Courtesy ACAP).

require, a forceful dynamic thrust is not in the majority in the typical clinical practice. Too forceful an application, especially during forced extension, can produce a torsion fracture of the neck of the femur in the elderly or dislocate the head of the femur in a youngster. At the same time, it must be kept in mind that the hip joint is much more stable than the shoulder and requires a greater force to overcome larger muscle and ligamentous restrictions. Clinical judgment is the directive.

Releasing Inferior Distraction Fixations

Hip Distraction: Patient Supine or Prone. A simple technique to achieve long-axis distraction (inferior, caudad motion) is conducted by grasping the supine patient's lower thigh in both hands and applying a pulling force caudad, thus applying a distraction force on the hip. To be effective, the patient's contralateral limb must be stabilized (manually or mechanically) in some manner. Some type of belt or harness to stabilize the patient's pelvis is often helpful. Once long-axis separation is restored, at least to a moderate degree, attention can be given to flexion, extension, abduction, and adduction hypomobilities.

Many clinicians apply the above technique with the contact hands placed above the ankle of the recumbent patient. With this procedure, the doctor must be able to perceive the difference between distraction at the knee and that of the hip. With practice, this can be learned and will be found easier to employ than the thigh contact.

Hip Distraction: Patient Laterally Recumbent. As an alternative technic, Faye recommends that the patient be placed laterally recumbent with the involved side upward. Stand oblique to the patient, and flex the patient's uppermost knee. The doctor-patient positions are similar to those used in making a lumbar adjustment. Place a thenar contact against the greater trochanter of the patient's femur (Fig. 9.7); and with your knee, apply traction on the patient's knee to distract the patient's hip joint. Your other hand should stabilize the patient's

trunk. Next, apply a stretch with both your thenar and knee contacts (Fig. 9.8). Once tissue slack is removed, add a dynamic impulse with your contact hand directed through the long axis of the patient's femur. Take special care not to apply too much force against the patient's knee; ie, concentrate your pressure for traction at the hip joint rather than an adduction force against the patient's knee.

Releasing Other Types of Hip Fixations

Following release of hip distraction, Faye uses Patrick's test (described previously) with a gentle springing action at the end of each maneuver to screen joint play mobility. A short dynamic impulse is added if an impediment to normal mobility is found. He also teaches that extension mobility appears

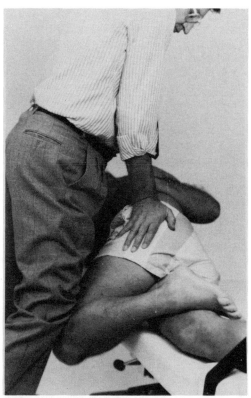

Figure 9.8. Hip distraction with patient laterally recumbent, involved side upward.

to have great significance and recommends the following adjustments to normalize restricted hip mobility:

1. *Extension.* Flex the uninvolved hip against the supine patient's chest while stabilizing the involved hip so that it will not raise from the table (Fig. 9.9). This maneuver will produce extension of the restricted hip. This technic, states Mennell, is often beneficial in cases of osteoarthritis of the hip.

2. *Flexion.* Stand at the side of the table obliquely facing the supine patient. Flex the patient's involved hip, and place the patient's leg over your shoulder (Fig. 9.10). With both hands, grasp high on the anterior aspect of the patient's proximal thigh (as near as possible to the head of the femur) and apply a pulling force that arcs downward to force full hip flexion.

3. *P-A glide.* Place the patient prone. Flex the patient's knee on the involved side to a 90° angle with your stabilizing hand while your active hand against the patient's greater trochanter impulses downward (Fig. 9.11).

4. *Posterior joint play.* Faye advises that the supine patient be positioned with the hip flexed to 90°. Stand on this side, and cup both hands over the patient's ipsilateral knee (Fig. 9.12). Using your upper body weight, press down along the long axis of the femur to push the head of the femur posteriorly. There should be a pain-free springy movement. Continue to test this backward springing at various points during circumduction. There is often a painful "hitch" that is relieved by an impulse into the restriction(s) found.

Rehabilitative Exercise

The following bed exercise is recommended in chronic cases. The patient positions himself laterally recumbent (near the edge of the bed) so that the involved side is up-

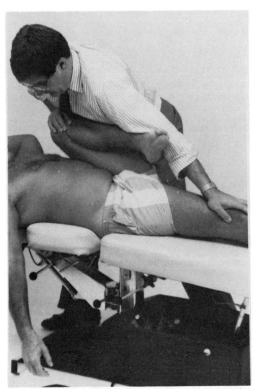

Figure 9.9. General testing of right hip extension with the patient supine.

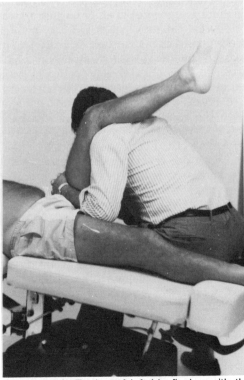

Figure 9.10. Testing of left hip flexion with the patient supine.

ward. The patient should be facing toward the remainder of the bed. A small pillow is then placed between the upper thighs, and the underlying uninvolved hip and knee is moderately flexed. The patient then slightly extends the limb and allows the leg to drop over the edge of the bed, thus producing hip adduction in moderate extension. The patient should then actively abduct the limb a few inches and let it drop by its own weight several times. This exercise will stretch lateral periarticular soft-tissue restrictions to external rotation and inferior distraction.

THE KNEES

Besides being the largest joint in the body, the knee (Fig. 9.13) is an unique joint because it is located between the body's longest bony segments (lever arms); thus, it is pre-disposed to direct trauma, leverage forces, and often unequaled pathologies and biomechanical faults. As with spinal segments, the inclusion of cartilaginous pads between weight-bearing joint surfaces makes for an interesting study of biped load transmission, injuries, and sites of articular derangements.

The long muscles of the thigh tend to have a restrictive effect on the mobility of the knee and patella. Although each may be treated locally, Gillet states that they are often shown to be secondary to articular and ligamentous fixations in the pelvis. The muscles of the knee, their functions, and their spinal level of innervation are shown in Table 9.4.

Biomechanical Considerations

The normal biomechanics of the knee are frequently altered by fixations that may be the cause or the effect of pathologic changes.

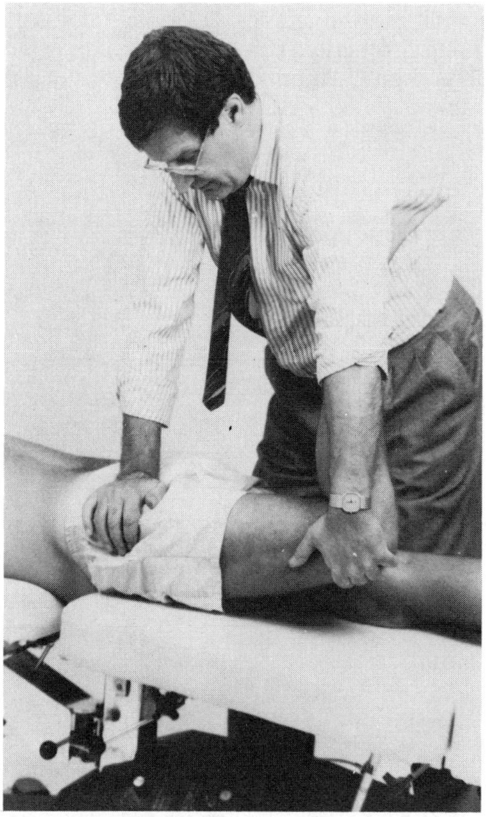

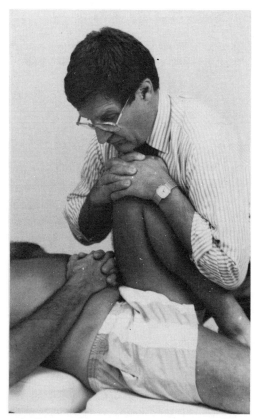

Figure 9.11. Testing P-A glide of the left hip with the patient prone.

Figure 9.12. Evaluating posterior joint play of the left hip with the patient supine.

Any of the three joints of the knee may be involved: the femorotibial, the patellofemoral, or the proximal tibiofibular joint.

Restricted rotation of the tibia (Fig. 9.14) on the femur during flexion-extension can produce severe dysfunction during weight-bearing. The tibia normally rotates internally during knee flexion and externally during extension. These rotatory movements of the tibia are governed by the ligaments and menisci of the knee and the action of the patella. The stability of the knee is provided almost fully by its ligamentous complex, especially those on the medial and lateral aspects. However, never underestimate the role of the popliteus muscle.

Diagnostic Considerations

Motion palpation of the knees is usually conducted immediately following the standard orthopedic/neurologic examination, including gross range of motion evaluation, muscle strength grading, reflexes, and light touch and pain perception.

Knee Pain

Common causes of knee pain are shown in Table 9.5. The priority consideration during physical examination when knee pain is the chief complaint are pain and tenderness and their localization, heat, motion restrictions, swelling, and the integrity of ligamentous stability. Although the knee has little soft-tissue protection, this same attribute offers helpful bony landmarks that are easily palpable.

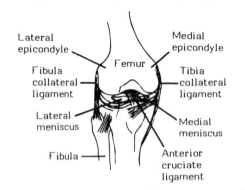

Figure 9.13. Drawing of the major anterior structures of the interior of the knee (Courtesy ACAP).

Table 9.4. Muscles of the Knee

Muscle	Major Functions	Spinal Segment
Gastrocnemius	Flexion	S1-S2
Gracilis	Flexion, medial rotation	L2-L3
Hamstrings	Flexion, rotation	L5-S2
Biceps femoris	Flexion, external rotation (long head)	S1-S2
Semimembranosus	Flexion, medial rotation	L5-S1
Semitendinosus	Flexion, medial rotation	L5-S2
Plantaris	Flexion	L5-S1
Popliteus	Flexion, medial rotation	L4-S1
Quadratus femoris	Extension	L4-S1
Rectus femoris	Extension	L2-L4
Sartorius	Flexion, medial rotation	L2-L3
Tensor fasciae latae	External rotation	L4-S1
Vastus muscles	Extension	L2-L4

Note: Spinal innervation varies somewhat in different people. The spinal nerves listed here are averages and may differ in a particular patient; thus, an allowance of a segment above and below those listed in most text tables should be considered.

Genu Varum: Bowed-Leg(s)

If the medial malleoli are touching and the knees are not when the patient is standing, the space between the knees determines the degree of genu varum. There will also be (1) excessive external rotation of the femur and internal rotation restriction, (2) excessive internal rotation of the tibia and external rotation restriction, (3) lateral patella deviation due to femur rotation, (4) anteversion of the femoral neck, and (5) an in-toeing gait. One study has shown that angular deformity of only 10° will triple the weight-bearing per unit of force in the knee.

Bilateral genu varum (Fig. 9.15) is common in early childhood, and spontaneously corrects itself 95% of the time, states Mercier, during further growth and maturation. Acquired causes include postural dysfunction, rickets, Paget's disease, scurvy, fibroid dysplasia, Blount's disease, degenerative arthritis, and various other bone diseases). In adults, genu varum is more common among males.

Genu Valgum: Knock-Knee(s)

If an abnormal space is found between the malleoli when the knees are touching when

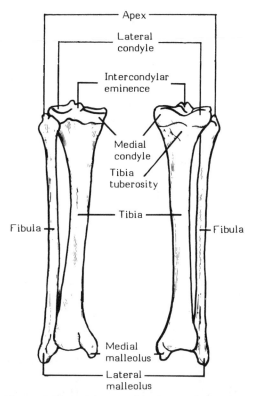

Figure 9.14. *Left,* bones of the leg as viewed from the anterior; *right,* as viewed from the posterior (Courtesy ACAP).

Table 9.5. Common Causes of Knee Pain

Acute Knee Pain	Chronic Knee Pain
Arthritis	Bursitis
Baker's cyst	Degenerative joint disease
Bursitis	Fixations
Contusion	Genu recurvatum
Dislocation	Genu valgum
Fixation	Genu varum
Fracture	Gout (rare)
Hydarthrosis	Hemarthrosis
Meniscal slip	Meniscal fragmentation/erosion
Loose bodies within joint	Patellar chondromalacia
Osgood-Schlatter disease	Pellegrini-Stieda disease
Osteochondritis dissecans	Psychogenic origins
Osteonecrosis	Referred pain (hip, lumbosacral spine)
Sprain/strain	Semilunar cartilage cyst
Synovitis	Tumor
Tendinitis	
Tumor	

the patient is standing with the kneecaps straight ahead, a degree of genu valgum exists that may be more marked on one side than the other. There will also be (1) excessive internal rotation of the femur and external rotation restriction, (2) excessive external rotation of the tibia and internal rotation restriction, (3) medial patella deviation due to femur rotation, and (4) foot pronation. This distortion results in a short leg causing pelvic imbalance if the condition is unilateral. Be aware, however, that people with a high degree of joint flexibility can hyperextend their knees along with femoral rotation—giving a false appearance of structural deformity.

Bilateral genu valgum is common in late childhood but typically corrects itself prior to the age of 8 or 9 years. Acquired causes include postural dysfunction and metabolic diseases. In adults, genu valgum is more common among females.

Genu Recurvatum: Hyperextension

Genu recurvatum is a state of exaggerated hyperextensibility. It is usually associated with a joint overstress producing A-P instability of the knee. In adolescence and early adulthood, contact sports, high jumping, or any activity that may induce anterior leg trauma or strenuous "take offs" from a locked knee may be the precipitating factor. If such is true, continuing such activities would be contraindicated (usually permanently). Faye mentions that this condition is

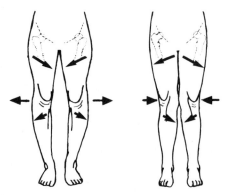

Figure 9.15. Drawings of genu varum, *left;* genu valgum, *right* (Courtesy ACAP).

often seen in retired professional athletes who have previously undergone multiple surgeries on the knee.

Tibial Rotation and Torsion

When the patient's kneecaps face straight ahead and the feet point distinctly outward, a positive sign of *tibial external rotation* on the femur exists. This sign is usually more pronounced on one side than the other. If the feet appear normally positioned but the patellae are rolled inward medially, a positive sign of *tibial torsion* exists.

Various causes have been shown to be at the root of tibial rotation and torsion. The most common etiologies reported are congenital defect, spastic paralysis, poliomyelitis, tibial subluxation-fixation, scurvy, and as a consequence of tibial fracture.

Internal Tibial Torsion Test. To confirm a suspicion of internal tibial torsion, have the patient sit on a table with the knee flexed at 90°. The tibial tubercle will palpate as if facing straight anteriorly. The examiner grasps the malleoli by the thumb and index finger to determine the position of the ankle joint. In normal adults, about 20°—30° of external tibial torsion is present and the lateral malleolus will be posterior to the medial malleolus. If internal tibial torsion exists, the lateral malleolus will be anterior to its medial mate.

External Tibial Torsion Sign. This is a markedly posterior position of the lateral malleolus relative to the medial malleolus in weight-bearing and supine positions. An everted heel and flat arch are commonly associated.

Therapeutic Considerations

In the average unathletic individual (child or adult), it is common to find (1) strong but tight hip flexors, (2) weak and tight hip extensors, and (3) weak and tight hip abductors and adductors. This imbalance leads to progressive biomechanical faults in the pelvis, knees, ankles, and feet.

Little can be accomplished once bone remodeling has occurred. However, much can be done in preventing further malformation by a long-term regimen of soft-tissue therapy, strengthening muscles showing weakness, stretching muscles and ligaments exhibiting shortening, maintaining fixation-free motion, nutritional concern, and assuring adequate innervation. Surgical reconstructure is rarely considered except in extreme cases.

These distortions of the knee underscore the need for early chiropractic preventive care, for many permanent genu distortions seen in adulthood could have been prevented by early treatment. Invariably, they begin as easy to correct fixations. For example, it will often be found during late childhood that genu varum (bowed leg) presents with fixation at the medial aspect of the femorotibial joint resulting in a compensatory hypermobility at the lateral condyle of the distal femur. This alteration in biomechanics tends to abduct the distal aspect of the femur.

Sitting habits are also contributory factors in the development of bowed legs. Children often sit on any type of support with their knees abducted, as if sitting on a barrel. Similarly, they often sit on the floor in a cross-legged manner. In both positions, the lateral aspect of the joints are stretched and the medial aspect of the joint are rarely mobilized.

In genu valgum (knock-knee), the converse is true. Here, mobility restriction will often be found at the lateral aspect of the femorotibial joint resulting in a compensatory hypermobility at the medial condyle of the distal femur. This alteration in biomechanics tends to adduct the distal end of the femur.

In bowed-legs, knock-knees, tibial rotation, or tibial torsion, associated patellar fixations are almost always the effect rather than the cause of the ipsilateral condylar hypomobility and contralateral hypermobility. This observation does not suggest that their release is not important to rehabilitation.

Significant Neurologic and Orthopedic Tests

Although most of the following tests were originally designed to bring out pathologic disturbances, many can also be used or modified slightly to elicit mobility fixations.

Anterior Drawer Sign. The anterior and posterior cruciate ligaments provide A-P stability to the knee joint. These intracapsular ligaments originate from the tibia and insert onto the inner aspects of the femoral condyles. To evaluate anterior stability, place the patient supine and flex the knees to 90° so that the feet are flat on the table. The examiner should sit sideways so that his hip can stabilize the patient's feet from moving during the tests. The examiner positions his hands around the knee being examined, similar to but lower than the bony palpation starting position; ie, thumbs pointing superiorly over the lateral and medial joint lines with fingers wrapped around the lateral and medial insertions of the hamstrings. In this position, the examiner pulls the tibia forward. When a distinct sliding forward of the tibia from under the femur is noted, it indicates a torn anterior cruciate ligament. Slight anterior sliding, however, is often normal. A positive sign should be confirmed by repeating the maneuver with the patient's leg internally rotated 30° and externally rotated 15°. The reason for this is that even if the anterior cruciate ligament (Fig. 9.16) is torn, external rotation should reduce forward movement of the tibia; if it does not, both the anterior cruciate and the anteromedial joint capsule may be torn. Likewise, even if the anterior cruciate ligament is torn, internal rotation should reduce forward movement of the tibia. If it does not, both the anterior cruciate and the anterolateral joint capsule may be torn. The medial collateral ligaments may also be involved in loss of A-P stability.

Posterior Drawer Sign. With the patient supine and the knees flexed, the stability of the posterior cruciate ligament is tested in the same manner as the anterior cruciate except the tibia of the flexed knee is pushed backward rather than pulled forward. Thus, it can be done in one continuous movement with the anterior drawer test. When a distinct sliding backward of the tibia from under the femur is noted, it indicates a torn posterior cruciate ligament. A posterior drawer sign is less common than its anterior counterpart.

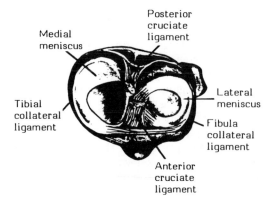

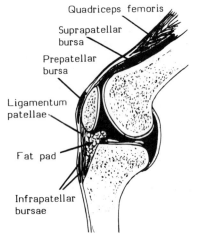

Figure 9.16. *Top,* schematic of the superior surface of the tibia showing the menisci. *Bottom,* schematic of the knee joint depicting the bursae and their structural relationships (Courtesy ACAP).

Helfet's Test. This test is designed to detect the presence of an intraarticular "loose body" that disturbs the normal biomechanics of the joint. To test normal knee locking, a dot is made with a skin pencil in the center of the patella and another is made over the tibial tubercle when the knee is flexed. The knee is then passively extended and the motion of the dot relative to the patella is observed. A positive Helfet test occurs when there is lack of full lateral movement of the dot. Palpation of the tibial tubercle during this passive test allows for more subtle determination of disturbed joint mechanics. Aside from intra-articular bodies, both a lack of rotational joint

play at the tibiofemoral articulation and imbalance in the tone of the internal and external rotators of the tibia could promote the pathomechanics observed during the test. It should also be noted that all but two of these muscles find their origin in the pelvis.

Q-Angle Sign. The patient is placed in the supine position with the knees extended in a relaxed position, and the quadriceps (Q) angle of the knee is measured. The Q-angle is formed by a line drawn along the long axis of the femur that is intersected by a line drawn through the center of the patella and the tibial tubercle (Fig. 9.17). To make a recording, a goniometer is centered on its side over the patella with one arm aimed at the ipsilateral ASIS and the other arm placed in line with the center of the patellar tendon. This angle is normally 10° in men and 15° in women. In external tibial rotation and/or genu varus, however, the Q-angle can be markedly increased; ie, the angle increases as the tibial tubercle is displaced laterally or when the distal femur and proximal tibia are angled toward the midline.

Anterolateral Rotary Instability Test. The leg of the supine patient is grasped with one hand and secured under the examiner's arm. The examiner's other hand is placed over the lateral proximal aspect of the patient's leg, and the leg is extended. A valgus stress is applied and the leg internally rotated as the knee is flexed. During flexion of the knee, the lateral tibial plateau can be felt to subluxate anteriorly in relation to the lateral condyle. The iliotibial tract tightens, lateral crepitation may be felt, and a slight resistance to flexion may be perceived. When the knee is in about 35° of flexion, the iliotibial band tightens, passes behind the transverse axis of rotation, and the tibial plateau is suddenly reduced, often with a "clunking" sensation both felt and heard.

Losee's Test. With the patient supine and the knee flexed, the examiner applies valgus stress to the tibia with one hand while the head of the fibula is pushed anterior with the other hand. If an anterior subluxation occurs at the lateral tibial plateau when the knee approaches full extension, anterolateral rotatory instability is indicated.

Hyperextension Stress Test. The patient is placed prone with the knees extended in

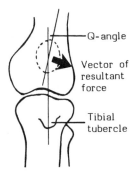

Figure 9.17. The Q-angle (Courtesy ACAP).

the relaxed position. The examiner places a fist under the distal thigh of the involved side, flexes the patient's knee to about 30° with the other hand, and then allows the leg to drop without assistance when the muscles are relaxed. Most knee lesions limit extension to some degree. Thus, if extension is limited or the rebound is abnormal during this "knee drop" test (as compared to the contralateral knee), some type of knee disorder should be suspected and may possibly be localized.

Hyperflexion Stress Test. With the patient in the supine position, the examiner places one hand on the involved knee and the other on the ipsilateral ankle. The patient's knee is moderately flexed, the thigh is brought towards the patient's abdomen, and the patient's heel is slowly pushed toward the patient's buttock. Unless the patient is considerably obese, the normal knee can be flexed without pain so that it touches the buttock. If knee pain or severe discomfort is induced by this maneuver, a subtle localized knee lesion may be brought out.

Lateral Stability Stress Tests. The collateral ligaments provide medial and lateral stability to the knee joint (Fig. 9.18). To examine sideward stability, the patient is placed supine and the knee is flexed just enough to free it from extension. To test the integrity of the medial collateral ligament, valgus stress is applied to open the knee joint on the medial side. The lateral collateral ligament is tested by applying stress to open the knee joint on the lateral side. In these maneuvers, the ankle is secured with one hand, the other hand is placed on the opposite side of the knee of the ligaments being tested, and pres-

sure is applied toward the ligaments being tested. More knowledge can be gained, however, if the examiner locks the patient's ankle between his arm and chest and uses this hand to palpate the ligaments in question and the underlying joint gap during the test.

External Rotation-Recurvatum Test. The patient is placed supine, and the examiner grasps the patient's heel with one hand and supports the calf with the other hand. The knee is allowed to pass from about 10° flexion into full extension. A positive test occurs when the knee assumes a position of slight recurvatum, the tibia rotates externally, and there is increased tibia vara. Such a sign indicates injury to the arcuate complex, lateral half of the posterior capsule, and a degree of injury to the posterior cruciate ligament.

Posterolateral Rotary Instability Test. Posterolateral rotary instability arises from a posterior subluxation of the lateral tibial plateau in relation to the lateral femoral condyle, accompanied by abnormal external tibial rotation. To test for posterolateral rotary instability, the external rotation-recurvatum and a posterior drawer test are performed. Excessive posterior sag of the lateral tibial plateau with external tibial rotation should be noted. This type of instability results from laxity of the arcuate complex, the lateral half of the posterior capsule, and a degree of failure of the posterior cruciate ligament.

Wilson's Sign. The patient is placed supine with the legs in an extended, relaxed position. This is a two-phase test: (1) The knee of the involved side is flexed to a right

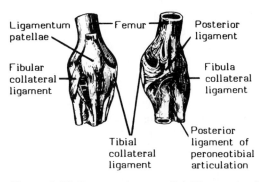

Figure 9.18. Some major superficial ligaments of the knee area. *Left,* anterior view; *right,* posterior view (Courtesy ACAP).

angle, the leg is firmly rotated internally, and then the knee is slowly extended while maintaining the leg in internal rotation. If osteochondritis of the knee is present, the patient will complain of pain in front of the medial condyle of the distal femur. (2) However, if the leg is then externally rotated, the pain will subside.

Effusion Test. If a joint is greatly swollen from a major effusion, the patient is placed in a relaxed supine position. The limb is relaxed, and the knee is slowly extended. The patella is then pushed into the trochlear groove and released quickly. This will force fluid under the patella to the sides of the joint and then to return under the patella. This rebound is referred to as a *ballottable patella.* Minimal effusion, however, will not ballot the patella. In cases of minor effusion, it is necessary to "milk" the fluid from the suprapatellar pouch and lateral side to the medial side of the joint. Once the fluid has been moved medially, tapping over the fluid will return it to the lateral side. Refer to Figure 9.16.

Meniscus Tests

Apley's Compression Test. The patient is placed prone with one leg flexed to 90°. The examiner stabilizes the patient's thigh with a knee and grasps the patient's foot. Downward pressure is applied to the foot to compress the medial and lateral menisci between the tibia and femur (Fig. 9.19). The examiner then rotates the tibia internally and externally on the femur, holding downward pressure. Pain during this maneuver indicates probable meniscal or collateral damage. Medial knee pain suggests medial meniscus damage; lateral pain, lateral meniscus injury.

Apley's Distraction Test. Apley designed this test to follow the compression test as an aid in differentiating meniscal from ligamentous knee problems. With the patient and the examiner in the same position as in the compression test, the examiner applies traction (rather than compression) while the leg is rotated internally and externally. This maneuver reduces pressure upon the menisci but stretches the medial and lateral ligaments of the knee.

Bounce-Home Test. The patient is placed supine. The examiner cups one hand under patient's heel and slightly flexes the patient's knee with the other hand. While the patient's heel is held, the patient's knee is allowed to passively drop gently toward the top of the table in full extension, normally with an abrupt stop. If this full extension is not achieved and passive pressure elicits a "rubbery" resistance to extension, a motion block is indicated. This lack of full extension points to a torn meniscus, intracapsular swelling, or a loose fragment within the knee joint.

Childress' Test. This is a two-phase test: (1) The patient is asked to stand with the feet separated about 12—18 inches apart, assume a "knock-kneed" position by rotating the thighs inward, and then attempt to squat as low as possible. Pain, joint restriction, or a clicking sensation suggests a lesion of the medial meniscus. (2) The test is then conducted with the patient assuming a "bowed-leg" position by rotating the thighs outward before squatting. Pain, joint restriction, or a clicking sensation when attempting

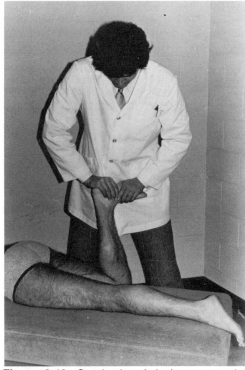

Figure 9.19. Conducting Apley's compression test (Courtesy ACAP).

to squat suggests a lesion of the lateral meniscus.

Steinmann's Sign. In meniscus disorders, tenderness moves posteriorly when the knee is flexed and anteriorly when the knee is extended. This displacement of tenderness is said not to occur in degenerative osteoarthrosis.

McIntosh's Test. The patient is placed supine, the lower extremity is supported at the heel with one hand, and the other hand is placed laterally over the proximal tibia just distal to the patella. The examiner's caudad hand applies valgus stress and internally rotates the tibia as the knee is gradually moved from full extension into flexion. During flexion of the knee, the lateral tibial plateau can be felt to subluxate anteriorly in relation to the lateral condyle. Lateral crepitation may be felt, and a slight resistance to flexion may be perceived. When the knee is at about 35° flexion, the iliotibial band tightens, passes behind the transverse axis of rotation, and the tibial plateau is suddenly reduced, often with a "clunking" sensation that can often be both felt and heard.

Hughston's Jerk Sign. This is a modification of McIntosh's test. With the patient supine, the foot is grasped with one hand while the other hand rests over the proximal lateral aspect of the leg just distal to the patella. The knee is flexed to 90°, and valgus stress is applied as the tibia is rotated internally. The knee is then gradually extended. The lateral tibial plateau is initially in a reduced position to the femoral condyle; however, as the knee is extended to about 35° of flexion, the lateral tibial plateau suddenly subluxates forward in relation to the femoral condyle with a jerking sensation. The lateral plateau slowly obtains its reduced position, which completes on full extension as the knee is extended.

Slocum's Test. This is another modification of McIntosh's test. The patient is placed in the lateral recumbent position with the involved knee uppermost. The under extremity is flexed at 90° at both the hip and knee. The pelvis is rotated slightly posterior about 30°, and the weight of the extremity is supported by the inner aspect of the foot and heel. This position causes valgus stress at the knee and a slight internal rotation of the leg. The examiner then grips the distal thigh with one hand and the proximal leg with the other hand and presses back of the fibula and femoral condyle with the thumbs. The knee is then gently pushed from extension into flexion and, as the iliotibial tract passes behind the transverse axis of rotation at about 35°, the lateral tibial plateau, which has subluxated forward, is reduced with a palpable "clunk" or "giving way" sensation.

McMurray's Test. In this two-part test, the patient is placed supine with the thigh and leg flexed until the heel approaches the buttock. One hand of the examiner is placed on the patient's knee, the other hand on the patient's ankle. The examiner internally rotates the patient's leg, then slowly extends the leg. Then the examiner externally rotates the leg and slowly extends the leg. The test is positive if at some point in the arc a painful click or snap is heard. This sign can be significant of meniscus injury. The point in the arc where the snap is heard locates the site of injury of the meniscus; eg, if noted with internal rotation, the lateral meniscus will be involved. The higher the leg is raised when the snap is heard, the more posterior the lesion is in the meniscus. If noted with external rotation, the medial meniscus will usually be involved. Unfortunately, false positive and false negative signs are not uncommon.

Dynamic Palpation and Releasing Fixations

Femorotibial Joint Motion Restrictions

When examining joint motion in the knee, special care must be taken that normal motion is not confused with the exaggerated motion resulting from joint instability.

Distraction Fixation. With the patient prone, stand perpendicular to the involved knee. Flex the patient's knee to a right angle, place your cephalad knee gently in the patient's popliteal space to stabilize the patient's femur, grasp the patient's leg distally (proximal to the ankle) with both hands, and apply an upward pulling force directed through the vertical axis of the tibia. If mobility is restricted, add a short dynamic impulse.

Restricted A-P Glide. Faye recommends that the patient be placed supine with the hip on the involved side flexed to a right angle. Place your foot on the table so that the patient's calf may rest on your thigh (Fig. 9.20). Keep the patient's knee flexed at 90°, and then push down on the neck of the tibia to test end play. This procedure will test A-P glide but not P-A glide. If A-P motion restriction is perceived, remove soft-tissue slack and apply a short dynamic impulse against the fixation.

Restricted P-A Glide. With the patient supine, flex the involved hip and knee so that the plantar surface of the patient's foot rests firmly on the table. Sit on the table, obliquely facing the patient, so that your cephalad thigh rests lightly against the patient's foot for stabilization. Grasp the proximal tibia and fibula with both hands as to elicit a drawer sign, and then apply a pulling force directed toward your sternum (Fig. 9.21). If a mobility restriction is found, hold the trac-

tion for several seconds, and then add a short dynamic impulse (pull). Faye adapts this maneuver to use with the patient prone.

A common home therapy is to have the sitting or supine patient bring the involved flexed knee toward the abdomen after inserting a rolled towel against the popliteal space, grasp the anterior surface of the leg distally with both hands, and apply firm pressure (directed toward the buttock) several times.

Restricted Internal or External Rotation. With the patient supine, flex the knee to be tested to a right angle, and rest the patient's calf on your thigh. Grasp the patient's lower leg with your active hand, and palpate the lateral and medial aspects of the knee joint simultaneously with the thumb and index finger of your stabilizing hand (Fig. 9.22). Rotate the tibia internally and then externally. Note the degree of end play. If mobility is restricted, add a short dynamic rotatory impulse at the end of free motion.

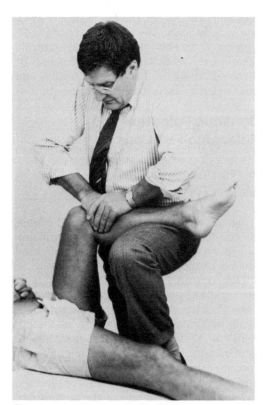

Figure 9.20. Position for evaluating A-P glide of the tibia on the femur with the patient supine.

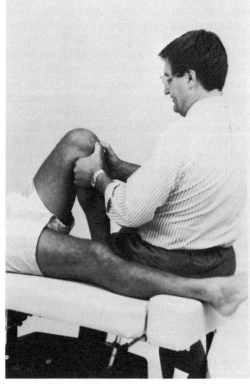

Figure 9.21. Position for evaluating P-A glide of the tibia on the femur with the patient supine.

Two additional technics are described below:

1. As a general maneuver with the patient in the testing position, grasp the proximal aspect of the tibia in both hands, rotate the tibia against the fixation, and then circumduct the tibia on the femur in clockwise and counterclockwise directions.

2. The following technic is beneficial when a more forceful technic is indicated. The doctor and patient positions are similar to those described above except that a towel is inserted between your knee and the distal aspect of the patient's thigh. The patient is then instructed to grasp his thigh near the knee and apply a pull during the correction. Wrap your medial arm around and under the patient's lower leg, so that it is firmed in an arm lock, and grasp your lateral elbow. Your other forearm will be adducted across your chest so that you can grip your medial arm. In this position, you can firmly rotate the patient's tibia internally or externally by laterally bending your trunk to the left or right. Apply pressure against the resistance,

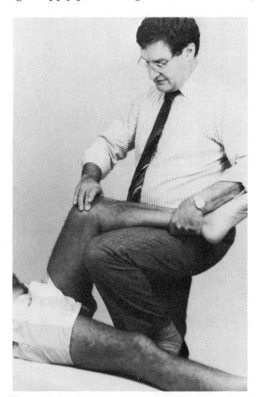

Figure 9.22. Position for evaluating internal and external rotation of the left tibia on the femur.

add traction, and then impulse to release the fixation. This is a forceful adjustment, described by Schultz, that is usually considered contraindicated in the elderly or very young.

Restricted Medial or Lateral Horizontal Glide. Place the patient supine with the involved knee slightly flexed. Stand perpendicular to the involved knee, crouch down, slip your caudad hand under the proximal aspect of the patient's tibia, and grasp the medial surface of the patient's leg just below the knee joint. Place the palm of your other hand against the lateral surface of the patient's thigh just above the knee joint. In this position, you will be able to pull the patient's tibia laterally with one hand while you push the patient's femur medially with your other hand to test horizontal glide (shear) in one direction. Reverse the positions of your hands to test horizontal glide in the other direction. A correction is made by testing and then applying a short impulse against the fixation. See Figure 9.23.

Restricted Medial or Lateral Side Tilt. Place the patient supine with the knee slightly flexed. Note that there is no perceptible knee tilt when the knee is in full extension (locked). Steady the patient's femur with one hand and toggle the tibia medially and laterally by abducting and adducting the distal aspect of the patient's leg. Positive joint end play should be perceived during both abduction and adduction of the leg on the thigh. If a springy end feel is absent, the adjustment is performed as follows: When tilt is absent medially, bring the patient's moderately flexed knee into full extension while simultaneously applying pressure against the inside of the patient's lower leg. If tilt is absent laterally, bring the patient's moderately flexed knee into full extension while simultaneously applying pressure against the outside of the patient's lower leg. This adjustment can easily be adapted as an alternative adjustment for restricted medial or lateral horizontal glide.

Menisical Displacements

On occasion, a patient will exhibit a locked knee in which either the medial or lateral meniscus is displaced. In such cases, the joint should be manipulated to create extension and medial or lateral deviation to allow the respective meniscus an opportunity to "reduce" spontaneously. A medial displacement is corrected by impulsing to the medial side of the knee from the lateral side as the knee is allowed to drop into extension.

Failure to unlock or repeated relocking is an indication for surgical correction. Recovery time, if there is no need for surgery, is slow even with the most cooperative and exercise-conscious patient.

If a meniscus displaces as a whole, manipulative correction is usually successful. However, if the meniscus is fragmented, surgical referral should be discussed with the patient as locking will usually tend to recur with progressing frequency. However, it is difficult to determine whether fragmentation exists by physical means.

Faye feels that recent studies will soon cause a change in the general interpretation of knee tests; ie, it has been observed that "overreading" signs is commonplace. "Manip-

ulation and rational physiologic therapeutics followed by exercise should and will prevent much unnecessary surgery."

Patella Fixations

The patella is a "free-floating" sesamoid. Thus, no true end point will be perceived as in a synovial joint nor can there be a true "articular" fixation. Soft-tissue (partial) fixations are common, however.

Patellofemoral Joint Motion Restrictions

When the knee is locked in full extension, patellar mobility normally exhibits free excursion superiorly, medially, inferiorly, laterally, and diagonally, and in circumduction. Only superior (cephalad) excursion is under voluntary control (quadriceps contraction).

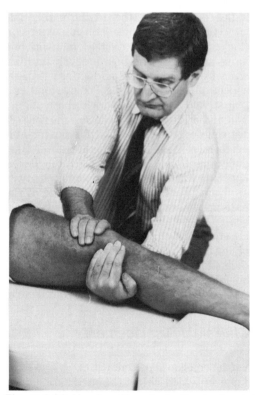 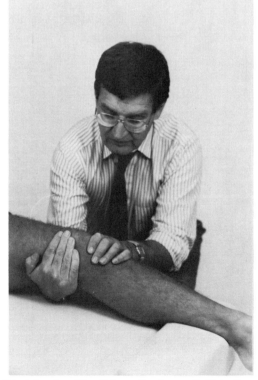

Figure 9.23. Hand positions for testing horizontal glide laterally of the tibia on the femur (*left*); testing horizontal glide medially of the tibia on the femur (*right*).

If any of these movements are lost, knee function is disabled. Thus, patella mobility must be assured prior to any attempt to release a knee fixation. Correction is made by applying a short impulse against the restricted plane. Some clinicians use a web contact, others apply a thumb and index finger contact, and still others prefer a double-thumb contact. If strong restriction is felt during excursion inferiorly, quadriceps stretching exercises are usually indicated.

Significant Clinical Tests

Clarke's Sign. The supine patient extends the knee and relaxes the quadriceps. The examiner places the web of a hand against the superior aspect of the patella and depresses it distally. The patient then actively contracts the quadriceps as the examiner compresses the patella against the condyles of the distal femur. The sign is positive if the patient cannot maintain contraction without producing sharp pain.

Fouchet's Test. The patient is placed supine with the limbs extended in the relaxed position. If firm pressure on the patella produces pain and focal tenderness at the margin of the patella, chondromalacia of the patella should be suspected.

Patella Apprehension Sign. The patella displaces laterally with vigorous quadriceps contraction. When a person strongly extends the flexed knee with the leg externally rotated, the patella may dislocate if its attachments are weakened. If a patella is prone to dislocation, any attempt by the examiner to produce such a dislocation will be met with by sharp patient resistance. In testing, the patient is placed in the relaxed neutral supine position, and the examiner applies increasing pressure against the patella. If a chronic weakness exists, the patient will become increasing apprehensive as the patella begins to dislocate.

Patella Wobble Sign. A patient in the sitting position is instructed to extend a knee while the examiner cups a palm over the patella. If erratic patellar motion is felt during the last phase of extension, an irregular retropatellar growth or some type of incomplete obstruction is indicated (eg, hypertrophied infrapatellar synovial folds, hardened fat pad).

Perkin's Tests. The patient is placed in a relaxed supine position. The examiner locks the top of the patella between the thumb and first finger and applies pressure towards the patient's foot while the patient is asked to tighten the quadriceps by hyperextending the knee. As the patella moves proximally, its movement should be smooth and gliding. An alternative method is for the examiner to place a firm double hand contact over the anterior knee, lean over the limb, and displace the patella from side to side while simultaneously applying pressure from the anterior to the posterior. Induced pain, grating, or crepitation (palpable or audible) during this maneuver is a positive sign, suggesting roughening as in chondromalacia patellae, osteochondral defects, or when degenerative changes within the trochlear groove occur (eg, retropatella arthritis).

Proximal Tibiofibular Joint Motion Restrictions

Gillet reports that proximal tibiofibular fixation is quite common. Normally, the joint between the proximal heads of the tibia and fibula opens slightly when the foot is inverted. This gap can be palpated just inferolaterally to the patellar tendon. In addition, the head of the fibula will shift slightly cephalad when the foot is actively dorsiflexed. These movements will not be felt if the joint is locked; ie, the knee must be at least slightly flexed. Gillet reports that "fixation at this joint is often linked to an L5 or sacral subluxation." Faye reminds us that Gillet's use of the term *subluxation* here means lumbosacral or sacroiliac fixation or inflammation due to hypermobile overstress.

Mennell states that the only joint-play movement at the tibiofibular joint is A-P glide: maximum at knee midflexion, minimal at full knee extension. Gillet, as mentioned, includes a perceptible inferior to superior glide.

Tibiofibular A-P Glide. Place the patient supine, flex the knee to be tested to an angle that would allow the patient's foot to rest flat against the table. Clasp the patient's proximal fibula between your thumb and index finger, and pull and push the fibula forward and backward (Fig. 9.24). It should move easily. If mobility is restricted, add a dynamic impulse at the end of free motion. During the adjustment, it is usually beneficial to reinforce your contact finger or thumb.

An alternative technic when mobility is restricted P-A is to position the patient prone, flex the knee to a right angle, and apply the index finger of a flattened hand contact as close as possible against the head of the fibula. Push deep within the lateral aspect of the popliteal space. Deliver a short impulse directed anteriorly while moderately flexing the patient's leg over your contact hand. The features of this type of fixation, states Faye, are sometimes confused with shin splints.

Inferior to Superior Glide. Position the patient supine with the knee to be tested extended. Place one or more palpating fingers as close as possible to the proximal fibulotibial articulation. With your other hand, dorsiflex the patient's ipsilateral foot (Fig. 9.25). Normally, a slight motion should be perceived; ie, the head of the fibula translating cephalad. If fixation is found, add a short

dynamic impulse against the plantar surface of the dorsiflexed foot that is directed up the shaft of the fibula.

If the distal fibulotibial joint is lax, the above technic will tend to drive the distal fibula inferiorly on the tibia rather than the proximal fibula superiorly. Thus, it might be more efficient to alter the technic. Schafer places the patient in the lateral recumbent position with the involved limb upward. A reinforced pisiform contact is applied to the inferior aspect of the patient's external malleolus, and the impulse is directed, in a plane almost parallel to the table, cephalad through the shaft of the fibula.

THE ANKLES

For most clinical purposes, the lower leg, ankle, and foot can be considered to work as a dynamic unit. The ankle itself is a complex hinge joint.

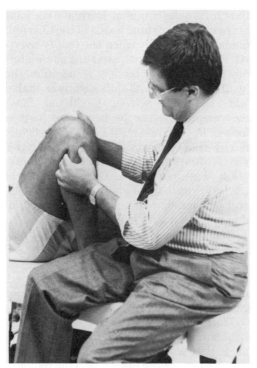

Figure 9.24. Evaluating glide of the proximal aspect of the fibula on the tibia with the patient supine.

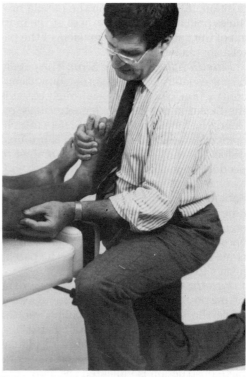

Figure 9.25. Testing inferior to superior glide of the proximal aspect of the fibula on the tibia.

The anatomical point where the ankle stops and the foot begins is a subject of varying opinions. Most authorities report that the ankle is formed by the tibia, fibula, and talus, with the subjacent foot including all structures distal to the talus.

Biomechanical Considerations

Body weight is transmitted downward from the knee through the tibia to the ankle and foot in the upright position, and the forces generated are greatly multiplied during walking, running, jumping, etc. Thus, the ankle and foot are uniquely affected by traumatic forces from above and below and static deformities infrequently seen in other areas of the body.

The stability of the complex series of joints that comprise the ankle and foot is primarily maintained by an expansive network of ligaments. In comparison to the knee, the integrated biomechanical actions within the ankle and foot are complex. The reader should refer to specific texts on the subject.

Diagnostic Considerations: Ankle Pain

Motion palpation of the ankles is usually conducted immediately following the standard orthopedic/neurologic examination, including gross range of motion evaluation, muscle strength grading, reflexes, and light touch and pain perception.

Common causes of ankle pain are shown in Table 9.6. The patient's history, localization of pain and tenderness, evidence of swelling, motion limitation, surface temperature, hemotologic findings, and associated systemic signs will aid differentiation.

Significant Neurologic and Orthopedic Tests

Toe-In Sign. Excessive toe-in, especially in children, may be the result of excessive internal rotation of the tibia caused by a fixed point at either end of the tibia. Common points of fixation are at the malleoli in the ankle or the tibial tubercle below the knee. The ankle mortise normally faces 15° externally; in internal tibial torsion, the ankle mortise faces anteriorly or internally.

Draw Sign. Tears of the anterior tibiofibular (talofibular) ligament produce joint instability, allowing the talus to slide forward (subluxate) on the tibia. To test for instability and subluxation of the tibia and talus, place one hand on the anterior aspect of the sitting patient's lower tibia and grip the heel within your other palm. When the calcaneus and talus are pulled anteriorly and the tibia is simultaneously pushed posteriorly, the anterior tibiofibular ligament should allow no forward movement of the talus on the tibia. The test is positive if the talus slides anteriorly from under the cover of the ankle mortise. Sometimes the abnormal bone move-

Table 9.6. Common Causes of Ankle Pain

Acute Pain	*Chronic Pain*
Arthritis/synovitis	Acquired Flatfoot
Bone bruise	Congenital fault (eg, calcaneovalgus)
Contusion	Degenerative joint disease
Dislocation	Fixation
Fracture	Peripheral vascular disease
Osteomyelitis	Postural foot disorder
Strain/sprain	Rheumatoid arthritis
Talar osteochondritis	Spur
Tarsal tunnel syndrome	Tuberculosis
Tendinitis	Tumor (rare)

ment can be heard as well as felt during the maneuver.

Dorsiflexion Test. Limitation of the gastrocnemius or soleus muscle restricting ankle dorsiflexion can be differentiated by this test. Have the patient sit on the examining table with the knees flexed and relaxed. Grasp the foot and flex the knee to slacken the gastrocnemius, then dorsiflex the ankle. If this can be achieved, the gastrocnemius is the cause of the restriction. If the soleus is at fault, it will not be affected by knee flexion; ie, it will be the same in either knee flexion or extension.

Talar Slide Test. This test evaluates ankle joint play (translation) in the horizontal plane. With the patient in either the prone or supine position, the doctor stands to the side and faces the ankle to be tested. The examiner's cephalad hand grasps the patient's lower leg just above the malleoli and the caudad hand grasps the heel just below the malleoli. A pull is made with the upper hand on the lower leg while the lower hand pushes the heel horizontally. Then a push is made with the upper hand while the lower hand pulls the heel horizontally. Excessive lateral or medial motion with pain indicates ligamentous instability. See Figure 9.26.

Lateral-Medial (Eversion-Inversion) Stability Tests. Gross lateral instability re-sults when both the anterior tibiofibular and calcaneofibular ligaments are torn (Fig. 9.27). To test lateral stability, stabilize the patient's leg and invert the heel back and forth, noting if the talus rocks loosely in the ankle mortise. Medial instability is the result of a tear or stretch of the deltoid ligament. To test medial stability, stabilize the patient's leg and evert the heel back and forth, noting any gapping at the ankle mortise.

Repetitive Heel Raise Test. The standing patient is asked to raise the heels (ie, toe stand) repetitively several times. If this induces ankle pain and/or instability, a posterior compartment syndrome or a subluxation complex should be suspected. When this exercise is unable to be performed because of weakness and ankle pain is absent, a gastrocnemius weakness or neurologic deficit should be suspected.

Beery's Sign. This sign is positive if a patient with a history of lower trunk discomfort and fatigue is fairly comfortable when sitting with the knees flexed but experiences discomfort in the standing position. It is typically seen in spasticity or contractures of the posterior thigh and/or leg muscles.

Claudication Test. If lower extremity claudication is suspected, the patient is instructed to walk on a treadmill at a rate of 120 steps per minute. If cramping, and sometimes a skin color change, occurs, the approximate level of the local lesion can be identified. The time span between the beginning of the test and the occurrence of symptoms is used to record the "claudication time," which is usually recorded in seconds.

Thompson's Test. To detect a rupture of the Achilles tendon, the patient kneels on a chair with the feet extended over the edge. The middle third of the calf is squeezed. If the Achilles tendon is ruptured, especially the soleus portion, the squeeze will not cause the normal plantar flexion response.

Simmond's Test. The patient is placed prone and the knee is flexed to a right angle. The examiner grasps the center of the leg with both hands and applies strong pressure so that the calf muscles are squeezed against the tibia and fibula. Normally, the foot will plantarflex slightly; if not, a ruptured Achilles tendon is indicated. This test is a common variant of Thompson's test.

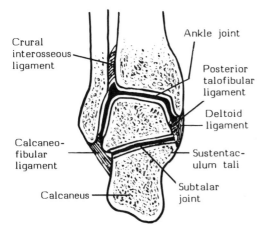

Figure 9.26. Coronal section through the left ankle joint viewed from the posterior (Courtesy ACAP).

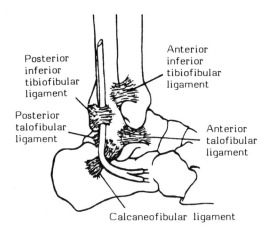

Figure 9.27. Schematic of some major ligaments of the ankle viewed laterally (Courtesy ACAP).

Tarsal Tunnel Syndrome

Tinel's Foot Test. With the patient prone and the knee flexed to a right angle, the posterior tibial nerve is percussed as it passes behind the lateral malleolus. If this induces paresthesias in the foot, tarsal tunnel syndrome is indicated.

Ankle Tourniquet Test. A sphygmomanometer cuff is wrapped around the suspected ankle, inflated to a point slightly above the patient's systolic blood pressure, and maintained for 1—2 minutes. An increase in foot pain suggests tarsal tunnel syndrome or a similar circulatory deficit.

Dynamic Palpation and Correction

Ankle Fixations: General Considerations

Two primary areas of possible motion restriction exist in the ankle area: above and below the talus. The talus is the key structure in the ankle. It supports the weight of the tibia superiorly, articulates with the non-weight-bearing fibula laterally, and rests primarily on the anterior two-thirds of the calcaneus inferiorly.

The Distal Tibiofibular Joint

A-P/P-A Glide. Place the patient in the lateral recumbent position with the ankle to be tested upward, and stand perpendicular to the patient's ankles. To judge A-P mobility, grasp the patient's involved heel with your caudad hand and the distal aspect of the patient's lower leg with your cephalad hand. Place both of your thumbs against the anterior surface of the patient's external malleolus, and push forward to test A-P mobility of the distal aspect of the fibula on the tibia (Fig. 9.28). To test P-A mobility, move your fingers so that their tips can be placed against the posterior aspect of the external malleolus and pull forward. If a mobility restriction is felt, remove soft-tissue slack and add a short dynamic impulse. If more force is necessary to release P-A mobility than can be obtained with the fingertips, move to the opposite side of the table, apply a double thumb

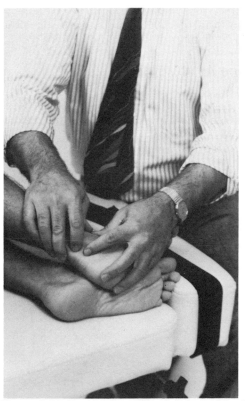

Figure 9.28. Position for testing A-P/P-A glide of the distal fibula on the tibia.

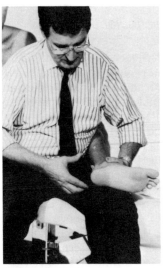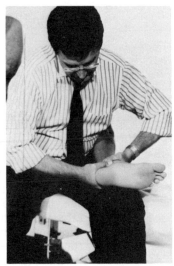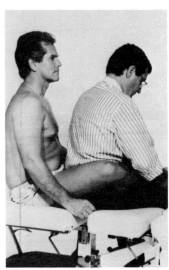

Figure 9.29. Position for evaluating and releasing long-axis extension of the left ankle mortise. *Left,* positioning the patient's ankle; *center,* applying the contacts; *right,* doctor and patient positions shown from a right lateral view.

contact against the external malleolus, and direct your impulse anteriorly. Fixations of the distal tibiofibular joint are often involved in complaints of knee and deep foot pain.

The Ankle Mortise

Being a hinge joint, the ankle mortise is designed to allow primarily plantar flexion and dorsiflexion. Only a slight amount of rotation is normally allowed.

Long-Axis Extension. Test ankle mortise distraction with the patient's hip and knee

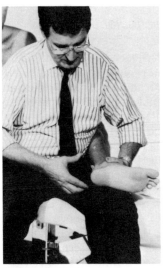

Figure 9.30. The subtalar joint can be likened to a mitered hinge joint (Courtesy ACAP).

flexed to a right angle. Grip the patient's heel and talus in both hands while sitting with your back against the patient's thigh (Fig. 9.29). Push the patient's foot away to distract the ankle. You should feel the mortise separate. If not, add a short dynamic impulse.

A-P/P-A Glide. Position the patient supine on the table with hip and knee flexed and the ipsilateral heel firmly resting against the tabletop. With the patient's foot at a right angle to the patient's leg, toggle the tibia backward to test A-P glide and forward to test P-A glide. If mobility restriction is found, add a corrective impulse.

The Subtalar Joint

Subtalar joint motion occurs about an axis that lies oblique to the three axes around which usual ankle flexion-extension, abduction-adduction, and rotation occur (Fig. 9.30). Long-axis extension, talar rock on the calcaneus, medial tilt, and lateral tilt are the primary considerations in the subtalar joint.

Talar Rock. Talar rock should not be confused with plantar flexion of the mortise joint. With the patient supine, support the foot to be tested from the plantar surface and push the tibia downward to produce full plantar flexion, then push further to increase plantar flexion by producing talar rock (Fig. 9.31). A corrective adjustment to release restricted P-A glide is made with the patient prone, thrusting downward on the calcaneus.

Long-Axis Extension. Distraction within the subtalar joints is evaluated in a manner similar to that described for the mortise joint (Fig. 9.32). It is actually a summation effect. The adjustment is also similar except the contact hands are placed to affect the more distal joints.

Medial and Lateral Side Tilt. With the patient supine, cup the calcaneus in both hands and apply inversion and eversion forces to test medial and lateral side tilt (Fig. 9.33). To release immobility, hold the heel in one hand, take up all soft-tissue slack, invert or evert the heel as is necessary, and apply a short dynamic impulse (Fig. 9.34).

Talocalcaneal Glide. To test P-A glide of the calcaneus on the distal tibia, stand perpendicular to the limb being examined, grasp the distal aspect of the patient's leg with your

cephalad stabilizing hand, and cup the patient's heel in your active caudad hand (Fig. 9.35). Pull upward with your active hand while maintaining pressure against the patient's leg with your stabilizing hand. Reverse the shearing forces to test A-P glide.

Achilles Tendinitis

A palpable tender area about the size of a quarter that is located 2 inches above the heel suggests Achilles tendinitis. The inflammation, which usually incorporates a tendosynovitis, can occur from overuse, calcaneal or talocalcaneal dysfunction, lack of warm-up prior to exercise, ill-fitting shoes, and direct trauma against the tendon. Foot and ankle manipulation, ice massage, low-volt currents, stretching with the knee slightly flexed, and PNF are usually beneficial.

THE FEET

The bony complex of a foot incorporates 27 articulations. The forefoot consists of the five metatarsals and the phalanges. The midfoot consists of the cuneiform, navicular, and cuboid bones. The hindfoot (rearfoot) includes the talus and calcaneus. See Figure 9.36.

The causes of foot pain may be traumatic (eg, posttraumatic dysfunction), inflammatory, neuropathic, circulatory, or postural. Common etiologies are shown in Table 9.7.

Biomechanical Considerations

The bones of the feet provide the foundation for the kinematic chain that extends from the occiput to the soles of the feet. Thus, the articulations of the foot and ankle serve an important role in holistic biomechanical integrity. See Figure 9.37.

The foot and ankle combine a complex series of joints and controlling forces and integrate them to meet the demands of static and dynamic situations. The segments of the foot and ankle must be flexible enough (free of fixation) to accommodate to different surfaces yet be stiff enough to provide

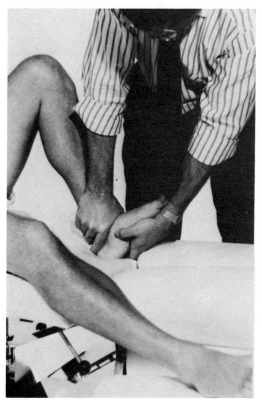

Figure 9.31. Conducting the talar rock test.

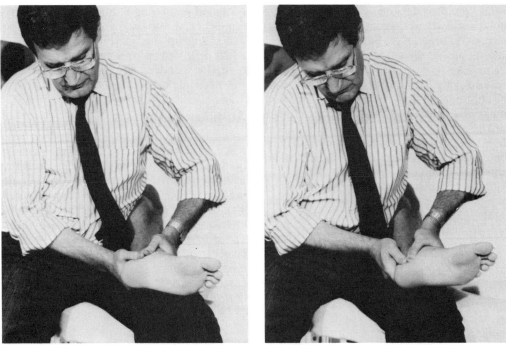

Figure 9.32. Position for evaluating subtalar long-axis extension. *Left,* securing the contacts; *right,* applying long-axis extension.

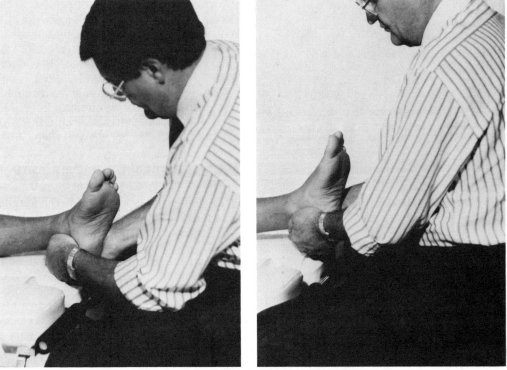

Figure 9.33. Positions for evaluating subtalar medial and lateral side tilt.

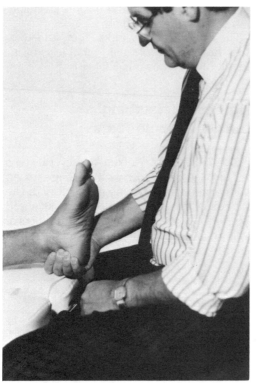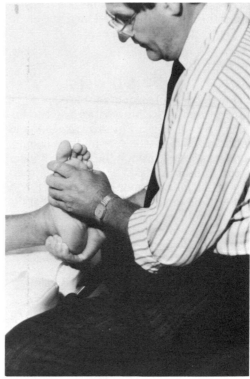

Figure 9.34. Positions for releasing restricted medial and lateral subtalar side tilt.

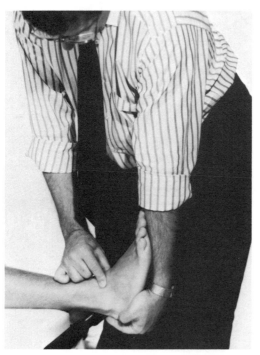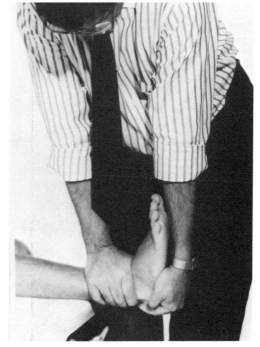

Figure 9.35. Position for evaluating talocalcaneal glide.

the required torque for locomotion. Disruption of the mechanics of the kinematic chain leads to pathologic function.

Terminology

Descriptors of foot motion have yet to be standardized. Most authorities use the following terminology: *Plantar flexion* and *dorsiflexion* (Fig. 9.38) are motions about a horizontal axis (through the ankle) that lies in the frontal plane. *Eversion* means rotation about an axis running in the A-P/P-A plane of the foot. *Adduction* of the foot occurs around a vertical axis. *Pronation* refers to combined dorsiflexion, eversion, and abduction of the foot; and *supination* is the

result of combined plantar flexion, inversion, and adduction of the foot.

The muscles of the ankle, foot, and toes, their functions, and their spinal level of innervation are shown in Table 9.8.

Significant Neurologic and Orthopedic Tests

Toe Walk Test. Walking for several steps on the base of the toes with the heels raised will normally produce no discomfort to the patient. With the exception of a localized forefoot disorder (eg, plantar wart, neuroma) or an anterior leg syndrome (eg, shin splints), an inability to do this because of low

Table 9.7. Common Causes of Foot Pain

Rearfoot Pain

Achilles strain/tendinitis	Fracture
Apophysitis	Plantar fascitis
Bursitis	Spur

Midfoot Pain

Fixation	Sprain/strain
Flat-foot syndrome	Subluxation
Fracture	Subtalar arthritis
Köhler's disease	Tarsal coalition
Plantaris rupture	

Forefoot Pain

Cellulitis	Morton's neuroma
Corn	Peripheral neuropathy
Degenerative joint disease	Phlebitis
Fixation	Plantar neuroma
Freiberg's disease	Plantar wart
Gout	Subluxation
Metatarsalgia	Synovitis

Toe Pain

Blister	Hammer toe
Corns	Osteochondritis
Fixation	Peripheral vascular disease
Fracture/dislocation	Strain/sprain
Hallux rigidus/valgus/varus	Subluxation

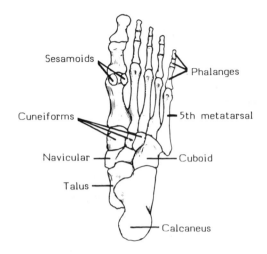

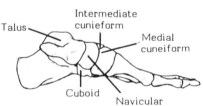

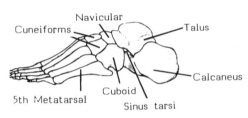

Figure 9.36. *Top,* bones of the foot and ankle viewed from above; *center,* the foot viewed laterally; *bottom,* the foot viewed medially (Courtesy ACAP).

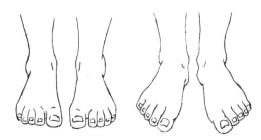

Figure 9.37. *Left,* normal foot alignment; *right,* excessive toe-out, which may be either the cause or the effect of chronic ankle pronation (Courtesy ACAP).

back pain or weakness can suggest an S1—S2 lesion.

Heel Walk Test. A patient should normally be able to walk several steps on the heels with the forefoot dorsiflexed. With the exception of a localized heel disorder (eg, calcaneal spur) or contracted calf muscles, an inability to do this because of low back pain or weakness can suggest a L5 lesion.

Plantar Tension Test. The patient is placed supine and the involved foot and toes are dorsiflexed so that the plantar fascia is tensed. If pain occurs or if bead-like swellings and irregularities are found as the examiner deeply runs his thumb vertically along the plantar surface, plantar fascitis is suggested.

Strunsky's Test. This test is designed essentially for the recognition of lesions of the metatarsal arch. See Figures 9.39 and 9.40. Under normal conditions when the toes are grasped and quickly flexed, the procedure is painless. Pain results if there is any inflammatory lesion of the metatarsal arch. This test is often positive in tendinitis of the toe extensors.

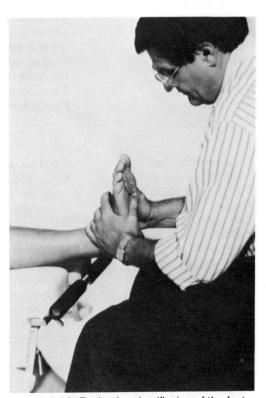

Figure 9.38. Evaluating dorsiflexion of the foot.

Metatarsus Varus Sign. With the patient seated on a table with the knees relaxed and flexed at 90°, note the posture of the relaxed bare foot. The lateral border of the foot will appear convex and the medial border concave if metatarsus varus is present.

Morton's Test. This test is positive when deep transverse pressure across the heads of the metatarsals, especially between the 2nd and 3rd metatarsal, causes a sharp pain in complaints of metatarsalgia (Fig. 9.41).

Neuroma Squeeze Test. If needle-like shooting pains occur when the forefoot is gripped and slowly squeezed, the probability of neuroma should be considered.

Dynamic Palpation and Correction of Fixations in the Feet

Gillet looks to the feet as the functional base of the spine. He feels that the cause of many frequently recurring fixations in the spine and pelvis can be traced to a mobility restriction in the feet. Several authorities

Table 9.8. Muscles of the Ankle, Foot, and Toes

Muscle	Major Functions	Spinal Segment
	THE ANKLE AND FOOT	
Extensor digiti longus	Dorsiflexion	L4-S1
Extensor hallucis longus	Dorsiflexion	L5-S1
Flexor digiti longus	Plantar flexion, foot inversion	L5-S1
Flexor hallucis longus	Plantar flexion	L5-S2
Gastrocnemius	Plantar flexion	S1-S2
Peroneus brevis, longus	Plantar flexion, foot eversion	L5-S1
Peroneus tertius	Dorsiflexion, foot eversion	L4-S1
Plantaris	Plantar flexion	L5-S1
Soleus	Plantar flexion	S1-S2
Tibialis anterior	Dorsiflexion, weak foot inverter	L4-L5
Tibialis posterior	Plantar flexion, foot inversion	L5-S1
	THE TOES	
Abductor digiti quinti	Small toe abduction	S1-S2
Adductor hallucis	Hallux adduction-flexion of great toe	L5-S2
Dorsal interossei	Abduction-flexion of toes 2-4	S1-S2
Extensor digiti brevis	Toe extension	L5-S1
Extensor digiti longus	Toe extension of lateral four toes	L4-S1
Extensor hallucis longus	Hallux extension	L5-S1
Flexor digiti	Flexion of lateral toes	L5-S2
Flexor hallucis brevis	1st metatarsophalangeal flexion	L5-S1
Flexor hallucis longus	Hallux flexion	L5-S2
Interossei	1st metatarsophalangeal flexion	S1-S2
Lumbricales	Flexion of toes	L5-S2
Plantar interossei	Abduction-flexion of lateral three toes	S1-S2
Quadratus plantae	Assist flexion of lateral four toes	S1-S2

Note: Spinal innervation varies somewhat in different people. The spinal nerves listed here are averages and may differ in a particular patient; thus, an allowance of a segment above and below those listed in most text tables should be considered.

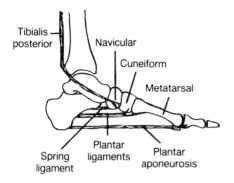

Figure 9.39. Drawing showing the major structures responsible for maintaining the longitudinal arch of the foot (Courtesy ACAP).

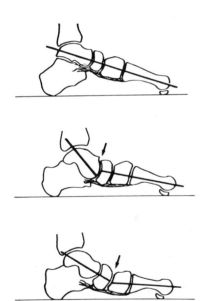

Figure 9.40. *Top,* schematic of the normal longitudinal arch; *center,* flattened arch due to talonavicular subluxation; *bottom,* flattened arch due to naviculocuneiform subluxation (Courtesy ACAP).

agree with this observation.

Motion palpation examination of the feet is usually conducted immediately following the standard orthopedic/neurologic examination, including gross range of motion evaluation, muscle strength grading, reflexes, and light touch and pain perception.

The foot is a common site of single or multiple fixations that can frequently be linked to spinal fixations. Gillet also states that fixations of the distal phalangeal joints are uncommon and fixations in those joints more proximal are common. He believes that the priority joint play motion to evaluate for possible fixations are midfoot (proximal metatarsal) and forefoot (distal metatarsal) A-P/P-A glide and rotation. Hindfoot mobility is evaluated indirectly during the evaluation of ankle mortise and subtalar mobility. See Figure 9.42.

The metatarsophalangeal joint of the great toe is a common site of fixation, especially where plantar flexion is restricted. The intermetatarsal ligaments are frequently shortened. Partial or complete fixations are also found at the cuneiform-metatarsal, cuboid-metatarsal, cuneiform-navicular, intercuneiform, cuneiform-cuboid, navicular-cuboid, talus-navicular, and talus-cuboid articulations. Keep in mind that a high stiff arch that does not reduce somewhat during weight bearing is just as abnormal as a flattened arch.

Complexes

Studies conducted by Gillet and associates have shown a distinct relationship between phalangeal fixations and upper cervical fixations, metatarsal fixation and C3—C7 fixations, metatarsal-tarsal fixations and thoracic fixations, intermetatarsal and costospinal fixations, cuneiform-navicular or cuboid-calcaneus and lumbar fixations, and talus fixations and L5 fixations. These empiric findings are awaiting further confirmation.

Gillet reports two curious observations regarding the feet:

1. One foot is nearly always in greater fixation than the other, and the correction of this foot will often produce a partial or even total correction of the fixations in the other foot before adjusting it. "If such fixations correct spontaneously," states Gillet, "leave them alone."

2. If all articulations of the foot are mobilized each time during the examination of a foot, it is Gillet's opinion that this procedure tends to *produce* secondary fixations in the spine through the awakening of local irritation.

Ligamentous Fixations in the Feet

Ligamentous fixations in the feet have a strong tendency to recur continually. It is here that we see the greatest effect of lack of exercise. In everyday living, the joints of the feet (usually bound in tight shoes that must constantly stand and walk on hard surfaces) are rarely forced to their full ranges of motions. See Figure 9.43.

Most accredited chiropractic colleges teach many good adjustive technics that can be applied to fixations in the feet; however, few colleges at this writing teach how to locate fixations in the feet.

The foot adjustments customarily taught can be either totally or partially effective. It is important, however, that axial distraction be incorporated into adjustive alternatives as the separation of jammed joint spaces is especially important in correcting biomechanical faults of the foot. The pull must be firm, short, and fast, for we are usually dealing with tough fibrosed tissue rather than elastic muscle fibers.

Motion Palpation and Correction of Fixations in the Feet

The examination and release of fixations in the interphalangeal and metatarsophalangeal joints of the foot are similar to those described for the interphalangeal and metacarpophalangeal joints of the hand. Please review those sections if the techniques are not fresh in mind.

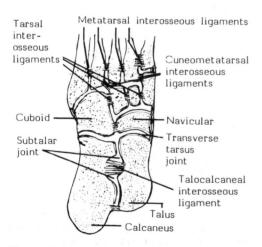

Figure 9.41. One method of applying Morton's test.

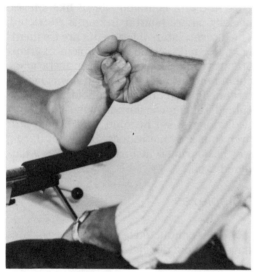

Figure 9.42. Schematic of an oblique section of the foot showing the intertarsal joints and their related structures (Courtesy ACAP).

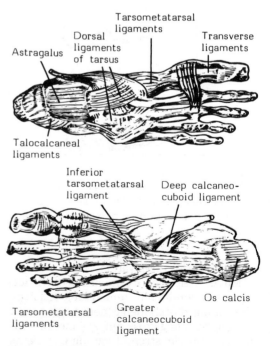

Figure 9.43. *Top,* major ligaments of the dorsal aspect of the foot; *bottom,* major ligaments of the plantar aspect of the foot (Courtesy ACAP).

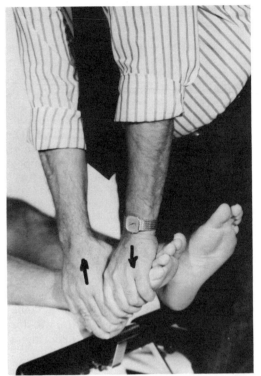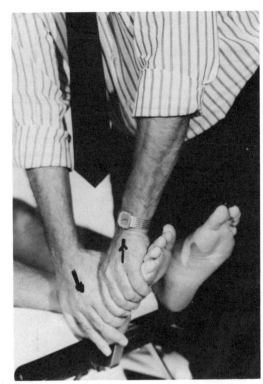

Figure 9.44. Evaluating A-P and P-A tarsometatarsal glide.

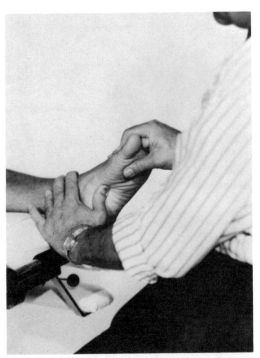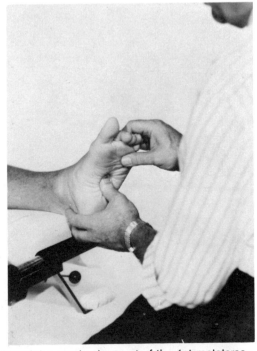

Figure 9.45. *Left,* evaluating plantar-to-dorsum glide of the proximal aspect of the 1st metatarsophalangeal joint; *right,* the 2nd metatarsophalangeal joint.

A-P/P-A Tarsometatarsal Glide

With the patient supine, position yourself perpendicular to the foot to be tested. Grasp over the top of the patient's forefoot with your active caudad hand and over the patient's tarsals with your cephalad hand (stabilizer). The curve of the patient's foot should fit comfortably within the webs of both hands. With the bases of the patient's metatarsals firmly stabilized, push downward and then lift upward with your active hand to produce A-P and P-A motion between the metacarpal bases and the articulating tarsals (Fig. 9.44). If motion resistance is perceived, impulse against the fixation.

To test specific plantar-to-dorsum glide of the metatarsal heads, place a firm thumb contact against the plantar surface of the metatarsal head, grasp the distal aspect of the metatarsal with your other hand, and then flex the patient's forefoot over your contact thumb (Fig. 9.45).

Tarsometatarsal Rotation

Sit facing the patient's foot, and rotate the patient's forefoot as a whole into eversion and then inversion so that the bases of the metatarsals will rotate on the articulating tarsals (Fig. 9.46). This maneuver will also elicit intermetatarsal restrictions. If fixation is found, it can usually be released with the classic figure-8 maneuver. The position to evaluate talonavicular and calcaneocuboid transverse mobility is shown in Figure 9.47.

Midtarsal A-P/P-A Glide

The technique to evaluate midtarsal glide is the same as that described above for tarsometatarsal glide except that the hands are moved cephalad so that the evaluating force can be directed at the midtarsal articulations (Fig. 9.48). The test for plantary to dorsum glide of the metatarsals, cuneiform, na-

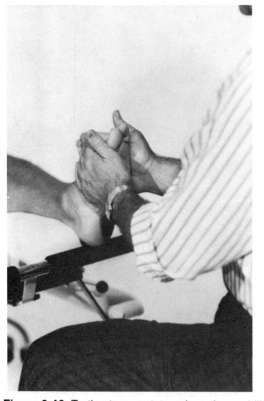
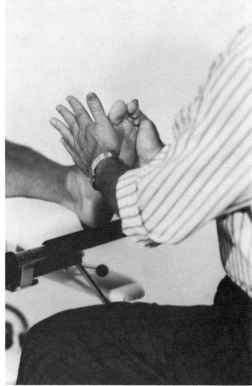

Figure 9.46. Testing tarsometatarsal rotation mobility.

vicular, and cuboid can also be conducted with the patient standing (Fig. 9.49).

The Phalangeal-Metatarsal Joints

Sit facing the supine patient's feet. Place your contact thumb just below the distal metatarsal head to be evaluated (Fig. 9.50, left). Crook the index finger of your other hand, and place the apex of the crooked finger under the metatarsal head with your thumb placed over the proximal phalanx (Fig. 9.50, right). Push forward with your contact thumb while simultaneously plantar flexing the phalanx. This will test plantar-to-dorsum mobility of the phalaneal-metatarsal joint being evaluated. If mobility is found to be restricted, impulse upward from the plantar contact with your index finger while simultaneously gently stretching the patient's toe with your thumb contact to separate the phalangeal-metacarpal joint.

Long-Axis Extension of the Metacarpal-Phalangeal Joint of the Great Toe

The hallux becomes painful if plantar flexion is forced excessively. To evaluate long-axis extension, stand at the lateral side of the involved foot. With your caudad hand, place

your thumb on the dorsal surface of the involved foot with your index finger firmed against the plantar surface of the great toe. These fingers are relaxed, but they are squeezed with your active hand. With this double-handed contact, lean away from the

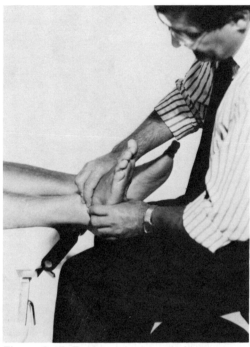

Figure 9.47. Testing calcaneocuboid transverse mobility.

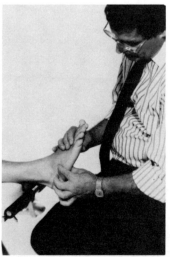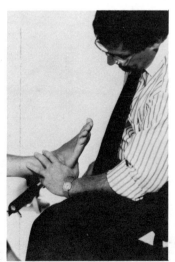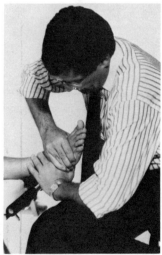

Figure 9.48. Testing cuboid A-P/P-A glide. *Left,* isolating the contact point; *center,* securing the contact thumb; *right,* applying the mobilizing force.

patient is apply long-axis traction to the metacarpophalangeal joint (Fig. 9.51). Add a short sharp mobilizing impulse if mobility is restricted.

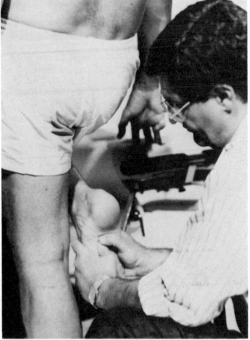

Figure 9.49. Testing midtarsal plantar-to-dorsum mobility with the patient standing.

Plantar Fascitis

Plantar fascitis is a frequent cause of foot pain. It is especially common in runners and basketball players. The medial tuberosity of the calcaneus will be extremely tender. Besides the standard treatment for inflammation, beneficial management usually includes a medial heel wedge, possibly a higher heel, and/or a cut-out orthotic. See Figure 9.52. All foot and ankle joint-play movements should be tested, and any fixations found should be released. Faulty mechanics often set up the overstresses that lead to inflamed tissues.

INTEGRATED TREATMENT APPROACH

Orthotics

Orthotics means the development, manufacture, and application of a body part device (usually applied or attached to an external surface) such as a splint, brace, or support. The practice is ancient, but the term is relatively new, as are technologic advances in this field.

Extremity orthoses include devices used

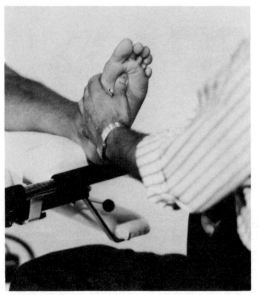
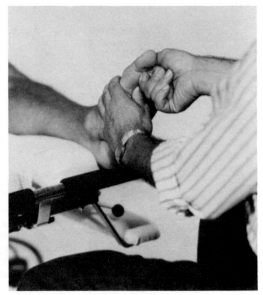

Figure 9.50. Evaluating plantar-to-dorsum mobility of the 2nd phalangeal-metatarsal joint.

in postfracture, postsprain, and postparalysis disorders. They may also be helpful during the management of metabolic disorders that tend to weaken bone. The basic principle in fitting many orthoses is the *3-point pressure principle;* ie, two pressure forces at the ends of the device that are resisted by an opposite force at or near the midpoint.

Indications for orthoses generally include one or more of the following benefits: (1) pain relief (eg, unloading a joint, immobilization), (2) protection of weak, unstable, or healing segments, (3) provide assistance in maintaining equilibrium, and (4) applying forces that tend to correct a structural deformity or normalize unequal muscle pull.

Once carefully fitted to avoid excessive pressure, circulatory impairment, and irritation, an appliance must be monitored frequently and adjusted to meet changing conditions in both the appliance and the patient. Thus, on each subsequent office visit, check the appliance before it is removed and after it has been reapplied.

If a deficit exists at the distal end of the body's axial kinematic chain, corrective and supportive foot orthotics can become an important aspect of treatment. The two most common foot appliances used in chiropractic during the management of articular disorders are (1) internal or external heel or sole lifts to permanently correct an anatomical short leg or shift body weight temporarily and (2) molded shoe inserts to support a flexible fallen arch and/or improve the alignment of a pronated ankle.

Rehabilitative Exercises

If it appears difficult to correct fixations in the feet, or should they fail to be released from visit to visit, Gillet recommends the following exercise: Instruct the patient to rise on the toes by raising the heels, stretching upward as far as possible. Then slowly settle down on the soles, bend the knees, and squat down as far as possible without raising the heels from the floor. Doing this a few times each morning and evening, will do much to keep the feet supple and not allow serious fixations to develop.

Bibliography

Apley AG: The diagnosis of meniscal injuries. *Journal of Bone and Joint Surgery,* 29:78-84, 1946.

Baltzell LG, Mackey RH (eds): *Firth's Technic Notes,* publishing data not shown, 1967. Available from National College of Chiropractic, pp 51-57, 63-71.

Basmajian JV, Stecko G: The role of muscles in arch support of the foot. *Journal of Bone & Joint Surgery,* 54A:1184-1190, 1963.

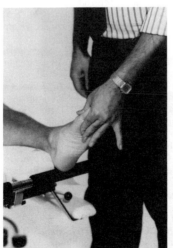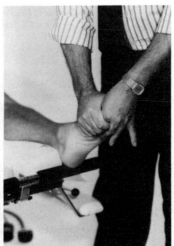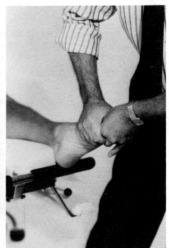

Figure 9.51. Position for evaluating and releasing long-axis extension of the metacarpophalangeal joint of the great toe. *Left,* applying the contact finger and thumb; *center,* reinforcing the contact; *right,* applying long-axis extension.

Bierman W, Ralston MJ: Electromyographic study during passive and active flexion and extension of the knee of the normal human subject. *Archives of Physical Medicine & Rehabilitation,* 46:71-75, January 1965.

Black J, Dumbleton JH (eds): *Clinical Biomechanics: Case History Approach.* New York, Churchill Livingstone, 1981, pp 87-88.

Bowerman JW: *Radiology and Injury in Sport.* New York, Appleton-Century-Crofts, 1977, pp 119-140,

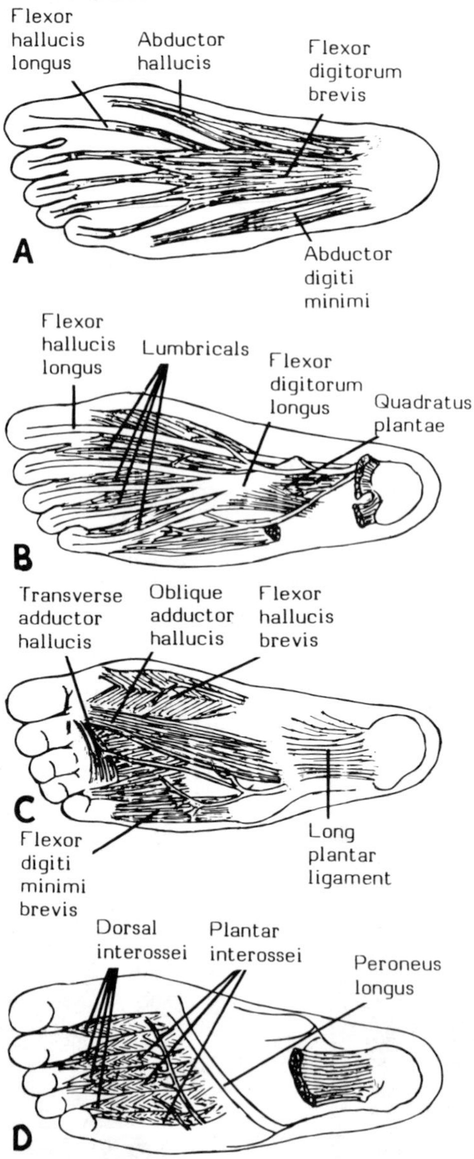

Figure 9.52. A, superficial muscles of the foot; B, second layer of muscles; C, third layer of muscles; D, deepest layer of muscles (Courtesy ACAP).

182, 219, 231, 273.

Branch WT Jr: *Office Practice of Medicine.* Philadelphia, W.B. Saunders, 1987, pp 931-951.

Brantigan OC, Voshell AF: The mechanics of the ligaments and menisci of the knee joint. *Journal of Bone and Joint Surgery,* 23(1):44-66, January 1941.

Cailliet R: *Foot and Ankle Pain.* Philadelphia, F.A. Davis, 1979, pp 1-39, 42-56, 81-93, 99-106, 109-110, 112, 117-124, 129, 216-231.

Cailliet R: *Knee Pain and Disability.* Philadelphia, F.A. Davis, 1973, pp 4-47, 62-71, 73-82, 110-131, 244-245, 250.

Cyriax J: *Textbook of Orthopaedic Medicine;* vol one, Diagnosis of Soft Tissue Lesions, ed 8. London, Bailliere Tindall, 1982, pp 297-298.

D'Ambrosia RD: The hip. In D'Ambrosia RD: *Musculoskeletal Disorders: Regional Examination and Differential Diagnosis.* Philadelphia, J.B. Lippincott, 1977, pp 298-403, 406-411, 428-430, 434-438.

Dempster WT: The range of motion of cadaver joints: the lower limb. *University of Michigan Medical Bulletin,* 22:364-379, 1956.

Denham RA: Hip mechanics. *Journal of Bone & Joint Surgery* (British), 41:550-557, 1959.

Faye LJ: *Motion Palpation and Clinical Considerations of the Lower Extremities.* Huntington Beach, CA, Motion Palpation Institute, 1986, pp 1, 8-18, 20-35.

Faye LJ: Motion Palpation and Manipulation of the Extremities [Cassette tape program]. Huntington Beach, CA, Motion Palpation Institute, 1981, 6 tapes.

Faye LJ: Motion Palpation and Manipulation of the Foot and Ankle [Videotape]. Los Angeles, Dynaspine, 1983.

Faye LJ: Motion Palpation and Manipulation of the Knee and Hip [Videotape]. Los Angeles, Dynaspine, 1983.

Galway R, et al: Pivot shift: a clinical sign of symptomatic anterior cruciate insufficiency. *Journal of Bone and Joint Surgery,* 54B:763-764, 1974.

Gertler L: *Illustrated Manual of Extravertebral Technic,* ed 2. Bayside, NY, published by author, 1978, pp 8-28, 41-50.

Giammarino MA: The adolescent knee. *Roentgenological Briefs,* ACA Council on Roentgenology, date not shown.

Gillet H, Liekens M: *Belgian Chiropractic Research Notes.* Huntington Beach, CA, Motion Palpation Institute, 1984, pp 17, 85-88, 90-92, 159-162, 164.

Gillet H: Feet, hands, cranium, etc. *Bulletin of the European Chiropractors Union,* 26(3):28-30, 1978.

Goodheart GJ: The psoas muscle and the foot pronation problem. *Collected Published Articles and Reprints.* Montpellier, OH, Williams County Publishing, 1969, pp 72-74.

Goodrich TM: Analysis and treatment of common lesions of the knee. *ACA Journal of Chiropractic,* January 1963.

Gowitzke BA, Milner M: *Understanding Scientific Basis of Human Movement,* ed 2. Baltimore, Williams & Wilkins, 1980, pp 23, 33.

Greenawalt MH: Feet and the dynamic science of chiropractic. *ACA Journal of Chiropractic,* May 1983.

Greenawalt MH: *Spinal Pelvic Stabilization,* ed 2,

Dubuque, IA, Foot Levelers, 1978, pp 7-13, 29-31, 34-35, 38-44, 63-72.

Grice AS, Fligg DB: Class Notes: Introductory Concepts to Clinical Analysis of Joint Movement and Muscle Testing. Department of Biomechanics/Kinesiology, BK101. Toronto, Canadian Memorial Chiropractic College, date not shown, pp 8-22, 25-69, 72-78, 80-84.

Grossman RB, Nicholas JA: Common disorders of the knee. *Orthopaedic Clinics of North America*, 8: 619-640, 1977.

Hadler NM: *Medical Management of the Regional Musculoskeletal Diseases*. New York, Grune & Stratton, 1984, pp 229-247, 251-270, 282, 285-289.

Harrington IJ: Biomechanics of joint injuries. In Gonzna ER, Harrington IJ (eds): *Biomechanics of Musculoskeletal Injury*. Baltimore, Williams & Wilkins, 1982, pp 56-66.

Helfet AJ, Gruebel Lee, DM: *Disorders of the Lumbar Spine*. Philadelphia, J.B. Lippincott, 1978, pp 24-25.

Insall JN: Patellar pain. *Journal of Bone and Joint Surgery*, 64A:147-152, 1982.

James SL: The knee. In D'Ambrosia RD: *Musculoskeletal Disorders: Regional Examination and Differential Diagnosis*. Philadelphia, J.B. Lippincott, 1977, pp 440-446, 450-462, 464-469, 472-485.

Janse J, Houser RH, Wells BF: *Chiropractic Principles and Technic*. Chicago, National College of Chiropractic, 1947, pp 564-609.

Jones RJ: The human foot: an experimental study of its mechanics and the role of its muscles and ligaments in the support of the arch. *American Journal of Anatomy*, 68:1-41, 1941.

Kapandji IA: *Physiology of the Joints: Lower Limb*, ed 2. New York, Churchill Livingstone, 1981, vol II, pp 10-23, 72-80, 88-92, 96, 98-208, 216.

Karpovich PV, Wilklow LB: Goniometric study of the human foot in standing and walking. *Industrial Medicine and Surgery*, 29:338-347, 1960.

Kelly ED: A comparative study of structure and function of normal, pronated and painful feet among children. *Research Quarterly*, American Association of Health and Physical Education, 18:291-312. 1947.

Kennedy JC, Fowler P: Medial and anterior instability of the knee. *Journal of Bone and Joint Surgery*, 53A: 1257-1270, 1971.

Kessler RM, Hertling D (eds): *Management of Common Musculoskeletal Disorders*. Philadelphia, Harper & Row, 1983, pp 368-379, 394-410, 425-442, 448-478.

Kettelkamp DB: Management of patellar malalignment. *Journal of Bone and Joint Surgery*, 63A:1344-1347, 1981.

Kettlekamp DB: Clinical implications of knee biomechanics. *Archives of Surgery*, 107:406-410, 1973.

Klein KK: The knee and the ligaments. *Journal of Bone & Joint Surgery*, 44A:1191-1193, 1962.

Klyop GW, et al: Iliotibial band syndrome. *The Physician and Sports Medicine*, 9(10):13, December 1981.

LaBan MM, et al: Electromyographic study of function of iliopsoas muscles. *Archives of Physical Medicine & Rehabilitation*, 46:676-679, 1965.

LeVeau B: *Williams and Lissner: Biomechanics of Human Motion*, ed 2. Philadelphia, W.B. Saunders, 1977, pp 76-77, 98-102, 106-115.

Lowman CL: Feet and body mechanics. *Journal of Health and Physical Education*, 11:137, 1940.

MacIntosch DL: The pivot shift and the anterior cruciate. Paper presented at the New York State Orthopaedic Society Meeting, New York, 1979.

Maitland GD: *Peripheral Manipulation*. London, Butterworths, 1976, pp 102-129.

Marshall J, et al: The anterior drawer sign: what is it? *American Journal of Sports Medicine*, 3:152-158, 1975.

Marshall J, Rubin R: Knee ligament injuries. *Orthopaedic Clinics of North America*, 8:651-665, 1977.

Mendler HM: Relationship of hip abductor muscles to posture. *Journal of American Physical Therapy Association*, 44:98-102, 1964.

Mercier LR: *Practical Orthopedics*. Chicago, Year Book Medical, 1980, pp 180-183, 185-193, 230-233, 235-236, 341, 243-248.

Michael RH, Holder LE: The soleus syndrome: a cause of medial tibial stress (shin splints). *The American Journal of Sports Medicine*, 13(2):87, March-April 1985.

Morehouse LE, Cooper JM: *Kinesiology*. St. Louis, C.V. Mosby, 1950, pp 45-47, 76-100.

Morrison JB: The mechanics of the knee joint in relation to normal walking. *Journal of Biomechanics*, 3:51-61, 1970.

Nachemson AL: Electromyographical studies of the vertebral portion of the psoas muscle (with special reference to its stabilizing function of the lumbar spine). *Acta Orthopaedica Scandinavica*, 37:177-190, 1966.

Nash JM: personal correspondernce, Pasadena, TX, 1985.

Ng YS: The significance of psoas myospasm in the lordotic compared to the kyphotic sacrolumbar spine. *ACA Journal of Chiropractic*, October 1978.

Nobel CA: Iliotibial band friction syndrome in runners. *American Journal of Sports Medicine*, 8:232-234, August 1980.

O'Connell AL: Electromyographic study of certain leg muscles during movements of the free foot and during standing. *American Journal of Physical Medicine*, 37:289-301, December 1958.

Ogden JA: Subluxation and dislocation of the proximal tibiofibular joint. *Journal of Bone and Joint Surgery*, 56A:145, 1974.

Pace JB, Nagle D: Piriform syndrome. *Western Journal of Medicine*, 124:435-439, 1976.

Reider B, Marshall JL, Warren RF: Clinical characteristics of patellar disorders in young athletes. *American Journal of Sports Medicine*, 9:270-274, 1981.

Rosse C, Clawson DK (eds): *The Musculoskeletal System in Health & Disease*. Hagerstown, PA, Harper & Row, 1980, pp 277-291, 293-300, 303-309.

Salter RB: Injuries of the ankle in children. *North American Clinical Orthopaedics*, 5:147, 1974.

Schafer RC (ed): *Basic Chiropractic Procedural Manual*, ed 4. Arlington, VA, American Chiropractic Association, 1984, pp 291-301.

Schafer RC: *Chiropractic Management of Sports and Recreational Injuries*. Baltimore, Williams & Wilkins, 1982, pp 474-475, 478-482, 484-486, 492-495.

Schneider RC, Kennedy JC, Plant ML (eds): *Sports Injuries: Mechanisms, Prevention, and Treat-*

ment. Baltimore, Williams & Wilkins, 1985, pp 764-783, 793-794.

Schultz AL: *Athletic and Industrial Injuries of the Knee.* Mitchell, SD, published by author, 1951, pp 54-101, 104-109.

Scott WN, Nisonson B, Nicholas JA (eds): *Principles of Sports Medicine.* Baltimore, Williams & Wilkins, 1984, pp 245-263, 291-299, 303-336, 342-361.

Sheffield FJ, et al: Electromyographic study of the muscles of the foot in normal walking. *American Journal of Physical Medicine,* 35:223-236, 1956.

Shephard E: Tarsal movements. *Journal of Bone & Joint Surgery,* 33B:258-263, 1951.

Shoji H: The foot and ankle. In D'Ambrosia RD: *Musculoskeletal Disorders: Regional Examination and Differential Diagnosis.* Philadelphia, J.B. Lippincott, 1977, pp 487-494, 500-502, 511-513, 520-521.

Singleton MC, LeVeau BF: The hip joint: structure, stability, and stress. *Physical Therapy,* 55:957-973, 1975.

Slocum D, et al: Clinical test for anterolateral rotatory instability of the knee. *Clinical Orthopaedics,* 118: 63-69, 1976.

Smidt GL: Biomechanical analysis of knee flexion and extension. *Journal of Biomechanics,* 6:79-92, 1973

Smith JW: The forces operating at the human ankle joint during standing. *Journal of Anatomy,* 91:545-564, 1957.

Smith JW: Muscular control of the arches of the foot in standing: an electromyographic assessment. *Journal of Anatomy,* 88:152-162, 1954.

Smith JW: Observations on the postural mechanism of the human knee joint. *Journal of Anatomy.* 90:236-261, 1956.

Soderberg GL: *Kinesiology: Application to Pathological Motion.* Baltimore, Williams & Wilkins, 1986, pp 175-198.

Stierwalt DD: *Extremity Adjusting.* Davenport, IA, published by author, 1975, pp 26-38.

Torg J, et al: Clinical diagnosis of anterior cruciate ligament instability in the athlete. *American Journal of Sports Medicine,* 4:84-92, 1976.

Van Dusen LG: *Chiropractic Relationship to Gravitational Force.* Sodus, NY, published by author, 1968, pp 73-85, 89, 97-99.

Wiles MR: Geriatric knee pain: diagnosis and treatment. *Journal of Manipulative and Physiological Therapeutics,* 2:93-98, 1979.

Williams JGP, Sperryn PN (eds): *Sports Medicine,* ed 2. Baltimore, Williams & Wilkins, 1976, pp 258, 434-497.

Williams M, Lissner HR: Biomechanical analysis of knee function. *Physical Therapy,* 43:93-99, 1962.

Index